Minimally Invasive Techniques in Pediatric Urology

Ciro Esposito
Ramnath Subramaniam
François Varlet • Lorenzo Masieri
Editors

Minimally Invasive Techniques in Pediatric Urology

Endourology, Laparoscopy and Robotics

Springer

Editors
Ciro Esposito
Pediatric Surgery Department
University of Naples Federico II
Napoli, Italy

François Varlet
Pediatric Surgery Department
University of Saint-Etienne
Saint-Etienne, France

Ramnath Subramaniam
Paediatric Urology Department
Leeds Teaching Hospitals NHS Trust
Leeds, UK

Lorenzo Masieri
Department of Clinical and
Experimental Medicine
University of Florence
Firenze, Italy

ISBN 978-3-030-99279-8 ISBN 978-3-030-99280-4 (eBook)
https://doi.org/10.1007/978-3-030-99280-4

This Springer imprint is published by the registered company Springer Nature Switzerland AG
The registered company address is: Gewerbestrasse 11, 6330 Cham, Switzerland

To Marina, my wife, my best friend, my love, for her precious support in the last 40 years.
To my father, the best pediatric surgeon I've ever met, I thank him for his continuous teaching and for transferring to me his love for children we care for every day.
To my mentors, Giovanni Esposito, Philippe Montupet, Jean Michel Guys, Michel Carcassonne, Arnaud Delarue, and Franco Corcione, who showed me the way to follow.

With Gratitude
Ciro Esposito

For all sick children! The world of MIS is amazing and allows for very good and less aggressive treatment in a wide range of urological diseases. It was an honor for me to contribute to the development of this book. I thank my dear pediatric surgeons and friends who have supported me for over 30 years. And thanks also to my wife and children who have waited for me so often, I love you!

François Varlet

It has been my pleasure to team up with Ciro, Francois, and Lorenzo as the editorial team for this textbook of minimally invasive surgery. Significant progress has been made to harness the power of technology for the benefit of our patients to improve their experience during treatment with minimally invasive techniques allowing early postoperative recovery and reduce hospital stay. Robotics is making significant strides in the minimally invasive approach to major procedures in children.
I am grateful to my wife and my children for their unconditional love and support.

Ramnath Subramaniam

It has been an honor for me to contribute as editorial team member to this important book. The topic is minimally invasive surgery in Pediatric Urology, and it was a big pleasure for me to contribute to the diffusion of Laparoscopy and Robotic Surgery in children.
I dedicate my work to all my patients, to my wonderful Team, to my Teachers, and to my Parents, my Wife, and my Sons.
"those who don't read a good book has no advantage over those who don't read" (M.Twain)

Lorenzo Masieri

Foreword

After asepsis and anesthesia, minimally invasive surgery is a new revolution. All areas of surgery have been involved and pediatric urology is no exception. In this magnificent and comprehensive treatise, the preface of which I have the honor to write, Ciro Esposito, Ramnath Subramanian, François Varlet, and Lorenzo Macieri have brought together no less than three generations of experts from all parts of the world. All areas are covered, from the kidney to the bladder through the ureter and the genitals, from oncology to the treatment of stones, including incontinence, malformative uropathies, disorders of sexual development, and foetoendoscopy. The reader will be able to appreciate in this work how the audacity, the tenacity, and the skills of the pioneers made it possible to open up new paths in the human body. We must also underline the essential role of the industry which has developed over the years ever smaller, more suitable and efficient instruments. Not to mention the robot, which makes laparoscopic procedures available to a greater number of us, procedures which were sometimes a technical feat and could wear out the operator and his cervical spine. The robot that initially allows access to difficult regions with exceptional quality of vision also allows high precision gestures. The way is open, the boundaries of the impossible have once again receded, and this overview of the current possibilities of minimally invasive surgery in pediatric urology shows how much our practices have evolved. The benefit for our patients sometimes remains to be established and other roads remain to be mapped out; but to this day, the contributors to this work are to be thanked for showing us the extent of the road traveled over the past decades.

Henri Lottmann
Pediatric Surgery and Urology Department
Necker-Enfants Malades Children University Hospital
Paris, France

Contents

Part II Kidney

Part I

General

1 Laparoscopic Approach in Pediatric Urology

Jean-Stephane Valla, Ciro Esposito, Maria Escolino, and Philippe Montupet

Learning Objectives

- To describe the general principles of the laparoscopic approach.
- To present the current indications and long-term outcome of the technique.
- To report the available evidence in the current pediatric literature about this subject.
- To describe the tips and tricks of the technique and all innovative technologies available to improve surgical treatment of pediatric urological pathologies.

1.1 Introduction

Since the introduction of diagnostic laparoscopy for the evaluation of impalpable testes, laparoscopic urological surgery in children has developed steadily from a simple diagnostic maneuver to an integral part of complex reconstructive procedures [1]. Pediatric laparoscopy has benefited from improvements in technology and instrumentation, as well as from an increase in the number of trained laparoscopic surgeons. The benefits of laparoscopy include increased magnification and visualization of the operative field, reduced postoperative morbidity, shorter convalescence, and improved cosmesis [2].

The principle of laparoscopic surgery is to create a working space into the abdominal cavity by CO_2 insufflation (pneumoperitoneum), which allows the visualization of the abdominal content and instrument insertion and manipulation for diagnostic and therapeutic purposes.

This chapter aims to provide a comprehensive overview of current indications, technique, and outcomes of laparoscopic transperitoneal surgery for treatment of urological pathologies in the pediatric population.

1.2 Preoperative Preparation

Before each laparoscopic procedure, it is necessary to evaluate the age and weight of the patient, eventual associated comorbidities, previous abdominal surgeries with respect to possible adhesions, or enlarged organs (liver, spleen, urinary bladder). A bowel preparation with simethicone, enema, and liquid diet may be useful

J.-S. Valla
Pediatric Surgery Unit, CHU Lenval, Nice, France
e-mail: jeff.valla@gmail.com

C. Esposito · M. Escolino (✉)
Pediatric Surgery Unit, Federico II University of Naples, Naples, Italy
e-mail: ciroespo@unina.it; maria.escolino@unina.it

P. Montupet
Pediatric Surgery Unit, CHU Bicêtre, Paris, France
e-mail: philippe.montupet@me.com

C. Esposito et al. (eds.), *Minimally Invasive Techniques in Pediatric Urology*,
https://doi.org/10.1007/978-3-030-99280-4_1

especially in newborns and infants, in whom the working space may be very limited. All patients undergoing procedures, including bowel or urinary tract opening, should receive intraoperative antibiotic prophylaxis.

All patients receive a general anesthesia with oro-tracheal intubation and myorelaxation. A nasogastric tube should be always placed in order to keep empty the stomach during the procedure and prevent aspiration during increase of intra-abdominal pressure. The bladder should be always emptied before surgery and positioning of Foley bladder catheter is recommended in case of demanding laparoscopic procedures.

1.3 Positioning

Regarding patient's position, it varies according to the type of procedure. In renal surgery, the patient is placed in the standard lateral or semi lateral kidney position, rotating the operative side up by 30°–45° axially using silicone pads underneath the patient (Fig. 1.1). In surgeries of pelvic/lower abdomen organs, the position of the patient should be supine.

Regarding trocars' number, three ports are commonly placed in most laparoscopic procedures: a 5- or 10-mm trocar is inserted trans-umbilically for the optic. After pneumoperitoneum induction, two 5- or 3-mm operating trocars are introduced under visual control. In some cases, an additional trocar may be inserted to retract the liver or the spleen or for other reasons. The ports' positioning varies according to the type of procedure. In upper urinary tract surgery, the optic port is placed trans-umbilically and two working ports are inserted along the midclavicular line in the upper and lower abdomen (Fig. 1.2). In surgeries of pelvic/lower abdomen organs, the optic port is placed trans-umbilically and two working ports are inserted in the right and left iliac fossa, respectively (Fig. 1.3). In general, a triangulation between the optic port and the working ports should be preferably respected in order to achieve a better ergonomics.

Regarding the surgical team's position, the surgeon and the assistant usually stand on one side of the patient and the screen is placed ergonomically opposite the surgeon in order to achieve adequate visualization.

1.4 Instrumentation

There are two basic types of instruments used in pediatric laparoscopic urology: those used to gain access to the patient, and those used to perform the surgical procedure. Access can be gained via closed technique with the Veress needle or open Hasson technique. The Veress needle, which can be disposable or reusable, works with the mechanism of safety telescopic blunt-tip trocar. The sharp needle penetrates the abdominal wall and the central blunt-tip trocar is extended after penetrating the resistance. Working ports are tubular cannulas with an extractable trocar that is removed after trans-parietal introduction of the working port. The working ports may be disposable or reusable as well. The optic port diameter ranges between 12 and 5 mm, whereas the working ports may have a 3 or 5-mm diameter. For the open access using the Hasson technique, conventional instruments are used.

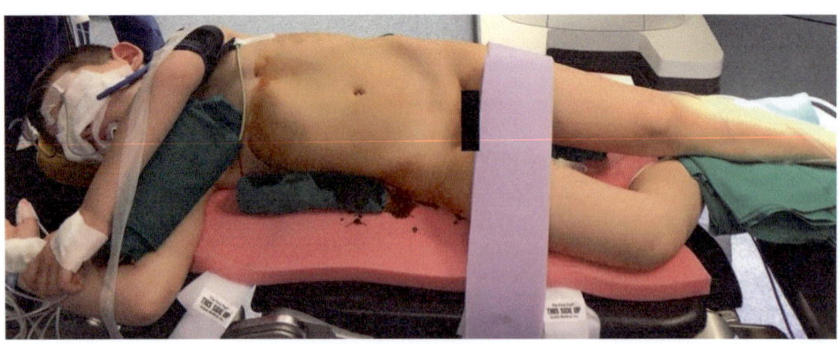

Fig. 1.1 Patient's position in kidney surgery

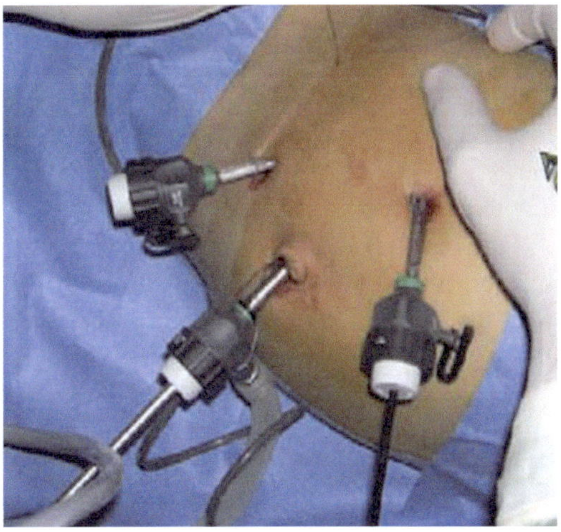

Fig. 1.2 Ports' position and triangulation in upper urinary tract surgery

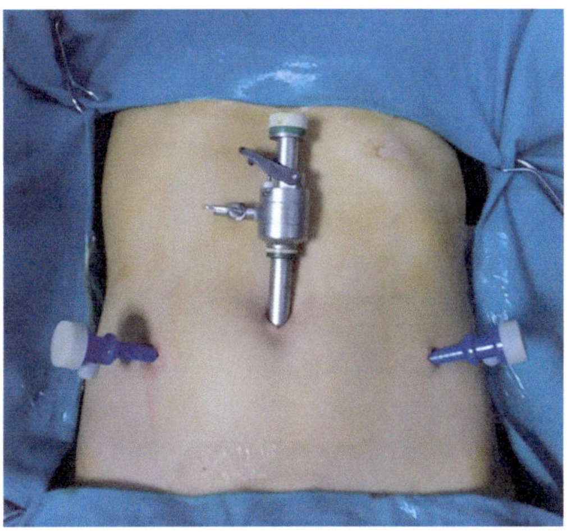

Fig. 1.3 Ports' position and triangulation in lower urinary tract surgery

The surgical instruments for pediatric laparoscopy include scissors, needle drivers, graspers, forceps, clamps, retractors, cautery devices, clip appliers, that come in sizes of 5- and 3-mm. These instruments are now made with shorter shaft lengths, specifically for pediatric indications. There are also different types of sealing devices that can be adopted especially in challenging procedures in order to reduce bleeding risk during tissue dissection or vessel control and are selected according to the surgeon's preference.

1.5 Technique

1.5.1 Creation of Pneumoperitoneum

1.5.1.1 Closed Method Using Veress Needle

An infra-umbilical incision that copies the inferior arc of the navel is performed using a scalpel. The fascia is exposed and incised longitudinally for Veress needle entry. The Veress needle is inserted perpendicularly through the fascia incision, while the anterior abdominal wall is elevated. After the "click" sound confirming its penetration, the needle is directed at an angle of 45° into the abdominal cavity. The insufflation tube is connected to the Veress needle and the peritoneal cavity is slowly insufflated, starting with gas flow values of 0.1–0.5 l/min and pressure values of 6–10 mmHg. The gas flow is then increased to 1–6 l/min with a mean pressure of 10–12 mmHg. At this point, the first port (5- or 10-mm) is inserted at the site of insufflation through the Veress needle, that is extracted after the pneumoperitoneum creation. The first port is used as optic port. Thereafter, other two working ports (3- or 5-mm) are inserted under vision. The cannula with the trocar is grasped so that the index finger acts as a break in order to prevent inadvertent deep penetration into the abdominal cavity. The trocar tip is directed into the small incision in the fascia and is inserted perpendicularly through the abdominal wall, using twisting movement and concurrent pressure. The sharp trocar is removed and the cannula is inserted deeper into the abdominal cavity.

1.5.1.2 Open Hasson Method

This method of creation of pneumoperitoneum should be preferred to the closed method using the Veress needle in case of patients after previous abdominal surgery with high related risk of postoperative adhesions and also in newborns and infants with very limited working space. A trans-umbilical incision, that should be 1–2 mm longer than the port diameter, is made using the scalpel. Once the peritoneal cavity has been opened, a 5- or 10-mm cannula with blunt-tip trocar is inserted into the opening and is fixed with a circular suture, placed on the circumference of the fascial incision, which is further fixed at the insufflation valve of the cannula. Insufflation tube is connected and the pneumoperitoneum is gradually created. Thereafter, the working ports are inserted under vision, as previously described.

1.5.2 Port Extraction and Emptying of Pneumoperitoneum

At the end of laparoscopic procedure, the CO_2 pneumoperitoneum pressure is decreased and the operating field is checked for any bleeding. If needed, one of the working ports can be adopted to insert a drain tube into the abdominal cavity and place it under visual control using a grasper. Thereafter, the working ports are extracted, checking possible bleeding into the peritoneal cavity following the cannula extraction. The insufflation tube is disconnected from the cannula, and, maintaining the valve open, light compression of the rib arches and abdominal wall is performed to evacuate as much CO_2 as possible and the cannula is finally extracted. In case of specimen retrieval, it can be extracted directly or by a retrieval bag through the umbilical port incision after slightly enlarging it, if needed. The trocars' orifices are finally closed using resorbable sutures.

1.6 Postoperative Care

The duration of indwelling bladder catheter normally ranges from 24 to 72 h postoperatively, according to the type of laparoscopic procedure. The drain is commonly removed within 24–48 h postoperatively, provided that no urine leak is detected. Full oral feeding is usually resumed few hours postoperatively as tolerated. Pain control is commonly obtained with oral analgesic medication (paracetamol 15 mg/kg/8 h and/or tramadol 1–2 mg/kg/8 h).

Clinical and radiological follow-up is set up according to the type of pathology.

1.7 Results

Since the introduction of diagnostic laparoscopy for abdominal exploration of undescended testes, the indications for laparoscopy in pediatric urology have expanded rapidly.

Regarding upper urinary tract surgery, laparoscopic nephrectomy has become the gold standard for kidney removal in infants and children for benign indications and increasingly also for malignancies [3]. It has been proven to be safe, effective, and associated with a low complication rate, while offering reduced morbidity due to surgical trauma, superior cosmesis, and fast recovery [3]. In our 20-year experience, no conversions to open were reported, the average operative time was 47 min and the complications rate was very low (2.9%) [4].

Laparoscopic partial nephrectomy for benign indication is done for resection of a poorly or non-functioning moiety of a duplex system. Since Jordan and Winslow reported on laparoscopic partial nephrectomy in 1993 [5], it has increasingly gained acceptance despite the operation being considered to be challenging and therefore offers limitations in terms of widespread diffusion among pediatric urologists. However, with the increasing use of evolving hemostatic and dissecting devices that allowed easier obtaining of vascular control and thus a more straightforward resection, laparoscopic partial nephrectomy has gained more popularity among surgeons. More recently, Piaggio et al. [6] also reported low complication rates (one omental hernia and one urinoma) out of 14 young children who underwent laparoscopic partial nephrectomy.

Uretero–pelvic junction obstruction (UPJO) is the most common cause of hydronephrosis in infants and children. The gold standard in surgical care for UPJO has been open dismembered pyeloplasty through a retroperitoneal approach as described by Anderson and Hynes [3]. After the first pediatric laparoscopic pyeloplasty described by Peters in 1995 [3], a new era of reconstructive laparoscopic surgery of the upper urinary tract began. Laparoscopic dismembered pyeloplasty has become an established technique in children. It offers superior visualization of the anatomy, accurate anastomotic suturing, and thus precise reconstruction of the UPJ which promises good functional results. Therefore, laparoscopic transperitoneal dismembered pyeloplasty can be considered as the gold standard for surgical treatment of intrinsic UPJO [7]. It has been proven to be safe, effective, and associated with a low complication rate with excellent functional results. In addition, laparoscopy seems to be as safe and effective as primary pyeloplasty for redo-surgery in case of failed pyeloplasty [8]. For repair of UPJO in association with a horseshoe kidney, the laparoscopic transperitoneal approach has been demonstrated to offer superior visualization of the anatomy, thus providing excellent functional results [9]. This approach is also applicable for children below 1 year of age. There is sufficient evidence in literature that laparoscopic dismembered pyeloplasty is also a safe procedure in infants, providing the same functional outcomes as the open approach [10]. Transperitoneal laparoscopic approach for adrenalectomy has been reported to be safe and effective, with shorter convalescence, minimal blood loss, and excellent functional outcome when compared with open adrenalectomy [3]. In a series of 21 children undergoing laparoscopic adrenalectomy, Skarsgard et al. [11] reported a mean operative time of 101 min and a mean hospital stay of 1.5 days, with conversion to open adrenalectomy necessary for one patient with a left adrenal carcinoma and tumor thrombus extending into the renal vein. In a different study of 17 children with adrenal lesions (mean size 4.8 cm), Miller et al. [12] reported a transperitoneal laparoscopic approach, with a mean operating time of 120 min, a mean estimated blood loss of 25 ml, and a mean length of hospitalization of 35 h.

Regarding lower urinary tract surgery, the most widespread laparoscopic procedure in children is laparoscopic anti-reflux ureteral reimplantation [3]. Meanwhile, the so called laparoscopic extravesical ureteral reimplantation (LEVUR) has become an accepted alternative to endoscopic treatment of vesico–uretereal reflux (VUR) in pediatric patients. Current data in literature describe a success rate of up to 95% and a recurrence rate of VUR as low as of 4% in a patient population with VUR grade II–IV in a retrospective study [13]. The authors concluded that LEVUR offers an acceptable success rate and better sustainability compared to conventional open and endoscopic techniques. A recent systematic review assessed five studies with a total of 69 LEVUR procedures performed, reporting a 96% success rate [14].

Steyaert and Valla [1] reported that seminal vesicle cysts and urachus remnants also represent an excellent indication for this approach. They reported five cases (1 seminal vesicle and 4 remnants), all with excellent results. They also reported three cases of ureterocelectomy after failure of an endoscopic treatment. Exposure was excellent and posterior bladder wall closure could be achieved without difficulty. Bladder diverticula are also easily accessible using an extravesical approach. They also used a transperitoneal approach for treatment of an infra-iliac ureteral stone with longitudinal opening of the ureter, extraction of the stone, and closure by a running suture without stenting. Recovery was uneventful.

Children with neurogenic bowel or bladder occasionally require reconstructive surgery to improve their quality of life, self- confidence, and to become more independent. Hedican et al. [15] reported the first series of eight patients (mean age 13.4 years) undergoing a variety of laparoscopically assisted reconstructive procedures (including bladder augmentation, appendiceal Mitrofanoff procedure, and tapered ileal Mitrofanoff and Malone ACE). They concluded that laparoscopically assisted surgery allows for mobilization of bowel segments with reconstruction via a low midline or Pfannenstiel incision, allowing for a more rapid recovery and an improved cosmetic appearance [15]. Initial reports described pure laparoscopic bladder augmentation procedures, but currently the technical demands of these procedures are not generally acceptable [1, 4]. However, with increasing experience, laparoscopically assisted reconstructive surgery is being used by a growing group of pediatric urologists.

There is little evidence regarding laparoscopic complication rates in the pediatric population, particularly in the urologic literature. In 1996, Peters reviewed 5400 laparoscopic cases performed by 153 pediatric urologists, reporting a complication rate of 5.4% [16]. However, excluding misdirected insufflation, the incidence of complications decreased to 1.2%, of which 0.4% required surgical repair. Peters also concluded that the greatest predictor of complication rate was laparoscopic experience [16]. In 2003, Esposito et al. reviewed 701 laparoscopic procedures performed in eight institutions, reporting 19 (2.7%) complications, of which six required conversion to open surgery [17]. Interestingly, surgical team experience in this review was not related to complication rate.

Today, the learning curve for complex pediatric laparoscopy is decreasing, as trainees are entering the field with far more laparoscopic experience, gained during general urology residency. This will certainly advance the field; however, it is important to note that, as the level of complexity of laparoscopic procedures increases, the incidence of complications might also increase [18].

Tips and Tricks

- Laparoscopic surgery may be challenging in newborn and small infants, due to the limited working space. In such patients, pre-operative bowel preparation provides important benefits as it increases the working space by reducing bowel content and allows to perform the entire procedure, keeping the intra-abdominal pressure (IAP) under 8 mmHg, that is very important in this patient category.
- In regard to trocars, two main rules should be considered especially in newborns and small infants: preferable use of trocars with micro-threaded shaft in order to prevent their slipping during instrument change (Fig. 1.4) and positioning of the working trocars on the same line with the camera port in order to obtain a larger working space and avoid the clashing between the optic and the instruments. Another technical trick is to place a 5-mm balloon trocar in the umbilicus (Fig. 1.5); this type of trocar can be lifted up with no risk of dislodgement thanks to the intra-abdominal balloon, allowing a large view of the operative field and a low IAP. During trocars' insertion, it may be also helpful direct the trocar tip into the cannula containing the optic ("trocar in trocar") (Fig. 1.6).
- In case of Veress needle use, a free circular movement of the needle after insertion into the abdominal cavity confirms its correct positioning. Then, a syringe should be connected and aspirated; if aspiration is not possible, 5–10 ml of saline be injected. Instillation should be without resistance and without possibility of secondary aspiration.
- Use of sealing devices, such as Ligasure, TLS3 Starion, Harmonic scalpel, or bipolar energy devices, may be helpful tools to prevent bleeding risk and fasten the surgical procedure.
- Use of the recent technology of fluorescence imaging with indocyanine green (ICG) may be very helpful in selected procedures to improve intra-operative visualization of anatomic structures and facilitate surgery.

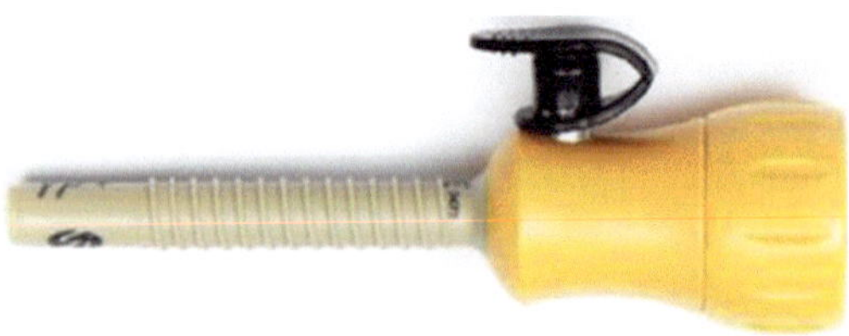

Fig. 1.4 Three-mm trocar with micro-threaded shaft

1.8 Discussion

The laparoscopic transperitoneal approach is the easiest approach to begin with as minimally invasive surgery (MIS) [1]. Laparoscopy is suitable even for retroperitoneal organs, particularly the kidneys. The advantages are the presence of a natural cavity and a more familiar space for minimally invasive surgeons. Potential disadvantages include the unnecessary opening of the abdominal cavity with the risk of bowel or vessel perforation during introduction of the trocars. Access to the kidney is also slightly more difficult due to the presence of the colon, pancreas, and/or the spleen. From a technical point of view, some hints should be followed: very accurate positioning of the patient using all possible positions of the operating table; use of a 30-degree scope; introduction of the operating instruments after exact localization of the pathology; the help of additional forceps or percutaneous sutures in order to suspend organs (colon, bladder) in order to facilitate surgery [1]. Currently, procedures such as laparoscopic exploration for undescended testicles and laparoscopic nephrectomy are accepted as the gold standard and are performed at most institutions. Other procedures, such as laparoscopic pyeloplasty and laparoscopic reconstructive surgery, have only recently been introduced and are primarily available at centers where surgeons have advanced laparoscopic experience [3].

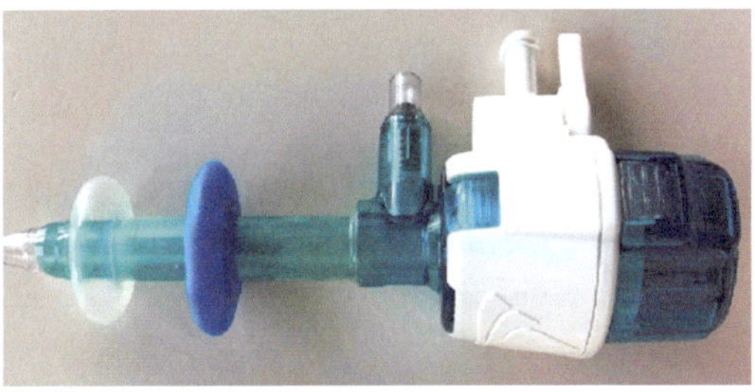

Fig. 1.5 Five-mm balloon trocar

A debated point is whether transperitoneal or retroperitoneal approach is of advantage for the patient. We recently published our 20-year experience with minimally invasive nephrectomy comparing both approaches: laparoscopy was significantly faster than the retroperitoneal approach and the complications rate was significantly higher with the retroperitoneal route [4]. Based upon our experience, transperitoneal approach should be always adopted in case of reflux nephropathy, allowing to perform a near total ureterectomy till up to the bladder dome and avoid leaving a residual distal ureteral stump. Laparoscopy is also preferable to retroperitoneoscopy in case of ectopic pelvic kidneys. Furthermore, retroperitoneoscopy is contraindicated in case of xanthogranulomatous pyelonephritis or other kidney infections, or in case of previous renal surgery [4].

In a multicentric study including 102 patients undergoing partial nephrectomy over a 5-year period either by a laparoscopic or a retroperitoneoscopic approach [19], we reported that overall complication rate was significantly higher for the retroperitoneoscopic group than for the laparoscopic group. In addition, the operating time for laparoscopy was significantly shorter

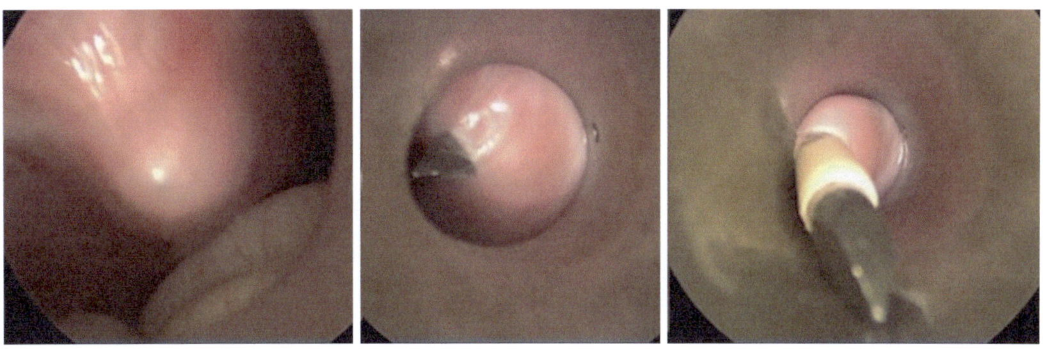

Fig. 1.6 The trocar may be safely inserted into the cannula containing the optic ("trocar in trocar")

compared to retroperitoneoscopy. We concluded that laparoscopic partial nephrectomy was faster and safer and technically easier to perform in children compared to retroperitoneoscopic partial nephrectomy mainly due to a larger working space. In addition, the possibility for complete ureterectomy in case of a refluxing system was considered to be an advantage along with laparoscopy [19]. Based upon our experience, the position of the diseased kidney, the presence or absence of a refluxing ureter, and the need for ureterocelectomy and bladder base reconstruction should be the main determining factors in the choice of type of approach in kidney surgery.

Use of new technologies is crucial to improve outcomes and large-scale applicability of technically demanding MIS procedures in pediatric urology. Different sealing devices (Starion, Ligasure, Ultracision), including the new generation of 3-mm devices (JustRight™ Vessel Sealing System), are now available and have been proved to be very useful tools during demanding surgical procedures, allowing for bloodless dissection and faster surgery compared with traditional monopolar energy [4, 19]. More recently, fluorescence imaging with indocyanine green (ICG) has been adopted in selected procedures to improve intraoperative visualization of anatomic structures and facilitate surgery [20]. The main applications in pediatric urology include varicocele repair with lymphography, partial nephrectomy, renal cysts deroofing, and renal tumors removal.

The main benefits of laparoscopic approach in pediatric patients have been reported in terms of decreased postoperative pain and analgesic requirement, fast mobilization and return to full daily activities, and short hospital stay. The last but no less important advantage of the laparoscopic approach is the excellent cosmetic outcome (Fig. 1.7).

As the field continues to develop, as new technologies continue to emerge and miniaturize to accommodate smaller children, and as more surgeons with laparoscopic experience enter the field, pediatric urologic laparoscopy will continue to progress [18]. The hope is that minimally invasive approaches become readily available to more children in the future, although one of the largest challenges facing pediatric urology is the ability to pass along the skills and knowledge of laparoscopic techniques to the wider community, such that all activity is not focused at centers with high caseloads.

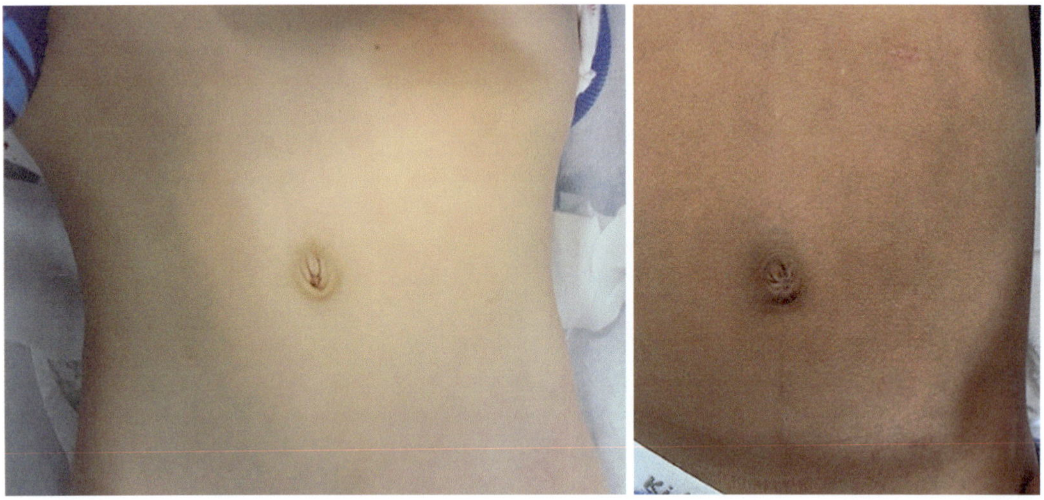

Fig. 1.7 Cosmetic outcome of laparoscopic surgery

Take-Home Points

- Laparoscopic techniques have expanded the field of pediatric urology from merely diagnostic procedures to include complex reconstructive surgeries.
- The benefits of laparoscopy include increased magnification and visualization of the surgical field, reduced postoperative morbidity, shorter convalescence, and improved cosmesis.
- New technologies, including surgical devices and fluorescence imaging using indocyanine green (ICG), are currently being adopted to improve surgical performance and outcome.
- As the field continues to develop with improvements in technology and the number of pediatric surgeons with backgrounds in basic laparoscopy increases, pediatric urologic laparoscopy will continue to progress.

References

1. Steyaert H, Valla JS. Minimally invasive urologic surgery in children: an overview of what can be done. Eur J Pediatr Surg. 2005;15:307–13.
2. Smaldone MC, Sweeney DD, Ost MC, Docimo SG. Laparoscopy in paediatric urology: present status. BJU Int. 2007;100:143–50.
3. Szavay PO. Applications of laparoscopic Transperitoneal surgery of the pediatric urinary tract. Front Pediatr. 2019;7:29.
4. Esposito C, Escolino M, Corcione F, et al. Twenty-year experience with laparoscopic and retroperitoneoscopic nephrectomy in children: considerations and details of technique. Surg Endosc. 2016;30(5):2114–8.
5. Jordan GH, Winslow BH. Laparoendoscopic upper pole partial nephrectomy with ureterectomy. J Urol. 1993;150:940–3.
6. Piaggio L, Franc-Guimond J, Figueroa TE, Barthold JS, Gonzalez R. Comparison of laparoscopic and open partial nephrectomy for duplication anomalies in children. J Urol. 2006;175:2269–73.
7. Symons SJ, Bhirud PS, Jain V, Shetty AS, Desai MR. Laparoscopic pyeloplasty: our new gold standard. J Endourol. 2009;23:463–7.
8. Moscardi PR, Barbosa JA, Andrade HS, et al. Reoperative laparoscopic ureteropelvic junction obstruction repair in children: safety and efficacy of the technique. J Urol. 2017;197:798–804.
9. Blanc T, Koulouris E, Botto N, Paye-Jaouen A, El-Ghoneimi A. Laparoscopic pyeloplasty in children with horseshoe kidney. J Urol. 2014;191:1097–103.
10. Fuchs J, Luithle T, Warmann SW, Haber P, Blumenstock G, Szavay P. Laparoscopic surgery on the upper urinary tract in children below one year of age – technical aspects and functional outcome. J Urol. 2009;182:1561–8.
11. Skarsgard ED, Albanese CT. The safety and efficacy of laparoscopic adrenalectomy in children. Arch Surg. 2005;140:905–8.
12. Miller KA, Albanese C, Harrison M, et al. Experience with laparoscopic adrenalectomy in pediatric patients. J Pediatr Surg. 2002;37:979–82.
13. Riquelme M, Lopez M, Landa S, et al. Laparoscopic extravesical ureteral reimplantation (LEVUR): a multicenter experience with 95 cases. Eur J Pediatr Surg. 2013;23:143–7.
14. Farina A, Esposito C, Escolino M, Lopez M, Settimi A, Varlet F. Laparoscopic extravesical ureteral reimplantation (LEVUR): a systematic review. Transl Pediatr. 2016;5:291–4.
15. Hedican SP, Schulam PG, Docimo SG. Laparoscopic assisted reconstructive surgery. J Urol. 1999;161(1):267–70.
16. Peters CA. Complications in pediatric urological laparoscopy: results of a survey. J Urol. 1996;155:1070–3.
17. Esposito C, Lima M, Mattioli G, et al. Complications of pediatric urological laparoscopy: mistakes and risks. J Urol. 2003;169(4):1490–2.
18. Sweeney DD, Smaldone MC, Docimo SG. Minimally invasive surgery for urologic disease in children. Nat Clin Pract Urol. 2007;4(1):26–38.
19. Esposito C, Escolino M, Miyano G, et al. A comparison between laparoscopic and retroperitoneoscopic approach for partial nephrectomy in children with duplex kidney: a multicentric survey. World J Urol. 2016;34(7):939–48.
20. Esposito C, Del Conte F, Cerulo M, et al. Clinical application and technical standardization of indocyanine green (ICG) fluorescence imaging in pediatric minimally invasive surgery. Pediatr Surg Int. 2019;35(10):1043–50.

Retropertioneoscopy Approach in Pediatric Urology

2

Fabio Chiarenza, Maria Escolino, Cosimo Bleve, Fulvia Del Conte, Vincenzo Coppola, Mariapina Cerulo, Giuseppe Autorino, and Ciro Esposito

Learning Objectives

- To describe step by step the general retroperitoneoscopic technique.
- To report the latest results of the major international papers about retroperitoneoscopy.
- To describe tips and tricks in retroperitoneoscopy and its uses in pediatric urology.

2.1 Introduction

Minimally invasive surgery (MIS) has gained popularity in the last three decades due to numerous advantages and has evolved and made remarkable progress. Compared to the adult population, the application of this approach in the pediatric population was somewhat delayed [1, 2].

However, since its advent, the use of laparoscopy and later retroperitoneoscopy in pediatric urology has revolutionized the diagnosis and treatment of many pediatric urological diseases.

The aim of a retroperitoneal approach is to strictly adhere to the principles of open urology for benign lesions and to ensure a high level of cosmesis after the surgical incisions are made [3].

In particular, retroperitoneoscopy has been used with excellent results on children for a wide range of urological procedures such as in renal, adrenal, upper and lower urinary tract surgery.

The main indications of the retroperitoneoscopic technique are

- Nephrectomy to treat benign diseases such as multicystic or dysplastic kidneys causing renal hypertension, nonfunctioning kidneys associated with obstructive uropathy or VUR, xanthogranulomatosis, pyelonephritis, protein-losing nephropathy, and occasionally, nephrolithiasis or nephropathy causing uncontrollable hypertension.
- Partial nephrectomy to treat renal duplication and a poorly functioning and chronically infected upper-pole segment. The retroperitoneal approach has already been described for upper and lower pole nephrectomy.
- Dismembered pyeloplasty to treat uretero–pelvic junction obstruction (UPJO) that is the most common disorder of the upper urinary tract in children.

F. Chiarenza · M. Escolino · C. Bleve
F. Del Conte · V. Coppola · M. Cerulo
G. Autorino · C. Esposito (✉)
Pediatric Surgery Unit, Federico II University of Naples, Naples, Italy
e-mail: fabio.chiarenza@ulssvicenza.it; maria.escolino@unina.it; cosimo.bleve@aulss8.veneto.it; fulvia.delconte@unina.it; vincenzocoppola1992@gmail.com; mariapina.cerulo@unina.it; autorino.giuseppe@gmail.com; ciroespo@unina.it

C. Esposito et al. (eds.), *Minimally Invasive Techniques in Pediatric Urology*,
https://doi.org/10.1007/978-3-030-99280-4_2

The aim of this chapter is to describe the basis of technique and find out the benefits of retroperitoneoscopy in the main frequent urological diseases in children.

2.2 Preoperative Preparation

The parents give their informed consent to the procedure. This is essential in pediatric population because the reported benefits of a retroperitoneoscopic approach have not been firmly established.

Children are prepared for surgery as usual without bowel preparation.

A standard anesthesia protocol is used after a premedication with midazolam: all children were mechanically ventilated after insertion of an appropriately sized endotracheal tube. Nitrous oxide is generally contraindicated to reduce bowel distension; a nasogastric tube is introduced for the same purpose and a bladder catheter is inserted to quantify diuresis.

Preoperative antibiotic dose is given according to the etiology: not necessary in case of dysplastic multicystic kidney, but necessary in case of destructed kidney by an obstructive or refluxing uropathy.

An intraoperative monitoring is performed with a pulse oximeter, non-invasive blood pressure monitor, and an electrocardiogram; end tidal carbon dioxide ($ETCO_2$) was monitored through a capnogram.

2.3 Positioning

The procedure is performed with the patient placed in lateral decubitus position (Fig. 2.1).

This access has been demonstrated as reliable for a large number of indications, particularly total nephrectomy, pyeloplasty, and pyelotomy [4–6]. Its direct access to the renal vessels without violating the peritoneal cavity is the main advantage of the lateral retroperitoneal method, and if an urgent open conversion is needed, it offers the best exposure to control great vessels.

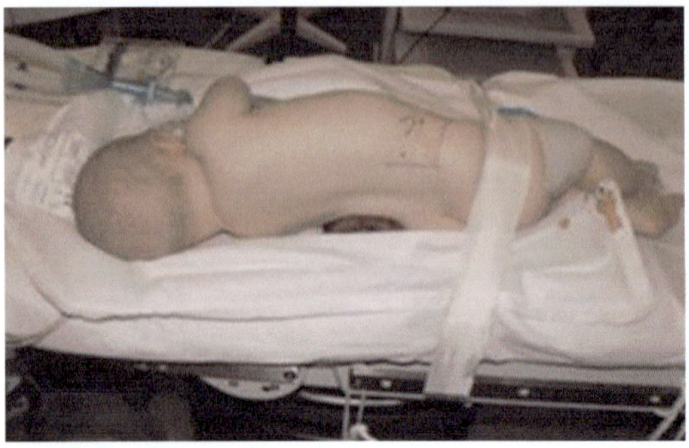

Fig. 2.1 Patient position

Normally, the surgeon and assistant face the back of the patient. The video column stands on the other side, the cables are fixed to the superior part of the operative field (Fig. 2.2). If a total ureterectomy is needed at the same time, the position of the surgeon and his assistant, and the position of the video column may change during the procedure; the installation must be planned accordingly.

2.4 Instrumentation

The choice of the telescope and of the cannulas must be adapted to each case: for example to remove a dysplastic multicystic kidney in a normal child less than 2 years of age, a 5-mm telescope and two 3- or 5-mm normal cannulas for operating device seems the good option. At the opposite, in order to remove a large hydronephrotic infected kidney in an obese teenager, there is no other way for the primary access than a quite large skin incision (15/20 mm) and the use of a large cannula with balloon for the primary access.

A plastic bag is fixed to the dorsal part of the patient and instruments are put away in this bag: monopolar hook, bipolar forceps, harmonic scalpel, aspiration cannula.

In the recent years, thanks to the use of new hemostatic and synthesis devices that permit faster and safer procedures, the technique seems to be easier to perform.

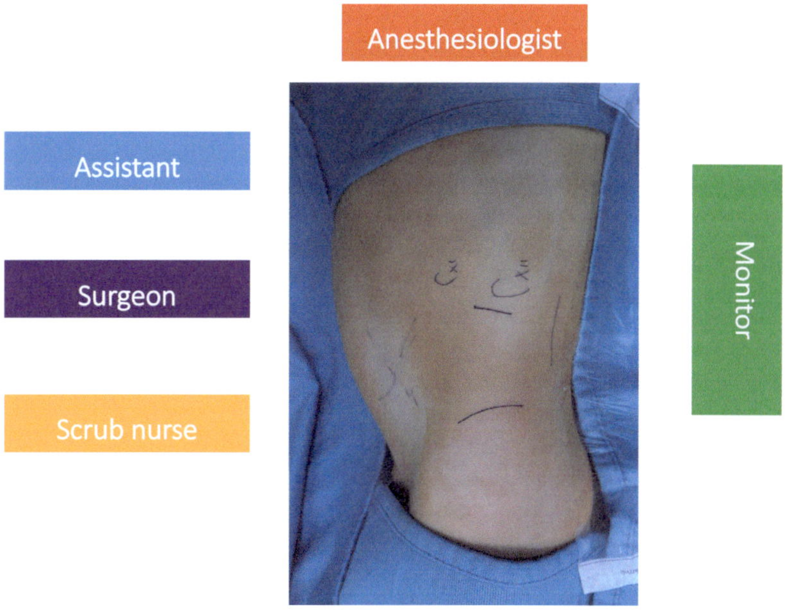

Fig. 2.2 Team position

2.5 Technique

An open technique is used to place the first port and access to retroperitoneal space. This is the key point of the technique because the majority of complications deal with access technique and the development of a working field [7]. After sterile preparation and draping, anatomical landmarks are palpated (11th, 12th ribs, iliac crest, sacrospinalis muscle) and the surgeon mentally localizes the lateral peritoneal reflexion.

The skin incision (8–15 mm long) is made just below the 12th rib tip at the posterior axillary line, in the area where the muscular wall is the thinnest (Fig. 2.3). If the incision is oversized, resultant gas leak could be managed with large retaining sutures or large cannulas with fascial retention balloons. A muscle splitting dissection is used to gain access into the retroperitoneal space; dissecting forceps, retractors, and Metzenbaum scissors are usually sufficient to bluntly divide the external oblique, internal oblique; after piercing the white transversalis fascia with the tip of scissors, the dissection is stopped when the yellow perirenal fat become visible. Two stay sutures are placed on each side of the muscular layers (2/0 short curved needle – semicircular 16 mm-). In case of large (15 mm) incision, it is sometimes possible to recognize the Gerota's fascia to incise it in order to begin CO_2 insufflation directly in the perirenal space; most often, the Gerota's fascia is not visible; so the working space is created in the retroperitoneal space, and the Gerota's fascia will be opened posteriorly in the following step.

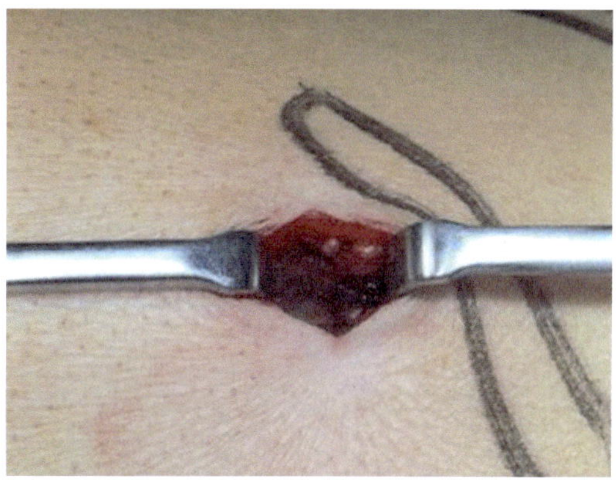

Fig. 2.3 First trocar access

Then a small gauze is introduced in the retroperitoneal space and manipulated carefully to create the space. The surgeon must keep the dissection in close touch with the posterior muscular wall to avoid peritoneal perforation. The primary blunt port (5–10 mm – disposable or reusable) is placed and secured to create a seal for the retropneumoperitoneum. CO_2 insufflation is started (8–10 mm in infant – 12–15 in children). A 0° or 30° lens is inserted. The working space, already created by the gauze, is progressively enlarged by moving the tip of the telescope, used as a palpator to free retroperitoneal fibrous tissues, behind the kidney. This allows to expose the anatomical landmarks: quadratus lumborum, psoas muscles, posterior part of the kidney. The thick lateral and posterior abdominal wall, closely attached to the bony boundaries, cannot be distended by insufflation as well as the anterior abdominal wall; this explains why a good curarization is essential so a sufficient operating space can only be achieved by pushing away peritoneum and intra-abdominal organs and by dissecting the lateral peritoneal reflection at least to the anterior axillary line [8].

Placement of accessory ports. Two additional ports (3 or 5 mm) are placed under direct vision: the posterior port is introduced first, in the costo–spinal angle, at the junction of the lateral border of the erector spinae muscle with the underside of the 12th rib; the inferior port just above the iliac crest, but it must not be placed too close to the iliac crest because the bony relief could restrict the device's mobility.

This port placement allows to achieve a triangulation of ports in order to maximize exposure and minimize instrument conflict in a small working space.

To exit retroperitoneal space, after performing a procedure and after a possible extraction, the port and telescope is reintroduced to check the hemostasis at low pressure, particularly near the hilum. If needed, a drain is introduced through the inferior cannula; ports are removed under direct vision. The closure of fascia is easy because of the two stay sutures placed at the beginning of the procedure. Port sites can be injected with bupivicaine and lidocaine. The skin is close with subcuticular stitches and/or adhesive strips.

2.6 Postoperative Care

In the postoperative period, the patients can keep a normal decubitus.

They can restart full oral feeding a few hours after surgery. The analgesic requirement (Paracetamol every 6 h) is generally limited to the first 24 postoperative hours.

In case of drainage, the drain is removed at day 1 or day 2 post-op. An ultrasound is performed at 1 week and 1 month post-op. to check the lumbar area. The following annual controls are focused on the remaining kidney..

Tips and Tricks

- **Dense perirenal adhesions:** 10 years ago at the beginning of our experience, dense perirenal adhesions due to previous nephrostomy, repeated perinephritis, xanthogranulomatous pyelonephritis were considered as contraindication for retroperitoneoscopic nephrectomy [9–12]. Now, we try a retroperitoneoscopic attempt and most of the time we succeed [10–13].
- **Horseshoe/ectopic kidneys:** we and others [14] have performed nephrectomy for horseshoe or ectopic sigmoid kidney, using the same lateral approach or a modified 45° flank position. Aberrant vascular anatomy is common in these cases and a careful dissection and clamping before division is mandatory especially in case of sigmoid ectopic kidney. The ultrasonic scalpel is very useful to cut between healthy and destructed parenchyma.

  Sometimes the kidney is "invisible" before operation. If it is suspected to be located in the lower part of the abdomen, it seems preferable to use an intraperitoneal approach [15]. But if the "invisible" kidney is suspected to be located around the normal place, the retroperitoneal approach could be successfully used as in one of our cases.

- **Giant hydronephrosis:** destructed kidney with giant hydronephrosis are usually soft with low pressure in it. Careful open approach allows to avoid entering the renal cortex or pelvis during the initial trocar placement. After having dissected the posterior part, decompressing the renal pelvis with an aspirative needle under visual control greatly improves exposure of anatomical elements, and a large working space is naturally created.

2.7 Discussion

Retroperitoneoscopic surgery in children is feasible and safe if performed by well-trained surgeons. Between transperitoneal and retroperitoneal approach, the choice should be made according to each case; however, in our opinion, pure pediatric urologist would favor the retroperitoneoscopic access to reach the upper urinary tract and the kidney, because this is the "natural" way even if it is more difficult to learn at the beginning.

Operative urological minimal access surgery has recently expanded its range of indications due to improved laparoscopic technology and an increased interest in minimally invasive therapeutics. In other words, the indications have evolved from diagnostic procedures 20 years ago, then to ablative procedures 10 years ago, and now to reconstructive surgery [3].

Nowadays, minimally invasive surgery for pediatric nephrectomies is established as routine practice. Transperitoneal and retroperitoneal are the two approaches for performing either total or partial nephrectomy [11, 12]. During transperitoneal laparoscopy, the surgeon must mobilize the hepatic flexure of the colon in order to expose the right kidney, and the splenic flexure to expose the left kidney. This approach is easier compared to retroperitoneoscopy, since it allows plenty of space, but it has an inherent risk of adhesion formation or intestinal perforation.

Faster access and easier dissection of the parenchyma can be achieved with the retroperitoneal approach [1].

As for the repair of ureteropelvic junction obstruction, the retroperitoneal approach is now an acceptable method [10]. The cosmetic result is superior in retroperitoneoscopy, and the need for reoperation is also reduced in comparison with the transperitoneal approach [1].

In conclusion, it is possible to state that retroperitoneoscopy is the technique of choice for reaching the urinary tract in children, as it can be performed on them safely and effectively. Still, this procedure is more challenging and requires excellent imaging of the retroperitoneal space, especially when partial nephrectomies are involved [12].

Retroperitoneoscopic approach offers several potential advantages. The main advantage is its more direct and rapid exposure without peritoneal cavity transgression and without dissection and handling of intraperitoneal structures which could be injured during these maneuvers.

The working space is not obscured by intestinal loops; therefore, the risk of postoperative paralytic ileus, shoulder pain, omental evisceration, and intestinal adhesions is eliminated.

References

1. Antoniou D, Karetsos C. Laparoscopy or retroperitoneoscopy: which is the best approach in pediatric urology. Transl Pediatr. 2016;5(4):205–13.
2. Esposito C, Valla JS, Yeung CK. Current indications for laparoscopy and retroperitoneoscopy in pediatric urology. Surg Endosc. 2004;18(11):1559–64.
3. Valla JS. Retroperitoneoscopic surgery in children. Semin Pediatr Surg. 2007;16(4):270–7.
4. El Ghoneimi A, Valla JS, Steyaert H, Aigrain Y. Laparoscopic renal surgery via a retroperitoneal approach in children. J Urol. 1998;160:1138–41.
5. Franks M, Schneck FX, Docimo SG. Retroperitoneoscopy in children. In: Caione P, Kavoussi LR, Micali R, editors. Retroperitoneoscopy and extraperitoneal laparoscopy in pediatric an adult urology. Berlin: Springer; 2003. p. 103–18.
6. Gaur DD. The accurate placement of the balloon for retroperitoneal dissection by the percutaneous method, insuring that it expands in the right plane. BJU Int. 1999;84:1095.

7. Peters GA. Complications of retroperitoneal laparoscopy in Pediatric Urology: prevention, recognition and management. In: Caione P, Kavoussy LR, Micali R, editors. Retroperitoneoscopy and extraperitoneal laparoscopy in pediatric and adult urology. Berlin: Springer; 2003. p. 203–10.
8. Micali S, Caione P, Virgini G, Capozza N, Scarfini M, Micali F. Retroperitoneal access in children using a direct vision technique. J Urol. 2001;165:1229–32.
9. Turrà F, Escolino M, Farina A, Settimi A, Esposito C, Varlet F. Pyeloplasty techniques using minimally invasive surgery (MIS) in pediatric patients. Transl Pediatr. 2016;5(4):251–5. https://doi.org/10.21037/tp.2016.10.0.
10. El-Ghoneimi A, Farhat W, Bolduc S, Bagli D, McLorie G, Aigrain Y, et al. Laparoscopic dismembered pyeloplasty by a retroperitoneal approach in children. BJU Int. 2003;92(1):104–8; discussion 108.
11. Esposito C, Escolino M, Corcione F, Draghici IM, Savanelli A, Castagnetti M, et al. Twenty-year experience with laparoscopic and retroperitoneoscopic nephrectomy in children: considerations and details of technique. Surg Endosc. 2016;30(5):2114–8. https://doi.org/10.1007/s00464-015-4472-7.
12. Lee RS, Retik AB, Borer JG, Diamond DA, Peters CA. Pediatric retroperitoneal laparoscopic partial nephrectomy: comparison with an age matched cohort of open surgery. J Urol. 2005;174:708–11.
13. Merrot T, Ordorica FR, Steyaert H, Ginier C, Valla JS. Is diffuse xanthogranulomatous pyelonephritis a contra-indication to retroperitoneoscopic nephroureterectomy? Surg Lap Endosc. 1998;8:366–9.
14. Leclair MD, Camby C, Capito C, DeWindt A, Podevin G, Heloury Y. Retroperitoneoscopic nephrectomy of a horseshoe kidney in a child. Surg Endosc. 2003;17:1156.
15. Yeung CK, Liu KW, Ng WT, Ttan HL, Tam YH, Lee KH. Laparoscopy as the investigation and treatment of choice for urinary incontinence caused by small "invisible" dysplastic kidney with infrasphincteric ureteric ectopia. BJU Int. 1999;84:324.

Prone Approach in Pediatric Urology

3

Sara Lobo, Naser Al-Soudan Al-Anazi, and Imran Mushtaq

Learning Points
- To describe, step by step, the posterior prone retroperitoneoscopic approach.
- To describe some tips and tricks to optimise and improve outcomes.
- To illustrate the approach with a video of the technique.

3.1 Introduction

Minimally invasive surgical (MIS) procedures for the treatment of several renal conditions, benign and malignant, are gradually replacing open surgery. Nephrectomy, partial nephrectomy and nephroureterectomy have now become standard procedures by MIS in centres where expertise is available [1]. After the landmark publication of Gaur describing the retroperitoneoscopic approach, many surgeons favour this approach, using one or more instrument ports. The single instrument port laparoscopic (SIMPL) technique has been shown to be safe and effective for unilateral and synchronous bilateral retroperitoneoscopic nephrectomy in the paediatric population [2, 3]. The purpose of this chapter is to describe the posterior prone retroperitoneoscopic which, depending on the experience of surgeon, complexity of the clinical case and type of procedure, can be utilised with one or more instrument ports.

S. Lobo (✉) · N. A.-S. Al-Anazi · I. Mushtaq
Department of Pediatric Urology, Great Ormond Street Hospital for Children NHS Foundation Trust, London, UK
e-mail: sara.lobo@gosh.nhs.uk; Naser.Alanazi@gosh.nhs.uk; mushti@gosh.nhs.uk; Imran.mushtaq@gosh.nhs.uk

3.2 Preoperative Preparation

The preoperative investigations vary according to the type of procedure to be performed, but should always include a thorough review of the imaging and clinical history to allow an understanding of the anatomy, a reliable estimation of the surgical time and any possible complications.

On the day of the surgery, preoperative antibiotics should be administered at anaesthetic induction, according to the urine culture results. A urethral catheter may be required in certain cases. Some surgeons may prefer to perform a cystoscopy ± retrograde studies prior to the main procedure to confirm the anatomy.

3.3 Positioning

The patient is placed fully prone, close to the edge of the operating table. Cotton wool bolsters are placed under the chest (folded) and beneath the anterior superior iliac spine (rolled) allowing the

C. Esposito et al. (eds.), *Minimally Invasive Techniques in Pediatric Urology*,
https://doi.org/10.1007/978-3-030-99280-4_3

abdomen to be dependent. Pressure points are protected in an appropriate manner. Mild lateral flexion of the patient to the contra-lateral side can help to open up the working space in smaller infants [4].

Marking of the landmarks should only be done once the patient is in the final position. The midline spine is marked, as well as the 11th and 12th ribs, the iliac crest and the lateral edge of the erector spinae muscles. As demonstrated in the video, the camera port site is marked half-way along the line between the 12th rib and the iliac crest lateral to the erector spinae muscles. The first instrument port is positioned at the intersection of the line running from the tip of 11th rib and a line drawn laterally from the camera port. If a second instrument needs to be used, the port insertion site is located midway between the camera port and the midline spine.

3.4 Instrumentation/Room Layout/Equipment

- The position of team members and instrumentation is shown in Fig. 3.1.
- Retroperitoneal dissecting balloon: size 8.5 sterile surgical glove, 12 Fr Jacques catheter, a silk suture, a 3-way tap and a 50 ml Luer-lock syringe.

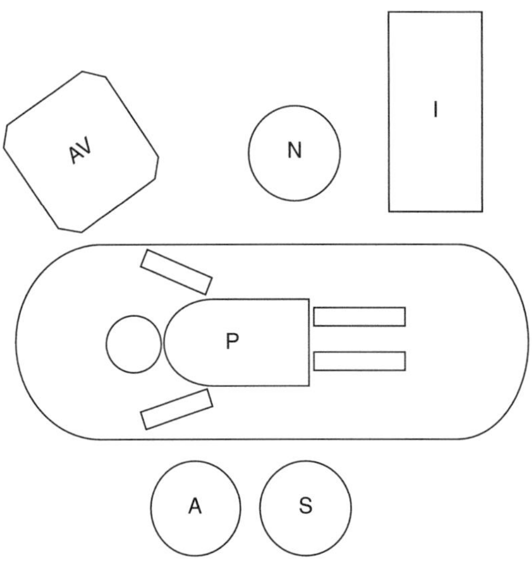

Fig. 3.1 Schematic representation of the room setup (*A* assistant; *AV* audio visual equipment; *I* instrument trolley; *N* scrub nurse; *P* patient; *S* surgeon)

3.5 Technique

3.5.1 Camera Port

Local anaesthesia is infiltrated before a 7 mm transverse incision is made. A small artery clip is used to separate the fascia and adipose tissue to the level of the muscles. The closed artery clip is then pushed under control through the thoracodorsal and transversalis fascia. 'A discreet popping sensation' can be felt as the instrument penetrates these layers. After, a larger artery clip is opened and closed to create an adequate and reliable tract through the muscle layers to the level just outside the Gerota's fascia.

3.5.2 Balloon Blunt Dissection

A dissecting balloon is created by securing the middle finger of a sterile glove to the end of a 12 Fr Jacques catheter with a silk tie (to create an airtight seal). The catheter is connected to a three-way tap and a 50 ml syringe and the balloon is tested. It is important to ensure that the balloon is fully deflated after the test, and the tip of the catheter must be at the tip of the glove finger.

The deflated dissecting balloon is lubricated and inserted into the retroperitoneal space. The balloon is slowly inflated to develop the retroperitoneal space, which, depending upon the size of the patient, will require 100–200 ml of air. A lateral bulge is often visible and confirms that the balloon is in the correct location and is not intraperitoneal. The balloon is left inflated for 30 s to promote haemostasis, and then deflated and removed.

The Hasson port is inserted, and insufflation is begun with a pressure of 10–12 mmHg. A 30-degree laparoscope is recommended for retroperitoneoscopic surgery to utilise maximal visualisation.

3.5.3 Working Ports

Local anaesthesia is infiltrated under vision and can aid in determining the direction of port insertion. An incision is made at the pre-marked site. A bladeless trocar with stability sleeve is recommended to reduce the risk of accidental dislodgement.

3.6 Postoperative Care

For all the procedures performed by this approach, the patient can start fluids and diet on return to the ward and to minimise risk of bacteraemia after the procedure, antibiotics should be continued to cover the immediate postoperative period (intravenous or oral). The patient is discharged when mobilising and clinically well, with adequate control of pain with simple analgesia.

3.7 Results and Applications

The posterior prone retroperitoneoscopic approach is reliable and adaptable for all type of renal surgery, as well as adrenal surgery. The SIMPL nephrectomy in particular has shown additional advantages comparing to other techniques for the same procedure [2]. A single instrument port in addition to one camera port is adequate to complete a nephrectomy and avoids instruments becoming entangled within the restricted retroperitoneal working space. The SIMPL nephrectomy facilitates the procedure as the surgeon can control the dissection more intuitively as he/she is holding the camera themself. The decreased number of incisions improves the cosmetic result and reduces pain. One disadvantage is that is does not allow complete ureterectomy in cases where this may be desirable, and in such cases a second groin incision may be required to achieve this.

Tips and Tricks

- When patient is positioned, the chest and pelvis need to be raised to allow the abdomen to lie in a dependent manner, which facilitates ventilation and allows the abdominal contents to move away from the kidney.
- A mild lateral flexion of the spine of the patient to the contra-lateral side opens up the working space, facilitating access to the retroperitoneum.
- To create the right tract for the balloon insertion is crucial. During the step of gently introducing the artery clip into the thoracolumbar fascia, two 'pops' should be felt (corresponding to the posterior and anterior layers being crossed). The aim is to inflate the balloon outside Gerota's fascia.
- The home-made dissecting balloon should be adjusted for patient size/age (a 4 cm balloon length is adequate for children aged <5 years and small children; a 7 cm length for aged >5 years or with a high body mass index – Fig. 3.2).
- For children with high body mass index or in pubertal age, two glove fingers with one inside the other, should be used to accommodate the higher pressure within the balloon.
- Despite a very low risk of peritoneal tear, it can occur in the following situations: if dissecting balloon is inflated too quickly and in children on peritoneal dialysis, where the peritoneum is often thin and friable.
- If a dissecting balloon rupture occurs, the ruptured balloon must be carefully examined for lost fragments, which should be sought and removed from the patient.
- Attention to meticulous haemostasis is paramount. Even small amounts of blood in the relatively small working space can absorb the light and impair the vision.

3.8 Discussion

The retroperitoneoscopic approach has several advantages over the transperitoneal laparoscopic approach to the kidney. It minimises the risk of

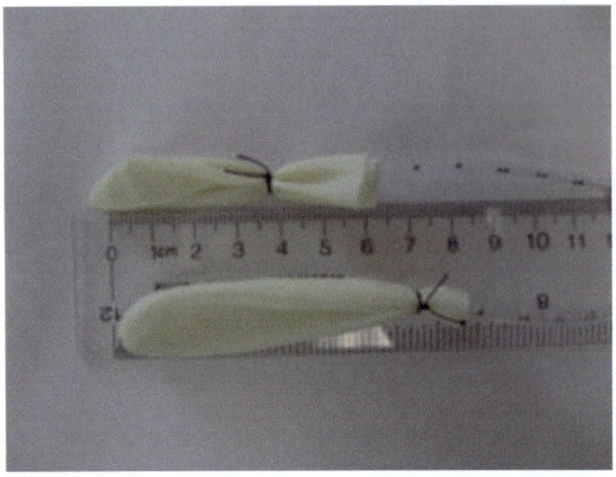

Fig. 3.2 Balloon dilator length adjusted for patient size/age (upper balloon for smaller children; lower balloon for children aged >5 years or with high body mass index) [3]

injury to intra-abdominal organs and promotes quicker recovery [5]. Compared to other approaches for retroperitoneoscopic surgery, the posterior prone retroperitoneoscopic technique minimises the risk of a peritoneal tear, and allows direct and rapid access to the kidney and renal hilum.

Take-Home Points

- The posterior prone retroperitoneoscopic technique can be used in several renal procedures safely and effectively.
- For total nephrectomies, the SIMPL technique (one single working instrument) can be used in the majority of the cases in experienced hands.
- Careful patient positioning and marking of the landmarks are essential for the success of the procedure and should not be underestimated.
- Complete ureterectomy is not achievable by this approach.

References

1. Cerulo M, Escolino M, Turrà F, Roberti A, Farina A, Esposito C. Benefits of Retroperitoneoscopic surgery in pediatric urology. Curr Urol Rep. 2018;10:33–8.
2. Garg S, Gundeti M, Mushtaq I. The single instrument port laparoscopic (SIMPL) nephrectomy. J Pediatr Urol. 2006;3:194–6.
3. Msezane LP, Mushtaq I, Gundeti M. An update on experience with the single-instrument port laparocopic nephrectomy. BJU Int. 2008;103:1406–9.
4. Mushtaq I. Laparoscopic nephrectomy and heminephrectomy. In: Spitz L, Coran AG, editors. Operative Pediatric Surgery; Springer, London. 2006. p. 767–78.
5. LeClair MD, Vidal I, Suply E, Podevin G, Héloury Y. Retroperitoneal laparoscopic heminephrectomy in duplex kidney in infants and children. Eur Urol. 2008;56:385–91.

4 Robotics in Pediatric Urology

Abhishek Deshpande and Mohan Gundeti

4.1 Introduction

Minimally invasive and robotic surgery techniques have rapidly become more widely utilized in the field of urology and pediatric urology. Laparoscopy was first introduced in pediatric urology in 1976 by Cortesti et al. for the evaluation of impalpable testes [1] and has since been used for many urological procedures. The first documented use of robotic-assisted surgery occurred in 1985, when the PUMA 200 robot was utilized for positional accuracy during a CT guided brain tumor biopsy [2]. In 1991, the same system was used by Davies et al. to perform a transurethral resection of the prostate (TURP) [3]. Nine years later, the da Vinci surgical system received FDA approval, representing a landmark moment in the sustainability of robotic surgery. One of the earliest uses of robotic surgery in pediatrics was by Peters and Borer in conducting a robotic pediatric pyeloplasty with symptomatic ureteropelvic junction (UPJ) in the United States 2002. In 2005, Gundeti et al. reported a pediatric retrocaval ureter correction utilizing robotic-assisted laparoscopy at Guy's Hospital in London, U.K [4].

Laparoscopic methods in children have many limitations, including a limited range of motion with four degrees of motion which is amplified by the small body habitus in younger patients. The use of robotic-assisted laparoscopic surgery can allow for improved visualization in small areas, increased range of motion with seven degrees of motion, as well as reduction or elimination of hand tremor. Additionally, robotic-assisted techniques can aid the surgeon in increasing dexterity and precision of movement, allowing for better control of instruments in small working spaces and improved ability to perform advanced suturing skills [5, 6]. Due to these advantages, such systems can act as a bridge between pure laparoscopic and robotic systems in addition to better facilitating pediatric patients. Over the past 20 years, robotic surgery has gained a foothold in urology as the standard of care for many different procedures due to the advantages of a stable, magnified, three-dimensional view, tremor filtering, motion scaling, and other bene-

A. Deshpande (✉)
University of Illinois College of Medicine, Chicago, IL, USA
e-mail: apdeshp2@uic.edu

M. Gundeti
Pediatric Urology (Surgery), The University of Chicago Medicine and Biological Sciences, Chicago, IL, USA

MFM (Ob/Gyn), The University of Chicago Medicine and Biological Sciences, Chicago, IL, USA

Pediatrics, The University of Chicago Medicine and Biological Sciences, Chicago, IL, USA

Pediatric Urology, Comer Children's Hospital, Chicago, IL, USA
e-mail: mgundeti@surgery.bsd.uchicago.edu

C. Esposito et al. (eds.), *Minimally Invasive Techniques in Pediatric Urology*,
https://doi.org/10.1007/978-3-030-99280-4_4

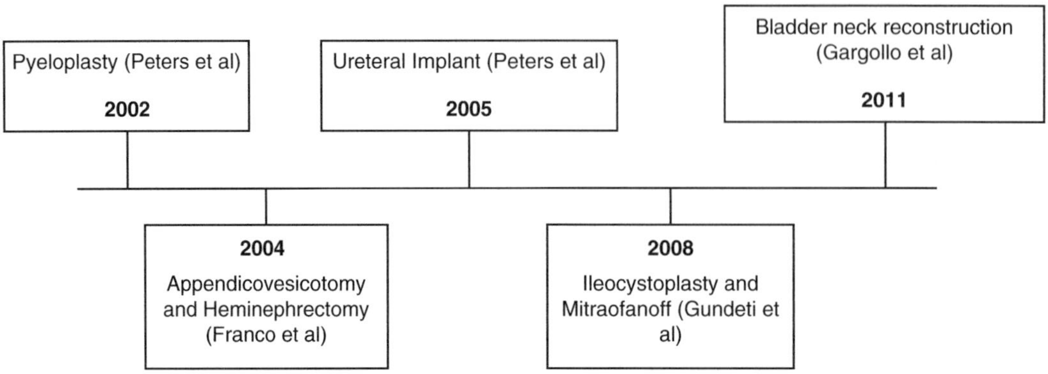

Fig. 4.1 Progression of the most commonly performed robotic urological procedures in pediatrics since 2002

fits. Overall, robotic surgical systems can also provide substantial benefits to patients for specific procedures in terms of a reduction in postoperative bleeding, complications, as well as cosmetic factors.

Robotic surgery was developed as a method to enhance the natural capabilities of a surgeon. In general, these devices often have a console which allows the surgeon to control movement and view the surgical field, a cart that includes mechanical arms, cameras, and surgical instruments, and a separate unit which may support other hardware and software components [7]. Some systems may be classified as "supervisory-controlled," wherein the surgeon positions a specific tool at a correct position and the robot autonomously performs a specific function (e.g., cutting bone for an implant). In "tele-surgical" (also known as master-slave) systems such as the da Vinci, the robot is operated by a surgeon at a specific distance. Finally, "shared-controlled" systems refer to robots which can be tele-operated but also resist a surgeon's movement if deemed unsafe or non-beneficial [8].

4.2 Procedural Evolution

Robotic surgery in pediatric urology has continued to progress in complexity and scope. While pyeloplasty for UPJ obstruction remains the most common robotic procedure in pediatric urology, other widely performed procedures include ureteral reimplantation, renal ablative procedures, continence procedures such as catheterizable channels (e.g., appendicovesicotomy, Ace channel) and bladder neck reconstruction. Increasingly, oncological applications like renal bladder tumors in children have also utilized robotic-assisted laparoscopy. Recently, the first complete intracorporeal robotic-assisted laparoscopic augmentation ileocystoplasty and Mitraofanoff appendicovesicotomy was performed by Gundeti et al. [9]. A timeline of the development of pediatric robotic urological procedures is shown in Fig. 4.1.

4.3 System and Instrumentation

The da Vinci robotic system has been the current standard of care for use in pediatric urology since its introduction in 2000. The system has had four iterations, including the Si system launched in 2009, which became the first model to offer high fidelity 3D vision and dual-surgeon console capacity. In 2014, the Xi system was launched with four robotic arms and the ability to attach the endoscope to any arm as well as have overhead instrument arm configuration [10]. The portfolio also includes the X with reduced cost and the newly developed single port with smaller profile and one robotic arm, though the single port is not yet FDA approved for pediatric use. However, the smaller profile of pediatric patients has posed challenges to use of the robot. Robotic instruments have been tailored to facilitate pediatric surgery through the

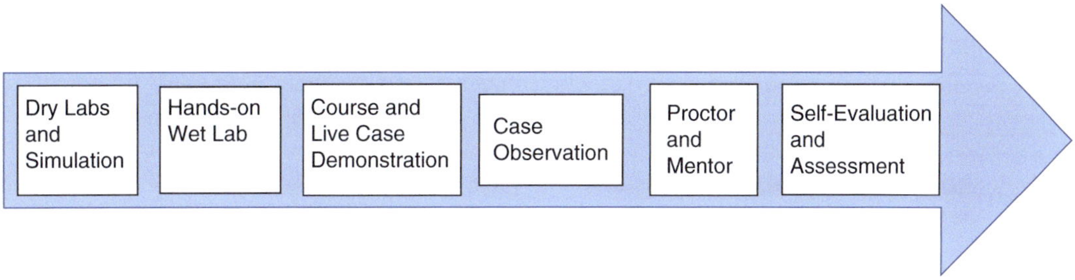

Fig. 4.2 Suggested approach for robotic surgery training

introduction of 5 mm instruments as opposed to the 8 mm instruments widely used in adults. However, although these have been introduced, in some manner, they have been counterintuitive due to different mechanisms. Despite its smaller profile, the 5 mm instruments are mechanically different as they function as a pulley system compared to the 8 mm instruments which work as a hinge joint. Due to this difference, studies have shown that the working distance for the 5 mm is actually greater and that the 8 mm instruments work better in terms of performance for parietal space constraints and reducing instrument collisions [11]. There is a need for future advancement in miniaturization for appropriate pediatric use.

4.4 Training and Credentialing

Like other surgical techniques, the use of robotic surgery in practice requires comprehensive training and development of expertise, often beginning in residency training and continuing through a surgeon's career. Currently, the training paradigm for robotic surgery consists of a stepwise approach consisting of pre-clinical training as well as clinical training recommended by many groups [12, 13]. Pre-clinical training largely consists of building familiarity with the da Vinci surgical system as well as "dry lab" practice using models and virtual reality simulation to train tasks such as suturing and knot tying. Training should also include "wet lab" practice using porcine models or cadavers so trainees can become familiar with higher-level skills and procedure-specific techniques. As trainees progress, the clinical component of surgical training should include clinical observation, acting as a bedside assistant to the acting surgeon, as well as time on the surgeon console. This gradual, step-wise approach emphasizing a transfer of skills has been studied widely with promising results (see Fig. 4.2) [14, 15]. Lee et al. published training and credentialing initiatives outlining a competency-based, stepwise curriculum to demonstrate proficiency in completing basic procedural skills [16]. Several organizations, including the American Urology Association (AUA) and British Association of Urological Surgeons (BAUS) have developed training guidelines. However, guidelines for the use of robotic surgery in pediatric patients are limited. Practicing urologists can utilize industry-developed programs through Intuitive Surgical, AUA-organized continuing medical education courses, or other training programs to develop their skills using the robot. A five-day pediatric robotic surgery mini-fellowship (PRM) was recently developed at the University of Chicago, which is provided through two modules, including upper and lower urinary tract surgery [17]. The modules consisted of hands-on inanimate training, animate skills training, as well as clinical case observations and discussions. Results from surveys from worldwide surgeons who adopted these modules indicated that a significant number of them were likely to incorporate robotic surgery in their practice and/or start a robotic program [17]. Such fellowships can provide training opportunities for surgeons who are already in practice as well as provide more specific pediatric skill competencies. Live case demonstrations can also be a useful didactic tool for teaching techniques and promoting discussion, though ethics consultations and appropriate patient selection is required [18].

4.5 Adoption of Robotic Surgical Practice

Surgical innovation should be met with appropriate assessment and evaluation. As laid out by the IDEAL criteria, emerging technologies should be evaluated utilizing thorough analysis of databases, prospective evaluation, and finally large-scale randomized control trials (RCTs) [19]. As robotic surgery continues to be used in more procedures and with a broader scope, more RCTs are required to demonstrate long-term effectiveness, safety, as well as compare alternative devices as more become approved for use. In order to overcome variations in surgical RCTs, it is recommended that surgeons maximize flexibility in delivery to allow for variation in surgeon and institution practices and use broad patient-eligibility criteria, among other potential solutions [20]. However, conducting RCTs can be difficult in later periods of practice adoption; thus, emphasis can be placed on prospective studies [21, 22].

Previously described by Everett Rogers, technological innovation is commonly adopted through an S-shaped curve, beginning slowly with early adopters before accelerating quickly to late adopters [23]. Based on recent trends in adoption, it is our speculation that pediatric urology is at a later portion of this S-shaped curve [24, 25]. For innovative surgical technologies, certain common characteristics include a procedure appeal to patients, compatibility with current practice, and support in available facilities. Critical dynamics for rapid adoption include a low cost to surgeons of learning and performing the procedure and the perceived benefit of the technology by all stakeholders [23].

Medical simulation as well as emerging technology such as virtual reality can be used to aid training and practice specific skills. Specifically, virtual reality simulators lower the high costs associated with training on robotic surgical systems as well as provide more opportunities to increase training time. Numerous trainers have been developed, including the Mimic dV-Trainer, Robotic Surgical Simulator (RoSS), SimSurgery Educational Platform, as well as other virtual reality-based simulators. Systematic review of these models have shown that they demonstrate face, content, and construct validity and provide an effective training environment for trainees [26]. Virtual reality simulators can reproduce the feel and visualization of performing procedures on the da Vinci Surgical System and may be especially beneficial for users who are early in their training.

Various simulation-based curriculums have been developed and validated for trainees seeking to learn robotic skills. The fundamental skills of robotic surgery (FSRS) was incorporated into the RoSS virtual reality simulator and shown to be effective in improving basic robotic surgery skills [27]. The simulation-based robotic surgery basic skills training curriculum (BSTC) was also developed as a 4-week offering and demonstrated improved robotic surgical skills among novice as well as experienced surgeons [28]. In addition, the fundamentals of robotic surgery (FRS) was an online robotic surgical skills program developed through funding from the Department of Defense as well as Intuitive Surgical. The curriculum was designed by a cohort of over 80 international experts and is intended to be used for initial accreditation, with validation trials currently ongoing [29]. Intuitive Surgical also offers an online training program for the da Vinci system called the Technology Training Pathway [30].

Credentialing for robotic surgery privileges is often defined by individual institutions, in contrast to credentialing programs by professional organizations [31]. The Crowd Sourced Assessment of Technical Skills (CSATS) has been utilized as an assessment of surgical skills through intraoperative video review, with previous studies showing that it correlates with expert reviews and may predict patient outcomes [32, 33].

4.6 Setting up a Robotic Program

Starting a pediatric robotic surgery program requires institutional support and a plan that accounts for training, costs, and case volume for procedures (see Fig. 4.3). Due to the significant initial costs of the robotic console, those who wish to implement robotic surgery in their practice should ensure that there is enough caseload to offset the cost. Previous studies have shown that approximately 3–5 cases per week are required to make a program profitable over a 5-year period in the U.S [34]. Pediatric urology programs should be part of a comprehensive, multispecialty, and/or adult robotic surgery program to help share costs and increase utilization of the equipment. Additionally, cost-effectiveness can vary at the individual hospital level due to local regulations as well as different modalities of cost analysis.

Implementation of robotic surgery equipment should be focused on modifying operating rooms (OR) as well as educating specific teams in the OR dedicated to robotic surgery. A robotic operating room coordinator and robotic program director should also be assigned to train other members in setting up, undocking, and general troubleshooting the device and coordinate the business and clinical components of the program, respectively. Marketing should focus on outreach to primary care pediatricians and advocacy groups to expand the referral base as well as increase patient education. Primary care physicians can become more involved through continuing medical education programs as well as other events [35].

4.7 Application and Future Direction

Robotic surgery continues to progress as a field with an increasing amount of technological innovation, new products, as well as new features to add to surgeons' abilities. The da Vinci surgical system, developed by Intuitive Surgical, has dominated the market since its FDA approval in 2000, with over five million surgeries conducted using the system [30]. However, the introduction

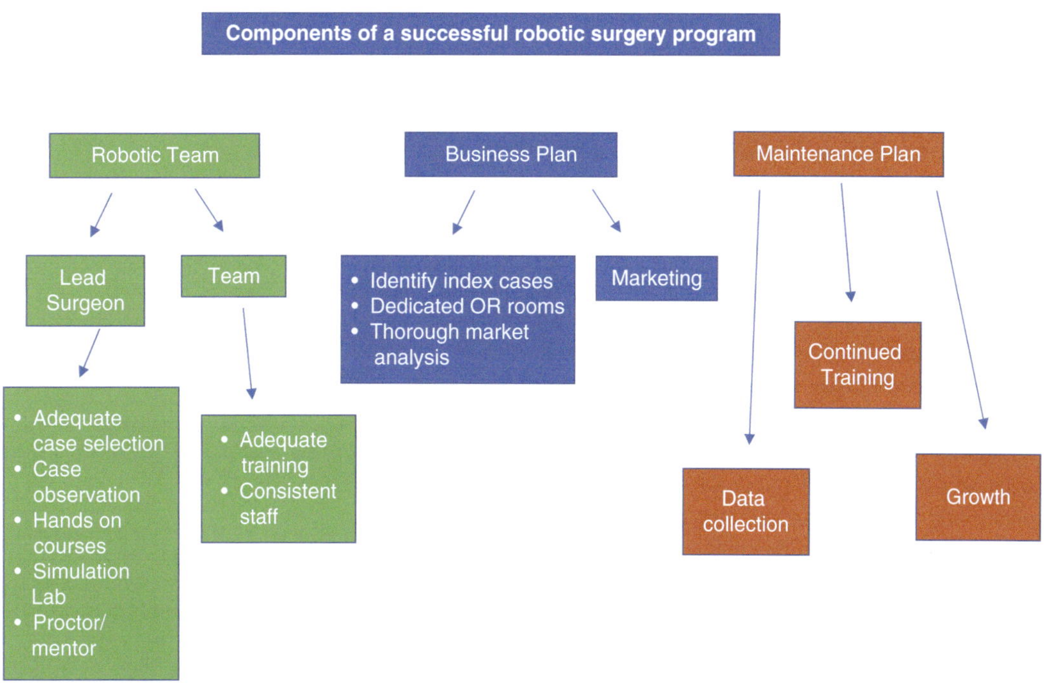

Fig. 4.3 Elements of a successful robotic program

of other competitors will provide more options for surgeons. For instance, Cambridge Medical launched its Versius system in the U.K. in 2020 which provides a more modular system with robotic arms mounted on individual carts [36]. The system also can provide haptic feedback on its joystick controllers, offers laparoscopic instruments at smaller sizes down to 5 mm, and can be utilized in non-robot dedicated ORs due to its smaller size profile. Multiple other robots are available or in development, including the SurgiBot-SPIDER system, which was developed to be used for underserved populations due to its low cost, and the MiroSurge system developed in Germany, which is a telemanipulated robot [36].

4.8 Safety Net and Digital Surgery

Moving forward, additional features which can provide benefits to patients and surgeons include the addition of safety triggers which can guide dissection and avoid injury to major vessels or nerves by detecting close proximity. In addition, intraoperative safety can also be improved with crowd sourcing. A review by Dai et al. found that crowd-based feedback can provide more consistent, beneficial, and less costly feedback to trainees, thus allowing for improved technical skills [37]. Telerobotic surgery, with surgeons operating a console from a distant location, can provide access to rural patients who may not otherwise have robotic surgery available to them. Such systems have been utilized in Canada and remain under study in the United States [38, 39]. Currently, telerobotic systems are limited by time delay between master and slave system, posing issues at the place of operation [40]. In addition, regulatory differences between two locations must also be dealt with in order to allow for telerobotic surgery to occur. However, these can be overcome with recent advances in wireless infrastructure to reduce latency and increasing regulatory scrutiny over telerobotic practice. The incorporation of machine learning and artificial intelligence can also individualize treatment for patients and help train surgeons by analyzing movement data and gaze tracking. Three-dimensional printing can also be utilized to aid surgeons in preoperative planning and designing specific implants or equipment to be used during surgery.

Automation and use of robotics cannot replace the human element in surgery, but can provide substantial benefits to patients, surgeons, and healthcare systems by improving efficiency and safety. As a specialty, pediatric urology continues to adopt the use of robotics to increasing effect to better serve patients with varied needs.

References

1. Cortesi N, Ferrari P, Zambarda E, Manenti A, Baldini A, Pignatti MF. Diagnosis of bilateral abdominal cryptorchidism by laparoscopy. Endoscopy. 1976;8(1):33–4.
2. Kwoh YS, Hou J, Jonckheere EA, Hayati S. A robot with improved absolute positioning accuracy for CT guided stereotactic brain surgery. IEEE Trans Biomed Eng. 1988;35(2):153–60. https://pubmed.ncbi.nlm.nih.gov/3280462/.
3. Davies BL, Hibberd RD, Ng WS, Timoney AG, Wickham JE. The development of a surgeon robot for prostatectomies. Proc Inst Mech Eng Part H. 1991;205(1):35–8.
4. Gundeti MS, Duffy PG, Mushtaq I. Robotic-assisted laparoscopic correction of pediatric retrocaval ureter. J Laparoendosc Adv Surg Tech. 2006;16(4):422–4. https://www.liebertpub.com/doi/abs/10.1089/lap.2006.16.422.
5. Clarke S. Paediatric robotic surgery and urology: where are we? J Pediatr Endosc Surg. 2019;1(2):49–52. https://doi.org/10.1007/s42804-019-00008-x.
6. Van Batavia JP, Casale P. Robotic surgery in pediatric urology. Curr Urol Rep. 2014;15(5):402.
7. Computer-Assisted Surgical Systems | FDA [Internet]. [cited 2020 Jul 6]. https://www.fda.gov/medical-devices/surgery-devices/computer-assisted-surgical-systems.
8. Boyraz P, Dobrev I, Fischer G, Popovic MB. Robotic surgery. In: Biomechatronics. Amsterdam: Elsevier; 2019. p. 431–50. https://linkinghub.elsevier.com/retrieve/pii/B978012812939500015X.
9. Gundeti MS, Eng MK, Reynolds WS, Zagaja GP. Pediatric robotic-assisted laparoscopic augmentation ileocystoplasty and Mitrofanoff appendicovesicostomy: complete intracorporeal--initial case report. Urology 2008 Nov;72(5):1144–1147; discussion 1147.
10. Robotics in GU oncology: current status, future directions – Urology Times – IoT – Internet of Things [Internet]. [cited 2020 Jul 19]. https://iot.ng/index.

php/2020/05/22/robotics-in-gu-oncology-current-status-future-directions-urology-times/.
11. Ballouhey Q, Clermidi P, Cros J, Grosos C, Rosa-Arsène C, Bahans C, et al. Comparison of 8 and 5 mm robotic instruments in small cavities: 5 or 8 mm robotic instruments for small cavities? Surg Endosc. 2018;32(2):1027–34. https://doi.org/10.1007/s00464-017-5781-9.
12. Moles JJ, Connelly PE, Sarti EE, Baredes S. Establishing a training program for residents in robotic surgery. Laryngoscope. 2009;119(10):1927–31.
13. Chitwood WR, Nifong LW, Chapman WHH, Felger JE, Bailey BM, Ballint T, et al. Robotic surgical training in an academic institution. Ann Surg. 2001;234(4):475–86.
14. Mirheydar H, Jones M, Koeneman KS, Sweet RM. Robotic surgical education: a collaborative approach to training postgraduate urologists and endourology fellows. J Soc Laparoendosc Surg. 2009;13(3):287–92.
15. Rashid HH, Leung Y-YM, Rashid MJ, Oleyourryk G, Valvo JR, Eichel L. Robotic surgical education: a systematic approach to training urology residents to perform robotic-assisted laparoscopic radical prostatectomy. Urology. 2006;68(1):75–9.
16. Lee JY, Mucksavage P, Sundaram CP, McDougall EM. Best practices for robotic surgery training and credentialing. J Urol. 2011;185(4):1191–7. http://www.jurology.com/doi/10.1016/j.juro.2010.11.067.
17. Andolfi C, Patel D, Rodriguez VM, Gundeti MS. Impact and outcomes of a pediatric robotic urology mini-fellowship. Front Surg. 2019;6:1–5.
18. Andolfi C, Gundeti MS. Live-case demonstrations in pediatric urology: ethics, patient safety, and clinical outcomes from an 8-year institutional experience. Investig Clin Urol. 2020;61:S51–6.
19. McCulloch P, Altman DG, Campbell WB, Flum DR, Glasziou P, Marshall JC, et al. No surgical innovation without evaluation: the IDEAL recommendations. In: The Lancet, vol. 374. Amsterdam: Elsevier; 2009. p. 1105–12. http://www.thelancet.com/article/S0140673609611168/fulltext.
20. Cook JA, McCulloch P, Blazeby JM, Beard DJ, Marinac-Dabic D, Sedrakyan A, et al. IDEAL framework for surgical innovation 3: randomised controlled trials in the assessment stage and evaluations in the long term study stage. BMJ. 2013;346:f2820. https://www.bmj.com/content/346/bmj.f2820.
21. Boysen WR, Akhavan A, Ko J, Ellison JS, Lendvay TS, Huang J, et al. Prospective multicenter study on robot-assisted laparoscopic extravesical ureteral reimplantation (RALUR-EV): outcomes and complications. J Pediatr Urol. 2018;14(3):262.e1–6. https://pubmed.ncbi.nlm.nih.gov/29503220/.
22. Boysen WR, Ellison JS, Kim C, Koh CJ, Noh P, Whittam B, et al. Multi-institutional review of outcomes and complications of robot-assisted laparoscopic extravesical ureteral reimplantation for treatment of primary vesicoureteral reflux in children. J Urol. 2017;197(6):1555–61. http://www.jurology.com/doi/10.1016/j.juro.2017.01.062.
23. Wilson CB. Adoption of new surgical technology. Br Med J. 2006;332:112–4.
24. Cundy TP, Harley SJ, Marcus HJ, Hughes-Hallett A, Khurana S. Global trends in pediatric robot-assisted urological surgery: a bibliometric and progressive scholarly acceptance analysis. J Robot Surg. 2018;12(1):109–15.
25. Cundy TP, Marcus HJ, Hughes-Hallett A, Khurana S, Darzi A. Robotic surgery in children: adopt now, await, or dismiss? Pediatr Surg Int. 2015;31:1119–25.
26. Abboudi H, Khan MS, Aboumarzouk O, Guru KA, Challacombe B, Dasgupta P, et al. Current status of validation for robotic surgery simulators a systematic review. BJU Int. 2013;111(2):194–205.
27. Stegemann AP, Ahmed K, Syed JR, Rehman S, Ghani K, Autorino R, et al. Fundamental skills of robotic surgery: a multi-institutional randomized controlled trial for validation of a simulation-based curriculum. Urology. 2013;81(4):767–74.
28. Foell K, Finelli A, Yasufuku K, Bernardini MQ, Waddell TK, Pace KT, et al. Robotic surgery basic skills training: evaluation of a pilot multidisciplinary simulation-based curriculum. Can Urol Assoc J. 2013;7(11–12):430.
29. Chen R, Rodrigues Armijo P, Krause C, Siu KC, Oleynikov D. A comprehensive review of robotic surgery curriculum and training for residents, fellows, and postgraduate surgical education. Surg Endosc. 2020;34(1):361–7. https://doi.org/10.1007/s00464-019-06775-1.
30. Intuitive | Products Services | Education Training [Internet]. [cited 2020 Jul 6]. https://www.intuitive.com/en-us/products-and-services/da-vinci/education
31. Kearns J, Gundeti M. Pediatric robotic urologic surgery-2014. J Indian Assoc Pediatr Surg. 2014;19:123–8.
32. C-SATS How it Works—C-SATS [Internet]. [cited 2020 Jul 19]. https://www.csats.com/how-it-works
33. Canalichio KL, Berrondo C, Lendvay TS. Simulation training in urology: state of the art and future directions. Adv Med Educ Pract. 2020;11:391–6. https://doi.org/10.2147/AMEP.S198941.
34. Palmer KJ, Lowe GJ, Coughlin GD, Patil N, Patel VR. Launching a successful robotic surgery program. J Endourol. 2008;22(4):819–24.
35. Murthy PB, Schadler ED, Orvieto M, Zagaja G, Shalhav AL. Gundeti MS. Setting up a pediatric robotic urology program: a USA institution experience. Int J Urol. 2018;25(2):86–93. https://doi.org/10.1111/iju.13415.
36. Khandalavala K, Shimon T, Flores L, Armijo PR, Oleynikov D. Emerging surgical robotic technology: a progression toward microbots. Ann Laparosc Endosc Surg. 2020;5(0):3. http://ales.amegroups.com/article/view/5499/html.

37. Dai JC, Lendvay TS, Sorensen MD. Crowdsourcing in surgical skills acquisition: a developing technology in surgical education. J Grad Med Educ. 2017;9:697–705.
38. Anvari M, McKinley C, Stein H. Establishment of the world's first telerobotic remote surgical service: for provision of advanced laparoscopic surgery in a rural community. Ann Surg. 2005;241(3):460–4.
39. Boysen WR, Gundeti MS. Use of robot-assisted surgery in pediatric urology—have we reached the limits of technology? ASSI Urol Sets. 2018:19–20.
40. Avgousti S, Christoforou EG, Panayides AS, Voskarides S, Novales C, Nouaille L, et al. Medical telerobotic systems: current status and future trends. BioMed Eng. 2016:15.

5 Endoscopic Approach for Urinary Tract Pathologies

Marcello Cimador, Maria R. Di Pace, Marco Pensabene, Fabio Baldanza, and Maria Sergio

Learning Objective
- Outline the real indications for the endoscopic procedure in pediatric urology.
- Describe the instrumentation suitable for the endoscopy.
- Describe the most used endoscopic techniques.
- Report the results of endoscopic treatment.
- Share tips and tricks of how to act endoscopically.

5.1 Introduction

The endoscopy of the lower urinary tract represents a minimally invasive diagnostic and therapeutic tool for a broad range of pathological anomalies in pediatric ages. From in utero fetal surgery to preterm infant, newborns and toddlers, endoscopic treatment is feasible by refined and very small caliber instruments.

In most cases, different congenital urological malformations (obstructive or refluxing) need endoscopic approach for achieving a permanent success by minimally invasive procedures. Furthermore, some anatomical defects can be comprehensively detected by endoscopy only. A deeper knowledge of pathophysiology of bladder and lower urinary tract anomalies has significantly widened indications to the endourological techniques. The use of bulking agents for the treatment of urinary incontinence as well as vesicoureteral reflux is the most relevant representative case.

Till date, the most common indications for endoscopy in pediatric urology are the following:

- Transurethral incision of posterior urethral valves (PUV).
- Transurethral incision of ureterocele.
- Injection of bulking agents:
  - Vesicoureteral reflux (VUR).
  - Bladder neck incontinence.
- Ureteral stents insertion for vesicoureteral junction anomalies.
- Stones removal.
- Vesicoureteral junction (VUJ) balloon dilatation.
- Bladder infiltration.
- Bladder malignancies.
- Ambiguous genitalia.

In this chapter, we shortly describe how to safely approach some of the urological anomalies endoscopically.

M. Cimador (✉) · M. R. Di Pace · M. Pensabene
F. Baldanza · M. Sergio
From Pediatric Surgery & Urology Unit, Department of PROMISE, Università di Palermo, Palermo, Italy
e-mail: marcello.cimador@unipa.it

C. Esposito et al. (eds.), *Minimally Invasive Techniques in Pediatric Urology*,
https://doi.org/10.1007/978-3-030-99280-4_5

5.2 Preoperative Preparation

Preoperative preparation can be different in relation to sex, age, type, and severity of disease.

Every endoscopic procedure should be performed under general anesthesia, therefore a preliminary clinical evaluation with a cardiopulmonary and renal function assessment is always implemented.

Before any urological endoscopy, even if prenatal diagnosis is available, it is necessary to wait for extrauterine life adaptation and postnatal imaging. Endoscopy is not ordinarily a procedure performed in urgency.

Broad-spectrum antibiotic prophylaxis is mandatory before any endoscopic procedure, as emptying of the bowels is required. Since the urethra in newborn is thin and tiny, it is recommended to insert a dilating 8 Fr transurethral catheter at least 24 h before the procedure.

Informed consent is shared with parents before the signature.

5.3 Positioning

All patients undergoing endoscopic procedures are placed in supine decubitus position. The table should be arranged in light Trendelenburg incline, to better expose genitalia. Depending on the age, usually after 1 year of age, the leg support can be used. In babies under 1 year of age, the frog-like position is appropriate and a small roller should be placed under the back for avoiding any compression by intestine on the bladder.

The surgeon stands in the center between the patient's legs, while the assistant is beside the patient ready to perform an ultrasound scan, if required.

5.4 Instrumentation

For pediatric diagnostic and therapeutic endoscopy, a cystoscopic suite that permits fluoroscopic or ultrasonographic visualization should be the ideal working environment.

Till date, a wide version of cystoscopes is available to pediatric urologists. Miniaturization provides very thin scopes with a working channel for ancillary instruments for newborn to the older child. Furthermore, cystoscopic view has been strongly improved by digital video camera, which allows better visualization and magnification of the field.

It is recommended to have in place different size of cystoscope for adapting instruments at the best. In both male and female newborns, a 5 Fr cystoscope ensures optimal observation, avoiding any injury to the urethra. This 5 Fr cystoscope is usually used only for make diagnosis. To have an adequate working channel, a larger cystoscope is needed, 8 Fr at least.

For management of posterior urethral valves, a 9 Fr resectoscope is required and many loops and cautery ends can be used. In addition, using any 8–11 Fr cystoscope, hooked and straight blades for cold incision are available.

Ancillary instruments are available in size from 3 to 5 Fr through rigid scopes, graspers for foreign bodies, biopsies forceps, and electrodes. 3 Fr and 5 Fr Bugbee electrodes are available for fulguration of valves and ureterocele.

Nowadays, equipment for pediatric endoscopy is still developing, and probe for ultrasound, laser probes, electrohydraulic probes are available for a 5 Fr working channel. Lastly, a 7.5 Fr flexible cystoureteroscopes are available too.

5.5 Technique

Before the insertion of the cystoscope, a careful examination of the external genitalia should be done to identify morphologic anomalies which could hinder the execution of endoscopy (labial adhesion, ectopic end or duplex urethral meatus, meatal stenosis, and more).

The cystoscope should be always gently inserted under direct vision. It is recommended to introduce de-ionized water for injection at low pressure and at a warm temperature to prevent potential hypothermia. Sodium-chloride solution should be avoided during procedures in which cautery is expected. It would be ideal to keep a bladder low filling compared to its capacity especially performing ureterocele puncture, subureteral injection for VUR, PUV ablation. In all cases, the surgeon starts the procedure by performing an exploratory cystoscopy to observe the anatomy and report any variation of the same.

- **Transurethral incision of posterior urethral valves**: when possible, the endoscopic incision is considered the primary treatment modality. Endoscopic fulguration can be performed using Bugbee electrode through a 5 Fr cystoscope with a 3 Fr working channel. Different ways for fulguration can be performed with a 9 Fr resectoscope using a Collings knife electrode or a cutting loop; in these procedures, valves are incised at 5, 7, and 12 o'clock position. In type 3 valve obstruction, the diaphragm can be easily ablated with a Bugbee electrode in a circumferential way. In infants, in whom a transurethral procedure is not possible due to smallest urethral caliber, antegrade ablation can been performed by a 9.5 Fr cystoscope through a suprapubic opening.
- **Transurethral incision of ureterocele**: ureterocele is approached within the bladder neck by cutting or puncture of the lower part of itself. After the incision, ureterocele can be explored by a cystoscope direct view. Ectopic ureterocele prolapsing in the urethra should be double punctured at the inferior border and at the top of the dome. Ureterocele incision can be performed with cautery by a 3 Fr Bugbee or with the use of laser. A simultaneous ultrasound scan can show the collapse of ureterocele in real time (Figs. 5.1 and 5.2).
- **Injection of bulking agents for VUR**: intraureteral and/or sub-ureteral endoscopic injection of bulking agents is widely used for management of VUR. A 9–11 Fr offset lens of cystoscope with a 4 Fr working channel allows a straightforward route to pass a stiff or flexible needle for injection of a bulking agent. This latter should create a mound which does not lose significant volume and efficacy over time. Bladder filling is a key-point performing the procedure, since a fully filled bladder may make it difficult to take the agent in an exact subureteral place. Injection of the bulking agent can be done by a single or multiple punctures in submucosal intra-ureteral space or in sub-ureteral position, just 1 cm below the ureteric meatus. Intra-ureteral and sub-ureteral injection can be carried out simultaneously to achieve the best antireflux mechanism. Following the Kirsh technique in intra-ureteral injection, the orifice can be dilated by hydrodistention having irrigation of fluid inside the ureter and in the meanwhile injecting the agent. In our more recent experience, intraoperative simultaneous ultrasound scan allows to control the bulking agent injection up to 1 cm in height of the mound (Fig. 5.3).
- **Injection of bulking agents for urinary incontinence**: several congenital defects causing bladder incontinence can be managed by endoscopic injection of bulking agents. Endoscopic injection has the aim of increasing neck resistance and therefore stimulating bladder growth. The procedure consists of injection of bulking agents in the submucosal space of the urethra just beneath the bladder neck. A 9–11 Fr offset lens cystoscope with a 5 Fr working channel allows to inject the agent firstly at 4 and 8 o'clock positions, but sometimes multiple punctures are needed. After the procedure, a small catheter is inserted to the bladder to avoid forcing the modeled bladder neck.
- **Bladder stones removal**: transurethral stone fragmentation can be performed in children with patent urethra. Fragmentation can be achieved using rigid endoscopic instruments with electrohydraulic-combined ultrasonic and pneumatic or holmium laser lithotripsy.
- **Other procedures**: stenotic uretero–vesical junction can be endoscopically managed using stent insertion or balloon dilation. In both cases, the aim of the procedure is to model and dilate the junction. Choice of stent depends on age and size of the patient and length of ureter. In the most of cases, the tight junction is patent to the 3 Fr J-J stent only. The stent insertion, taken in place for a period of 6 months at least, can avoid ureteric surgery by modeling

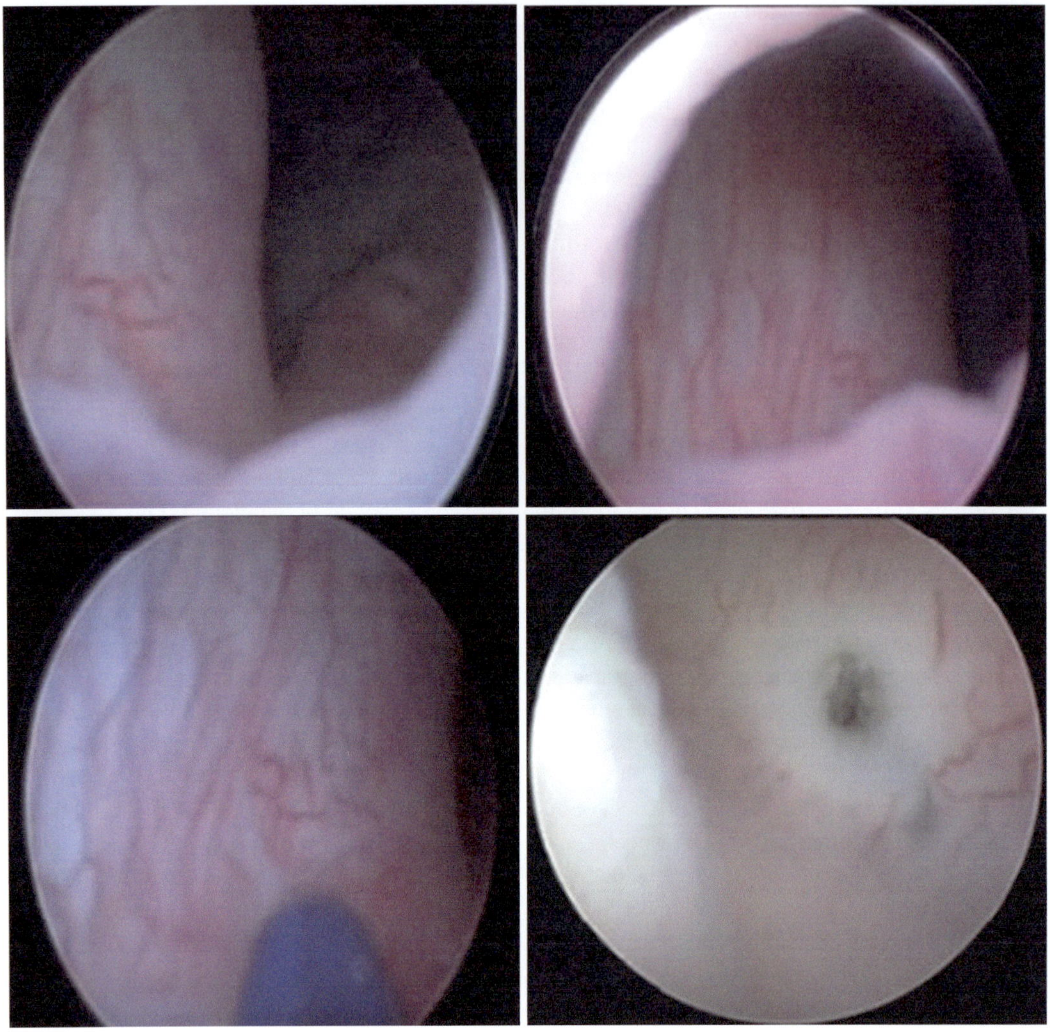

Fig. 5.1 Clockwise: a right ureterocele opened by Bugbee electrode

the junction. Very tight junction can be early managed with easily and feasible pneumatic balloon dilatation. Side effects of this procedure are either recurrent urinary infection and vesico–uteric reflux.

– **Bladder infiltration**: in some cases of overactive bladder (both neurogenic or non- neurogenic bladder) resistant to administration of anticholinergics, multiple puncture (up to 40 punctures) of botulinum toxin through a cystoscope could be effective in reduction of symptoms.
– **Tumors**: bladder malignancies in children are rare. In a few cases, the endoscopic procedure is used to identify the lesion that has been noted on imaging scan. The most commonly noted lower urinary tract tumors in children are rhabdomyosarcomas of the bladder or prostate. With the cystoscopy, it is easy to outline the preoperative extent of tumor and to obtain biopsies to confirm diagnosis. Cystoscopy may be needed for follow-up in patients who have undergone bladder-sparing procedures.
– **Ambiguous genitalia**: endoscopy is routinely performed to plan reconstruction in children with ambiguous genitalia. Endoscopy of the various perineal orifices may help to deter-

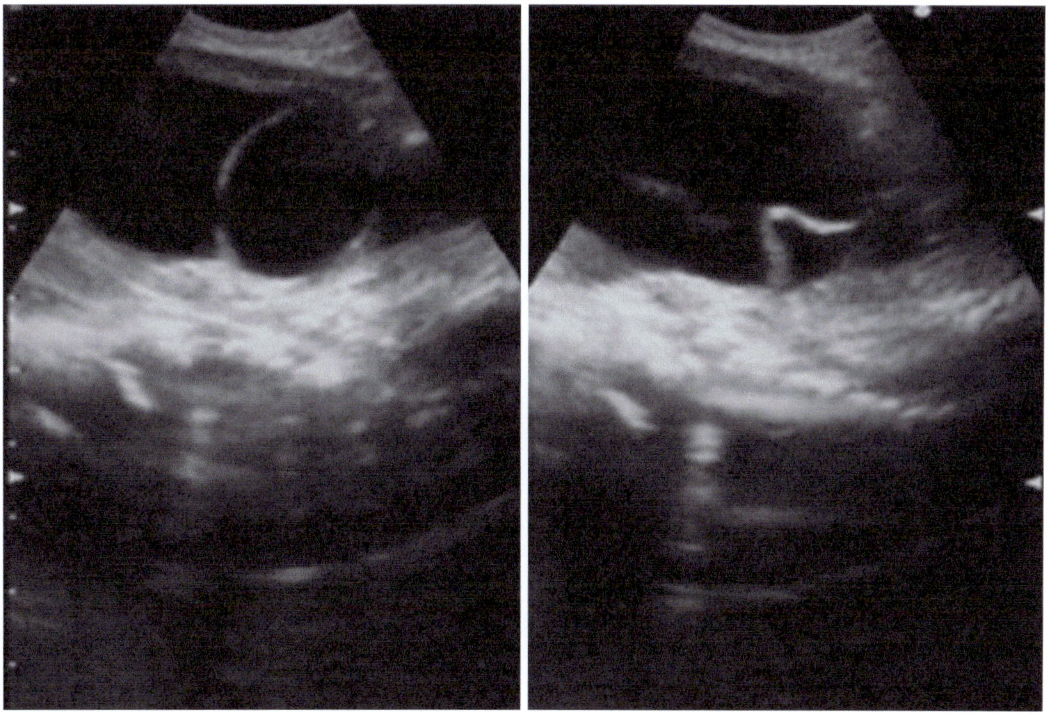

Fig. 5.2 US image of the collapsing ureterocele after fulguration

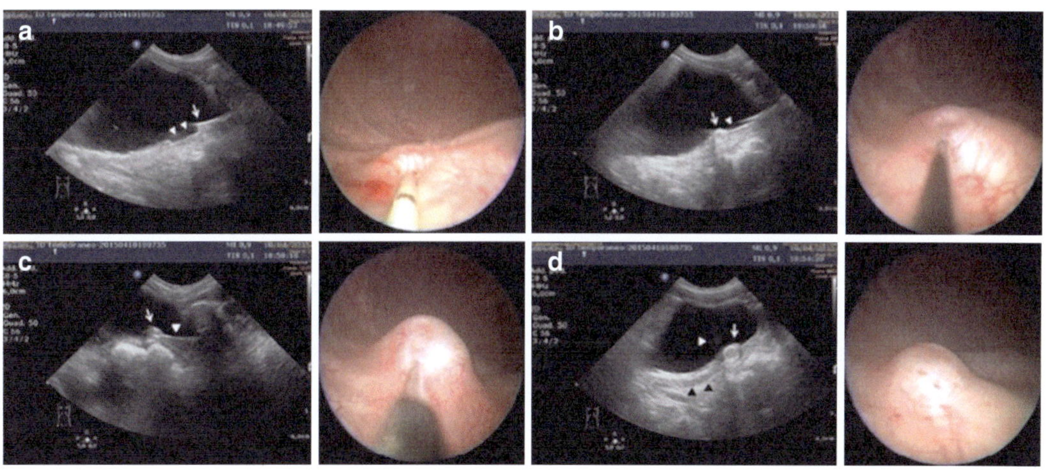

Fig. 5.3 Main steps of surgical procedure compared to IO-US: on the left IO-US views and on the right endoscopic appearance. (**a**) Initial catheterization (arrow cystoscope, arrowheads ureteral catheter); (**b**) optimal ureteral placement and initial mound formation (arrow initial mound; arrowhead needle); (**c**) needle injecting Dx/HA positioned (arrow mound; arrowhead needle); (**d**) final mound appearance (arrow mound; white arrowhead ureteral jet; arrowheads ureteral course)

mine the relationships among the components of the urogenital tract. The location of the vaginal entry into the urogenital sinus in girls with virilization secondary to congenital adrenal hyperplasia is used to determine the type of procedure required for reconstruction. The vaginal orifice in the urethra in these children may be noted as a small orifice at the tip of the verumontanum. This opening can at times be entered with the smaller cystoscopes and vaginoscopy performed. Catheterization of the vagina with a Fogarty balloon catheter is helpful for identification of the vagina during vaginoplasty.

5.6 Postoperative Care

Usually, patients begin feeding orally 6 h after surgery. During the first post–operative day, paracetamol is administered as needed (dosage 10–15 mg/kg at 6-h intervals).

The patient undergoes antibiotic therapy for the procedure performed, during the bladder catheter maintenance time and according to the underlying pathology for an appropriate time.

The duration of hospitalization depends on the underlying pathology and the type of procedure performed. Patients are discharged on first postoperative day after VUR treatment, ureterocele puncture, stents insertion, or balloon dilatation.

The clinical follow-up is generally performed 10 days after endoscopy by ultrasound scan and urinalysis. The timing of further checks follows the basic pathology.

5.7 Results

We will report the main results from the international literature on the use of endoscopy for some of the urological anomalies already summarized in this chapter.

The effect of primary endoscopic fulguration versus any surgical diversion in patients affected by posterior urethral valves on long-term bladder and renal function remains controversial.

In a longitudinal study, 67 patients with PUV were divided into three groups, depending on the initial treatment: fulguration (n = 38, 56.7%), vesicostomy (n = 25, 37.3%), and ureterostomy (n = 4, 6%). Analyzing the urodynamic patterns, Puri et al. have found that good capacity and compliant bladders were the pattern in the fulgurated group; small-capacity bladders with hyperreflexia in the vesicostomy group; and good capacity, compliant bladders in the ureterostomy group [1].

A routine relook cystoscopy after primary fulguration of PUV to investigate residual obstructive valves is not standardized. In a retrospective study on a total of 127 PUV patients, 21 patients (20.8%) underwent endoscopic reevaluation after primary valves ablation due to the suspicion of inadequate bladder drainage based on clinical and radiological data, and residual valves or strictures were detected in 10 cases (9.9%) [2].

Puncture of the intravesical ureterocele is associated with high success rates, with minimal post- procedure reflux or need for later surgery. In a study of 41 neonates with a diagnosis of duplex system ureteroceles, we have found that there was no significant difference between intravesical and ectopic ureteroceles in the occurrence of VUR in the punctured moiety, rate of nonfunctioning upper poles, or need for secondary surgery [3].

In a recent study, data show that endoscopic puncture of ureterocele is a durable and long-term effective procedure in vast majority of the children [4].

Endoscopic treatment of vesico–ureteric reflux is widely considered an optimal choice compared with surgical approach in terms of reduced morbidity, shorter hospitalization, reduced costs, and increased patients' preference. A recent study reports that endoscopic treatment of VUR is feasible in patients less than 1 year of age. The authors show that the efficacy is lower when patients are treated at a later age, but it is, however, over 80% in their series. No complications related to the procedure itself or to the general anesthesia are reported [5]. We have recently demonstrated a strong correlation between mound height and result after endoscopic injection of dextranomer/hyaluronic acid in children with ultrasound intra-operative scan control and with a reabsorption rate of 23% at 6 months from treatment [6] (Fig. 5.1).

Only a few studies [7–10] report outcomes on endoscopic injection of bulking agents for persistent incontinence after sling and/or bladder neck revision in children with neurogenic bladder. To date, even if the minimally invasive procedure remains an important option, achievement of dryness after up to two treatments occurs in a very low percentage of patients [11].

Tip and Tricks

- Lower urinary tract endoscopy should be conducted by experts in pediatric urology. Despite being simple to perform, the technique requires adequate learning time to avoid complications linked to inadequate use of instruments, with potential injury and lifelong consequences.
- Accuracy in inserting the cystoscope and little instruments related to the procedure is of primary importance. Never force the urethral meatus with the cystoscope, nor the ureteral meatus with the stents. Therefore, it should be mandatory to insert the cystoscope under direct vision and under permanent jet of water.
- Taking care about bladder capacity and bladder filling can avoid dangerous increase in intravesical pressure while performing the procedures. Do not swipe the cystoscope on the bladder mucosa to avoid any bleeding, therefore movements should be slow and precise.
- After insertion of the bladder catheter at the end of the procedure, it is recommended to completely empty the bladder to prevent parents' alarm in the presence of blood in the urine.

5.8 Discussion

Endoscopic management of congenital and acquired diseases of the lower urinary tract has radically improved the approach in terms of minimally invasive and diagnostic accuracy in pediatric urology. A worldwide consensus has been reached on the preliminary use of endoscopy for the main indications already listed in this chapter.

Endoscopic treatment should be the primary choice for patients affected by PUV, ureterocele, VUR, especially in cases without factors preventing the use of that procedure.

Exploratory endoscopy preliminary to surgery on the lower and upper urinary tract is of great support for clarifying the anatomy and planning for the optimal treatment.

Through endoscopy we can acquire skills on the lower urinary tract conditions and external genitalia: appearance of bladder mucosa, positioning of the trigone, bladder volume capacity, ectopic ureteral orifice outlet, bladder neck assessment, and many others.

Take-Home Points

Even if the procedure is burdened by contained complications, we are used to carrying it out following some basic elements:

- Before the procedure.
  - stabilize the general condition of the patient (often hydro-electrolytic balance and creatinine levels),
  - insert a urethral catheter 24 h before, in males,
  - stimulate the evacuation,
  - look at the urine and postpone the procedure in case of urinary tract infection.
- During the procedure.
  - general anesthesia at all ages for any pathology,
  - maximum asepsis,
  - keep the intra-vesical pressures low or very low.
- After the procedure.
  - leave a urethral catheter,
  - start an antibiotic prophylaxis,
  - start a bladder training before removing the catheter.

References

1. Puri A, Grover VP, Agarwala S, Mitra DK, Bhatnagar V. Initial surgical treatment as a determinant of bladder dysfunction in posterior urethral valves. Pediatr Surg Int. 2002;18(5-6):438–43.
2. Oktar T, Salabas E, Acar O, Atar A, Nane I, Ander H, Ziylan O. Residual valve and stricture after posterior urethral valve ablation: how to evaluate? J Pediatr Urol. 2013;9:184–7.
3. Castagnetti M, Cimador M, Sergio M, de Grazia E. Transurethral incision of duplex system ureteroceles in neonates: does it increase the need for secondary surgery in intravesical and ectopic cases? BJU Int. 2004;93(9):1313–7.
4. Jawdat J, Rotem S, Kocherov S, Farkas A, Chertin B. Does endoscopic puncture of ureterocele provide not only an initial solution, but also a definitive treatment in all children? Over the 26 years of experience. Pediatr Surg Int. 2018;34(5):561–5.
5. Fuentes S, Gómez-Fraile A, Carrillo-Arroyo I, Tordable-Ojeda C, Cabezalí-Barbancho D. Endoscopic treatment of Vesicoureteral reflux in infants. Can we do it and should we do it? Urology. 2017;110:196–200.
6. Zambaiti E, Sergio M, Di Pace MR, Casuccio A, Cimador M. The fate of implant after endoscopic injection of dextranomer/hyaluronic acid in vesicoureteral reflux: time to partial reabsorption and stabilization. J Pediatr Urol. 2020;16(2):191.e1–6.
7. De Vocht TF, Chrzan R, Dik P, Klijn AJ, De Jong TP. Long-term results of bulking agent injection for persistent incontinence in cases of neurogenic bladder dysfunction. J Urol. 2010;183:719–23.
8. Guys JM, Breaud J, Hery G, Camerlo A, Le Hors H, De Lagausie P. Endoscopic injection with polydimethylsiloxane for the treatment of pediatric urinary incontinence in the neurogenic bladder: long-term results. J Urol. 2006;175:1106–10.
9. Kitchens DM, Minevich E, DeFoor WR, Reddy PP, Wacksman J, Koyle MA, et al. Incontinence following bladder neck reconstructioneis there a role for endoscopic management? J Urol. 2007;177:302–5.
10. Misseri R, Casale AJ, Cain MP, Rink RC. Alternative uses of dextranomer/hyaluronic acid copolymer: the efficacy of bladder neck injection for urinary incontinence. J Urol. 2005;174:1691–3. [discussion 1693e4].
11. DaJusta D, Gargollo P, Snodgrass W. Dextranomer/hyaluronic acid bladder neck injection for persistent outlet incompetency after sling procedures in children with neurogenic urinary incontinence. J Pediatr Urol. 2013;9(3):278–82.

Devices in Pediatric Endourology

6

Liza M. Aguiar, Anthony A. Caldamone,
and Hsi-Yang Wu

Learning Objectives

- To describe commonly used ureteral stents, wires, baskets, and devices used for retrograde ureteral access and antegrade renal access.
- To present the latest advances in these devices.
- To describe helpful tips and tricks for using these devices.

6.1 Introduction

The devices used for retrograde ureteral access and antegrade renal access have become progressively smaller in diameter, allowing for safer access to the pediatric urinary collecting system with less risk of ureteral stricture from the retrograde approach and bleeding from renal parenchymal dilation. The benefits of using ureteral access sheaths are to minimize ureteral trauma in cases where multiple passes of the ureteroscope are required due to a large stone burden, and maintenance of low intrarenal pressure from irrigation fluid, which decreases the risk of postoperative sepsis. After the initial description by Alken of percutaneous nephrolithotomy in 1981 [1], the miniaturization of percutaneous nephrostomy sheaths and needles has decreased the risk of bleeding from renal access and dilation, and the need for nephrostomy tamponade after surgery. In order to gain ureteral and upper tract access safely, wires are used to exchange devices and instruments during pediatric endourology cases. Ureteral stents are widely used to aid in drainage of the kidney in the setting of obstruction or postoperative healing.

Pediatric urologists are performing more endoscopic cases given the increasing incidence of pediatric stone disease. There are several stone retrieval devices to choose from, mainly used in the setting of stone extraction under direct visualization, although these devices can also be used to extract foreign bodies in the genitourinary tract. Baskets are now more flexible, less traumatic, and disposable.

This chapter aims to review these commonly used tools in pediatric endourology and provide insight on how best to use them in practice.

L. M. Aguiar · A. A. Caldamone · H.-Y. Wu (✉)
Division of Pediatric Urology, Hasbro Children's Hospital, Warren Alpert School of Medicine at Brown University, Providence, RI, USA
e-mail: Liza.Aguiar@Lifespan.org; liza_aguiar@brown.edu; ACaldamone@Lifespan.org; HWu6@Lifespan.org

C. Esposito et al. (eds.), *Minimally Invasive Techniques in Pediatric Urology*,
https://doi.org/10.1007/978-3-030-99280-4_6

6.2 Positioning and Preoperative Preparation

For combined retrograde intrarenal surgery and percutaneous nephrolithotomy, the Valdivia modified Galdakao position [2] allows for simultaneous placement of the percutaneous nephrostomy access, lithotripsy, and retrograde ureteroscopy.

Prior to a pediatric endourology case, it is important to consider the size of the patient as well as the sizing of instrumentation and tools that are available. This includes the size of the working channel, as many reusable and disposable instruments cannot thread through working channels that are less than 5 Fr. For any implants, such as ureteral stents, it is important to consider the indications, the appropriate size of the stent, and the length of time it will remain in place.

6.3 Instrumentation

6.3.1 Ureteral Access Sheath/Ureteral Dilator

Although the initial experience with ureteral access sheaths in children used an adult 14 Fr sheath [3], the most commonly used sheaths have a 9.5 Fr inner diameter and 11 Fr outer diameter and come in shorter lengths, so the working distance to the child is closer. Active dilation of the ureter and placement of both a safety and working wire can be done using a dual lumen coaxial dilator which tapers from 8 Fr when placed in the proximal ureter to 10 Fr in the distal ureter. Ureteral dilation balloons are rarely used as they dilate the orifice to 15 Fr (5 mm), which is larger than necessary.

6.3.2 Percutaneous Nephrolithotomy

The "all-seeing" needle comes in a 4.85 Fr size for micro-perc [4]. The mini-perc set, which is no longer commercially available [5], consisted of a 11 Fr peel-away sheath over an 8–10 Fr dual lumen dilator. As a substitute, Amplatz dilators can be used to dilate the nephrostomy tract to 12 Fr, an 8–10 dual lumen dilator used to place a working and safety wire, and a ureteral access sheath placed and trimmed to appropriate length. The Amplatz nephrostomy dilator set has an 8 Fr sheath that fits over the working wire, with sheaths that increase by 2 Fr up to 30 Fr. It is made of a stiff plastic material, polytetrafluoroethylene (PTFE). For larger patients, an Amplatz dilator set can be used to dilate the tract from 6 Fr after initial percutaneous access, up to the desired size. The metal Alken dilators have a knob on the smallest dilator, and since they are metal, they can be sterilized for reuse. Similar to the Amplatz dilator, the progressively larger dilators are placed over the initial dilator until the tract is of appropriate size.

6.3.3 Endopyelotomy Balloons

The Acusize Endopyelotomy catheter is no longer commercially available, it consisted of an 8 mm (24 Fr) balloon, which had a 100 mm cutting wire attached to one side [6]. The initial benefit of the Acusize was that it could be deployed in a retrograde fashion to treat ureteropelvic junction obstruction, so no percutaneous access was required. Due to a 65% success rate and progressive long-term failure, it has been replaced by laparoscopy pyeloplasty [7]. In cases where an antegrade endopyelotomy under vision after failed pyeloplasty is appropriate, balloons with an inflated diameter of 6 mm (18 Fr) are available to delineate the area of stenosis, which allows for incision of the ureteropelvic junction.

6.3.4 Ureteral Stent

Since its introduction in 1978, the double-J ureteral stent is widely used in pediatric urology to maintain patency of the ureter and help recover from ureteral injury [8]. Advances in development and design have been driven by the goal to decrease stent-related morbidity, including pain, encrustation, and biofilm. These advances have included using a loop-type end, rather than pigtail coil in the bladder, various coatings, and use of different biomaterials.

Most commercially available stents are polymeric double J ureteral stents. Silicone stents are also available and thought to be less apt to encrust as well as form a bacterial biofilm [8, 9]. In addition, they are associated with less stent-related symptoms compared to polyurethane ureteral stents [9]. Metallic stents are theoretically better for ureteric obstruction, given their rigidity and resistance to extrinsic compression [10]. For pediatric patients, removal of the ureteral stent often involves another anesthetic and cystoscopy. Magnetic stents can provide reduced general anesthetic exposure and cost savings, but these stents do require catheterization for removal [11].

Choosing the correct size of stent is important. The calculation of patient age +10 cm is commonly used for selecting ureteral stent length for a pediatric patient [12]. For torturous, dilated ureters, retrograde insertion of a measured ureteral catheter can be used to estimate the size prior to stent insertion. Stent size ranges from 3 to 8 Fr. Stents are typically passed over a wire for safe positioning. It is important to choose the correct wire diameter in order for the stent to pass over the wire (Table 6.1).

6.3.5 Wires

There are three main types of wires used in urology: hydrophilic straight and angled wires, hybrid wires, which have a distal hydrophilic tip and typically a nitinol core, and stiff wires. The hydrophilic wires are useful for bypassing difficult obstructions and for navigating tortuous ureters. They come in straight and angled tip. The angled tip can further facilitate passage through narrow, tortuous ureters. The hybrid wire provides the gentleness of a hydrophilic tip, enabling safe passage through the ureter, but also the stiffness that can facilitate straightening of the ureter and stabilization when advancing instrumentation over it. The extra stiff wires are most useful when passing dilating catheters and sheaths, as they are even more kink resistant. Complications associated with stiff wires include puncture and passage through the ureteral wall. Therefore, hydrophilic tipped wires are preferred for retrograde ureteral access. Wire diameters range from 0.018 to 0.038 in.

Table 6.1 Appropriate size wires for stents

Diameter of stent (fr)	Diameter of wire (in)
3	0.018
4	0.025
6	0.035
8	0.038

6.3.6 Baskets

There has been recent advances and innovation in disposable stone retrieval devices, including stone extraction baskets. Baskets were once made of reusable stainless steel, but are now single use and made of nitinol, making them more flexible and less traumatic. There are multiple types of baskets, with different characteristics and mechanisms of action (Table 6.2). There are newer, smaller 1.3–1.5 Fr baskets that are less likely to interfere with deflection of the flexible ureteroscope in the kidney and do not occlude the flow or irrigation through the working channel as much as larger baskets. Another recent innovation is the tipless basket that is less traumatic and can conform to the shape of the calyx while ensnaring a stone. End-engaging baskets do not completely envelope the stone, but rather grasp the stone circumferentially (Fig. 6.1). This allows for more precise grasping and easy release [13]. Although baskets are more commonly used for stone extraction, they can be used for stent removal during flexible cystoscopy, and for stents that have migrated proximally into the ureter.

6.4 Technique

6.4.1 Ureteral Access Sheath/Ureteral Dilator

After placement of the ureteral guidewire, place the 8–10 coaxial dilator to the mid-ureter under fluoroscopic guidance. Place the safety wire,

Table 6.2 Properties of different stone baskets

Basket shape	Manufacturer	Basket name	Special basket features
Tipless (4-wire round)	Bard	Skylite	
	Boston scientific	Zero tip	
	Coloplast	Dormia no-tip	
	Cook	NCircle	Also comes as delta (sturdier) version and helical (intertwined) configuration
	Olympus	Ultra-catch	Twisted wires to maintain shape, rotation control handle
	Sacred heart	Halo	Rotation control handle
		Vantage	Rotation control handle
Tipless (end engaging)	Boston scientific	Dakota	OpenSure handle capable of secondary opening to ensure release
	Cook	NGage	
Tipless (unique)	Coloplast	Dormia no-tip	Twisted wire with flower design
	Olympus	X-catch NT	Cross-paired wires for increased radial dilating force, basket changes to multiple sizes, rotatable handle
	Sacred heart	Halo	
Tipped	Cogentix medical/ Laborie	Flat/helical	
	Coloplast	DormiaN. Stone	
	Cook	NForce	
	Sacred heart	Apex	
Miscellaneous	Bard	EXPAND212	2-1-2-1 wire design for increased wire coverage over stone
		Dimension	Able to articulate position of basket at handle
	Boston scientific	Escape	2-in-1 basket designed to hold stone and allow simultaneous lithotripsy
		Graspit	Shaped like grasping forceps, has serrated nitinol wire edges
		OptiFlex	Rotation control knob on handle, extendable cage diameter
	Cook	NCompass	16 wire meshed construction designed for small stone fragment retrieval
		NTrap	Woven meshed wires extend beyond stone, preventing retropulsion of fragments

Adapted from: Khaleel SS, Borofsky MS. Innovations in Disposable Technologies for Stone Management. *UrolClin North Am*. 2019;46(2):175–184 [15]

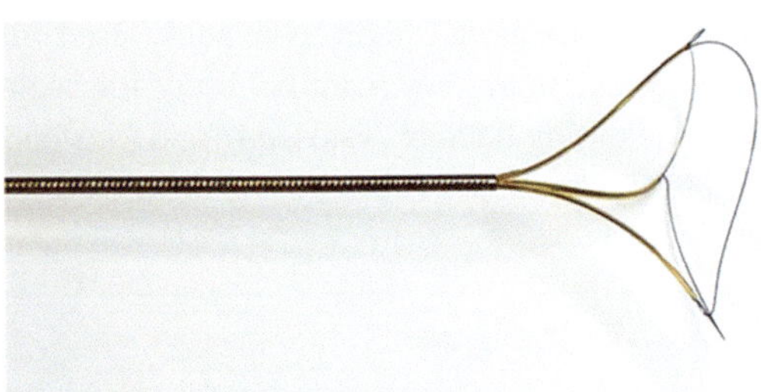

Fig. 6.1 End-engaging basket

remove the 8–10 dilator, coil the safety wire, and place the appropriate length ureteral access sheath to the mid-ureter. Remove the inner portion of the access sheath; if the sheath is too long, trim the portion outside the patient before starting ureteroscopy.

6.4.2 Percutaneous Nephrolithotomy

For mini-perc and standard PCNL, after obtaining initial access, use Amplatz dilators to dilate the nephrostomy tract to 12 Fr. Place an 8–10 dual lumen dilator to position an additional safety wire down the ureteropelvic junction into the proximal ureter. Trim the appropriate size ureteral access sheath to the correct length and pass this over the working wire, remove the inner portion of the access sheath. For micro-perc, the entire procedure is done through the needle by passing the laser fiber through the central channel. A limitation of micro-perc is that stones cannot be extracted at the time of surgery, so it is more similar to shock wave lithotripsy, in that the stone fragments need to pass spontaneously [4].

6.5 Results

6.5.1 Ureteral Access Sheath/ Ureteral Dilator

Despite initial concerns about causing distal ureteral strictures from dilation, the stricture rate is <1% in most series, showing that properly applied active or passive dilation is safe, even in small children [14]. However, the caveat is that all patients who had placement of a ureteral access sheath previously underwent placement of a ureteral stent to allow for passive dilation. If you are attempting a one-step dilation on a ureter that feels tight, placement of a stent is the safer course. Stone-free rates after a single procedure remain in the 80% range with low complication rates [14].

6.5.2 Percutaneous Nephrolithotomy

Standard PCNL in children provides a stone-free rate of 80–90% [2], while mini-perc has an 85% stone-free rate [5]. Micro-perc showed an 89% stone-free rate for stones with a mean size of 14 mm in a study population of 2 children and 8 adults [4], with an identical 88% stone-free rate in 8 children [2]. Micro-perc seems to be ideal for lower pole stones <20 mm.

6.5.3 Endopyelotomy Balloon

Follow-up of primary endopyelotomy (both Acusize and antegrade ureteroscopic) with 34 months showed a 65% success rate, whereas, in secondary endopyelotomy at 61 months, the success rate was 94%. Time to failure for primary Acusize incision ranged from 1.5 to 131 months [7].

Tips and Tricks

- **Ureteral access sheath/ureteral dilator**. If the 8–10 dilator cannot be passed, it is safer to place a stent and return in 2 weeks after the ureter has passively dilated to proceed with ureteroscopy, rather than risk creating a ureteral stricture. Similarly, if the ureteral access sheath cannot be passed easily, the decision on whether to proceed without the sheath should be made based on the stone burden and if relatively few passes would be required.
- **Percutaneous nephrolithotomy sheath**. Keeping the sheath in place when removing the nephroscope is the biggest challenge. The risk of dislodgement can be decreased by using an offset nephroscope or cystoscope without a curved beak, so that the sheath stays in the tract if the scope needs to be withdrawn to remove stone fragments. Confirm that the diameter of the stone fragment will fit through the nephrostomy sheath before removing the scope and the basket. If the sheath is pulled out, placing the inner portion of the sheath over the safety wire and passage of both the inner and outer sheaths into the tract allows for replacement of the outer sheath.
- **Stents, wires, and baskets**. Become familiar with the instruments available to you, especially size and caliber of working channel, so you can appropriately choose the proper size stent, wire, or other device. For dilated/tortuous ureters, measuring the ureteral length with a ureteral catheter can help with choosing the appropriate size of the stent. For stents that are in place for a short time, leaving the string attached to the distal coil of the stent to facilitate in office removal is an option, avoiding an additional anesthetic and cystoscopy.

6.6 Discussion

Percutaneous nephrolithotomy achieves a higher stone-free rate after a single procedure, but carries a higher risk of bleeding due to dilation of the tract, which is improved with the development of the mini-perc. The micro-perc allows for the possibility of a truly tubeless nephrolithotomy through a small tract, but is most beneficial in lower pole stones less than 2 cm in size. Retrograde ureteroscopy in children sometimes requires three procedures under anesthesia: placement of the ureteral stent, ureteroscopy, and stent removal. Therefore the risk/benefit balance for patients may shift based on each surgeon's comfort with micro-perc, which could allow for combined access with ureteroscopy, if needed.

The use of ureteroscopy for treatment of pediatric stone disease has increased dramatically over the past two decades, as it has been established as safe and efficacious. Advances in technology, including smaller instruments, have facilitated the application of these minimally invasive techniques to the pediatric population. In order for most endourology cases to be done safely, wires are used to exchange instruments in the kidney and ureter. In addition, stents are used to drain the kidney before and after these procedures. During a ureteroscopic procedure, baskets are commonly implemented in order to retrieve stone fragments. Ureteral access sheaths have made repetitive removal and reintroduction into the ureter to retrieve multiple stone fragments safer. The use of all of these devices requires a sound familiarity and understanding of the equipment as well as the specific tools available.

References

1. Alken P, Hutschenreiter G, Gunther R, Marberger M. Percutaneous stone manipulation. J Urol. 1981;125:463–6.
2. Caione P, Collura G, Innocenzi M, De Dominicis M, Nappo SG, Cappoza N. Percutaneous endoscopic treatment for urinary stones in pediatric patients: where we are now. Trans Pediatr. 2016;5:266–74.
3. Singh A, Shah G, Young J, Sheridan M, Haas G, Upadhyay J. Ureteral access sheath for the management of pediatric renal and ureteral stones: a single center experience. J Urol. 2006;175:1080–2.
4. Desai MR, Sharma R, Mishra S, Sabnis RB, Stief C, Bader M. Single-step percutaneous nephrolithotomy (Microperc): the initial clinical report. J Urol. 2011;186:140–5.
5. Jackman SV, Hedican SP, Peters CA, Docimo SG. Percutaneous nephrolithotomy in infants and preschool age children: experience with a new technique. Urology. 1998;52:697–701.
6. Chandoke PS, Clayman RV, Stone AM, McDougall EM, Buelna T, Hilal N, Chang M, Stegwell MJ. Endopyelotomy and endoureterotomy with the Acusize ureteral cutting balloon device: preliminary experience. J Endourol. 1993;7:45–51.
7. Kim EH, Tanagho YS, Traxel EJ, Austin PF, Figenshau RS, Coplen DE. Endopyelotomy for pediatric ureteropelvic junction obstruction: a review of our 25-year experience. J Urol. 2012;188:1628–33.
8. Finney RP. Experience with new double J ureteral catheter stent. J Urol. 1978;120:678–81.
9. Gadzhiev N, Gorelov D, Malkhasyan V, Akopyan G, Harchelava R, Mazurenko D, Kosmala C, Okhunov Z, Petrov S. Comparison of silicone versus polyurethane ureteral stents: a prospective controlled study. BMC Urol. 2020;20:10.
10. Chow PM, Chiang IN, Chen CY, Huang KH, Hsu JS, Wang SM, Lee YJ, Yu HJ, Pu YS, Huang CY. Malignant ureteral obstruction: functional duration of metallic versus polymeric ureteral stents. PLoS One. 2015;10:e0135566.
11. Mitchell A, Bolduc S, Moore K, Cook A, Fermin C, Weber B. Use of a magnetic double J stent in pediatric patients: a case-control study at two Canadian pediatric centers. J Pediatr Surg. 2020;55:486–9.
12. Palmer JS, Palmer LS. Determining the proper stent length to use in children: age plus 10. J Urol. 2007;178:1566–9.
13. Bechis SK, Abbott JE, Sur RL. *In vitro* head-to-head comparison of the durability, versatility and efficacy of the NGage and novel Dakota stone retrieval baskets. Transl Androl Urol. 2017;6:1144–9.
14. Berrettini A, Boeri L, Montanari E, Mogiatti M, Acquati P, De Lorenzis E, Gallioli A, De Marco EA, Minoli DG, Manzoni G. Retrograde intrarenal surgery using ureteral access sheaths is a safe and effective treatment for renal stones in children <20 kg. J Ped Urol. 2018;14:59.e1–6.
15. Khaleel SS, Borofsky MS. Innovations in disposable Technologies for Stone Management. Urol Clin North Am. 2019;46:175–84.

7 Instruments for Pediatric MIS Urology (Laparoscopy, Endourology, Robotics)

Mario Mendoza Sagaon and Ernesto Montaruli

Learning Objectives

- General knowledge of the most frequent instruments of MIS in pediatric urology.
- Choice of most suitable device for endourology, laparoscopy and robotics procedures.
- To describe tips and trick of instruments during MIS procedures.

7.1 Introduction

Technology in pediatric surgical procedures continues to evolve. Particularly in the domain of urology, minimal invasive surgery is becoming popular and well accepted in the pediatric surgical community. The evolution and arrival of new technology, including instruments, telescopes, ultrasonic and laser generators, electronic devices, etc. require that pediatric surgeons and pediatric urologists get continuously updated and familiarized with this new technology. Thus, in order to obtain the best results in minimally invasive pediatric urology procedures, accurate knowledge of the instruments is fundamental. Each instrument used during endourology, laparoscopic or robotic interventions, deserves its detailed knowledge to obtain the best results during the intervention and to be able to cope with the complications that can occur during these procedures.

The first part of this chapter will be dedicated to the description of the instruments used for endourological surgery, including cystoscopy and ureterorenoscopy. The second part of the chapter will describe commonly instruments used during pediatric laparoscopic urological procedures and finally, we will describe the particularities of urological robotic surgery instruments.

7.2 Endourology Instruments

Endourological exploration of the urinary tract is a standard procedure of the pediatric urologist. It may be performed in a variety of circumstances and requires three conditions: (1) a cavity filled with fluid; (2) an endoscope of the right diameter and (3) a light source connected to an external unit. Usually, a digital camera is used to connect the eyepiece to the external unit. The images are sent to the endoscopic tower to be processed and subsequently to a monitor to be viewed. Typically, xenon or halogen light source deliver cool light to

M. M. Sagaon (✉) · E. Montaruli
Department of Pediatric Surgery and Pediatric Orthopedic Surgery, Pediatric Institute of the Southern Swiss, Bellinzona, Switzerland
e-mail: mario.mendozasagaon@eoc.ch; ernesto.montaruli@eoc.ch

C. Esposito et al. (eds.), *Minimally Invasive Techniques in Pediatric Urology*,
https://doi.org/10.1007/978-3-030-99280-4_7

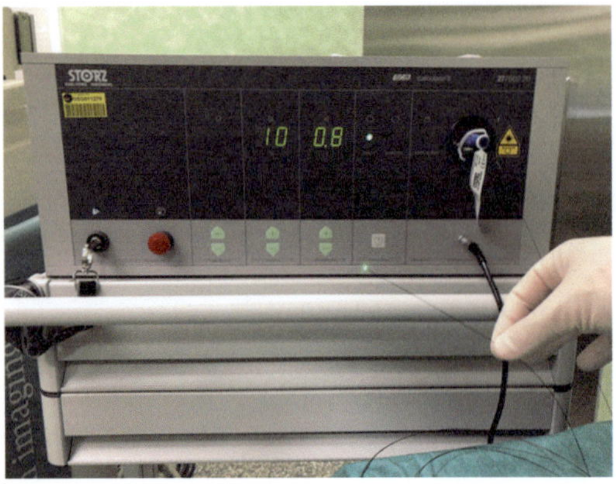

Fig. 7.1 Laser light source generator delivers cool light to the endoscope by a fine fiber-optic cable

the endoscope by a fiber-optic cable (Fig. 7.1). The most used irrigation fluids are sterile water, saline or glycine solutions. Usually, an electrolytes-free solution must be preferred if the use of electrocautery is expected.

Cystourethroscopy could be performed using a rigid or flexible endoscope. Each of these tools has specific advantages based on the clinical situation.

Rigid endoscopes offer better image quality than the flexible system based on optical fibers. Furthermore, the rigid cystoscope has a larger working channel and allows the introduction of different types of instruments, greater irrigation flow (Fig. 7.2). In addition, they allow easier handling and better stability during the surgical procedures. Rigid cystoscopes require precise assembly before use. Usually they have a mark on the end that identifies the cystoscope size and the working channel width.

The flexible video ureteroscope (Fig. 7.2) has the advantage of allowing an easier examination of the upper urinary tract and allowing a complete inspection of the bladder. Thanks to its flexibility, it is often used to explore the upper urinary tract and treat urological pathologies located above the level of the iliac vessels. In pediatric age, it is used for endoscopic treatment of nephrolithiasis. Some type of laser probes, such as the holmium laser, are used to vaporize the stones [1]. This procedure has excellent results even in the pediatric age [2]. It is important to be aware that flexible cystoscopes are much more delicate and fragile than the rigid ones, but with a correct handling and maintenance, a long life of these devices could be achieved [3].

Pediatric endoscopes have sizes ranging from 8 to 12 Fr, while cystoscopes for adults with a caliber from 16 to 25 Fr may be used on teenagers. Obviously the size of the endoscope will depend on the age of the patient and the procedure to be performed and therefore on the need to introduce different types of tools. However, it should not be forgotten that a small cystoscope is less traumatic in the urinary tract. Additionally a portable fluoroscopic system is required in order to control localization of lithiasis, position of catheters, intraoperative contrast studies, etc. (Fig. 7.3).

7.3 Laparoscopic Instruments

Laparoscopy is an essential tool in diagnostic investigations and in the treatment of multiple pediatric urological diseases. Laparoscopy requires four essential components: (1) laparoscopic telescopes, (2) an external light source with a fiber-optic cable, (3) a camera with a monitor connected to a tower to process images and (4) a system of CO_2 insufflation.

Laparoscopic telescopes are commonly available in different sizes. In the pediatric population, the most commonly used are of 3, 5 and 10 mm diameters. The optics can have a different angle depending on the type of procedure performed. The 0°, 30° and 70° optics are the most commonly used. Semi-flexible laparoscopes that allow a 90° exploration are less used (Olympus, Karl Storz Endo CAMeleon). Finally, there are laparoscopes that integrate a working channel to reduce the number of trocars needed for other instruments, but they have the inconvenience that they are of 10 mm diameter and the quality of the image may be affected by the concomitant presence of the working channel. Laparoscopic lens fogging is a frequently encountered problem and some solutions are available [4].

Correct positioning and orientation of the optic and the camera is essential to obtain good quality images. It should be remembered that

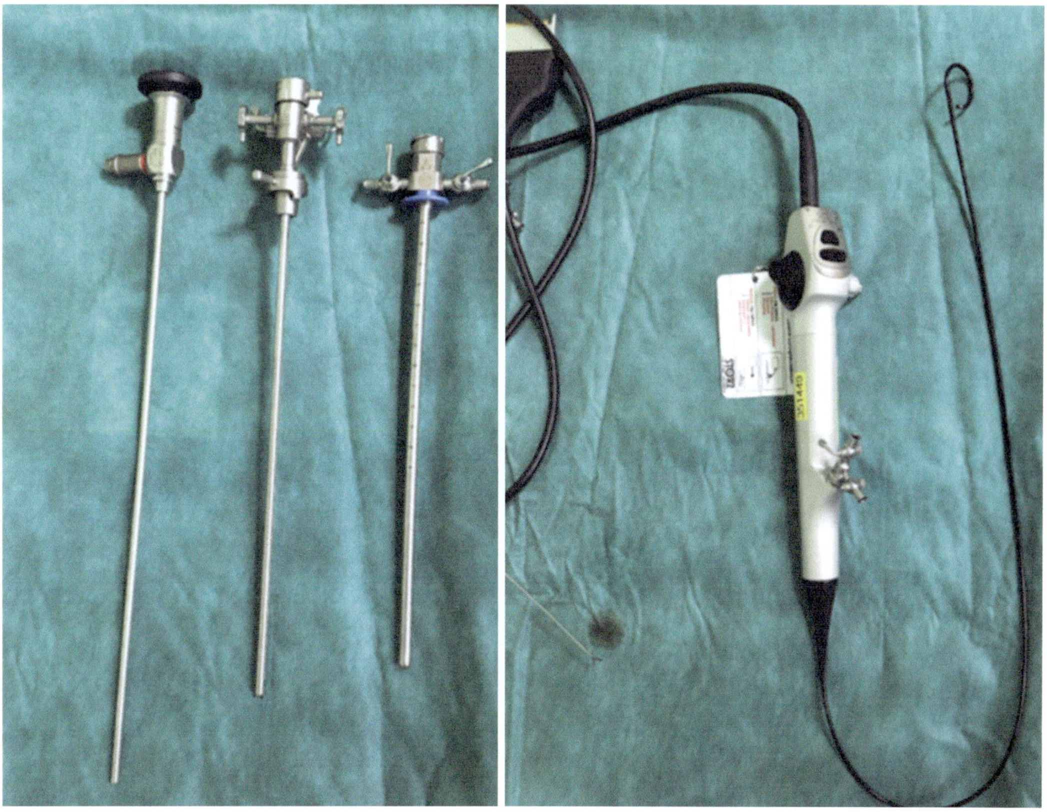

Fig. 7.2 Rigid cystoscope and flexible video ureteroscope

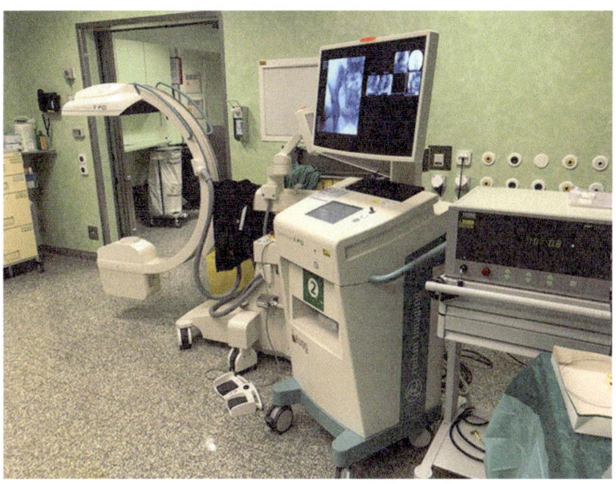

Fig. 7.3 Portable fluoroscopy system

during the procedure the camera must be oriented at 0° with the optics in order to avoid image rotations, which can disrupt the procedure.

The light source is essential for good quality images. Halogen or Xenon light sources are usually used. The access to the abdominal cavity during laparoscopic operations can take place in different ways of trocar placement, and triangulation may be achieved when possible. Surgical approach can be transperitoneal, extraperitoneal and retroperitoneal. These techniques require an access route [5] and adequate equipment, and will not be discussed in this chapter.

In pediatric laparoscopic urology, the 5 and 3-mm instruments are generally used (Fig. 7.4). They offer 4 degrees of freedom: (1) in/out, (2) external pitch (up/down), (3) external yaw (left/right) and (4) rotation (clockwise/counterclockwise).

The instruments used during a laparoscopic urologic procedure are those for grasping and retraction, for blunt and sharp dissection, incising, hemostasis (electrocautery or ultrasonic energy), suturing, clipping, specimen retrieval, suction and irrigation.

The most frequently used instruments for cutting and hemostasis are: monopolar hook, mono-

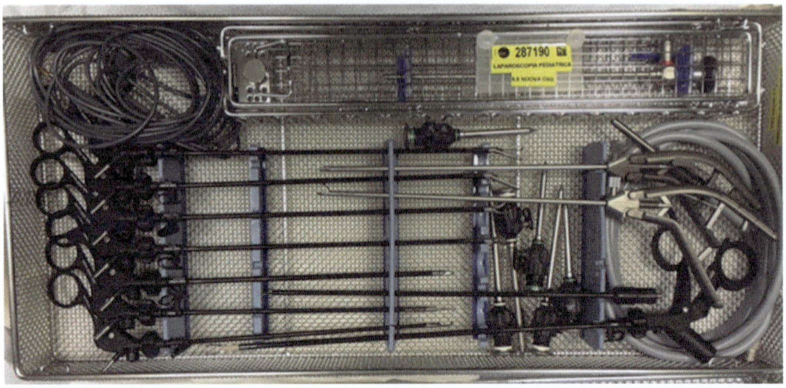

Fig. 7.4 3-mm laparoscopic instruments

polar scissors, laparoscopic scalpels, electrocautery and ultrasonic devices and lasers. The scissors can be single-use or reusable and the tip can be fixed or rotating. Laparoscopic scalpels are often used for pyelotomy procedures (Fig. 7.5). The electric scalpel is employed much more often in comparison to the mechanical one, which can have different tips depending on its use. Care should be taken that the end of the scalpel is always protected by an inert envelope to avoid injury to other organs during cauterization. There are different types of ultrasonic coagulation and sealing vessels tools that permit to avoid intracorporeal knotting [6, 7]. The technology of these devices is based on a low voltage radio frequency generator. Finally, laser instruments, based mainly on CO_2 and Helium technology, can be used for cutting and hemostasis thanks to the use of light impulse energy through optical-fibers. Argon coagulation is reserved predominantly for hepatobiliary surgery [8].

A fundamental principle during a laparoscopic operation is the gentle and accurate manipulation of the organs and their dissection and suture. The force applied during tissue palpation plays an important role to reduce organ damage [9]. Several tools make this task easier. In pediatrics, dissectors and laparoscopic graspers have dimensions that can vary from 3 to 10 mm with a liner, pointed or curved design, traumatic or more often atraumatic, locking or non-locking.

Laparoscopic needle holders have a locking mechanism which facilitates their use during laparoscopic suturing procedures. Mechanical staplers have certainly accelerated surgical procedures and become reliable to the mechanical stress [10].

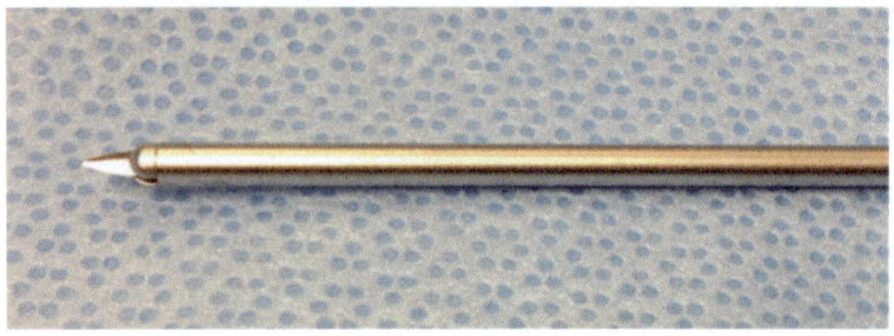

Fig. 7.5 Laparoscopic knife

Several tools become useful when making vascular dissections and occlusion, in this case clips devices are indispensable. There are different sizes of clips according to the type of procedure and the tissue thickness. During or before ending an operation, the abdominal cavity must be clean. In this regard, there are different types of laparoscopic disposable or non-disposable aspirators/irrigation devices.

Specimen retrieval bags permit to extract full organs or fragments of them during a laparoscopic procedure. The bags have different sizes and are made of different materials. These devices may request an enlargement of the abdominal wall incisions to permit the organ extraction.

7.4 Robotic Instruments

Robotic surgery is gaining in popularity in pediatric urology due to the advantages of the three dimensional vision and the EndoWrist® technol-

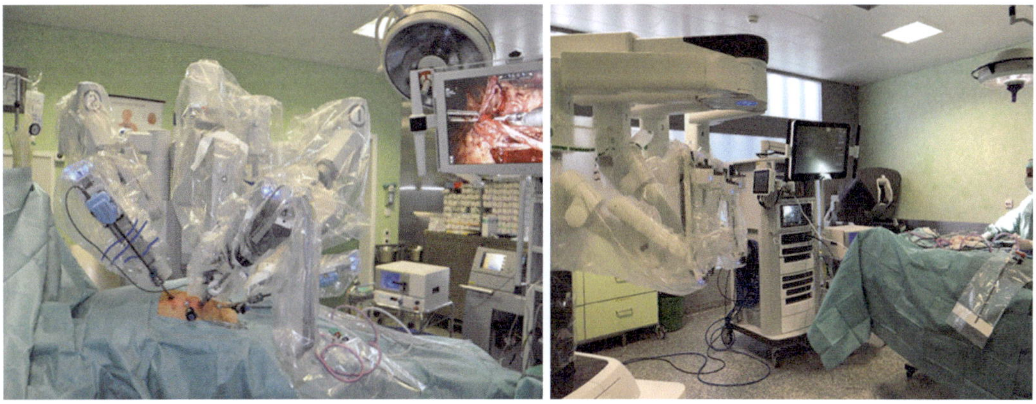

Fig. 7.6 Si and Xi da Vinci® platforms

ogy instrumentation that offer a wide range of motion, allowing great dexterity and precision through a minimal invasive approach. In addition, the robotic console offers better ergonomics for the surgeon during the procedures.

Many robotic urological procedures in children have been reported with excellent results, including pyeloplasty, nephrectomy and heminephrectomy, uretero-vesical reimplantation, renal tumor excision, bladder augmentation, nephrolithiasis, etc. [11]. Some limitations of this technology are the higher costs, the low availability of the platform and lack of haptic feedback. Although an advised limitation in neonates and infants due to the size of the robotic instruments and the deficiency of distance necessary between the ports of the robotic arms in order to avoid instrument clashes, some authors have reported good results in infants of less than 10 kg [12].

Currently there are two platforms of the da Vinci® system available, the Si and the Xi (Fig. 7.6). Older versions have been discontinued by Surgical Intuitive Inc., Sunnyvale, USA. The new system da Vinci® Xi offers the innovation of a crystal clear 3-D HD vision, integrated generator for electrocoagulation and ultrasonic energy, robotic vessel sealers, robotic staplers and single port technology. Another important benefit of the Xi platform is that the structure of the surgical cart allows easier docking and a multi-quadrant access, avoiding the necessity of re-docking.

The surgeon and all the surgical team must be familiarized with the structure, components and function of the three main units of the da Vinci® platform: the surgeon's console, the surgical cart and the vision cart in order to benefit of the best capabilities of the platform and to guarantee the best surgical results. Moreover, knowledge that the platform will give strategies for troubleshooting in case of technical problems.

It is advised to create adequate checklists of the different robotic urologic procedures. These checklists should include (1) patient's position, (2) surgical cart and visual cart position for the setting of the docking, (3) availability of the robotic instruments (including staplers, ultrasonic devices or clips) and their position in the robotic arms as well as the position of the monopolar or bipolar cables, (4) additional laparoscopic instruments, (5) additional urologic devices such as stents, catheters, drains, specimen retrieval bags, etc.

Robotic telescopes are available in 8 and 12 mm, 0° and 30° for the Si platform and only 8 mm with the video camera integrated, 0° and 30° for the Xi platform.

Robotic instruments exist in 5 and 8 mm for the Si platform and only 8 mm for the Xi platform [13]. Around 39 instruments of 8 mm are available with a wide variety of graspers, scissors, dissectors, needle drivers that can articulate the tip up to 90° and allow 7 degrees of freedom (in/out, rotation; external and internal wristed pitch [up/down]; external and internal wristed yaw [left right]; and Grip) (Fig. 7.7). Moreover, some of these instruments can be

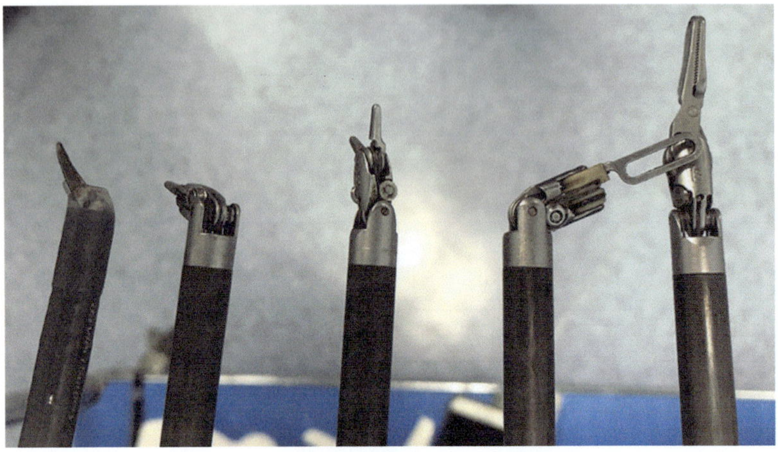

Fig. 7.7 Robotic 8-mm instruments

associated with monopolar or bipolar cauterization. In general, the 8-mm instruments have a lifespan of ten uses. Generally, for most of the pediatric urologic procedures, only three of the four robotics arms of the surgical cart are used, and the five or six more instruments used are the bipolar forceps, the grasper, the monopolar scissors, the needle drivers (2x) and the monopolar hook.

Regarding 5-mm instruments, these are only available in the Si platform. They are limited to ten instruments (hook, spatula, needle drivers, two forceps, two graspers, non-articulated ultrasonic shears and two cold scissors) and in comparison to the single articulation tip in the 8-mm instruments, the 5-mm have three joints, creating a snake-like curvature and will require more space to wrist. In addition, no bipolar instruments are available and they have a lifespan of 20 uses [14].

In general, the cost of each instrument during a robotic procedure is estimated to be between 250 and 300 Euro. To reduce these costs, it is advised the use of additional laparoscopic working ports of 3, 5 or 10 mm that can be used for insertion/extraction of surgical devices (sutures, catheters, wirelines, etc.), suction and irrigation, retrieval of specimens, additional retraction, clip applying, use of staplers, etc. (Fig. 7.8). Moreover, a good preoperative strategy and a checklist will permit to avoid using unnecessary robotic instruments for a certain procedure.

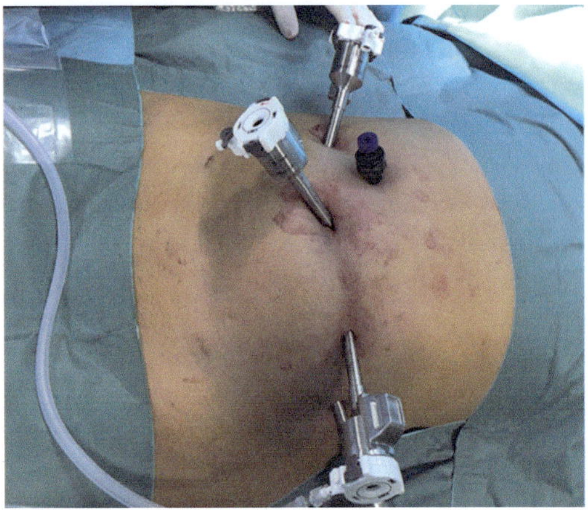

Fig. 7.8 Robotic and supplementary laparoscopic trocars

Evolution of robotic technology is necessary to create smaller instrumentation and develop robotic miniaturization in order to improve minimal invasive procedures, where pediatric surgery will benefit, particularly in the domain of neonatal surgery.

In conclusion, continuing evolution of technology in the domain of minimal invasive surgery requires continuous update and knowledge of new instrumentation, devices, generators, robotic platforms as well as development of new skills of the surgeon and his/her surgical team. This will allow the surgeon to take advantage of all the benefits that the new technology offers and to face troubleshooting when necessary.

References

1. Breda A, Ogunyemi O, Leppert JT, Schulam PG. Flexible ureteroscopy and laser lithotripsy for multiple unilateral intrarenal stones. Eur Urol. 2009;55(5):1190–6. https://doi.org/10.1016/j.eururo.2008.06.019.
2. Chedgy EC, Griffin SJ, Dyer JP, Somani BK. Ureteroscopy for Paediatric renal tract stones - outcomes from a tertiary European Centre. Urol Int. 2015;95(3):320–3. https://doi.org/10.1159/000380857.
3. Lin CC, Wu LS, Huang SS, Lin CF, Chen WH, Wu CT. Surgical technique to achieve high durability of flexible ureteroscopes: a single hospital experience. Biom J. 2018;41(6):385–90. https://doi.org/10.1016/j.bj.2018.10.002.
4. Manning TG, Perera M, Christidis D, et al. Visual occlusion during minimally invasive surgery: a contemporary review of methods to reduce laparoscopic and robotic lens fogging and other sources of optical loss. J Endourol. 2017;31(4):327–33. https://doi.org/10.1089/end.2016.0839.
5. Kaistha S, Kumar A, Gangavatiker R, Br S, Sisodiya N. Laparoscopic access: direct trocar insertion versus open technique. J Laparoendosc Adv Surg Tech A. 2019;29(4):489–94. https://doi.org/10.1089/lap.2018.0408.
6. Li CC, Yeh HC, Lee HY, et al. Laparoscopic partial nephrectomy without intracorporeal suturing. Surg Endosc. 2016;30(4):1585–91. https://doi.org/10.1007/s00464-015-4382-8.
7. Pogorelić Z, Katić J, Mrklić I, et al. Lateral thermal damage of mesoappendix and appendiceal base during laparoscopic appendectomy in children: comparison of the harmonic scalpel (Ultracision), bipolar coagulation (LigaSure), and thermal fusion technology (MiSeal). J Surg Res. 2017;212:101–7. https://doi.org/10.1016/j.jss.2017.01.014.
8. Okada T, Sasaki F, Kurauchi N, et al. Laparoscopic liver biopsy using cup-shaped punch biopsy forceps and argon beam coagulator in children. Pediatr Surg Int. 2007;23(10):947–51. https://doi.org/10.1007/s00383-007-1976-9.
9. Alleblas CCJ, Vleugels MPH, Coppus SFPJ, Nieboer TE. The effects of laparoscopic graspers with enhanced haptic feedback on applied forces: a randomized comparison with conventional graspers. Surg Endosc. 2017;31(12):5411–7. https://doi.org/10.1007/s00464-017-5623-9.
10. Mitchell IC, Barber R, Fischer AC, Schindel DT. Experience performing 64 consecutive stapled intestinal anastomoses in small children and infants. J Pediatr Surg. 2011;46(1):128–30. https://doi.org/10.1016/j.jpedsurg.2010.09.076.
11. Narula VK, Melvin WS. Robotic surgical systems. In: Patel VR, editor. Robotic urologic surgery. 1st ed. Berlin: Springer; 2007. p. 5–14.
12. Kafka IZ, Kocherov S, Jaber J, Chertin B. Pediatric robotic-assisted laparoscopic pyeloplasty (RALP): does weight matter? Pediatr Surg Int. 2019;35(3):391–6. https://doi.org/10.1007/s00383-019-04435-y.
13. Borin JF. Chapter 1: Laparoscopic and robotic instrumentation for urologic reconstructive surgery in adults. In: Robotic and laparoscopic reconstructive surgery in children and adults. Berlin: Humana Press/Springer Science; 2011. p. 3–15.
14. Chandrasoma S, Koh CJ. Chapter 2: Instrumentation during pediatric robotic anastomoses and reconstruction. Humana Press/Springer Science: Berlin, 2011 pp 17–27.

8 Energy Sources in Pediatric MIS Urology

Peter Zimmermann and Martin Lacher

Learning Objectives
- To understand the basics of electrosurgery.
- To become familiar with the different electrosurgical systems.
- To know the current literature on the applications of electrosurgery used in pediatric MIS Urology.

8.1 Basics and Biophysics of Electrosurgery

Electrosurgery requires an electrosurgical unit (ESU), an active electrode, target tissue, and a return electrode [1]. The ESU takes alternating electrical current (AC) from a socket (with a frequency of 50 or 60 Hz) and converts it into AC with frequency ranges of 200 kHz to 50 MHz. These frequencies allow the desired thermal effects without muscle fasciculation, nerve stimulation, and interferences with the conductivity of the heart muscles resulting in cardiac arrest and death by electrocution. The ESUs can generate different waveforms like low-voltage continuous mode, interrupted high-voltage mode, and various blended modes [2, 3]. The conversion of the generated flowing electric energy to thermal energy when it encounters the resistance of the target tissue leads to different tissue effects. Depending on the voltage and active time of the electrode, the effects are cutting, coagulation, desiccation, and fulguration [4].

P. Zimmermann (✉) · M. Lacher
Department of Pediatric Surgery, University of Leipzig, Leipzig, Germany
e-mail: Peter.Zimmermann@medizin.uni-leipzig.de; Martin.Lacher@medizin.uni-leipzig.de

8.2 Electrosurgical Technologies

8.2.1 Monopolar Electrosurgery

In monopolar electrosurgery, a focused alternating electrical current is delivered by a single small electrode at the tip of the surgical instrument to the target tissue. To complete the electrical circuit, a dispersive electrode is placed on the patient, remote from the surgical site [3]. Due to low costs, easy availability, and the variety of tissue effects, monopolar electrosurgery remains a popular modality in MIS. Monopolar electrosurgery is the only electrosurgical modality responsible for tissue vaporization (tissue destruction and/or transection) and fulguration (tissue destruction and small vessel hemostasis) (Fig. 8.1) [1]. However, its limitations are the need for a dispersive electrode, the possibility of stray current injuries and the inability to seal vessels larger than 1–2 mm in diameter.

C. Esposito et al. (eds.), *Minimally Invasive Techniques in Pediatric Urology*,
https://doi.org/10.1007/978-3-030-99280-4_8

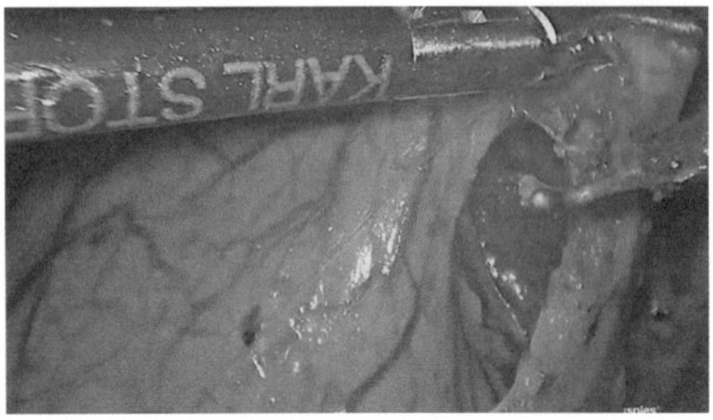

Fig. 8.1 Dissection of the ureteropelvic junction with monopolar hook cautery during laparoscopic transabdominal dismembered pyeloplasty

8.3 Conventional and Advanced Bipolar Electrosurgery

8.3.1 Conventional Bipolar Electrosurgery

In bipolar electrosurgery, both electrodes are at the tip of the surgical instrument itself. The electric current flows from one electrode to the other through the tissue held by the two electrodes to achieve the desired effect. The advantages over monopolar electrosurgery include the fact that the current does not flow through the patient's body. However, in comparison to monopolar electrosurgery, coagulation takes longer, which may lead to tissue adherence to the electrodes and the risk of incidental tearing of adjacent blood vessels. Another disadvantage of bipolar electrosurgery is that the electrodes cannot cut tissue [1, 3].

8.4 Advanced Bipolar Electrosurgery

In advanced bipolar electrosurgical systems, the delivered electrical energy is highly pulsatile, which allows tissue cooling during activation in order to decrease lateral thermal diffusion [4]. Computerized feedback control systems on tissue impedance and temperature adjust the current and voltage for an optimal tissue vascular sealing and indicate the achievement of the desired tissue effect by an alarm or deactivation system. This protects against prolonged activation, avoiding high tissue temperatures, and reduces the risk for lateral thermal diffusion. Advanced bipolar devices allow the sealing of vessels up to a diameter of 7 mm (Table 8.1) [5, 6, 9]. Moreover, most advanced bipolar devices have an incorporated retractable blade between the jaws of the instrument for tissue transection.

8.5 Ultrasonic Instruments

The basic principle of ultrasound devices is the creation of ultrasonic waves without electrosurgical current. Ultrasonic instruments produce tissue effects by generating mechanical vibrations of frequencies greater than 20 kHz. This mechanical energy, combined with the generated thermal energy, leads to protein denaturation and formation of a coagulum, sealing vessels up to 7 mm in diameter (Table 8.1) [4]. The advantages of ultrasonic instruments are less lateral thermal diffusion, less tissue necrosis and carbonization, and less amount of smoke generated. An ultrasonic generator provides the mechanical energy necessary to produce the desired tissue effects to the instrument. The "min" mode provides fine oscillations that are ideal for vascular sealing; however, the lateral diffusion is greater. In the "max" mode, higher mechanical energy leads to wider oscillations resulting in rapid transection with less hemostasis. Like in advanced bipolar electrosurgery devices, a feedback control system regulates the energy according to tissue conditions coupled with an alarm system indicating the achievement of the desired effect [7].

8.6 Hybrid Technology (Bipolar + Ultrasound)

Hybrid technology combines the principles of advanced bipolar systems and ultrasonic systems. With such multi-functional instruments, it is possible to seal and cut vessels up to 7 mm in size with minimal thermal spread (Table 8.1).

Table 8.1 Selection of currently available vessel sealing device (VSD) technologies [1, 5–8]

Trade names (commonly used)	LigaSure™	Harmonic™	ThunderBeat system™
Manufacturer	Medtronic/Covidien, Boulder, CO, USA	Johnson & Johnson Plaza, New Brunswick, New Jersey, U.S.	Olympus Medical Systems Corporation, Shinjuku, Tokio, Japan
Year of availability 1998 2003 2005	1998	2003	2012
Technology	Pulsed bipolar energy	Ultrasonic technique	Ultrasonic and bipolar technique
Vessel seal (max. diameter in mm)	7	7	7
Mean time to seal (in vessel of 2–7 mm in s)	3.24 ± 0.32	3.3 ± 1.0	2.43 ± 0.76
Mean burst pressure (in arteries of 5–7 mm in mmHg)	615 ± 40	454 ± 50	734 ± 64
Sufficient safety margin (mm)	5	5	5

Different clinical trials have shown superiority of this technique over the existing electrosurgery devices [8, 10].

8.7 Applications in Pediatric Minimally Invasive Urological Surgery

Esposito et al. analyzed complications encountered during 701 urologic procedures performed at eight urological centers in Italy [11]. Nineteen complications (2.7%) were recorded, of which six required conversion to open surgery. Bleeding or dissection problems occurred in eight cases in which monopolar coagulation was used. For this reason, the authors recommended the use of advanced bipolar or ultrasonic instruments instead of monopolar electrocautery to reduce the risk of bleeding and of thermal injuries during delicate dissections. In another study, Esposito et al. reported their results of 149 nephrectomies in children using MIS (laparoscopic and retroperitoneoscopic). They concluded that the use of hemostatic devices like LigaSure™ or Harmonic™, instead of monopolar electrosurgery, reduces the risk of bleeding and shortens the operation time [12].

In a prospective study, Metzelder et al. compared the use of LigaSure™ with the use of clips or ligations during laparoscopic transabdominal nephrectomy in ten consecutive pediatric patients in each group. They showed that the use of LigaSure™ in laparoscopic transabdominal nephrectomy is safe, effective, and facilitates significantly lower operating times compared to clip application and intracorporeal suturing [13]. In a second study, the same group evaluated the feasibility of using LigaSure™ in laparoscopic transperitoneal hemi-nephroureterectomy in children with impaired renal duplex systems (Fig. 8.2). The authors reported an excellent feasibility of this procedure using this vessel-sealing device [14].

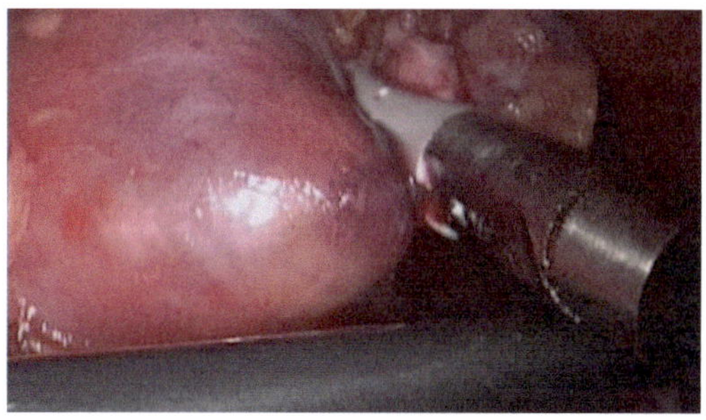

Fig. 8.2 Division of the renal parenchyma with LigaSure™ during right-sided transperitoneal laparoscopic heminephroureterectomy

These findings were confirmed by two other studies which reported their experience with transperitoneal laparoscopic heminephroureterectomy using LigaSure™ [15, 16].

Laparoscopic heminephroureterectomy, however, mainly in adults, has been performed in selected cases of renal tumors and where nephron preservation is essential. Comparable results without complications for nephron sparing tumor dissection either by cold scissors or by an ultracision device have been reported [17]. Of note, although the tissue margins of the specimen may be deformed by the effects of lateral thermal diffusion, the interpretation regarding a benign or a malignant character of the cells is not compromised [18].

Two studies by Marte et al. and Koyle et al. compared the use of the LigaSure™ vessel-sealing system with laparoscopic clip ligation in laparoscopic Palomo varicocele ligation (LPV) in children and adolescents. In both studies, the authors concluded that LPV using a vascular sealing device is a rapid, safe, and effective therapeutic option for the pediatric and adolescent patient with varicocele, which has excellent results [19, 20].

8.8 Discussion

With the introduction of minimally invasive techniques in pediatric surgery and urology, there is a growing demand for electrosurgical devices which maximize the desired tissue effects, while minimizing adverse events. Advanced bipolar electrosurgical systems and ultrasound systems have found their place in pediatric minimally invasive urological surgery. The use of these devices is safe, effective, and can help to reduce operating times and complication rates. However, they should be used with great care and a margin of at least 5 mm to adjacent organs is recommended to avoid any thermal damage.

Take-Home Points

- All electrosurgery devices should be used with great care due to lateral thermal diffusion.
- The maximum approved vessel diameter for sealing is 7 mm for each of the different systems.
- If advanced bipolar electrosurgery or ultrasonic systems are used, a margin of at least 5 mm to adjacent organs is recommended to avoid any thermal damage.

References

1. Lyons SD, Law KS. Laparoscopic vessel sealing technologies. J Minim Invasive Gynecol. 2013;20(3):301–7. https://doi.org/10.1016/j.jmig.2013.02.012.
2. Vilos GA, Rajakumar C. Electrosurgical generators and monopolar and bipolar electrosurgery. J Minim Invasive Gynecol. 2013;20:279–87.
3. Ihnát P, Ihnát Rudinská L, Zonča P. Radiofrequency energy in surgery: state of the art. Surg Today. 2014;44(6):985–91. https://doi.org/10.1007/s00595-013-0630-5.
4. Pandey D, Yen CF, Lee CL, Wu MP. Electrosurgical technology: quintessence of the laparoscopic armamentarium. Gynecol Minim Invasive Ther [Internet]. 2014;3(3):63–6. https://doi.org/10.1016/j.gmit.2014.06.003.
5. Newcomb WL, Hope WW, Schmelzer TM, et al. Comparison of blood vessel sealing among new electrosurgical and ultrasonic devices. Surg Endosc. 2009;23:90–6.
6. Okhunov Z, Yoon R, Lusch A, et al. Evaluation and comparison of contemporary energy-based surgical vessel sealing devices. J Endourol. 2018;32(4):329–37. https://doi.org/10.1089/end.2017.0596.
7. Devassy R, Hanif S, Krentel H, Verhoeven HC, la Roche LAT, De Wilde RL. Laparoscopic ultrasonic dissectors: technology update by a review of literature. Med Devices (Auckl). 2018;12:1–7. https://doi.org/10.2147/MDER.S113262.
8. Seehofer D, Mogl M, Boas-Knoop S, et al. Safety and efficacy of new integrated bipolar and ultrasonic scissors compared to conventional laparoscopic 5-mm sealing and cutting instruments. Surg Endosc. 2012;26(9):2541–9. https://doi.org/10.1007/s00464-012-2229-0.
9. Sutton C, Abbott J. History of power sources in endoscopic surgery. J Minim Invasive Gynecol. 2013;20(3):271–8. https://doi.org/10.1016/j.jmig.2013.03.001.
10. Milsom J, Trencheva K, Monette S, et al. Evaluation of the safety, efficacy, and versatility of a new surgical energy device (THUNDERBEAT) in comparison with harmonic ACE, LigaSure V, and EnSeal devices in a porcine model. J Laparoendosc Adv Surg Tech A. 2012;22(4):378–86. https://doi.org/10.1089/lap.2011.0420.
11. Esposito C, Lima M, Mattioli G, et al. Complications of pediatric urological laparoscopy: mistakes and

risks. J Urol. 2003;169(4):1490–2. https://doi.org/10.1097/01.ju.0000055256.43528.f6.
12. Esposito C, Escolino M, Corcione F, et al. Twenty-year experience with laparoscopic and retroperitoneoscopic nephrectomy in children: considerations and details of technique. Surg Endosc. 2016;30(5):2114–8. https://doi.org/10.1007/s00464-015-4472-7.
13. Metzelder ML, Kübler JF, Nustede R, Ure BM. LigaSure in laparoscopic transperitoneal heminephroureterectomy in children: a comparative study. J Laparoendosc Adv Surg Tech A. 2006;16(5):522–5. https://doi.org/10.1089/lap.2006.16.522.
14. Metzelder ML, Kübler J, Petersen C, Glüer S, Nustede R, Ure BM. Laparoscopic nephroureterectomy in children: a prospective study on Ligasure versus clip/ligation. Eur J Pediatr Surg. 2006;16(4):241–4. https://doi.org/10.1055/s-2006-924375.
15. Dingemann C, Petersen C, Kuebler JF, Ure BM, Lacher M. Laparoscopic transperitoneal heminephrectomy for duplex kidney in infants and children: a comparative study. J Laparoendosc Adv Surg Tech A. 2013;23(10):889–93. https://doi.org/10.1089/lap.2013.0194.
16. Aydogdu I, Silay MS. Transperitoneal laparoscopic heminephroureterectomy in pediatric population: a single-Centre experience using a sealing device [published online ahead of print, 2018 may 14]. Can Urol Assoc J. 2018;12(9):E409–14. https://doi.org/10.5489/cuaj.4992.
17. Wille AH, Tüllmann M, Roigas J, Loening SA, Deger S. Laparoscopic partial nephrectomy in renal cell cancer—results and reproducibility by different surgeons in a high volume laparoscopic center. Eur Urol. 2006;49(2):337–43. https://doi.org/10.1016/j.eururo.2005.11.016.
18. Phillips JM, Narula N, Deane LA, et al. Histological evaluation of cold versus hot cutting: clinical impact on margin status for laparoscopic partial nephrectomy. J Urol. 2008;180(6):2348–52. https://doi.org/10.1016/j.juro.2008.08.029.
19. Marte A, Sabatino MD, Borrelli M, et al. LigaSure vessel sealing system in laparoscopic Palomo varicocele ligation in children and adolescents. J Laparoendosc Adv Surg Tech A. 2007;17(2):272–5. https://doi.org/10.1089/lap.2006.0046.
20. Koyle MA, Oottamasathien S, Barqawi A, Rajimwale A, Furness PD 3rd. Laparoscopic Palomo varicocele ligation in children and adolescents: results of 103 cases. J Urol. 2004;172(4 Pt 2):1749–52. https://doi.org/10.1097/01.ju.0000138676.68054.67.

Endoscopic Suturing in Paediatric MIS Urology

9

Dariusz Patkowski

Learning Objectives
- To describe basic principles of perfect endoscopic suturing.
- To describe types of endoscopic knots and differences between them.
- To show a video with endoscopic suturing technique.
- To describe tips and tricks of endoscopic suturing.

The process of minimally invasive surgery techniques adaptation to paediatric urology was rather slow. The first procedures performed were mostly diagnostic shifting with time to operative one. With growing experience, more and more sophisticated operations were undertaken to broaden the spectrum of potential endoscopic procedures, mainly for reconstructive ones. Majority of the endoscopic procedures are mainly a kind of surgical resection that normally doesn't require advanced suturing as opposed to reconstructive surgeries involving advanced endoscopic suturing.

Suturing is one of the most difficult and challenging skills in endoscopic surgery. It requires a very good eye-hand coordination. There are many very experienced endoscopic surgeons doing great procedures that have no idea about the proper technique of endoscopic suturing as it is occasionally needed. When difficulties arise and it comes to suture placement, they struggle a lot with instruments, knots and tissue, making the procedure longer and risky, and finally they often decide to convert to open surgery. They try to follow their experience with knots-tying technique coming from open classical surgery. However, it usually doesn't work well in endoscopy.

Main reasons making endoscopic suturing particularly difficult are

- Restricted and small operative space, especially for newborns and infants.
- Precise needle positioning in needle holder with assistance of another instrument, not with surgeon's fingers.
- The control of needle movements in small space without touching and injuring surrounding structures.
- Fixed angle between instruments and target organ or tissue, impeding precise suture placement.
- Lack of direct tissue touch and feel.
- Two-dimensional picture and lack of operative field depth.
- Paradoxical instruments' movements.

D. Patkowski (✉)
Department of Paediatric Surgery and Urology, Wroclaw Medical University, Wroclaw, Poland
e-mail: dariusz.patkowski@umw.edu.pl

C. Esposito et al. (eds.), *Minimally Invasive Techniques in Pediatric Urology*,
https://doi.org/10.1007/978-3-030-99280-4_9

It is impossible to perform advanced endoscopic paediatric urology without proper knowledge about endoscopic suturing. There are many indications in paediatric urology for endoscopic suturing. The most frequent is placement ligatures around vessels (varicocelectomy, nephrectomy, ovariectomy). It is a good training option for residents, especially for varicocelectomy, instead of easy vessels clipping. Other indications are more demanding like pyeloplasty or ureter reimplantation or even more advanced reconstructive procedures.

A perfect endoscopic knot is the result of a small steps series. It is extremely imperative to repeat each step in the same way and order, with a continuous movement of instruments as slowly as possible to get the best result and reproducibility. It necessitates many hours of training on simulators to become an expert. As simulators are becoming available easier, more efficient training may be expected. More to say, endoscopic suturing requires very precise and advanced eye-to-hand coordination that it should begin any training in endoscopic surgery.

9.1 Techniques of Suturing

There are different techniques of making knots. It may be accomplished in extracorporeal and intracorporeal way and is compared in Table 9.1. It seems that intracorporeal suturing, apart from being more difficult, should be regarded as a standard for any endoscopic surgery.

Table 9.1 Comparison between extracorporeal and intracorporeal suturing techniques

	Extracorporeal	Intracorporeal
Precision	Low	High
Suture adjustment control	Low	High
Suture construction	Easier	Difficult
Thread length	Long, thread wasting	Short, economic
Construction time	Longer	Shorter
Risk of damage to very thin, delicate thread	High	Low

9.2 Suture Types

The proper selection of suture type is important from the endoscopic surgery viewpoint. A discussion about different suturing materials is beyond the scope of this chapter. Basically, it is a selection between a monofilament or braided thread, as both behave differently during endoscopic procedure. The main differences are showed in Table 9.2. It seems that braided thread is more practical for endoscopic surgery; however, for special indication, the monofilament should be considered (e.g., pyeloplasty).

Table 9.2 Thread types comparison

Type	Monofilament	Braided
Handling	Difficult	Easy
Memory	Yes	No
Sticking to tissue	No	Yes
Damage	Easy to be broken	Easy to be torn
Sliding	Easy	Less easy

9.3 Knots Types

There are different types of knots used in endoscopic surgery (Table 9.3). The elementary knot's role is to bring and keep tissue together. In author's opinion, the sliding knot is the most practical knot working in each situation. Using this knot, the surgeon can control the tension between tissues avoiding their disruption. If the tension seems to be high, one can stop tissue approximation and put another one or more sliding knots. The knots are closed gradually bringing the tissue's edges together. In this way, the traction force is distributed between sutures preventing tissue damage.

9.4 Instruments

The endoscopic suturing requires dissector, needle holder and scissors. Instead of dissector, one can use another needle holder or delicate fenes-

Table 9.3 Comparison between different types of knots

Name	Surgical knot	Square knot	Sliding knot
Structure	First double knot and second single opposite one	Two single opposite knots	Square knot converted into sliding and back to square one
Tension between tissue	Moderate	Small	The highest to withstand by tissue
Action	Must be closed with the first knot	Must be closed with the first knot, a risk to self-opening with tissue tension	Adjustable, possible several knots to place and to close step by step decreasing tissue tension

trated grasper. Available needle holders may be straight or angled right or left. Angled needle holders are more versatile and make handling the needle at appropriate plane against tissue easier. Some needle holders are designed to a special needle's size that is very important to bear in mind to avoid needle holder's damage.

9.5 Needle Delivery and Extraction

Depending on needle's size, it may be delivered inside through a trocar or abdominal wall. However, if a patient is obese, it may be difficult. In such a case, the needle should be straightened to accommodate trocar diameter.

9.6 Handling a Needle

A needle position in a needle holder's jaws is crucial for a perfect tissue piercing and a later construction of a perfect suture. It is frequently an underestimated part of endoscopic suturing. In open surgery, the surgeon adjusts the needle position with the aid of his fingers. In endoscopic surgery the instrument replaces his fingers, making it difficult and problematic. There are two main steps to achieve proper needle position in needle holder:

9.6.1 First Step: Needle Grasping

The needle is grasped with instrument by dominant surgeon's hand at the region between the half to second/third distance from the needle's edge. The needle arch should be grasped with the very tip of needle holder's jaws. If the needle is gripped deeply in the jaws, then jaw's tips will touch and move the surrounding structures in small operative space, making correct and precise tissue piercing difficult.

9.6.2 Second Step: Correcting Needle's Position

The needle's position is corrected separately in vertical and horizontal plane. The needle is kept with the needle holder by dominant hand. To correct the vertical position, the needle is turned left or right with the aid of second instrument while kept horizontally. To correct the horizontal position the needle's shaft kept by the needle holder is set upright and then the process is repeated by turning needle left or right to desirable position.

9.7 Making a Knot

The concept of making a knot is based on the shape of letter "C" both real or reversed as seen on the picture. One end of "C"-shape formed thread comes out from the tissue and the other one from the needle holder's jaws. The free second instrument is placed into the "C" shape part of thread from above. Depending on the knot type (single or double) one or two loops are created around the free instrument. Next, the thread end is grasped and is dragged out through one or two formed loops. The process is repeated in the opposite direction using the shape of reversed "C." The formed square knot before closing may be converted into the sliding one by pulling apart inner and outer line of knot on the same side. Such a sliding knot allows to bring the tissue edges step-by-step together, controlling the tension between them.

Tips and Tricks

- Always use the same suturing technique and repeat each step in the same way and order.
- Any modification of the suturing technique should be reserved for special intraoperative situation and for very experienced endoscopic surgeons.
- Always keep the instruments' tips inside the operative view, avoiding any movements without eye's control and vision.
- Always work using both hands; however, move one instrument at a time unless you have enough experience in endoscopic surgery.
- Move the instruments as slowly as possible like in "a slow-motion film." It makes the surgery faster, resulting in perfect motion and by avoiding ineffective, repeated and bad movements.
- The excessive thread's length is not a problem if you keep it out of operative field dragging it out through the tissue from one side of the operative field to the opposite end.
- Continuous training on simulator is the best way to achieve proficiency and automated manoeuvres in endoscopic suturing.

Pediatric Anesthesia in MIS Urology

10

Giuseppe Cortese, Costanza Tognon, Rosario Sara, and Giuseppe Servillo

Learning Objectives
- To define the systemic alterations of pneumoperitoneum.
- To present a perioperative management for minimally invasive urology surgery.
- To describe adequate administration of systemic complications during this surgery.

10.1 Introduction

The use of laparoscopic and robotic surgery in pediatric population has been rapidly increasing over the last 15–20 years, and has become a standard of care for many of the operations involving the thoracic and abdominal cavities like some urological surgical procedure [1].

The anesthesiology management of the pediatric patient in this operative setting is a new challenge for the anesthesiologist: though laparoscopic and robotic surgery don't have same concerns about anesthesia as open abdominal surgery, they usually introduce different ones, including physiologic effects of the pneumoperitoneum, absorption of CO_2, and positioning required for surgery (it has to be noticed, in fact, that some laparoscopic procedures can take longer than the open alternative). Moreover, although laparoscopy in children and adolescents seems to be similar to the one in adults, experience in adult surgery does not directly translate into safe surgery in younger patients. Pediatric procedures must be performed with a full understanding of the relevant anatomic and physiopathological variation during MIUS.

Laparoscopy requires the insufflation of a gas (CO_2) that is rapidly absorbed across the peritoneum and increases total body CO_2 content, determining changes in many physiological parameters. Carbon dioxide is an incombustible and high soluble gas that potentially produces excessive absorption, subcutaneous emphysema, intravascular embolization, pneumothorax or pneumomediastinum. Adequate surgical management of surgical access and gas pressure in association with anesthesiology strategies are able to reduce complications.

Indeed, minimally invasive surgery (MIS) does not mean minimally invasive anesthesia.

The application of minimally invasive technologies to urologic procedures in children

G. Cortese (✉) · R. Sara · G. Servillo
Department of Nephrology, Urology, General Surgery, Kidney's Transplantation, Anesthesia and Intensive Care – A.O, University of Naples "Federico II", Naples, Italy
e-mail: giuseppe.servillo@unina.it

C. Tognon
Department of Woman and Child's Health, University Hospital of Padua, Padua, Italy
e-mail: costanza.tognon@aopd.veneto.it

C. Esposito et al. (eds.), *Minimally Invasive Techniques in Pediatric Urology*,
https://doi.org/10.1007/978-3-030-99280-4_10

includes both upper and lower urinary tract procedures as complete nephrectomy, partial nephrectomy, pyeloplasty, ureterocalicostomy, ureteroureterostomy, anti-reflux surgery, creation of continent catheterizable channels, and augmentation cystoplasty [2].

MIUS often requires distension of the peritoneal cavity (except in a retroperitoneal approach), usually obtained by insufflation of CO_2: it can be performed blindly using a Verres needle or placing a port under direct vision through a small subumbilical incision. In infants and young children, insufflation pressures of 4–12 mmHg are typically sufficing to visualize intraperitoneal structures and create operating space as the prepubertal abdominal wall is more pliable and the peritoneal cavity is smaller than in adults. The insertion of the laparoscope, after the expansion of the abdominal wall, grants the surgeon the capability to easily observe intra-abdominal space, to place instruments ports and to perform the procedure. A robotic system occupies a lot of space in the operating room and is made by a surgeon's control console (remote from the patient), a stand for the optical system, and patient-side cart with robotic arms. After having created the pneumoperitoneum, the surgeon can place ports for the camera and robotic arms, then controls them from the console. An assistant is at the patient's side for suctioning, retraction, and passage of suture or sponges in and out of the abdomen.

10.2 Preoperative Evaluation

Any pediatric patient to be subjected to anesthesia is different and requires an individual assessment and management. The spectrum of patients is broad and ranges from healthy children in election operative setting to newborn with many systemic diseases for emergency surgery. The principle of management is similar, in the major part, to anesthesia in open surgery.

Anesthesiological evaluation should not be made on the day of surgery, but in a period of time to permit request for any exams and adequate time required for informed consent [3].

Complete physical examination and pathological anamnesis should be carried out to identify contraindication to laparoscopy, in particular, heart disease or pulmonary dysfunction. The hydration status, pharmacological therapy, and allergies should be registered. A primary target in this stage is the evaluation of comorbidities that may impact the ability to tolerate surgery. In anticipation of laparoscopy, preoperative evaluation has to be focused on those medical conditions that may affect the response to physiological changes associated with laparoscopy and surgical procedure.

Indeed, congenital abnormalities of the genitourinary tract, often treated with MIS, may be associated, for example, with heart malformations and can be easily used as a signal for the diagnosis of congenital heart disease. Insufflation of abdomen may pose an important risk in patients sensitive to decrease of ventricular preload. Management of these patients requires preoperative consultation with a pediatric cardiologist and intraoperative care by an anesthesiologist experienced in such conditions. Moreover, in a congenital malformation scenario, it's important to seek abnormalities in central nervous system, respiratory tract, and airways.

The need for laboratory investigation depends on the general status of the patient. The validity of laboratory exams is six months unless clinic or drugs news in the child's anamnesis. Blood tests necessary to submit a pediatric patient to anesthesia are specified in Table 10.1. A preoperative ECG is recommended. Thorax radiography is not recommended routinely.

The preoperative assessment must be completed by an adequate airway examination which must allow an appropriate decision on the airway management algorithm. The small diameter of the infant's airway explains many of the problems that might occur during orotracheal intubation or other techniques: the narrow superior airway is the principal factor in the choice of the tracheal intubation technique; from this choice depends the quality of child ventilation and the risk of postoperative pulmonary complications because the functional residual capacity is less than the adult and atelectasis ensues. A displace-

Table 10.1 Blood tests and exams recommended

Exams	Conditions
Electrolytes, hematocrit, hemoglobin, transaminase, glucose serum, cells blood count, creatinine, white blood cells count	Common use (not mandatory)
Coagulation panel (partial thromboplastin time, prothrombin time, INR), platelet count and blood group	Potential hemorrhagic surgery, anamnesis positive to coagulation problem
Pregnancy test	Female patients in fertile period
ECG	From birth to 6-month-old patients
Thorax radiography	Risk of bronco pulmonary dysplasia (BPD)
ECG + cardio examination	Risk of BPD, heart murmur, or obstructive sleep apnea (OSAS)

Table 10.2 Appropriate intake of food and liquids before anesthesia

Ingested material	Minimum fasting period, hours
Clear liquids: water, fruit juice without pulp, clear tea, black coffee	2
Breast milk	4
Nonhuman milk	6
Light meal (toast and clear liquids	6

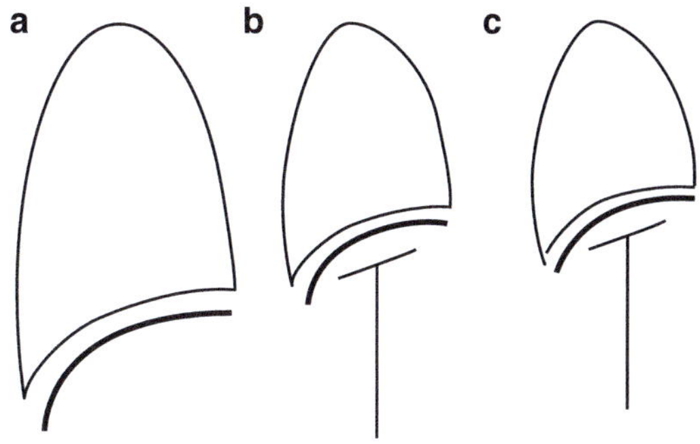

Fig. 10.1 Pneumoperitoneum causes a cephalic shift of the diaphragm, which reduces lung volumes, increases airway pressure and promotes atelectasis: these changes lead to deterioration of respiratory mechanics and gas exchange. (**a**) Normal; (**b**) pneumoperitoneum; (**c**) pneumoperitoneum plus Trendelenburg [15]

ment of the tracheal tube can occur during the change of the decubitus position or during surgery, because the infant's airway is very short. The tracheal and bronchial mucosa might suffer damage during intubation and a small lumen is easily obstructed by blood or secretions.

Recommendations for fasting are the same used in adults, with the addition of guidelines for breast milk and infant formula intake [4] (Table 10.2). Sometimes a bowel preparation is suggested to optimize the working space during laparoscopy [5].

The anesthesiologist should be very clear and exhaustive in providing information. Although some surgeons might minimize the procedure ("only three small holes"), parents must know that, along with the benefits, there are also some risks, whose frequency and severity must be explained. Minimally invasive surgery does not mean minimal risk [6].

10.3 Physiological Effect of Laparoscopy

10.3.1 Respiratory System

The pneumoperitoneum associated to the pushing up of the abdominal content (often in the Trendelenburg position) determinates a cephalad shift of the diaphragm (Fig. 10.1). The total thoracic compliance and functional residual capacity (FRC) decreases and raises airways resistance (Table 10.3).

A decrease in arterial oxygenation has been reported in adult population under gynecological surgery. The reduction of FRC and atelectasis may produce a ventilation/perfusion mismatch with hypoxemia [7]. End-tidal CO_2 can be increased from baseline value of 33–42 mmHg during surgery if the ventilator settings were not adjusted [8]. It is necessary to increase over the 30–60% ventilator rate to restore end-tidal CO_2 to baseline level. Greater than 90% of infants required at least one intervention in ventilator pattern to restore tidal volume and end-tidal CO_2 [9].

However, the respiratory changes rarely have a bad effect on the postoperative respiratory functional outcome. Respiratory acidosis may occur only in case of poor preoperative respiratory function or if residual drugs depress pulmonary drive.

Table 10.3 Respiratory system changes during laparoscopy

Parameters	Changes	Causes
FRC	Decrease	Displacement of diaphragm, positioning
PO2	Decrease	Atelectasis, preoperative respiratory function, vasoconstriction hypoxia induced
Lung compliance	Decrease	Elevation of diaphragm, intra-abdominal pressure increased
PCO_2	Increase	CO_2 absorption

Table 10.4 Cardiovascular system changes during laparoscopy

Parameters	Changes	Causes
SVR MAP	Increase	Hypercapnia, neuroendocrine response
Cardiac rhythm	Brady or tachyarrhythmia	Peritoneal stretch, vagal reflex, hypoxia, hypercapnia
Cardiac index	Decrease or stable	Increase in afterload, decrease in venous return, positioning, decrease in cardiac filling

10.3.2 Cardiovascular System

Cardiovascular changes are the result of the effect of pneumoperitoneum, the absorption of carbon dioxide and the blood volume shift by positioning.

Several studies have evaluated cardiovascular changes using echocardiography during laparoscopic surgery. The cardiac index decreases by 13% when intra-abdominal pressure value reaches 12 mmHg [10]. Authors have studied an increase in mean arterial pressure (MAP), vascular resistance (SVR) and central venous pressure (CVP) with the decrease of stroke volume (SV) [11] (Table 10.4).

The increase of IAP induces neuroendocrine response, with spread of catecholamine and the activation of angiotensin system. The result is an increase of MAP and SVR.

10.3.3 Additional Systemic Effects

Plasma renin and aldosterone increase over baseline values and these changes are similar to the ones in open surgery. Decreased renal plasma flow, glomerular filtration pressure may produce a reduction of urine output. These alterations in a healthy patient are well compensated. Permanent renal impairment is not evidenced [12].

Exposure of the peritoneal cavity to a large volume of cold and not humidified CO_2 may contribute to the development of hypothermia. Hypothermia with impact on the cardiovascular system and the coagulation pattern remains a possibility during long time surgery and especially in neonates.

Recent study has detected that, in pediatric population under laparoscopic surgery, cerebral blood flow and intracranial pressure (ICP) may be increased [13].

CO_2 reacts with peritoneal fluid, reduces peritoneal pH, and creates an acid environment to limit the inflammatory response. The level of intra-abdominal pressure and the type of gas chosen produce different degrees of inflammation. Low pressure CO_2 causes minor changes in peritoneum differently from high pressure and air insufflation. The amendments concern a greater number of inflammatory cells represented by eosinophils, mastocytes, and lymphocytes, but no clinical modifications were detected.

MIUS involves a faster postoperative rehabilitation that includes a rapid recovery of bowel function, a rapid removal of devices, rapid mobilization and pain relief [14].

10.4 Anesthesia Management

There is no dedicated anesthetic strategy to MIS in pediatric patients: the induction and maintenance are in line with the standard pediatric anesthesia. A flow chart summarizing the anesthetic management is provided (Fig. 10.2).

Even before premedicating, the anesthesiologist, according to standard American Society of Anesthesiologists (ASA), must make sure that: adequate 02 supply and ventilator are checked;

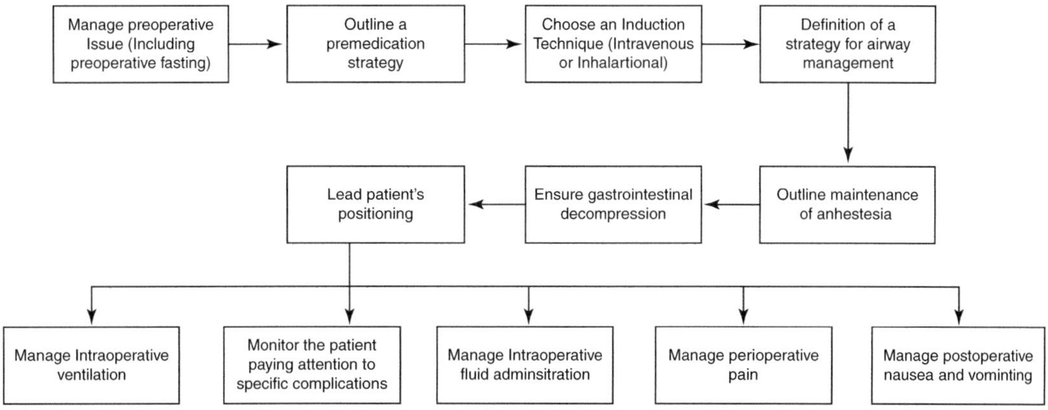

Fig. 10.2 A flow chart summarizing the anesthesiologic management [22]

size appropriate airway equipment (facial masks, laryngoscope blades, endotracheal and rhinotracheal tubes, stylet, any devices for difficult airways management) are present; all the basic drugs needed to support any phases of anesthesia have been prepared; pulse oximeter, ECG, noninvasive pressure, capnography, and stethoscope are present and functioning, defibrillator has been periodically checked and there are special equipment and drugs for the singular particular case.

However, capnography does not consistently reflect $PaCO_2$, especially in infants, because the respiratory rate is usually faster and the arterial to end tidal (a-et) CO_2 gradient is variable [15].

10.5 Premedication

Premedication of anesthesia in children presenting for MIUS should not be different from other types of surgery. Since the surgery robotic room is often distant from the ward (being a multidisciplinary room), the premedication must be done in condition of extreme control and safety. The choice depends on the anxiety level and physical global status. Commonly, midazolam 0.5 mg/kg orally half an hour before induction is a good choice. Midazolam rectally (0.5 mg/kg) or sublingually (0.3 mg/kg) or nasally (0.3 mg/kg) are alternative valid choices. A good alternative to midazolam in younger children, 8–20 kg, over 6 months, is the administration of clonidine, 4 mcg/kg. Atropine or glycopyrrolate may be included in premedication to prevent the reflex bradycardia induced by abdominal insufflation and to dry secretions.

At least one venous catheter must be placed; an additional device that is useful in case blood loss is expected. It is preferable to position the venous access above the diaphragm, as the pneumoperitoneum may limit the entry of fluid and drugs into the central circulation. Eutectic mixture of local anesthetics (EMLA) should be applied before positioning the intravenous access to reduce pain.

10.6 Anesthesia

Induction may be intravenous or inhalational: the choice largely depends on the ability of the child to tolerate placement of an IV catheter. In the clinical practice, this usually means that an inhalational induction should be preferred for children in pre-scholar age, and an IV induction for older ones. However, the decision has to be always individualized, based upon the child's anxiety level. When compared with inhalational agents, IV induction agents are able to achieve more rapidly a level of anesthesia deep enough for airway instrumentation. Among these, propofol is the agent of choice as it provides rapid onset and short duration of action, reduces the bronchospastic response to intubation, and has antiemetic effects. When inhalational induction is chosen, most potent inhalational agents have the advantage of decreasing airway responsiveness: sevoflurane is generally preferred for induction because it is the least pungent compared to isoflurane and desflurane. Desflurane is not generally used for inhalational induction because it is an extremely pungent volatile anesthetic that can produce an increase in secretions, coughing, airway resistance, and laryngospasm.

After induction, an orogastric tube should be placed to decompress the stomach and the gut, allowing minimizing of stomach injury and increasing intra-abdominal visibility.

In relation to airway management for pediatric laparoscopy, endotracheal intubation is often preferred rather than a supraglottic airway (SGA): it provides optimal control of ventilation for elimination of CO_2 and protection against aspiration. It is also true that some authors show that the ventilator efficacy of Proseal™ laryngeal mask is comparable to ventilation through endotracheal tube [16].

A protocol of rapid sequence induction must be considered in children with high risk for regurgitation and pulmonary aspiration. H2-receptor antagonists such as ranitidine must be administered to these patients.

Standard practice in pediatric anesthesia includes the use of an uncuffed endotracheal tube (ETT) if the child is younger than 8 years age: this can make it difficult to maintain minute ventilation during the laparoscopy. The use of a cuffed ETT instead can allow the use of positive end expiratory pressure (PEEP) and high peak pressure along the airways during pneumoperitoneum. This far, ETT intubation with minimum cuff inflation can limit difficulties with ventilation.

The use of SGAs for laparoscopy is controversial, and it has been used safely for short procedures. Maintenance of general anesthesia during laparoscopy may be based on inhalational or intravenous agents, as it's usually done for open abdominal procedures.

The anesthetic is supplemented with intravenous opioids (e.g., Fentanyl or remifentanil), if needed.

The use of nitrous oxide (N_2O) is controversial: concerns with regard to an increase in postoperative nausea and vomiting and bowel distention, N_2O diffuses into air containing closed spaces over time and can lead to bowel distention, being able to increase the technical difficulty of surgical maneuvers. Moreover, it could have deleterious metabolic and neurotoxic effects in pediatric populations [17].

Neuromuscular blocking agents are often administered during surgery to facilitate endotracheal intubation and to improve surgical conditions, but the literature about optimal level of neuromuscular blockade during laparoscopic surgery is inconsistent and the need of neuromuscular blockade may depend on the surgical procedure.

Most of cases require controlled ventilation: as modern ventilators make it possible to have small tidal volumes delivered smoothly, a lung-protective and volume-targeted ventilation can be assured to pediatric patients. In fact, even if pediatric surgical data about ventilation outcome are missing now, lung-protective ventilation cannot be less than beneficial for sure, as it's been observed in adults. The strategy uses a target tidal volume in a range of 6–7 ml/kg, predicting use of PEEP to prevent atelectasis and, in case, recruitment maneuvers to revert it.

Implementing such a strategy safely and effectively requires selecting the ventilation mode and monitoring the interaction between the ventilator and the patient to optimize the ventilator settings. Notwithstanding this theory is clear, applying it tends to be challenging because of the difficulty to have exact bodyweight and optimal PEEP level in a pediatric patient: in this case, bedside monitors are a priority need in order to let the operator choose the optimal ventilation strategy, adjust with a real time approach gas exchange, and also ventilator parameters (Fig. 10.3). Goals to achieve in this case are:

- Optimal arterial oxygen tension at the least inspired oxygen concentration.
- Acceptable arterial CO_2 tension.
- Delivered tidal volumes at the least inspiratory pressure.

Another factor to be looked at because of its postoperative outcomes is the fluid management.

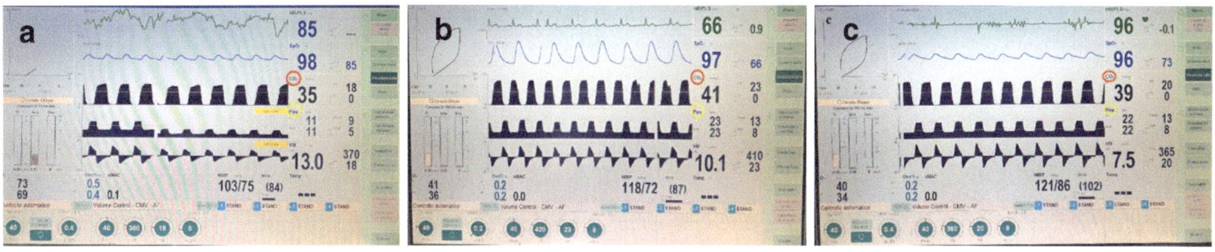

Fig. 10.3 Changes in ventilator outcomes during minimally invasive uro-surgery (MIUS). Image (**a**) shows the setting of ventilation at T_0 with the values of $etCO_2$ (red circle) and the airway pressures (P_{peak} and P_{plat}, yellow circle). Image (**b**) shows the changes on $etCO_2$ and airway pressures following laparoscopic gas insufflation with the same ventilator setting. Image (**c**) shows the changes in the ventilatory setting necessary to bring $etCO_2$ back into a suitable range

Perioperative fluid requirements, in fact, depend upon multiple factors such as preoperative volume status, perioperative conditions, patient's age, anesthetic management, and nature of the interventions (laparoscopic procedures are associated with less insensible fluid losses than open ones). First goal in fluid therapy is to maintain standard volemia: it's done by applying fixed volume algorithms to administer substantial amounts of fluid even if, as it's being observed, it can be easily obtained a decreasing of perioperative morbidity and then mortality by restricting intraoperative fluid administration. This is true both in adult and pediatric patients.

Laparoscopy has been identified as a risk factor for PONV, therefore routine prophylactic multimodal antiemetic therapy should be utilized in all patients undergoing laparoscopic\robotic surgery.

Postoperative pain after laparoscopic and robotic surgery is usually less than the corresponding open procedure, but the degree of pain depends on how the specific surgery has been performed. Pain after laparoscopy can often be managed effectively with acetaminophen, nonsteroidal anti-inflammatory drugs, dexamethasone, and opioids. Moreover, it could be useful to infiltrate the incision with local anesthetic at the time of wound closure.

The position of the patient during surgery may be quite extreme, therefore areas prone to pressure injury should be protected with specific padding.

Each patient must be heated sufficiently (liquids, ambient, devices), remembering that the newborn produces maximum heat loss from the head and trunk.

10.7 Postoperative Pain, Nausea, and Vomiting

Postoperative pain is the result of ports insertion in the abdominal wall, irritation of phrenic nerve and distention of peritoneum; its intensity may persist for 24 h. The multimodal regimen of local anesthetic infiltration of incision sites, locoregional analgesia, opioids, NSAIDS, and paracetamol reduces the incidence of substantial pain.

An example of this approach is the postoperative administration of intravenous fentanyl (1–2 γ/kg), iv paracetamol (15 mg/kg), iv morphine (0.1–0.2 mg/kg) and iv ketorolac (0.5 mg/kg)/ketoprofene (1–1.5 mg/kg). The paracetamol, intravenous or orally administered at regular intervals, is the choice drug for postoperative pain treatment. A rescue drug, excluding fentanyl and morphine, is tramadol (1/2 mg/kg when needed, three times a day).

A promising approach to the provision of postoperative analgesia after abdominal surgery is to block the sensory nerve supply to the anterior abdominal wall by placing a local anesthetic in the transversus abdominis plane (TAP).

There has been a growing interest in ultrasound-guided transversus abdominis plane (TAP) block as an alternative and valid postoperative analgesic method in pediatric patients undergoing lower abdominal surgery.

The TAP block was first described by McDonnell et al. in 2004 [18]. Ultrasonography-guided TAP block provides excellent pain relief in lower abdominal surgeries.

This regional anesthetic technique that blocks neural afferents of the anterolateral abdominal wall provides superior and long-lasting analgesia without the risk of respiratory depression of intravenous opioids.

A recent research concluded that the pain scores were considerably lower in the TAP block when compared with the local infiltration group in the initial 2 h and this technique reduces the intraoperative requirement of further anesthetic drugs, as evidenced by decreased hemodynamic response during surgical maneuvers.

Laparoscopy has been identified as a risk factor of postoperative nausea and vomiting (PONV), therefore routine prophylactic antiemetic therapy should be administered. Dexamethasone is superior to ondansetron in preventing postoperative nausea after 4–6 h of laparoscopic surgeries. However, both drugs are of equal efficacy in preventing postoperative vomiting up to 24 h after surgery [19].

10.8 Complications

Both adult and pediatric procedures share similar complications, including those related to the physiologic effects of the laparoscopic approach (e.g., hemodynamic and respiratory decompensation, gas embolism), surgical maneuvers (vascular or solid organ injuries), and patient positioning.

It's necessary for the anesthesiologist to be aware of potential problems and be ready for a quick approach to them.

The management of the complications (hypotension, hypertension, and arrhythmias) includes confirmation that IAP must be kept within definite limits of pressure, when all of treatable causes are excluded or resolved by the right supportive therapies (e.g., reduction or variation in the use of intraoperative anesthetics, fluid administration, pharmacologic interventions).

It may even be necessary to deflate the abdomen if therapies are not effective and, eventually, to migrate to an open procedure in agreement with the surgeon. Hypercarbia or hypoxia could be, instead, signs of respiratory failure related to the physiologic effects of the technique or to a surgical injury (e.g., Diaphragm injury).

Hypercapnia is handled with the increase of ventilation aiming to compensate for CO_2 absorption.

Hypoxia can occur as a result of reduction in FRC and atelectasis caused by pneumoperitoneum and surgical positioning, or because of different reasons occurring during any anesthetic procedure. First, the chest should be auscultated to rule out a selective intubation or a bronchospasm, then the initial treatment should include an increase of inspired oxygen concentration and, unless the patient is hypotensive, both recruitment maneuver and PEEP optimizing should be performed. If refractory hypoxemia occurs, pneumoperitoneum must be desufflated; CO_2 insufflation may also determine subcutaneous emphysema, capnothorax, capnomediastinum, capnopericardium, and gas embolism.

Subcutaneous emphysema, in most cases, tends to resolve without specific interventions just after the abdomen has been deflated. CO_2 absorption, in case of significant subcutaneous emphysema, may continue for several hours after surgery, but healthy patients are able to increase ventilation to eliminate CO_2: only patients with respiratory or cardiovascular problems should be observed in the post-anesthesia care unit until they resolve. Capnothorax, capnomediastinum, and capnopericardium, although rare, may be life-threatening because they can be associated with severe hemodynamic compromise. They should be a matter of suspicion in case of an unexplained increase of airway pressure, hypoxemia, and hypercapnia with subcutaneous emphysema of head and neck or inequality of chest expansion. Reduction of insufflation pressure, increase in PEEP, and hyperventilation are often sufficient to manage these syndromes.

Normally, venous gas embolism is common during laparoscopy, but it is almost always subclinical and it does not impair the patient's health status. Rarely, carbon dioxide embolism into artery or large vein may be a potentially fatal complication [20]. Clinical presentation is characterized by cardiovascular collapse (sudden drop in End-tidal CO_2, collapse of oxygen saturation, fall in blood pressure, and different arrhythmias) and variations of blood gas analysis, which can lead even to death, depending on the scale of the embolus. The aspiration of air through the central vein catheter, if it has been positioned, the Durant's position placement and cardio pulmonary resuscitation with 100% oxygen ventilation represent correct life-saving maneuvers. In case of suspected embolism, the abdomen should be deflated, ventilation and fraction-inspired oxygen increased to reduce dimensions of CO_2 bubbles, and then supportive therapies with fluids and vasopressors administration may be helpful.

Vascular, bowel, or bladder injury appears to be serious complications too: a survey of major complications of pediatric urological laparoscopy reported a rate of 1.2% [21]. These occur mostly during initial entry or subsequent placement of trocars into the abdomen, as it usually happens in adult laparoscopy. Bleeding may be less obvious during laparoscopy than during open procedures. The view of the surgical field, in fact, is limited, and blood can pool away from the surgical field when patients are in head-up or head-down position. Signs of hypovolemia (e.g., hypotension, tachycardia) should be suggesting occult bleeding, and needs to be brought to the surgeon's attention.

Positioning is generally similar for pediatric and adult populations: care should be mostly taken to cushion pressure points on the arms, wrist, and hand in order to avoid inadvertent nerve injury during the procedure. Indeed, the use of the memory mattress is the best choice to avoid this kind of injury.

10.9 Discussion

Minimally invasive uro-surgery can be an advantage in terms of speed, postoperative recovery time, better pain control, and approval of the patient.

However, it is clear that anesthesia associated with the changes brought about by the pneumoperitoneum may be an issue, if not properly handled.

It is therefore necessary to continue cooperation, research, and comparison between surgeons and anesthesiologists to ensure the best standard of care for the pediatric patient.

In recent years, in the adult population, some laparoscopic surgeries are being performed by the use of epidural or spinal anesthesia with excellent results. In the future, it is hoped that MIUS anesthesia management qualifies for an international scientific validation, backed by a growing quantity of RCTs.

Take-Home Points

- Before starting to manage pediatric anesthesia in an MIUS, it is mandatory to have the knowledge of the systemic changes of patient during surgery (pneumoperitoneum).
- An adequate preoperative assessment is critical for an anesthesiologic strategy to reduce the risks of the intervention.
- A multimodal approach to postoperative pain, nausea, and vomiting is nowadays mandatory.

References

1. Mattei P. Minimally invasive surgery in the diagnosis and treatment of abdominal pain in children. Curr Opin Pediatr. 2007;19:338–43.
2. Traxel EJ, Minevich EA, Noh PH. A review: the application of minimally invasive surgery to pediatric urology: upper urinary tract procedures. Urology. 2010;76:122–3.
3. Astuto M, Baroncini S, Borrometi F, Bortone L, Ceschin C, et al. Raccomandazioni per la valutazione

anestesiologica e la richiesta di esami preoperatori nei pazienti pediatrici. Gruppo di studio SARNePI.
4. Brady M, Kinn S, Ness V, et al. Preoperative fasting for preventing perioperative complications in children. Cochrane Database Syst Rev. 2009;(4):CD005285.
5. Rosenbaum A, Kain ZN, Larsson P, et al. The place of premedication in pediatric practice. Paediatr Anaesth. 2009;19:817–28.
6. Mukhtar AM, Obayah GM, Elmasry A, Dessouky NM. The therapeutic potential of intraoperative hypercapnia during video assisted thoracoscopy in pediatric patients. Anesth Analg. 2008;106:84–8.
7. Kalmar AF, Foubert L, Hendrickx JF, et al. Influence of steep trendelenburg position and CO_2 pneumoperitoneum on cardiovascular, cerebrovascular, and respiratory homeostasis during robotic prostatectomy. Br J Anaesth. 2010;104:433–9.
8. Manner T, Aantaa R, Alanen M. Lung compliance during laparoscopic surgery pediatric patients. Paediatr Anaesth. 1998;8(1):25–9.
9. Bannister CF, Brosius KK, Wulkan M. The effect of insufflation pressure on pulmonary mechanics in infants during laparoscopic surgical procedures. Pediatr Anaesth. 2003;13(9):785–9.
10. Sakka SG, Huettemann E, Petrat G, Meier-Hellmann A, Schier F, Reinhart K. Transesophageal echocardiographic assessment of hemodynamic changes during laparoscopic herniorrhaphy in small children. Br J Anaesth. 2000;84(3):330–4.
11. Meininger D, Westphal K, Bremerich DH, et al. Effects of posture and prolonged pneumoperitoneum on hemodynamic parameters during laparoscopy. World J Surg. 2008;32:1400–5.
12. Joris J, Lamy M. Neuroendocrine changes during pneumo-peritoneum for laparoscopic cholecystectomy. Br J Anaesth. 1993;70(Suppl.):24–9.
13. Tuna AT, et al. Effect of carbon dioxide insufflation on regional cerebral oxygenation during laparoscopic surgery in children: a prospective study. Rev Bras Anestesiol. 2015;66(3):249–53.
14. Michelet D, Andreu-Gallien J, Skhiri A, Bonnard A, Nivoche Y, Dahmani S. Factors affecting recovery of postoperative bowel function after pediatric laparoscopic surgery. J Anaesthesiol Clin Pharmacol. 2016;32(3):369–75.
15. Spinelli G, Vargas M, Aprea G, Cortese G, Servillo G. Pediatric anesthesia for minimally invasive surgery in pediatric urology. Transl Pediatr. 2016;5(4):214–21.
16. Sinha A, Sharma B, Sood J. ProSeal as an alternative to endotracheal intubation in pediatric laparoscopy. Paediatr Anaesth. 2007;17(4):327–32.
17. Baum VC. When nitrous oxide is no laughing matter: nitrous oxide and pediatric anesthesia. Paediatr Anaesth. 2007;17:824–30.
18. McDonnell JG, O'Donnell BD, Tuite D, Farrell T, Power C. The regional abdominal field infiltration (R.a.F.I.) technique: computerized tomographic and anatomical identification of a novel approach to the transversus abdominis neurovascular fascial plane. Anesthesiology. 2004;1:899.
19. Maitra S, Som A, Baidya DK, et al. Comparison of Ondansetron and dexamethasone for prophylaxis of postoperative nausea and vomiting in patients undergoing laparoscopic surgeries: a meta-analysis of randomized controlled trials. Anesthesiol Res Pract. 2016;2016:7089454.
20. Tognon C, De Corti F, Michelon S, Gamba PG. Carbon dioxide embolism during laparoscopic lymph-node in a girl: a rare occurrence. J Pediatr Surg Case Rep. 2014;2:377–9.
21. Cortese G, Tognon C, Servillo G, Gamba P. Anesthesia in pediatric minimally invasive surgery. In: Esposito C, Becmeur F, Steyaert H, Szavay P, editors. ESPES manual of pediatric minimally invasive surgery. Berlin: Springer; 2019.

Part II

Kidney

Endourologic Retrograde Balloon Dilatation of the Primary Ureteropelvic Junction Obstruction in Children

11

José María Angulo, Javier Ordoñez, Alberto Parente, Laura Burgos, Laura Pérez-Egido, Beatriz Fernández-Bautista, and Rubén Ortiz

Learning Objectives

- To describe the endourologic technique for the UPJO dilatation with high-pressure balloon.
- To present the long-term outcomes of the ERBD.
- To describe the advantages of the ERBD compared with other minimally invasive options in the treatment of the UPJO.
- To show a video with the ERBD technique.
- To describe tips and tricks of the ERBD and some key points of the endourologic approach.

Supplementary Information The online version contains supplementary material available at [https://doi.org/10.1007/978-3-030-99280-4_11].

J. M. Angulo (✉) · J. Ordoñez L. Burgos
L. Pérez-Egido · B. Fernández-Bautista · R. Ortiz
Pediatric Urology, Gregorio Marañón University Hospital, Madrid, Spain
e-mail: josemaria.angulo@salud.madrid.org; javier.orodnez@salud.madrid.org; laura.burgos@salud.madrid.org; lpereze@salud.madrid.org; bfbautista@salud.madrid.org; ruben.ortiz@salud.madrid.org

A. Parente
Pediatric Urology, Gregorio Marañón University Hospital, Madrid, Spain

Pediatric Urology Department, Reina Sofía University Hospital, Cordoba, Spain
e-mail: alberto.parente.sspa@juntadeandalucia.es

11.1 Introduction

Open pyeloplasty is still considered the gold standard procedure for the treatment of the ureteropelvic junction obstruction (UPJO) (with a success rate of over 94%) [1], but recent publications report an increasing effectiveness of the minimally invasive approaches [2–4]. The advantages of these techniques (reduction of postoperative pain, length of hospital stay, better cosmesis, etc.), together with their effectiveness and safety, are making them considered as the first therapeutic option in many cases.

Endourologic balloon dilatation for the treatment of UPJO was first described in 1982 [5], but experience and outcomes in children are limited. Pediatric sized instruments and technical improvement in the last years are making the endourologic approach a safe and effective treatment, as it has been reported in other urological conditions (primary obstructive megaureter [6], secondary UPJO [7, 8], etc.). But its role in the primary

C. Esposito et al. (eds.), *Minimally Invasive Techniques in Pediatric Urology*,
https://doi.org/10.1007/978-3-030-99280-4_11

UPJO has been questioned due to discrepancy in the success rates and outcomes published.

In the present chapter, we describe our experience in the management of primary UPJO treated by endourologic retrograde balloon dilatation (ERBD). It is established as the first line of treatment in our institution, and it is performed using low-profile, high-pressure balloons (HPB). In case of presenting an incomplete resolution of the stenosis, the dilatation is completed using a peripheral cutting balloon microsurgical dilatation device (Cutting Balloon™, CB).

11.2 Preoperative Preparation

All patients with UPJO are followed up with periodic ultrasound scans, beginning in the second day of life (if prenatal diagnosis is presented). Under conservative surveillance with low-dose antibiotic prophylaxis, this study is then repeated at 1 month of life and then, every 3 months. This exploration is useful in the measurement of the anteroposterior pelvis diameter, calyces, and renal parenchyma thickness, and it is also performed in order to discard any other associated malformations. Mercaptoacetyltriglycine (MAG-3) renal scans with furosemide washout is always performed, revealing an obstructive pattern. Also, a micturating cystourethrogram is performed to rule out the presence of vesicoureteral reflux.

Preoperative antibiotic prophylaxis is administered, usually amoxicillin-clavulanic acid 30 mg/kg, or a specific antibiotic according to the patient's urine culture. Patients receive general anesthesia with laryngeal mask, and no vesical catheter or nasogastric tube is used.

11.3 Positioning

Intervention is performed with the patient in lithotomy position (Fig. 11.1). In case of small infants, the patient's perineum is brought to the edge of the table and a towel roll of appropriate size is located below the flexed knees. This position is secured using adhesive tapes. In case of older children, the position is secured using leg supports attached to the table. The surgeon and the assistant stand on the feet or between the legs of the patient. The cystoscopy monitor is placed on the right side of the table, and the fluoroscopy at the head. The fluoroscopy C-arm is introduced from the left side of the patient.

11.4 Instrumentation

The cystoscopy is performed with a 9.5 Fr cystoscope with a 5 Fr instrumentation channel. A 4 Fr ureteral catheter is placed in the affected ureter, and a retrograde pyelography is then performed using a radiopaque contrast agent (iopamidol). In order to tutorize up the ureter to the renal pelvis, a hydrophilic guidewire (0.014″ Choice PT™, J-tip, Boston Scientific; or 0.018″ Radiofocus® Terumo) is used; in case of difficulties, we choose

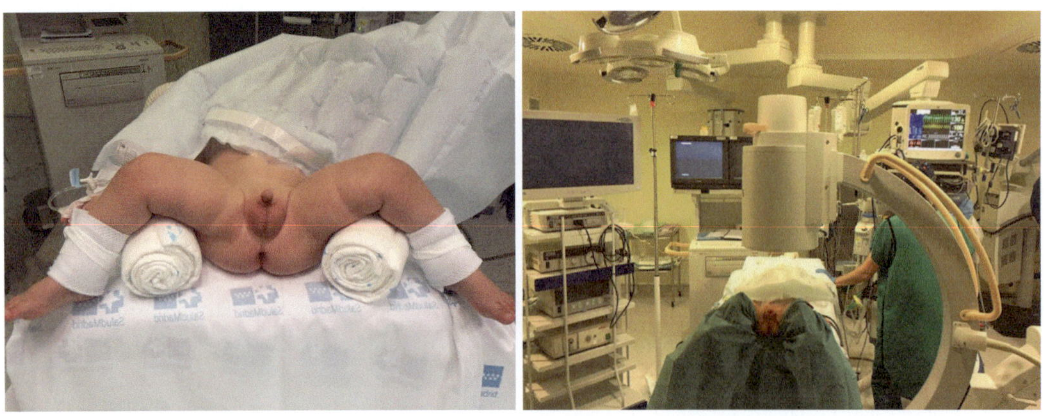

Fig. 11.1 Patient position

a 0.035″ hydrophilic guidewire, as it travels easier in the retrograde direction inside the ureteral lumen. The UPJ is dilatated with 3 Fr high-pressure, semi-compliant balloon catheters (HPB) (Fig. 11.2), with different nominal diameter (from 5 to 7 mm) according to the patient's weight (5 mm in patients <6 kg, 6 mm in 6–10 kg, and 7 mm in >10 kg) and 2 cm length (RX Muso™, Terumo). In case of being needed, a 2 cm length and a 3-, 4-, or 5-mm diameter Cutting Balloon™ (Boston Scientific, Natick, MA, USA) (Fig. 11.3) catheter is used (it combines the features of conventional balloon dilatation with advanced microsurgical capabilities). A double-J ureteral stent is always placed (3 Fr, 8–12 cm; Sof-Flex Multi-Length Ureteral Stents; CookMedical Europe™), and a transurethral bladder catheter (Foley catheter) is placed for 16–18 h after surgery.

11.5 Technique

The first step is to perform the cystoscopy and to introduce in the affected ureter a 4 Fr ureteral catheter. The retrograde pyelography is then performed. The ureter is tutorized up to the renal pelvis using a hydrophilic guidewire (0.014″ or 0.018″; in case of difficulties, a 0.035″ is preferred). Then, and under fluoroscopic guidance, the high-pressure balloon catheter is inserted over the guidewire and located in the UPJ. It is filled with radiologic contrast to its nominal pressure (14–16 atm) until the balloon notch or hourglass image disappears (Fig. 11.4). After successful dilatation procedure, a double-J ureteral stent is placed (3 Fr, 8–12 cm long) between renal pelvis and bladder. The transurethral bladder catheter is removed 16–18 h after surgery.

The Cutting Balloon™ (CB) catheter is reserved for those cases when the balloon notch or hourglass image of the high-pressure balloon does not completely disappear after 20 s at 16–18 atm. In those cases, a CB is inflated at the level of the UPJ to up to 12 atm. Dilatation is then completed using a HPB as described before, and double-J ureteral stents are always placed.

Double-J stents are removed 4–6 weeks after the dilatation procedure. In this intervention, the UPJ is assessed (calibration) in day-hospital regimen. This procedure consists of the inflation of a HPB at low pressure (6–8 atm) in the UPJ to check the absence of residual stenosis. If a residual stenosis is found in the fluoroscopy, a new dilatation is then performed using an HPB, placing a double-J with a 4/0 Prolene suture attached to its distal tip and exteriorized (transurethral). It is removed 1 week later in the outpatient clinic pulling out the suture. In the case of persistent stenosis despite HPB dilatation, and similar to the initial intervention, a CB dilatation is then performed, and the double-J stent is removed in the daycare center 4 weeks later.

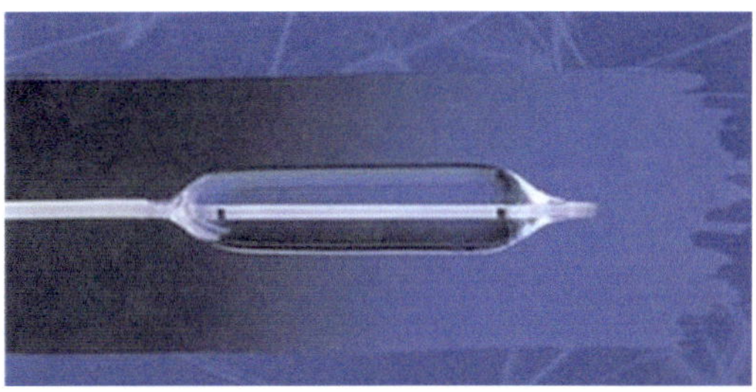

Fig. 11.2 High-pressure balloon. Balloon diameter: 5, 6, or 7 mm; balloon length: 2 cm

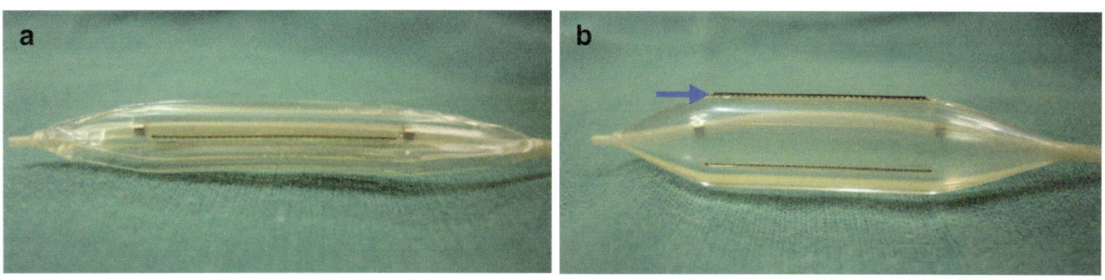

Fig. 11.3 Cutting-balloon. (**a**) Collapsed. (**b**) Filled with radiologic contrast. Arrow: Atherotomes (0.0127 cm tall microsurgical blades). Balloon diameter: 3, 4, or 5 mm; blade length: 6, 10, or 15 mm

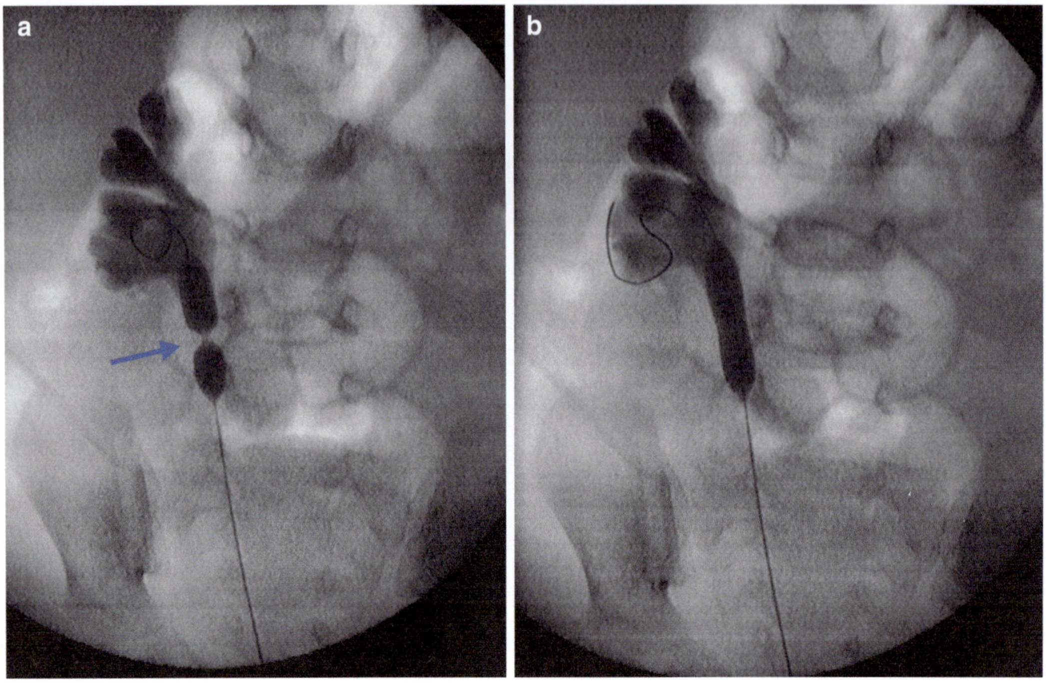

Fig. 11.4 UPJO dilatation under fluoroscopic guidance. (**a**) Inflation of the balloon (filled with fluoroscopic contrast) and location of the ureteropelvic junction obstruction (balloon notch, blue arrow). (**b**) Resolution of the narrowing after complete dilatation

11.6 Postoperative Control

Oral feeding is started as soon as the patient has recovered from the anesthetic procedure. For the initial intervention, analgesic requirements are limited to intravenous non-opioid drugs for less than 24 h, requiring no oral analgesics after discharge. The transurethral bladder catheter is removed 16–18 h after surgery, and the patient is discharged after spontaneous miction is observed. The "calibration" procedure is performed in day-hospital regimen.

After discharge, follow-up consists in regular clinical review and renal ultrasonography at 3, 6, and 12 postoperative months (thereafter, it is performed every 6 months). Anteroposterior renal pelvis diameter (APD, maximum pelvis diameter in a coronal view), pelvis/cortex ratio (relation between APD and minimum cortex thickness), and percentage of improvement of the APD are the main parameters used to predict the outcome. Postoperative MAG-3 diuretic renogram is performed only when a poor outcome is predicted at the six postoperative months attending to the ultrasonography parameters (when APD > 18.5 mm, PI<35% or PCR > 3.5). In case of UPJO recurrence, the procedure can be performed again in the same way.

11.7 Results

Our group recently performed a review of 112 patients with unilateral primary UPJO who underwent this technique. Mean surgical time for the initial intervention was less than 30 min (25 ± 10 min), and it was successfully performed in 90% of the cases. In 10% of the cases, a CB dilatation was needed. Causes of failure were the persistence of hourglass image (most common) or the failure to pass the guidewire to the renal pelvis. There were no intraoperative complications, and in more than 80% of the patients, hospital stay was 24 h. Causes of prolonged hospital stay (more than 48 h) were preoperative urinary tract infection, requiring antibiotics or pain and vomiting in less than 2% of the patients. Causes of readmission after discharge were pain and vomiting (4%), persistent hematuria (2%), and urinary tract infection requiring an early double-J stent removal (2%).

Mean operative time of the double-J stent removal and calibration was 18 ± 14 min and with no intraoperative complications registered. A residual stenosis was presented in 24% of the patients, requiring an HPB dilatation (21%) or a CB dilatation (3%). Despite initial success, a late recurrence was observed in 8% of the patients, requiring an additional intervention. Overall success rate for this technique was 76.7% (including those who required only one ERBD); this percentage raises up to 86.6% if those who required a second ERBD are included. Only seven (6.3%) patients required an open pyeloplasty, and two patients required a nephrectomy due to loss of renal function (one presented a preoperative differential renal function of 21%, and the other, a severe pre- and postoperative pyelonephritis).

Finally, there was a statistically significant improvement in the reduction of APD (25 ± 10 mm preoperative vs. 10 ± 5 mm at one postoperative year) and parenchymal thickness (4 ± 1.5 mm preoperative vs. 1.3 ± 1.0 mm at one postoperative year) on those patients who required one or two ERBD ($p < 0.05$, t-test). Mean percentage of improvement after 1 year was 55% ± 25%.

Tips and Tricks

- Adequation of the instruments to the patient size is essential. Technical improvement and pediatric sized instruments have increased the safety of this procedure. Using instruments over 4 Fr in a child under 2 years of age has a high probability of failure and injury.
- Specific and proper material is needed to increase the success percentage: different balloon types (high-pressure, cutting balloon) with different dimensions, guidewires, pediatric cystoscopes, double-J stents, etc.
- The learning curve is as needed as any other minimally invasive technique. Most part of our failures and recurrences were registered in the first half of the study, with a significative reduction of the number of failures in the last years.
- In case of difficulties with the endourologic approach, it is important to not force and prolongate the procedure. If we observe that the procedure is being too difficult and taking too long, it is preferable to change the approach in order to avoid a major complication. It is important to remember that the endourologic approach leaves the surgical field intact, so a pyeloplasty is always an option if the ERBD can't be performed with safety.

11.8 Discussion

The minimally invasive options for the treatment of the UPJO have become more attractive in the recent years, with promising results of the laparoscopic and robot-assisted pyeloplasty [2, 9]. But concerns about its application in small children, the need of specific technology and demanding training, and a higher cost make these options not universally applicable and available. Compared with these options, ERBD presents some advantages, as the reduction in the hospital stay and operative time (mean operative time of 240 minutes and 1.5–3.0 days of hospital stay in recent laparoscopic and robotic series [9, 10]), the aesthetic benefits of the absence of scars, less analgesic requirements, and its safe application in small infants. Furthermore, this technique does not alter the external anatomy of the ureter or renal pelvis, and the surgical field is intact in case of needing a pyeloplasty.

ERBD has proved good outcomes in the adult population [11], but previous publications in children showed inconsistent results [12, 13].

Some authors prefer the percutaneous anterograde approach, reporting successful results in UPJO recurrences after pyeloplasty [14]. In our opinion, due to the higher risk of complications, we prefer to reserve the anterograde percutaneous approach for patients with UPJO recurrence [8]. In the recent years, the improvement and adaptation of the endourologic tools to the pediatric population made the retrograde approach a safe, less invasive and feasible option even in infants (as we demonstrate with the low percentage of intraoperative complications).

Probably the main disadvantage of the procedure is that, in some cases (in up to 23% in our experience), a second dilatation procedure is needed to achieve a persistent resolution of the stenosis. This requires a second anesthetic procedure (general anesthesia), but in our experience, no anesthetic adverse event was recorded. This could be explained due to the short duration of the intervention (less than 30 minutes in the majority of cases) and the minimal invasiveness. Moreover, this technique requires a learning curve (as any other minimally invasive option). We have observed a higher number of recurrences and failures in the first years of its application than in the recent years.

The radiation exposure of the infants is an important concern in our practice. During the intervention, the operator reduces the effective dose to the minimum and it has promoted the use of radiation shields where possible. Furthermore, we have recently changed the postoperative image follow-up protocol (following recent recommendations [15, 16]), and a postoperative MAG-III diuretic renogram is only performed when an postoperative ultrasound worsening is observed.

In conclusion, even though the success rate is slightly lower than other minimally invasive options, we believe that the advantages of the ERBD approach make it a safe and valid option for the treatment of UPJO in infants. The success of this technique lies in the use of adequate material suitable for pediatric age (<4 Fr profile instruments, hydrophilic guidewires, balloon catheters, double-J stents, etc.). The complication rate is very low, being the most common event in urinary infection. This could be related with the double-J stent placement, but we strongly believe that its use is necessary in order to avoid an acute postoperative ureteropelvic junction obstruction [17]. Furthermore, the addition of the Cutting Balloon™ allowed a successful outcome on those patients with a persistent stenosis despite the high-pressure balloon dilatation. Finally, the success rate (76.7%, including those who required only one ERBD, and 86.6% if those who required a second ERBD are included) demonstrates the consistency of this technique in a significant number of patients and with a wide follow-up.

Take-Home Points

- Endourologic approach is the least invasive option for the treatment of the UPJO.
- ERBD requires experience with the endourologic approach, and the learning curve is long.
- The use of specific and pediatric-sized instrumentation is essential in order to avoid complications and to increase the success rate.
- The main advantages of this approach are the few analgesic requirements, short hospital stay and surgical time, the absence of scars, and the integrity of the surgical field in case of failure. A lower success rate (compared with pyeloplasty) and the probability of requiring a second procedure are the main disadvantages.
- The use of a double-J stent is important to avoid an acute obstruction of the ureteropelvic junction.
- In case of failure, a pyeloplasty can always be performed (the surgical field is intact).

References

1. O'Reilly PH, Brooman PJC, Mak S, Jones M, Pickup C, Atkinson C, et al. The long-term results of Anderson-Hynes pyeloplasty. BJU Int. 2001;87(4):287–9.
2. Avery DI, Herbst KW, Lendvay TS, Noh PH, Dangle P, Gundeti MS, et al. Robot-assisted laparoscopic pyeloplasty: multi-institutional experience in infants. J Pediatr Urol. 2015;11(3):139.e1–5. https://doi.org/10.1016/j.jpurol.2014.11.025.
3. Huang Y, Wu Y, Shan W, Zeng L, Huang L. An updated meta-analysis of laparoscopic versus open pyeloplasty for ureteropelvic junction obstruction in children. Int J Clin Exp Med. 2015;8(4):4922–31.
4. Parente A, Angulo JM, Romero RM, Rivas S, Burgos L, Tardáguila A. Management of ureteropelvic junction obstruction with high-pressure balloon dilatation: long-term outcome in 50 children under 18 months of age. Urology. 2013;82(5):1138–44.
5. Kadir S, White RI, Engel R. Balloon dilatation of a ureteropelvic junction obstruction. Radiology. 1982;143(1):263–4.
6. Ortiz R, Parente A, Perez-Egido L, Burgos L, Angulo JM. Long-term outcomes in primary obstructive megaureter treated by endoscopic balloon dilation. Experience after 100 cases. Front Pediatr. 2018;6(October):1–9.
7. Patel T, Kellner CP, Katsumi H, Gupta M. Efficacy of endopyelotomy in patients with secondary ureteropelvic junction obstruction. J Endourol. 2011;25(4):587–91.
8. Parente A, Angulo JM, Burgos L, Romero RM, Rivas S, Ortiz R. Percutaneous endopyelotomy over high pressure balloon for recurrent ureteropelvic junction obstruction in children. J Urol. 2015;194(1):184–9. https://doi.org/10.1016/j.juro.2015.01.074.
9. Tam YH, Pang KKY, Wong YS, Chan KW, Lee KH. From laparoscopic Pyeloplasty to robot-assisted laparoscopic Pyeloplasty in primary and Reoperative repairs for Ureteropelvic junction obstruction in children. J Laparoendosc Adv Surg Tech. 2018;28(8):1012–8.
10. Satyanarayan A, Peters CA. Advances in robotic surgery for pediatric ureteropelvic junction obstruction and vesicoureteral reflux: history, present, and future. World J Urol. 2019;(1) https://doi.org/10.1007/s00345-019-02753-3.
11. Jacobs BL, Lai JC, Seelam R, Hanley JM, Wolf JS, Hollenbeck BK, et al. The comparative effectiveness of treatments for Ureteropelvic junction obstruction. Urology. 2018;111:72–7. https://doi.org/10.1016/j.urology.2017.09.002.
12. Sugita Y. Retrograde balloon dilatation for primary pelvi-ureteric junction stenosis in children. Br J Urol. 1996;77(4):587–9.
13. Wilkinson AG, Rajan P, MacKinlay GA. Endoluminal balloon dilatation for pelvi-ureteric junction obstruction in children: an effective alternative to open pyeloplasty. J Pediatr Urol. 2005;1(4):301–5.
14. Veenboer PW, Chrzan R, Dik P, Klijn AJ, De Jong TPVM. Secondary endoscopic pyelotomy in children with failed pyeloplasty. Urology. 2011;77(6):1450–4. https://doi.org/10.1016/j.urology.2010.10.021.
15. Helmy TE, Harraz A, Sharaf DE, El Demerdash Y, Hafez AT, Gad H, et al. Can renal ultrasonography predict early success after pyeloplasty in children? A prospective study. Urol Int. 2014;93(4):406–10.
16. Rickard M, Braga LH, Oliveria JP, Romao R, Demaria J, Lorenzo AJ. Percent improvement in renal pelvis antero-posterior diameter (PI-APD): prospective validation and further exploration of cut-off values that predict success after pediatric pyeloplasty supporting safe monitoring with ultrasound alone. J Pediatr Urol. 2016;12(4):228.e1–6. https://doi.org/10.1016/j.jpurol.2016.04.003.
17. MacKenzie RK, Youngson GG, Hussey JK, Mahomed AA. Is there a role for balloon dilatation of pelviureteric obstruction in children? J Pediatr Surg. 2002;37(6):893–6.

12 Robotic Pyeloplasty

Alexander M. Turner, Salahuddin Syed, and Ramnath Subramaniam

Learning Objectives
- Treatment options for pyeloplasty.
- Advantages of MIS and robotic approach.

12.1 Introduction

Intrinsic or extrinsic compression of the pyeloureteric junction (PUJ), caused respectively, by fibrosis/stenosis of the proximal ureter or aberrant lower pole vessels, are common issues in paediatric urology. Whereas the former cause is largely detected by antenatal screening, the latter often presents as an older child with Dietl's crisis. Although many have theorised on the aetiology, we are no closer to a conclusion [1], but have excellent imaging options to predict outcome and guide therapy. Ultrasound is the mainstay of monitoring of the total antero-posterior diameter (TAPD) of the intra-renal pelvis and there are established international guidelines as the appropriateness and timing of investigations such as dynamic drainage scans (e.g. MAG-3) and retrograde studies to determine suitability for surgery.

A number of techniques have been described to treat pyeloureteric junction obstruction (PUJO) according to the cause, from the gold-standard Anderson-Hynes dismembered pyeloplasty and other 'plasty' techniques such as Y-V and Fenger, to the vascular hitch for crossing vessels, to stenting or performing balloon dilatation or endopyelotomy, with differing levels of success [2, 3].

The robotic pyeloplasty has become a natural progression from the development of open, then laparoscopic procedures to treat pyeloureteric junction obstruction (PUJO). With the Anderson-Hynes, laparoscopic results soon equalled those performed open with greater operative duration being traded for shorter inpatient stays and reduced post-operative analgesia [3]. The temporal and dextrous advantages of open surgery and the post-operative benefits of the laparoscopic approach, however, has made the robotic pyeloplasty the operation of choice and is now so well established that it is often used as a benchmark of robotic surgical training within the field of paediatric urology training [4]. Easily adapted from the laparoscopic approach from the surgical point of view, there is often a rapid learning curve in terms of robot time. As an important

Supplementary Information The online version contains supplementary material available at [https://doi.org/10.1007/978-3-030-99280-4_12].

A. M. Turner · S. Syed · R. Subramaniam (✉)
Department of Paediatric Urology, Leeds General Infirmary, Leeds, UK
e-mail: alexander.turner@nhs.net; salahuddin.syed@nhs.net; ramnath.subramaniam@nhs.net

C. Esposito et al. (eds.), *Minimally Invasive Techniques in Pediatric Urology*,
https://doi.org/10.1007/978-3-030-99280-4_12

training procedure, it is often a case which reveals the technical learning curve of robotics [5]. Personal preference will dictate which approach is used; those with access to smaller instruments may choose a retroperitoneal procedure, whereas transperitoneal access is equally acceptable and allows for wider spacing between instruments. One would expect minimally invasive surgery to follow the same route as open – retroperitoneally; after all, it allows a more direct route to the PUJ and removes intra-abdominal contents from the equation. In addition, any urine leak would be confined to the retroperitoneal space. However, spacing of the instruments, especially in smaller children, is a challenge, with clashing of the robotic arms a common issue. For this reason, the transperitoneal route has been adopted, especially as the use of stenting has helped reduce the rate of urinary leak [6].

12.2 Robotic Pyeloplasty

12.2.1 Patient Positioning and Planning

The author uses a transperitoneal approach with the patient in a mid-lateral position so omentum and bowel fall away from the field of view. The patient is placed on the operating table in a supine position. A padded buttress, attached to the operating table, is placed, with appropriate padding, on the upper arm and upper thigh of the contralateral side. Straps are also placed over the chest and knees to stop patient roll. A head ring can be used to keep the head steady. At this point, a test tilt is completed, where the operating table is tilted so that the patient is in the mid-lateral position with the affected kidney uppermost. Once patient safety has been assured, the table can return to a supine position and the operative field prepared from nipples to thighs, including the perineum, and drapes applied. Once the area is sterile, a Foley catheter is placed transurethrally into the bladder with a spigot, to retain any upper tract dilatation, to ease pelvic mobilisation. A clear, sterile drape covers the genitals. Intraoperative analgesia can be achieved with epidural, TAP or local anaesthetic means, dependent upon local protocol.

12.3 Incision and Port Placement

The camera port should be placed through an incision in the umbilicus (Fig. 12.1). The port is placed under direct vision, and insufflation achieved with appropriate flow rate and pressure. The camera can then be inserted to assess the anatomy. One working port should be placed in the midline of the epigastrium, as shown, and the other in the iliac fossa of the affected kidney. This should be at a distance equal to that of the umbilicus-epigastric ports and offset from the midline by approximately 5–10 degrees, avoiding the inferior epigastric vessels. Once the ports have been placed, the mid-lateral position can again be adopted in preparation for robot docking.

12.4 Robot Positioning

For this procedure, the robot is side-docked. The cart advances at an almost perpendicular angle to the operative table, although allowance of a few degrees of angulation towards the head allows for the slightly superior position of the renal pelvis above the transumbilical plane. The arms pass over the semi-laterally lying patient and reflect back to be docked with the ports (Fig. 12.2).

12.5 Procedure Steps

12.5.1 Step 1: Decide upon the Best Approach to the Pelvis

In a smaller child with virtually no intra-abdominal fat, a bulging renal pelvis may be apparent through the mesocolon and dissection through this structure is all that is necessary. The author prefers a DeBakey forceps in the left arm and a Plasmakinetic grasper in the right. However, a high, malrotated kidney or hostile, adipose

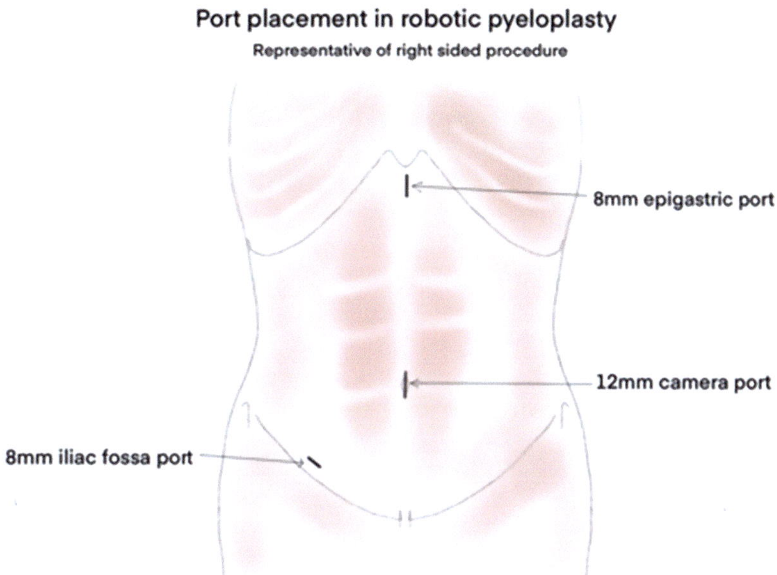

Fig. 12.1 Port placement

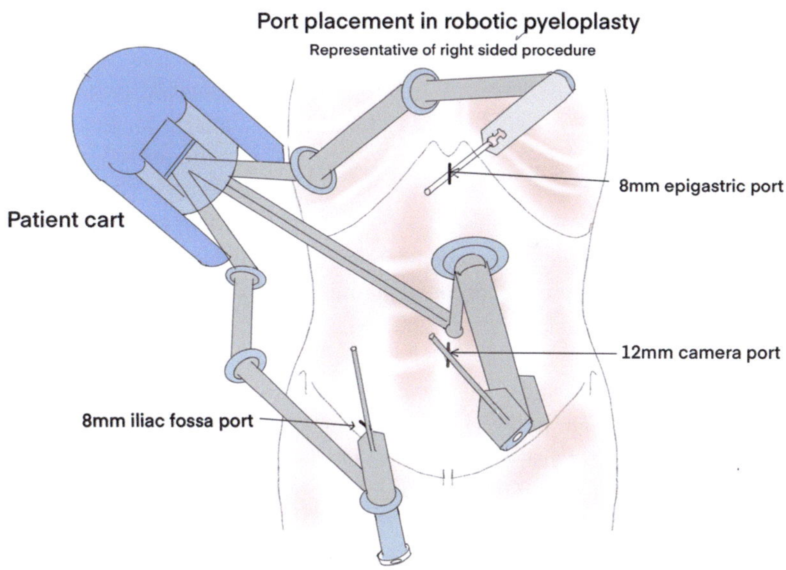

Fig. 12.2 Cart position

abdomen may mandate alternate approaches. Mobilisation of the colon either up to hepatic or splenic flexures may be necessary to improve field of view or to access a difficult kidney. The well-documented principle of locating the ureter and tracking upwards is easier in the retroperitoneal approach (Fig. 12.3).

12.5.2 Step 2: Establish the Clinical Problem

Once the pelvi–ureteric junction (PUJ) has been identified, the cause of the obstruction should be confirmed. Assessment of the calibre of the ureter, peristaltic effort and the presence of aberrant

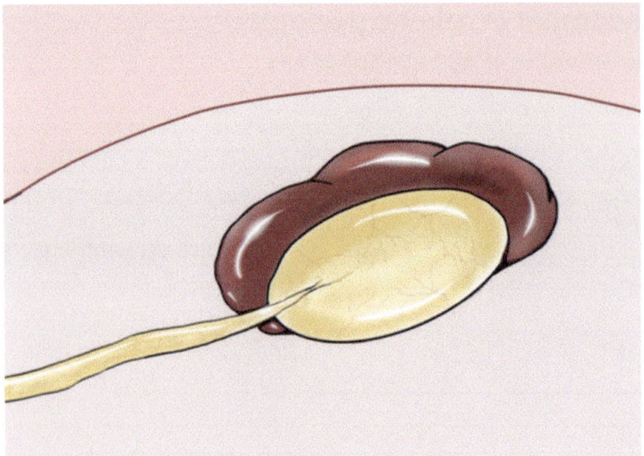

Fig. 12.3 Anatomy of the clinical problem

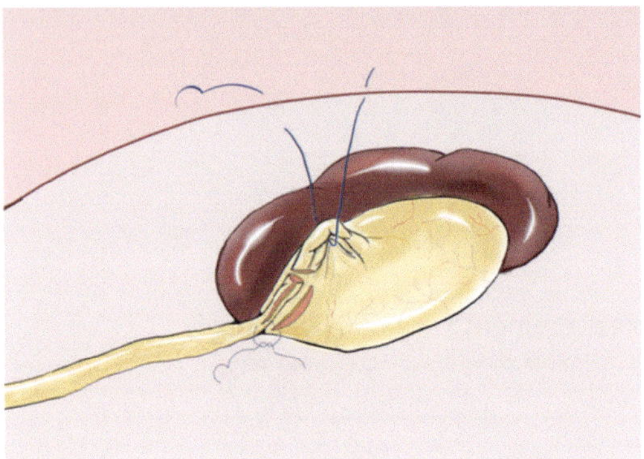

Fig. 12.4 Extracorporeal hitching suture at the PUJ for traction

lower pole vessels should be documented. To aid with mobilisation, an extracorporeal suture (e.g. 5/0 Prolene) on a straight or straightened needle should be passed into the abdominal cavity, leaving the long end outside. The suture is passed superficially through the PUJ, and back outside, to be clipped under tension by the assistant. This allows good visualisation of the pelvis, PUJ and ureter, and extraneous tissue can be removed to straighten the tissues (Fig. 12.4a, b).

12.5.3 Step 3: Incise Ureter and Pelvis

Switching to a bipolar scissor, a transverse cut is made in the postero-medial aspect of normal ureter, distal to the obstruction. Lack of urine flow confirms the obstruction. A spatulation should be made in this same plain, for a length of approximately 1–1.5 cm (the length of the scissor head). The most dependent portion of the pelvis should be identified and a longitudinal incision made, reducing the volume of the pelvis as necessary, but taking care not to enter the calyces laterally. Ensure the apex of the ureteric spatulation reaches the pelvis. Suction is usually required at this point to evacuate urine expressed under pressure from the pelvis.

12.5.4 Step 4: Anastomosis

The author uses a suture-cut robotic device for the anastomosis. The assistant passes a 5/0 PDS suture via the right working port using a manual needle holder, to be grasped and pulled into the abdomen by the DeBakey forceps on the left. The length of the suture should be stipulated beforehand and is determined by personal preference and how many throws are envisaged. The apex of the ureteric spatulation is sutured to the most dependent portion of the open pelvis using the 'outside-in, inside-out' method so the knot lies on the serosal surface. Correct lie of the knots is essential. The author's preference is to use four further interrupted sutures, two either side of the apex. A continuous suture is then used to anastomose the posterior wall of the ureter to the pelvis.

12.5.5 Step 5: Stenting the Ureter

Using an extracorporeal approach, the assistant inserts a device capable of admitting a Ch4.7 stent, such as a Ch5 suprapubic catheter cannula. This should be inserted at an angle so the cannula, once the needle is removed, is able to be brought close, and parallel to, the ureter, which is still hitched up. Before advancing the guidewire, it is a useful tip to measure the approximate distance from pelvis to bladder, so that one knows when the guidewire should have been expected to have passed through the vesicoureteric junction (VUJ) and also not to enable it to pass into the bladder neck. Once the guidewire is deemed to be in the bladder, the stent is passed through and, with the help of a pusher, traverses into the bladder. Lift the sterile drape regularly to expose the genitals to see whether the guidewire or stent has emerged from the urethra. Pressure over the bladder should result in a spurt of urine from the proximal stent fenestrations, and now the catheter spigot can be removed and the catheter attached to a urine bag.

12.5.6 Step 6: Complete the Anastomosis

The anastomosis of the anterior ureter can now be completed in a continuous fashion (Fig. 12.5). Once the first knot of the pelvic closure has been placed, the PUJO can be excised completely and removed via one of the working ports (Fig. 12.6). In turn, this loses the traction suture and so the short end of the pelvic suture can be lifted to ensure the view is not lost. Any residual urine can be aspirated before undocking the robot.

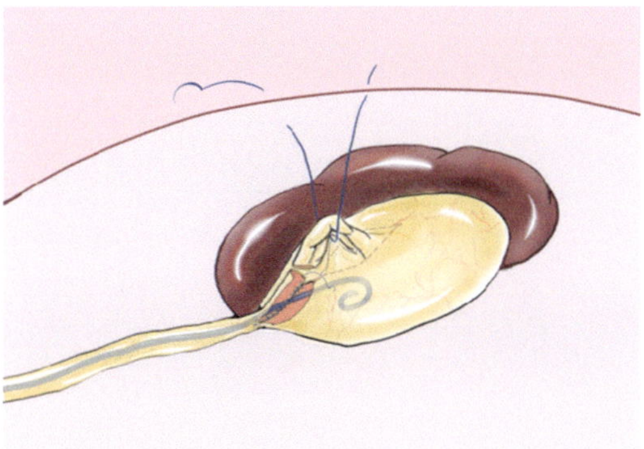

Fig. 12.5 Anastamosis of anterior leaflet of pelvis and ureter, with stent placement

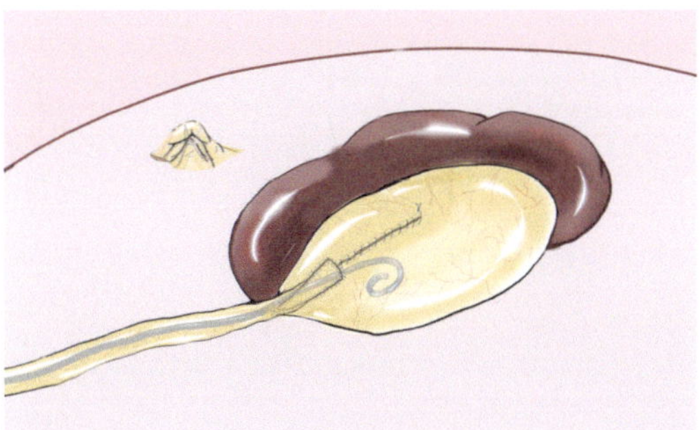

Fig. 12.6 Completed anastomosis and removal of PUJO

12.6 Post-Operative Actions

The patient can eat and drink when they feel well enough to do so. The urethral catheter is placed on free drainage overnight and rosé urine should be seen. Prophylactic antibiotics ± antimuscarinic should be used while the stent is in situ. Day one post-operatively, if all is well, the catheter is clamped for 3 h in an attempt to untangle any potential connection between catheter and stent, prior to removing the catheter. An X-ray is performed to confirm correct stent positioning. The patient is normally well enough to go home the day after surgery. Eight weeks later, the stent is removed with cystoscopy and follow up is by ultrasound assessment of the kidney.

12.7 Conclusion

In all but the smallest infants, where the open procedure has benefits in terms of duration of general anaesthetic and there are limitations in the size of instruments, robotic pyeloplasty is becoming the preferred option for those centres able to fund the devices [7]. Results for the robotic approach are also extremely promising, with shorter operative times than laparoscopy and equal success rates, length of stay and complications [3, 6]. By 2009, robotic surgery became the most-used modality to treat all PUJO and continues to grow in popularity [3].

References

1. Avanoglu A, Tiryaki S. Embryology and morphological (mal) development of UPJ. Front Pediatr. 2020;8:7–9. https://doi.org/10.3389/fped.2020.00137.
2. Corbett HJ, Mullassery D. Outcomes of endopyelotomy for pelviureteric junction obstruction in the paediatric population: a systematic review. J Pediatr Urol. 2015;11:328–36. https://doi.org/10.1016/j.jpurol.2015.08.014.

3. Autorino R, Eden C, El-Ghoneimi A, Guazzoni G, Buffi N, Peters CA, et al. Robot-assisted and laparoscopic repair of ureteropelvic junction obstruction: a systematic review and meta-analysis. Eur Urol. 2014;65:430–52. https://doi.org/10.1016/j.eururo.2013.06.053.
4. Tasian GE, Wiebe DJ, Casale P. Learning curve of robotic assisted pyeloplasty for pediatric urology fellows. J Urol. 2013. https://doi.org/10.1016/j.juro.2013.02.009.
5. Ashraf J, Krishnan J, Turner A, Subramaniam R. Robot docking time: cumulative summation analysis of a procedure-independent learning curve in pediatric urology. J Laparoendosc Adv Surg Tech. 2018;28:1139–41. https://doi.org/10.1089/lap.2017.0418.
6. Casale P. Robotic pyeloplasty in the pediatric population. Curr Urol Rep. 2009;10:55–9. https://doi.org/10.1007/s11934-009-0010-2.
7. Castagnetti M, Iafrate M, Esposito C, Subramaniam R. Searching for the least invasive Management of Pelvi-Ureteric Junction Obstruction in children: a critical literature review of comparative outcomes. Front Pediatr. 2020;8:1–6. https://doi.org/10.3389/fped.2020.00252.

Laparoscopic Approach for Uretero–Pyelo Junction Obstruction (UPJO)

13

Philipp Szavay

Learning Objectives

- To describe step by step the technique of laparoscopic transperitoneal dismembered pyeloplasty.
- To present long-term outcomes of laparoscopic transperitoneal dismembered pyeloplasty.
- To report the latest results in literature on laparoscopic transperitoneal dismembered pyeloplasty.
- To show a video with the technique of laparoscopic transperitoneal dismembered pyeloplasty.
- To describe tips and tricks of laparoscopic transperitoneal dismembered pyeloplasty.

13.1 Introduction

In 1995, Peters performed the first laparoscopic pyeloplasty in a child, thereby beginning the era of reconstructive pediatric laparoscopic urology. Uretero–pelvic junction obstruction (UPJO) is the most common cause of hydronephrosis in infants and children. The gold standard in surgical care for UPJO has been open dismembered pyeloplasty through a retroperitoneal approach as described by Anderson and Hynes. Laparoscopic dismembered pyeloplasty offers advantages such as superior visualization of the anatomy, accurate anastomotic suturing and thus precise reconstruction of the UPJ consecutively, promising good functional outcome. For the approach to minimally invasive pyeloplasty, the laparoscopic transperitoneal approach is a multiused, standardized approach as for a large variety of indications in pediatric surgery and pediatric urology, respectively. It offers a maximum capacity of working space – rather than retroperitoneoscopy – and is suitable for all ages and weight groups in the pediatric patient population, ranging from newborns to adolescents. It provides excellent overview, detailed visualization and augmentation, which make it the superior approach, particularly for complex anatomy and pathology, respectively.

Supplementary Information The online version contains supplementary material available at [https://doi.org/10.1007/978-3-030-99280-4_13].

P. Szavay (✉)
Department of Pediatric Surgery, Lucerne Children's Hospital, Lucerne, Switzerland
e-mail: philipp.szavay@luks.ch

C. Esposito et al. (eds.), *Minimally Invasive Techniques in Pediatric Urology*,
https://doi.org/10.1007/978-3-030-99280-4_13

13.1.1 Preoperative Preparation

Indications for pyeloplasty include:

- Differential renal function (DRF) of the affected side below 40%.
- Decrease of DRF, documented in more than just one examination, such as a renal scintigram and an MRI, respectively.
- Relevant urodynamic obstruction in renal scintigram and MRI, respectively.
- Recurrent urinary tract infection (UTI) and/or pyelonephritis.
- Subjective patient complaints, such as flank pain.
- Special anatomical condition such as horseshoe kidney along with obstruction.

The aim of surgery is to maintain DRF and to improve urinary drainage.

Preoperative diagnostic work-up include:

- Ultrasound.
- Diuretic renal scintigram and/or.
- MRI.
- Intravenous pyelography is widely considered to be obsolete and should be reserved for selected and complex indications only.

Preoperative preparation includes informed consent, obtained from all patients or their parents, prior to surgery. Laparoscopic pyeloplasty is performed under general anesthesia with muscle relaxation. A Foley catheter should be inserted prior to surgery in order to control urinary drainage as well as emptying the urinary bladder for improved working space and view. Perioperative single-shot antibiotic therapy is administered according to local guidelines. The patient is prepped and placed according to local standards and following the rules of asepsis.

For the positioning, the patient is placed in a (semi-) supine position, with a slight elevation of flank on the affected side. In order to provide a maximum of ergonomics, the screen is positioned on the side which will be operated on and lowered down towards the bottom to provide a natural sight-angle for the surgeon. Additional monitors may be placed meaningfully to facilitate the view for the assistant surgeon, scrub nurses, anesthetists and others, respectively. The surgeon's position is on the opposite side of the patient, while the assistant surgeon driving the camera is seated on the same side, with both the surgeons looking in direction to the side of the operating field. The scrub nurse is standing across at the patient's opposite side.

13.2 Technique

At the inferior site of the umbilicus, a cut down technique is preferred to access the peritoneum and installation of a 5 mm camera port, using a 30° scope. This will be followed by the placement of two 3 mm working ports under direct vision in the upper and lower abdomen of the affected side with respect to triangulation regarding the renal pelvis to operate on. Access to the affected kidney is obtained by either a retrocolonic or a trans-mesocolic approach through Gerota's fascia. After the incision of the fascia as well as of the trans-section fatty capsule of the kidney, a blunt/sharp dissection is carried out leading to the (dilated) renal pelvis. When the pyelon becomes visible, a direct attempt should be made to grasp it and further dissection is performed, using blunt and/or sharp techniques with the help of electrocautery, scissors, harmonic scalpel or similar devices, respectively. When the pyelon and the UPJ are sufficiently exposed, two transabdominal hitching sutures are placed to facilitate resection of the UPJ. Those should be placed with care, safely sparing the renal hilar vessels cranially and leaving enough space on the caudal and lateral aspects of the UPJ, in order to allow the resection of the UPJ in front of the hitching suture (see Fig. 13.1).

When the resection of the UPJ is completed, the ureter has to be incised; however, we prefer to not cut completely at a level well below the UPJ in order to assure an adequate lumen of the ureter. Then, on its lateral aspect, the ureter will be spatulated for a sufficient length of the ureteral wall and the consecutive side-to-side anastomosis (see Fig. 13.2).

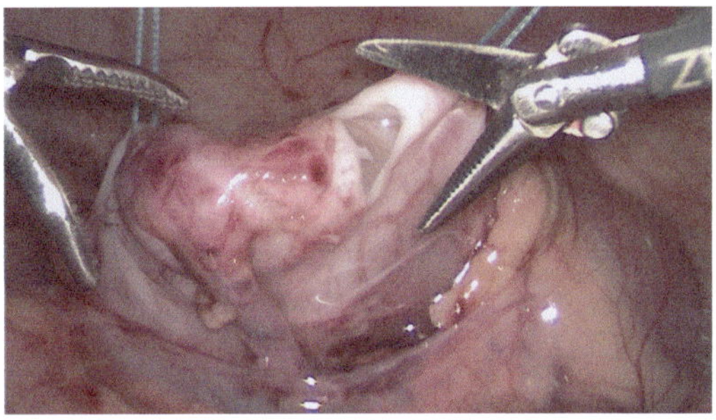

Fig. 13.1 Transabdominal hitching sutures, exposure and resection of UPJ

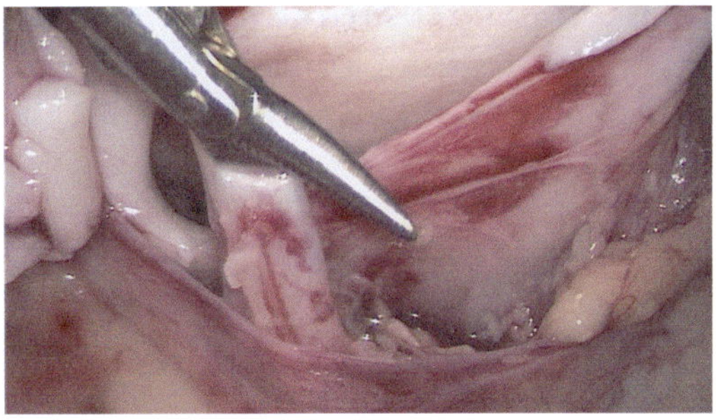

Fig. 13.2 Spatulation of the ureter

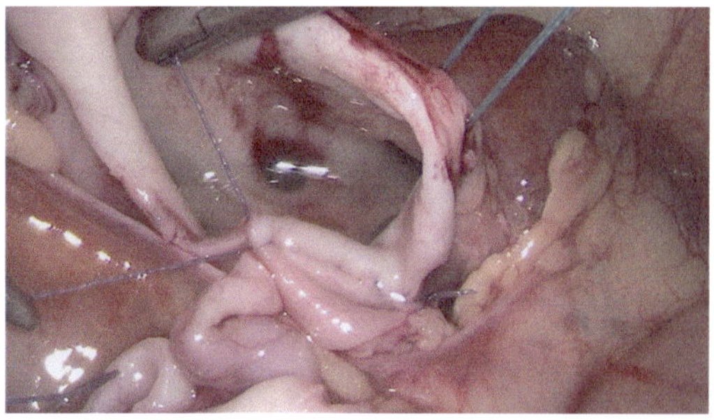

Fig. 13.3 Inverted single interrupted suturing on the dorsal side

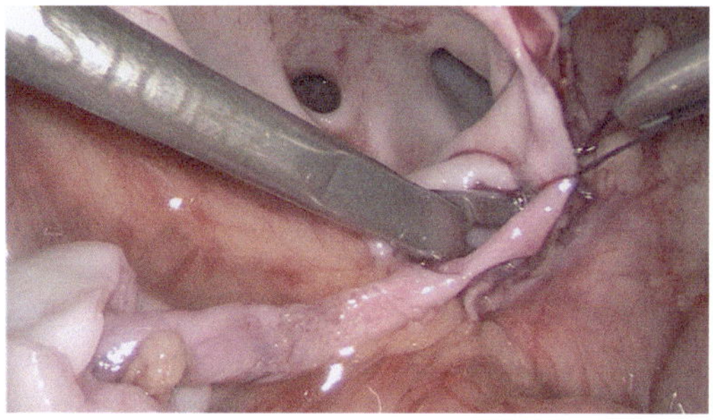

Fig. 13.4 Check for patency of neo-UPJ

While not cutting off completely the proximal part of the ureter along with the UPJ, the remaining tissue may provide as a "handlebar" for suturing of the anastomosis. This will facilitate the ureteral tissue to be picked up and grabbed and consecutively become compromised by edematous alterations. According to Anderson and Hynes, a side-to-side anastomosis is then carried out, starting on the dorsal side (see Fig. 13.3). This can be done with either single interrupted sutures or a running suture. Single-interrupted sutures may provide more safety in watertightness and may be more tissue-sparing as well. A running suture may allow a time-saving technique; however, it requires constant application of tension to the thread in order to avoid loosening, which might be the cause for urinary leakage later [1]. Meanwhile barbed sutures are available down to metric sizes of 5/0; those may facilitate a running suture in this setting. We prefer the use of braided sutures in sizes of 6/0 for infants and 5/0 for older patients. An inverting technique of suturing is required to avoid exposure of the threads to the lumen as this might cause crystallization with consecutive bacterial colonization. When completed, the back side of the patency of the neo-UPJ should be checked, before continuing the anastomosis of the front side (see Fig. 13.4).

The front side is then sutured in the same technique (see Fig. 13.5), the remaining pyelon can be closed using a "z-type" single interrupted suture or a running suture alternatively. The result should provide a wide-open side-to-side anastomosis with a patent neo-UPJ.

Whether to stent the anastomosis and, if so, what kind of stent to use is subject of ongoing discussion. We prefer to apply a transabdominal, transanastomotic stent technique before continuing with the front-sided anastomosis, a 6–8 Fr stent is poked into the abdomen with the use of a curved (custom-made) spear, then through the open renal pelvis and through an identified calyx, respectively, punctured through the renal parenchyma and the lateral abdominal wall, respectively (see Fig. 13.6). The tip of the catheter is then pulled into the abdomen and inserted into the distal ureter [2]. This allows removal of the

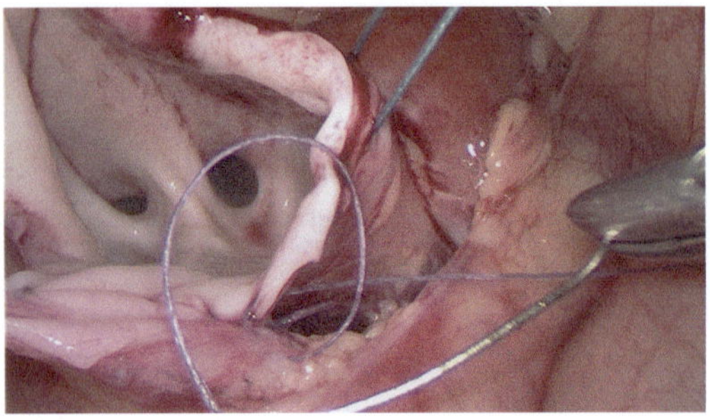

Fig. 13.5 Single-interrupted suture of the front side. The remaining UPJ is used as a "handlebar" (left)

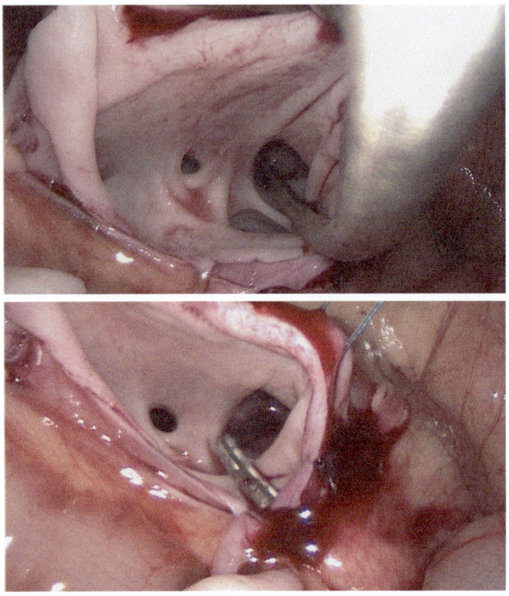

Fig. 13.6 Transabdominal, transanastomotic ureteral stent placement

stent from outside without requiring a second general anesthesia (see Fig. 13.7).

In addition, this enables retrograde irrigation intraoperatively in order to prove watertightness of the anastomosis at the end of the procedure. Other options for stenting include double-J stents, percutaneous nephrostomy stents and others. The procedure will be terminated by removal of the hitching sutures' reposition of the kidney. In a regular case, any other drainage will not be necessary. The specimen can be easily collected along with one of the working ports.

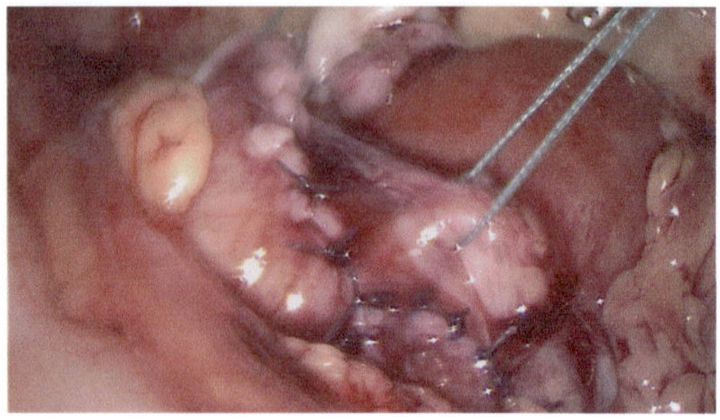

Fig. 13.7 Completed pyeloplasty

13.3 Postoperative Care

Patients are transferred to the ward following the recovery room. Analgesics are administered according to local regimens and guidelines in general following international recommendations such as the WHO "Treatment Guidelines on Pain." We recently changed the antibiotic treatment to a single-shot regimen perioperatively only. Oral feeds are allowed 4–6 h postoperatively and patients are back to full feeds on day one postoperatively in a regular case. Patients can be discharged from hospital on the second or third postoperative day, when drainage with the transureteral stent is secured. However, we leave the transanastomotic stent for 7 days, while the patient may prefer to continue staying in the hospital. The question whether to put a stent in and, if so, how long it should stay is left to the preference of the surgeon, as there is so far no evidence in favor for one of the mentioned methods. Postoperative clinical as well as ultrasound controls are scheduled for 4 weeks and 1 year postoperatively. At 3 months postoperatively, we routinely perform a Uro-MRI, aiming to assess differential renal function and urinary drainage postoperatively.

13.4 Results

In a publication already 10 years old, we could prove in a total of 70 patients, including 26 patients below 1 year of age, who underwent laparoscopic dismembered pyeloplasty, a median operating time of 140 min (range 95–220 min). The described stent placement was successful in all patients. There was only one intraoperative complication with an initially unnoticed accidental perforation of the sigmoid leading to septic peritonitis and a complicated postoperative course. Mean length of hospital stay was 7 days (range 6–14 days) at that time. During follow up, diuretic MAG-3_{Tc99} renography was repeated 3 and 12 months postoperatively. Therewith, the preservation of the differential function of the operated kidney could be documented with no significant difference in DRF from pre- to 12 months postoperatively ($P > 0.05$). All children investigated 1 year after operation showed a significant improvement in tracer clearance on diuretic MAG-3_{Tc99} renography ($P < 0.0001$). None of the patients had complaints during the postoperative course related to surgery or persistent hydronephrosis. Since then, numerous publications could prove the efficiency and excellent outcome of laparoscopic dismembered pyeloplasty, while operating times as well as the duration of hospitalization were continuously decreasing.

Tips and Tricks

- The application of transabdominal hitching sutures for exposure of the pyelon will help to resect the UPJ as well as to safely perform a patent anastomosis. The subtotal dissection of the proximal ureter, leaving the most proximal part of the ureter along with the UPJ and the resected part of the renal pelvis, respectively, in place until the anastomosis has been completed will allow using these tissues as a "handlebar," avoiding repeated picking up of the sensitive urothelium in the area of the anastomosis. The described placement of a transanastomotic ureteral stent will allow avoiding any secondary general anesthesia such as for the removal of a Double-J catheter through cystoscopy.

13.5 Discussion

Laparoscopic dismembered pyeloplasty has evolved to become the gold standard for the surgical treatment of intrinsic UPJO since first done in 1995 by Craig Peters [3]. It has been proven to be safe, effective and associated with a low complication rate with excellent functional results [4–15]. This is obviously also true for recurrent UPJO [16]. Laparoscopic dismembered pyeloplasty provides low morbidity due to the surgical trauma, superior cosmesis, fast recovery and quick return to daily and social activities. It has therefore surpassed open pyeloplasty in many centers as the standard surgical management for UPJO [14, 17].

Compared to open surgery, there have been implications coming along with minimal invasive approach techniques. The most remarkable one is probably the less reduction of the renal pelvis as compared to the original technique described by Anderson and Hynes. However, different authors considered a less reductive resection of the renal pelvis not to be determinative in terms of the functional result [18]. One striking advantage of transperitoneal laparoscopic pyeloplasty is that the approach is a standard procedure for many indications in both pediatric surgery and urology. In addition, it is applicable also for children below 1 year of age. There is sufficient evidence in literature that infants' laparoscopic dismembered pyeloplasty has also been proven to be a safe procedure, providing the same functional outcomes as the open approach [6, 15, 19]. Multiple studies were aiming to describe differences between open, laparoscopic and robotic pyeloplasties, respectively. All of these demonstrate that patients undergoing robotic-assisted laparoscopic pyeloplasty had a shorter hospital stay and less request for pain medication; however, there could be no difference shown in the success rates for open, laparoscopic and robotic-assisted laparoscopic pyeloplasty, respectively [4, 5, 11, 12].

Take-Home Points

- Laparoscopic dismembered pyeloplasty offers an evidenced-based standard of care for UPJO in children of all age and weight groups.
- Laparoscopic dismembered pyeloplasty provides low morbidity due to the surgical trauma, superior cosmesis, fast recovery and quick return to daily and social activities.
- Transabdominal hitching sutures will help better expos the renal pelvis and the UPJ.
- The described technique of a transanastomotic ureteral stent might be favorable in terms of atraumatic removal as well as of monitoring urinary drainage.

References

1. Shao P, Qin C, Ju X, Meng X, Li J, Lv Q, Zhang W, Xu Z, Yin C. Comparison of two different suture methods in laparoscopic dismembered pyeloplasty. Urol Int. 2011;87(3):304–8.
2. Obermayr F, Luithle T, Fuchs J. Laparoscopically guided external transanastomotic stenting in dismembered pyeloplasty: a safe technique. Urology. 2015;86(1):200–4.
3. Peters CA, Schlussel RN, Retik AB. Pediatric laparoscopic dismembered pyeloplasty. J Urol. 1995;153(6):1962–5.
4. Abdel-Karim AM, Fahmy A, Moussa A, Rashad H, Elbadry M, Badawy H, Hammady A. Laparoscopic pyeloplasty versus open pyeloplasty for recurrent ureteropelvic junction obstruction in children. J Pediatr Urol. 2016;12(6):401.e1–6.
5. Chan YY, Durbin-Johnson B, Sturm RM, Kurzrock EA. Outcomes after pediatric open, laparoscopic, and robotic pyeloplasty at academic institutions. J Pediatr Urol. 2017;13(1):49.e1–6.
6. Fuchs J, Luithle T, Warmann SW, Haber P, Blumenstock G, Szavay P. Laparoscopic surgery on the upper urinary tract in children below one year of age – technical aspects and functional outcome. J Urol. 2009;182(4):1561–8.
7. García-Aparicio L, Blazquez-Gomez E, Martin O, Manzanares A, García-Smith N, Bejarano M, Rodo J, Ribó JM. Anderson–Hynes pyeloplasty in patients less than 12 months old. Is the laparoscopic approach safe and feasible? J Endourol. 2014;28(8):906–8.
8. Gatti JM, Amstutz SP, Bowlin PR, Stephany HA, Murphy JP. Laparoscopic vs open pyeloplasty in children: results of a randomized, prospective, controlled trial. J Urol. 2017;197(3 Pt 1):792–7.
9. Juliano RV, Mendonça RR, Meyer F, Rubinstein M, Lasmar MT, Korkes F, Tavares A, Pompeo AC, Tobias-Machado M. Long-term outcome of laparoscopic pyeloplasty: multicentric comparative study of techniques and accesses. J Laparoendosc Adv Surg Tech A. 2011;21(5):399–403.
10. Peters CA. Laparoscopy in pediatric urology. Curr Opin Urol. 2004;14(2):67–73.
11. Piaggio LA, Corbetta JP, Weller S, Dingevan RA, Duran V, Ruiz J, Lopez JC. Comparative, prospective, case-control study of open versus laparoscopic pyeloplasty in children with ureteropelvic junction obstruction: long-term results. Front Pediatr. 2017;5:10.
12. Song SH, Lee C, Jung J, Kim SJ, Park S, Park H, Kim KS. Comparative study of pediatric open pyeloplasty, laparoscopy-assisted extracorporeal pyeloplasty, and robot-assisted laparoscopic pyeloplasty. PLoS One. 2017;12(4):e0175026.
13. Szavay PO, Luithle T, Seitz G, Warmann SW, Haber P, Fuchs J. Functional outcome after laparoscopic dismembered pyeloplasty in children. J Pediatr Urol. 2010;6(4):359–63.
14. Szavay PO. Applications of laparoscopic transperitoneal surgery of the pediatric urinary tract. Front Pediatr. 2019;7:29. https://doi.org/10.3389/fped.2019.00029. eCollection 2019.
15. Turner RM, Fox JA, Tomaszewski JJ, Schneck FX, Docimo SG, Ost MC. Laparoscopic pyeloplasty for ureteropelvic junction obstruction in infants. J Urol. 2013;189(4):1503–7.
16. Moscardi PR, Barbosa JA, Andrade HS, Mello MF, Cezarino BN, Oliveira LM, Srougi M, Dénes FT, Lopes RI. Reoperative laparoscopic ureteropelvic junction obstruction repair in children: safety and efficacy of the technique. J Urol. 2017;197(3 Pt 1):798–804.
17. Symons SJ, Bhirud PS, Jain V, Shetty AS, Desai MR. Laparoscopic pyeloplasty: our new gold standard. J Endourol. 2009;23(3):463–7.
18. Reismann M, Gratz KF, Metzelder M, Ure B, Glüer S. Excision of the dilated pelvis is not necessary in laparoscopic dismembered pyeloplasty. Eur J Pediatr Surg. 2008;18(1):19–21.
19. Neheman A, Kord E, Zisman A, Darawsha AE, Noh PH. Comparison of robotic pyeloplasty and standard laparoscopic pyeloplasty in infants: a bi-institutional study. J Laparoendosc Adv Surg Tech A. 2018;28(4):467–70. https://doi.org/10.1089/lap.2017.0262.

14 Retroperitoneal Laparoscopic Pyeloplasty in Infants and Children

Annabel Paye-Jaouen, Matthieu Peycelon, and Alaa El-Ghoneimi

Learning Objectives

- To describe step by step the technique of RLP.
- To present long-term outcomes of RLP.
- To report the latest results of the major international papers about RLP.
- To show a video with the technique of RLP.
- To describe tips and tricks of RLP.

14.1 Introduction

Pyeloplasty, as described by Anderson and Hynes (Fig. 14.1), is an effective procedure for long-term correction for children with significant ureteropelvic junction obstruction (UPJO) leading to impaired differential renal function. Many studies have shown the benefits of laparoscopic treatment of the UPJO compared to open surgery [1]. Retroperitoneal laparoscopic pyeloplasty (RLP) appears to offer more advantages compared to the transperitoneal laparoscopic approach [2]. In our team, Alaa El Ghoneimi has started the retroperitoneal approach for nephrectomy and then for urologic reconstructive surgery (pyeloplasty) since 1998 [3]. He first reported his preliminary experience in 22 patients in 2003, and this technique has been modified several times since [3, 4]. We first used 5/0 absorbable monofilament sutures for the ureteropelvic anastomosis and then with the development of 3-mm instruments we moved to 6/0 sutures. Another technique change was to decrease the number of trocars from 4 to 3. The youngest child who had an RLP in our department was of 6 weeks of age with a weight of 4.8 kg.

14.2 Preoperative Preparation

Investigations must include renal ultrasonography and functional imaging. We prefer the use of magnetic resonance urography than renal scintigraphy as it provides an anatomical view of the urinary tract. All patients and their parents have to sign a specifically formulated consent before the procedure. Patients receive a general anesthesia and require orotracheal intubation and myorelaxation. Antibiotic prophylaxis is done preoperatively with a 50 mg/kg dose of ceftriaxone.

Supplementary Information The online version contains supplementary material available at [https://doi.org/10.1007/978-3-030-99280-4_14].

A. Paye-Jaouen (✉) · M. Peycelon · A. El-Ghoneimi
Department of Pediatric Urology, Robert-Debré University Hospital, APHP, National Reference Center of Rare Urinary Tract Malformations (MARVU), University of Paris, Paris, France
e-mail: annabel.paye-jaouen@aphp.fr; matthieu.peycelon@aphp.fr; alaa.elghoneimi@aphp.fr

C. Esposito et al. (eds.), *Minimally Invasive Techniques in Pediatric Urology*,
https://doi.org/10.1007/978-3-030-99280-4_14

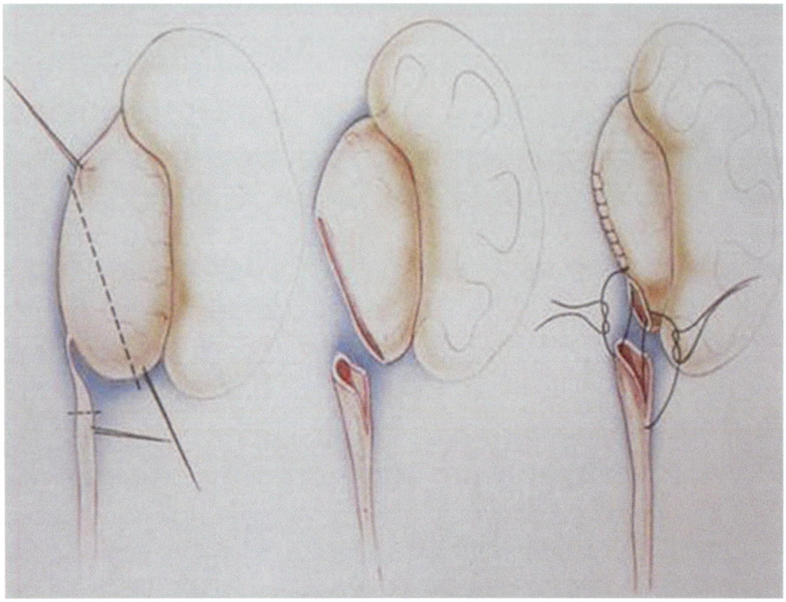

Fig. 14.1 Operative steps for a pyeloplasty described by Anderson and Hynes

14.3 Positioning

The retroperitoneal access is done by a lateral approach. The patient is placed in the lateral decubitus position, with a lumber padding to flex the patient and thus expose the area of trocars placement, between the last rib and the ileac crest (Fig. 14.2). Yeung used a different positioning according to the side of the kidney: semi-prone for the right side and semi-lateral for the left side [5].

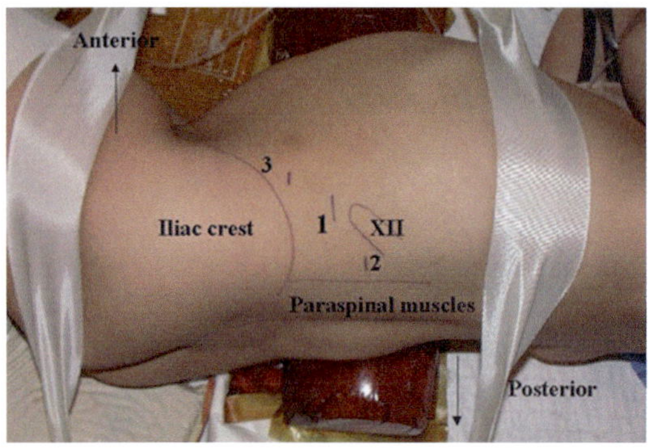

Fig. 14.2 Trocars placement for a pyeloplasty by retroperitoneoscopy

14.4 Instrumentation

Regarding the laparoscopic procedure, we adopt a 5-mm 0-degree optic trocar and two 3-mm assistant trocars. We use one atraumatic grasping forceps, one 2-mm scissors, one 3-mm bipolar forceps and one needle driver. The JJ stent or the pyelostomy tube is inserted through a 2-mm trocar.

14.5 Technique

Retroperitoneal access is achieved through a 10-mm incision, one finger from the lower side of the 12th rib (Fig. 14.2). The use of narrow retractors with long blades allows a deep dissection with short incision. The Gerota's fascia is approached by a muscle-splitting blunt dissection, then it is opened under direct vision and the first blunt 3-mm trocar is inserted directly inside the Gerota's fascia (Fig. 14.3). A working space is created by gas insufflation, and the first trocar is fixed with a purse-string suture that is applied around the deep fascia to ensure an airtight seal and to allow traction on the main trocar, if needed, to increase the working space. We prefer this type of fixation to the single-use self-retaining trocar, as we think that this type of trocar is relatively too big in children and may interfere with the mobility of instruments. The second 3-mm trocar

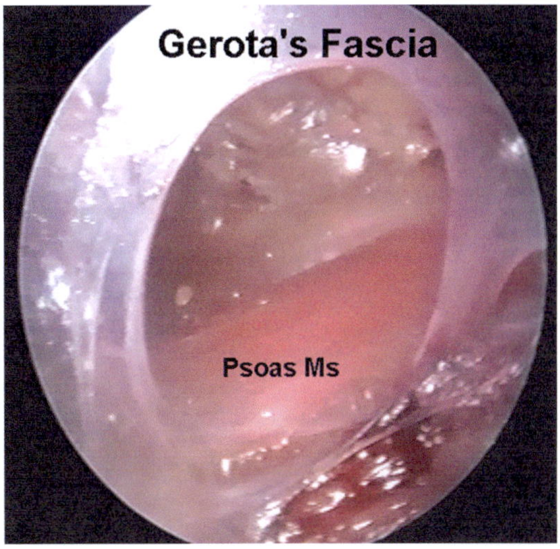

Fig. 14.3 Insertion of the first 3-mm trocar inserted directly inside the Gerota's fascia

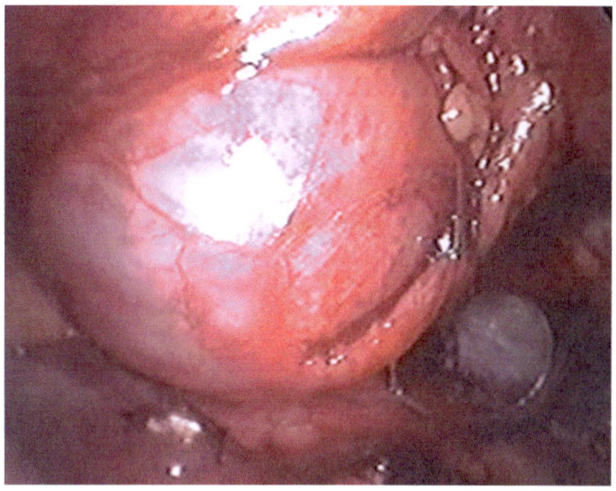

Fig. 14.4 Identification and minimal dissection of the ureteropelvic junction

is inserted posteriorly in the costovertebral angle, in front of the lumbosacral muscle. The third 3-mm trocar is located one finger above the top of the iliac crest. To avoid transperitoneal insertion of this trocar, the working space is fully created, and the deep surface of the anterior wall muscles is identified before the trocar insertion. Insufflation pressure does not exceed 12 mm Hg, and the Co2 flow rate is progressively increased from 1 to 3 l/min. Access to the retroperitoneum and creation of the working space are the keys to success in the retroperitoneal renal surgery. Age and low weight are not limiting factors for this approach. Young children have less fat and the access is even easier. We also used the retroperitoneal laparoscopic approach in other indications like nephrectomy in newborns less than 3 weeks old [6].

We currently use a 3-trocar technique [4]: the first one for the 5-mm laparoscope (at the tip of the 12th rib), the second is inserted in the costovertebral angle (and it will be used for the needle driver in case of a left pyeloplasty), and the third one is inserted at the top of the iliac crest (the needle driver is used here in case of right pyeloplasty). The kidney is approached posteriorly, and the renal pelvis is first identified. The ureteropelvic junction is identified and a minimal dissection is done to free the junction from connective tissue (Fig. 14.4). The anterior surface of the kidney should be left intact to keep it adherent to the peritoneum, which can play a role of "self-retraction" to avoid the kidney from dropping. Small vessels are divided using bipolar electrocoagulation. Care is taken not to section ureteral blood vessels. A stay stitch is placed at the junction. Aberrant crossing vessels are identified. The renal pelvis is partially divided using scissors at the most dependent part (Fig. 14.5) and gentle traction on the stay suture helps to define this point. Keeping the traction, the ureter is partially divided and incised vertically for spatulation. The traction suture helps to mobilize the ureter (Fig. 14.6) so the scissors can be in the correct axis of the ureter, usually introduced through the last trocar. The anterior surface of the kidney is left adherent to the peritoneum so that the kidney is retracted medially without the need for individual kidney retraction. The ureteropelvic anastomosis begins using a 6–0 absorbable suture with a tapered 3/8 circle needle, placed from the most dependent portion of the pelvis to the most inferior point or vertex of the ureteral spatulation (Fig. 14.7). The suture is tied using the intracorporeal technique with the knots placed outside the lumen. The same stitch is used to run the anterior wall of the anastomosis. The UPJ is kept intact for traction and stabilization of the suture line and removed just before tying the last suture on the pelvis. This stay suture may be fixed to the psoas muscle to give stability and to

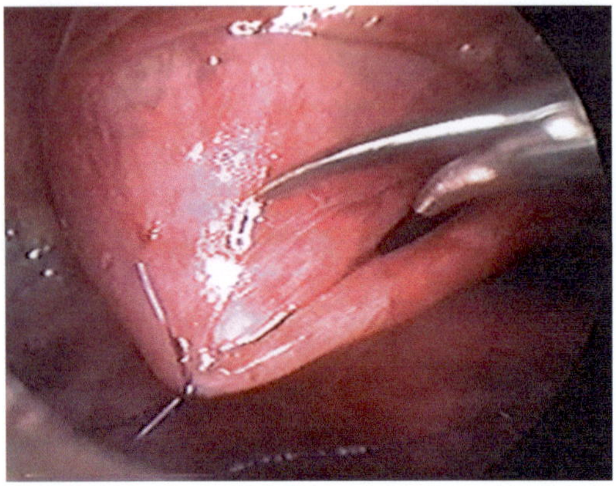

Fig. 14.5 Section of the renal pelvis at the most dependent part

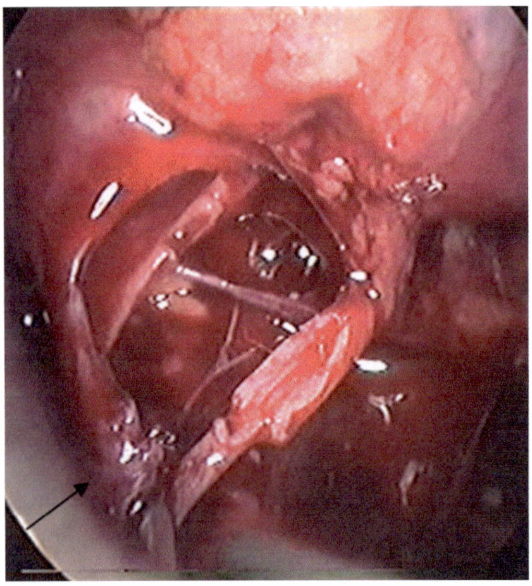

Fig. 14.6 Tip for a better ureter visualization and suture

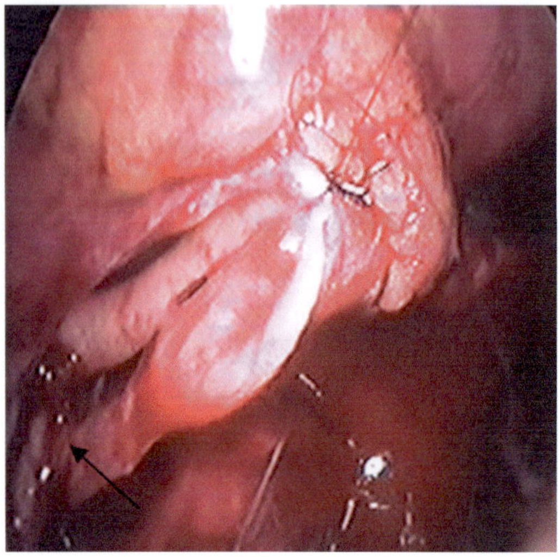

Fig. 14.7 Ureteropelvic anastomosis

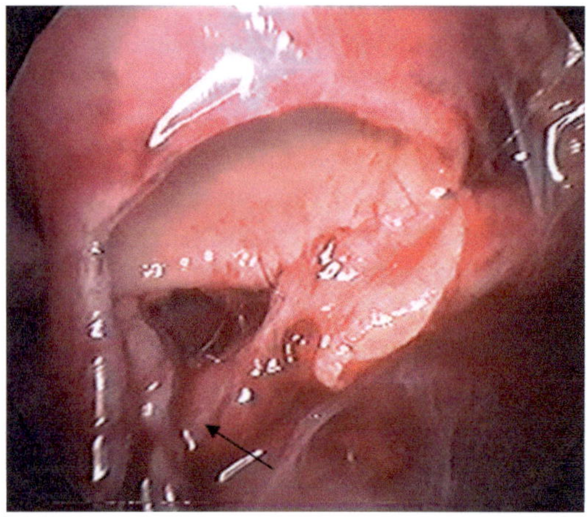

Fig. 14.8 Tip to facilitate the suturing process thanks to the stay suture on the psoas muscle

facilitate the suturing (Fig. 14.8). A double-pigtail stent or a transanastomotic pyelostomy stent is inserted through the costovertebral-angle trocar, and if there is doubt, its position in the bladder is assured under fluoroscopy. The posterior ureteropelvic anastomosis is then done. We still proceed with double-pigtail stent in the cases with intra-renal pelvis because of the technical difficulties to insert the pyelostomy stent in these cases. The pelvis is trimmed if needed. In case of aberrant crossing vessels (Fig. 14.9), the technique is slightly different. After placement of the stay suture, the ureter is completely divided and the UPJ and the pelvis are delivered anteriorly from the vessels with the help of the stay suture. Then the anastomosis is performed as described (Fig. 14.10).

We do not use a perirenal drain.

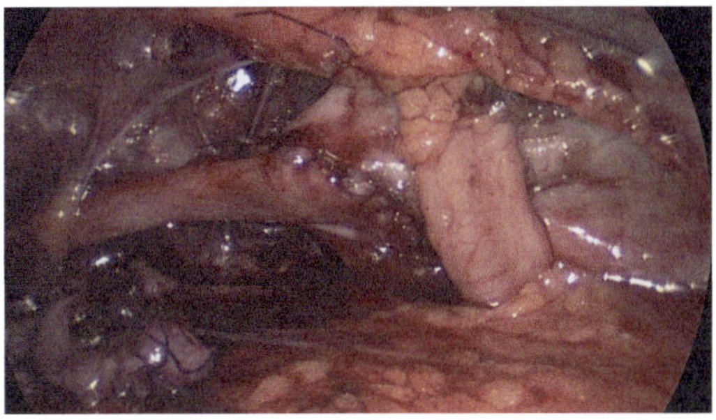

Fig. 14.9 Final aspect of the anastomosis

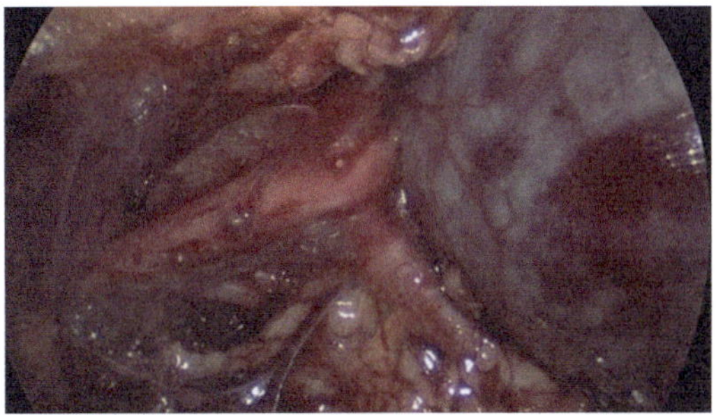

Fig. 14.10 Ureteropelvic junction aspect in case of aberrant crossing vessels

14.6 Postoperative Care

Patients start oral feeding 4 h postoperatively. Pain management is controlled with acetaminophen (15 mg/kg every 6 h) for 24 h after surgery. No postoperative antibiotics are given, and patients are discharged from hospital on day one. The bladder catheter is left for 24 h postoperatively. The JJ stent is removed between 4 and 6 weeks under general anesthesia, or under hypnosis for girls more than 6 years old.If the patient has a transanastomotic stent, this external stent is clamped on day one postoperatively and removed after 10 days in the outpatient clinic. The follow up included a renal ultrasound (RUS) 1 month after surgery; if no increased pelvic dilatation is described, RUS regimen is at 6 months, 1 year, every year for 5 years, every 5 years until puberty. An MR Urography is repeated if a preoperative impaired differential renal function was noted.

14.7 Results

This technique is feasible even in children less than 1 year old, but need well-experienced surgeons in pediatric laparoscopy. Even if operative time may be longer, no significant complication or worse outcomes have been reported so far. The largest monocentric experience with RLP in children has been published by El Ghoneimi et al.: 104 patients were included with a mean operative time of 185 min, and a 98% success rate [7]. They even started to perform this procedure for children under the age of one. Between 2012 and 2017, 144 RLP were performed, including 24 done in children less 1 year old and we compare the open surgery and RLP for UPJO repair in children less than 1 year of age. No conversion has been noted. Hospital stay and intravenous analgesic use were significantly lower in the RLP group in comparison to the open group, although operative time was significantly longer. Postoperative complication included urinary tract infection, subfascial hematoma, and gross hematuria without urinary retention. Complication rate was statistically identical in each group [8].

To avoid a second general anesthesia for the stent removal, we use nowadays, more often, a transanastomotic pyelostomy stent. Our experience using external ureteropelvic stenting after RLP was reported in 2011 on 22 patients with no complication. All stents were removed at the outpatient clinic on postoperative day 10 without any urinary leakage, while the double J stent need to be removed under general anesthesia between 4 and 6 weeks [9].

Tips and Tricks

- A good positioning for the lateral retroperitoneal approach is needed.
- The anterior surface of the kidney must be left adherent to the peritoneum.
- A stay suture can be fixed to the psoas muscle to give stability and to facilitate the running suture.
- Long-term follow-up is needed to assess the decrease of the renal pelvis and to check the renal function.

14.8 Discussion

Clear advantages of laparoscopic pyeloplasty over open surgery have been proven by retrospective and prospective studies [10, 11]. Early series were reported by Yeung et al. and El Ghoneimi et al. with good outcomes [4, 5]. More recently, larger series were reported by Zhou et al. and Subotic et al. and they concluded that RLP was a safe, efficient, and reproducible procedure in high volume and at expert laparoscopic centers [11, 12]. The largest series about RLP in children was published by El Ghoneimi et al.: 104 patients were included with a mean operative time of 185 min and a 98% success rate. They highlighted that this procedure is associated with a long learning curve and autonomy is achieved after about 30 procedures [7]. Qadri et al. supported the retroperitoneal approach, given advantages such as shorter operative time, less dissection needed, a higher sensitivity of detecting crossing vessels, a decreased risk of visceral injury, and an early start of oral feeds [13]. In a randomized clinical trial, Badawy et al. was in favor of the RLP because of shorter operative time, shorter hospital stay, and early resumption of oral feeding [14]. The retroperitoneoscopic approach allows a more rapid access to the renal pelvis, but this technique needs to be more delicate in maneuvering in a restricted workspace. As a consequence, an experienced surgeon with laparoscopic skills and working in a high volume center is recommended. This procedure is also feasible for infants younger than 2 years old. Zhang et al. reported their experience in 2019: 22 children underwent an RLP and 14 a transperitoneal LP with no difference between the two groups in terms of operative time [15]. A shorter postoperative hospitalization and faster oral feeding were noted in the RLP group [15]. El Ghoneimi et al. also reported recently 24 RLP on children under 1 year age with no conversion and only one failure [8]. Canon et al. reported no major difference between the RLP and the transperitoneal LP. The difference in operative time reflected eventually the learning curve for suturing and dissection [16]. Both techniques should be considered equal in the successful correction of the UPJO. We think in our center that it is important to learn and use both procedures.

RLP is really interesting in cases of anatomical variants as it can also be effective with retrocaval ureter in children, even if the anomaly was not detected preoperatively [17].

RLP is thus nowadays the gold standard procedure in many departments and, since 2003, in our team [6]. However, it is a challenging procedure and needs training in an experienced team (technical difficulties) [18]. The procedure is safe, gives as good functional results as open surgery, but with better cosmetic appearance and more comfortable postoperative course. Nowadays, the robotic-assisted laparoscopic pyeloplasty represents an attractive option to perform minimally invasive surgery in case of UPJO in children [19]. Suturing may be more precise and the learning curve seems to be shorter [20]. Our pediatric urology department still performs RLP in children less than 1 year age, but we use now the robotic approach for older children.

Take-Home Points

- A good experience in the retroperitoneal approach is required before starting an RLP.
- You should learn this procedure in a high-volume center using RLP routinely.
- This procedure is efficient in children younger than 1 year.
- A transanastomotic pyelostomy avoids a second general anesthesia.
- The patient can be discharged at day one postoperatively.

References

1. Huang Y, Wu Y, Shan W, Zeng L, Huang L. An updated metaanalysis of transperitoneal versus open pyeloplasty for ureteropelvic junction obstruction in children. Int J Clin Exp Med. 2015;8:4922–31.
2. Wu Y, Dong Q, Han P, Liu L, Wang L, Wei Q. Meta analysis of transperitoneal approach versus retroperitoneal approaches of laparoscopic pyeloplasty for ureteropelvic junction obstruction. J Laparoendosc Adv Surg Tech A. 2012;22:658–62.
3. Farhat W, Khoury A, Bagli G, Mc Lorie G, El Ghoneimi A. Mentored retroperitoneal laparoscopic renal surgery in children: a safe approach to learning. BJU Int. 2003;92:617–20.
4. El Ghoneimi A, et al. Laparoscopic dismembered pyeloplasty by a retroperitoneal approach in children. BJU Int. 2003;92:104–8.
5. Yeung CK, Tam YH, Sihoe JD, Lee KH, Liu KW. Retroperitoneoscopic dismembered pyeloplasty for pelvi-ureteric junction obstruction in infants and children. BJU Int. 2001;87:509–11.
6. El Ghoneimi A. Laparoscopic management of hydronephrosis in children. World J Urol. 2004;22:415–7.
7. Blanc T, Muller C, Abdou H, Peev S, Paye Jaouen A, Peycelon M, El Ghoneimi A. Retroperitoneal laparoscopic pyeloplasty in children: a long term outcome and critical analysis of 10 year experience in a teaching center. Eur J Urol. 2013;63:565–72.
8. Kallas Chemaly A, Peycelon M, Ali A, Grapin C, Carricaburu E, Philippe Chomette P, Enezian G, Paye Jaouen A, El Ghoneimi A. Reflective practice about retroperitoneal laparoscopy in comparison to open surgery for ureteropelvic junction obstruction repair in children less than 1 year of age. Front Pediatr. 2019;7:194.
9. Helmy T, Blanc T, Paye Jaouen A, El Ghoneimi A. And al. Preliminary experience with external ureteropelvic stent: alternative to double J stent in laparoscopic pyeloplasty in children. J Urol. 2011;185:1065–70.
10. Autorino R, Eden C, El Ghoneimi A, et al. Robot assisted and laparoscopic repair of ureteropelvic junction obstruction: a systematic review and meta analysis. Eur Urol. 2014;65:430–52.
11. Zhou H, Li H, Zhang X, et al. Retroperitoneoscopic Anderson-Hynes dismembered pyeloplasty in infants and; a 60-case report. Pediatr Surg Int. 2009;25:519–23.
12. Subotic S, Weiss H, Wyler S, et al. Dismembered and non dismembered retroperitoneoscopic pyeloplasty for the treatment of ureteropyelic junction obstruction in children. World J Urol. 2013;31:689–95.
13. Qadri SJ, Khan M. Retroperitoneal versus transperitoneal laparoscopic pyeloplasty; our experience. Urol Int. 2010;85:309–13.
14. Badawy H, Zoaier A, Ghoneim T, Hanno A. Transperitoneal versus retroperitoneal laparoscopic pyeloplasty in children: randomized clinical trial. J Pediatr Urol. 2014;11:019.
15. Zhang S, Li J, Li C, Xie X, et al. Evaluation of the clinical value of retroperitoneal laparoscopic pyeloplasty in the treatment of ureteropelvic junction obstruction in infants. Medicine. 2019;98(40):e17308.
16. Canon SJ, Jayanthi VR, Lowe GJ. Which is better—retroperitoneoscopic or laparoscopic dismembered pyeloplasty in children? J Urol. 2007;78(4Pt2):1791–5.
17. Peycelon M, Rembeyo G, Tanase A, Muller CO, Blanc T, Alhazmi H, Paye Jaouen A, El Ghoneimi A. Laparoscopic retroperitoneal approach for retrocaval ureter in children. World J Urol. 2019;38(8):2055–62.
18. Gopal M, et al. Management of ureteropelvic junction obstruction in children- a roundtable discussion. JPU. 2019;15:322–9.
19. Blanc T, Kohaut J, Elie C, et al. Retroperitoneal approach for ureteropelvic junction obstruction: encouraging preliminary results with robot assisted laparoscopic repair. Front Pediatr. 2019;7:209.
20. Castagnetti M, Iafrate M, Esposito C, Subramaniam R. Searching for the least invasive management of pelvi-ureteric junction obstruction in children: a critical literature review of comparative outcomes. Front Pediatr. 2020;8:252.

15 Uretero-Pelvic Junction Obstruction (UPJO) Treatment Using: One-Trocar-Assisted Pyeloplasty (OTAP)

Neil Di Salvo, Eduje Thomas, Tommaso Gargano, and Mario Lima

Learning Objectives

- To describe the historical process which led to the invention of the technique.
- To describe step by step the technique of One-Trocar-Assisted Pyeloplasty (OTAP).
- To present our experience with the technique, including results and complications.
- To show a video with the OTAP technique.

15.1 Introduction

During the past decades, several techniques have been designed to achieve the main goal of surgery in the uretero-pelvic junction obstruction (UPJO): preserving the renal function by allowing unobstructed drainage of the renal pelvis. Among these, the Anderson–Hynes dismembered pyeloplasty is the most adopted, being considered the mainstay in the surgical treatment of UPJO.

Minimally invasive surgery has evolved and has been introduced to reduce postoperative morbidity, length of hospitalization and aesthetic impact. Pyeloplasty can be carried out in a transperitoneal or retroperitoneal manner. The transperitoneal approach provides increased working space and readily identifiable anatomic landmarks, but requires adequate bowel mobilization [1]. The retroperitoneal approach is hampered by limited working space, but has the advantage of direct and rapid access to the ureteropelvic junction (UPJ) and less risk of bowel damage.

Craig Peters reported the first case of paediatric laparoscopic trans-mesenteric pyeloplasty in 1995 [2]; Furthermore, retroperitoneoscopic pyeloplasty, first attempted by C.K. Yeung in 2002, is often performed by paediatric urologists [3, 4].

In 2004, in the conception of a hybrid surgery, Mohammed Amin El Gohary described the first laparoscopic assisted pyeloplasty in children, using three ports to gain access to the UPJ [5]. The procedure entailed mobilization of the colon to expose the pelvis and upper ureter. The UPJ was brought to the flank via a 10 mm port and the procedure was completed as in the open technique. We developed his idea of extracting the UPJ, but we adopted the retroperitoneoscopic

Supplementary Information The online version contains supplementary material available at [https://doi.org/10.1007/978-3-030-99280-4_15].

N. Di Salvo · E. Thomas · T. Gargano · M. Lima (✉)
Paediatric Surgery Unit, IRCCS Sant'Orsola University-Hospital, University of Bologna, Bologna, Italy
e-mail: niel.disalvo@aosp.bo.it; eduje.thomas@studio.unibo.it; tommaso.gargano2@unibo.it; mario.lima@unibo.it

C. Esposito et al. (eds.), *Minimally Invasive Techniques in Pediatric Urology*,
https://doi.org/10.1007/978-3-030-99280-4_15

route, being more direct, instead of the laparoscopic one.

Due to our increasing experience in one trocar video assisted procedures, in 2005 we attempted a new technique, the One Trocar Assisted Pyeloplasty (OTAP) [6]. This technique combines the advantages of a minimally invasive retroperitoneoscopic approach with the high success rate of an open dismembered pyeloplasty. Since its introduction in 2005, OTAP has been adopted in many paediatric surgical units in Italy [7–9].

15.2 Surgical Technique

The patient is placed in lateral decubitus on the non-pathologic side, exposing the pathologic flank. A transurethral catheter is inserted. A 12 mm long incision is made on the prolongation of the 11th to 12th rib (Fig. 15.1). The Gerota fascia and the perirenal fat are reached anteriorly after blunt dissection through the muscles. A 10 mm balloon anchorage trocar is inserted, and we use a 10 mm 0° lens operative telescope with a 5 mm operative channel (Fig. 15.2).

The retroperitoneal working space is created through insufflation of CO_2 (Pressure 8–10 mmHg, Flow 0.5–1 l/min; according to the patient's size and weight) and moving the telescope with an Endo peanut (Coviden, Massachusetts, US); once the lower renal pole is identified, the pelvis and the proximal ureter are anteriorly approached targeting the UPJ (Video 15.1/Figs. 15.3 and 15.4). Small vessels are coagulated by unipolar cautery. The UPJ is then isolated with an "L" dissector and exteriorized through the lumbar incision, after previously placing a vessel loop for traction purposes (Fig. 15.5). In cases of massive hydronephrosis, the pelvis can be emptied with a needle to facilitate the procedure (Fig. 15.6). A stay suture is first given on the ureter in order to correctly orientate the UPJ thus avoiding twisting of the ureter.

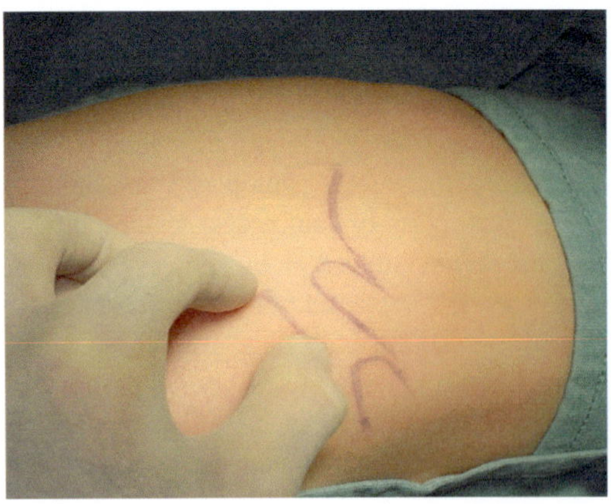

Fig. 15.1 Anatomical landmarks for a small incision

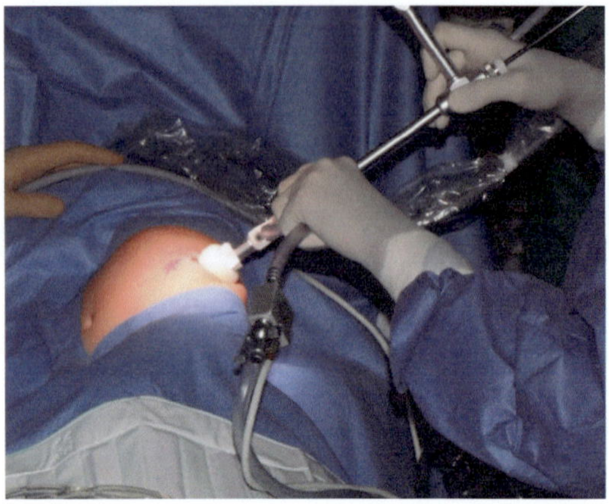

Fig. 15.2 Position of the surgical team during the retroperitoneoscopic phase

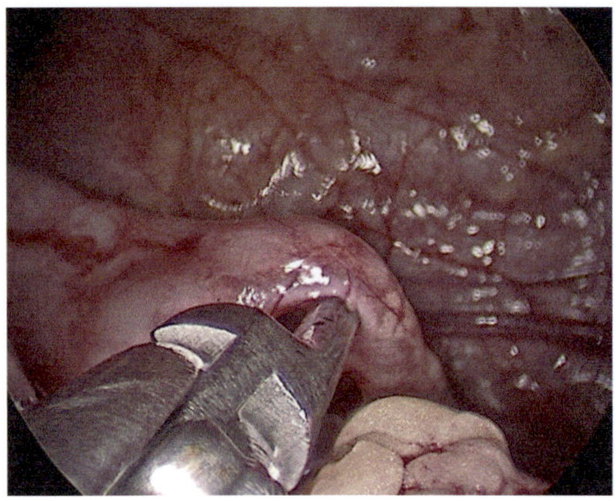

Fig. 15.3 Ureter identification during the retroperitoneoscopic phase. The L dissector, inserted in the operative channel of the operative telescope, can be seen

The Anderson–Hynes pyeloplasty is then performed in a traditional manner, using 6–0 or 7–0 PDS running sutures (Fig. 15.7). Before completing the pyeloplasty, an external uretero-pelvic

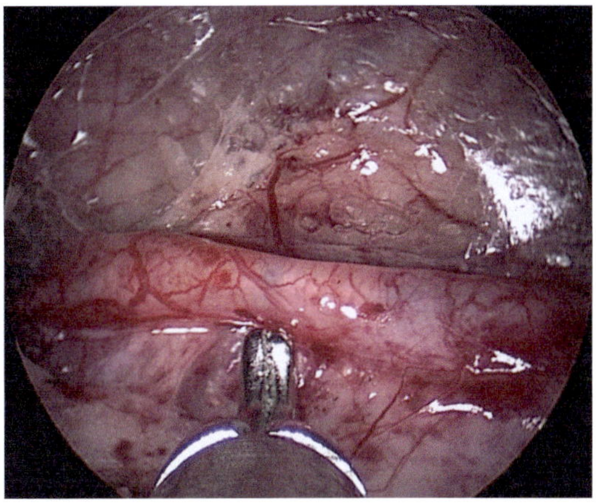

Fig. 15.4 Isolation of the UPJ with the L dissector

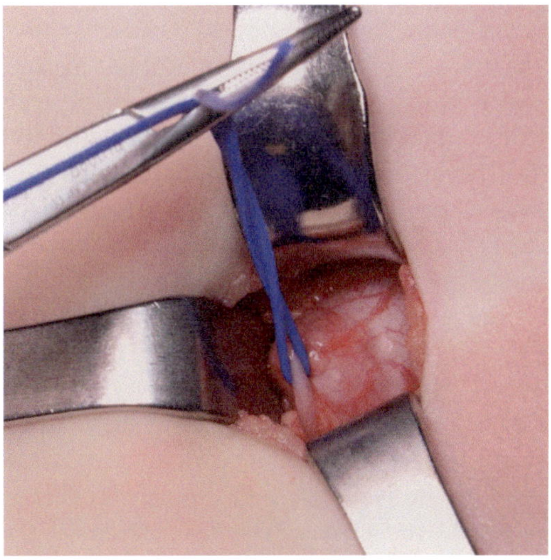

Fig. 15.5 The UPJ is brought out through the lumbar incision using a vessel loop, inserted during the retroperitoneoscopic phase

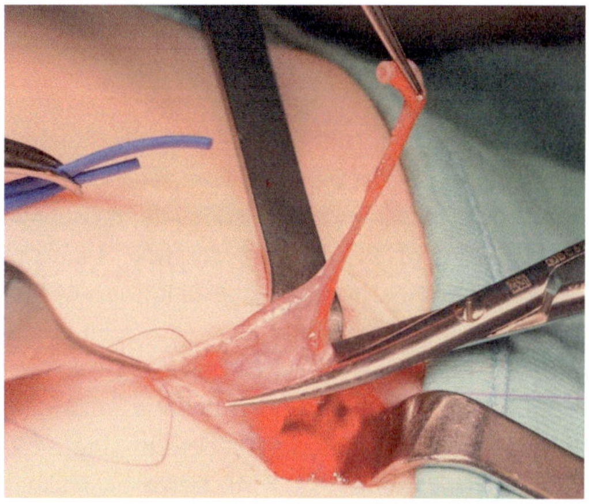

Fig. 15.6 The obstructed UPJ with part of the dilated pelvis and proximal ureter are removed

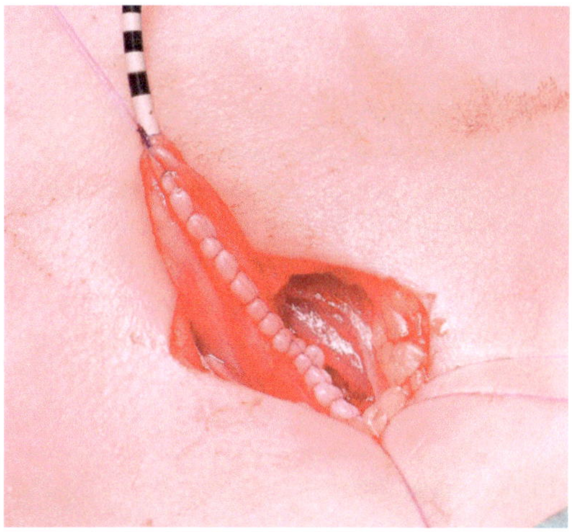

Fig. 15.7 Final aspect of the reconstructed pelvis, with an external ureteropelvic stent emerging from one end of the suture

stent is placed in anterograde manner, emerging from the end of the anastomosis. Alternatively, an internal ureteral stent (double J stent) can be anterogradely positioned and cystoscopically removed 3–4 weeks later. The pelvis is repositioned into the renal lodge and the anastomosis can be checked with a retroperitoneoscopic look. In case of extrinsic obstruction due to crossing vessels, these are uncrossed prior to completing the anastomosis. A soft Penrose drain is left in place near the anastomosis and the wound is closed by absorbable sutures.

During the postoperative period, a full course of antibiotics is administered. The transurethral catheter is removed on the first or second postoperative day, whereas the uretero-pelvic stent and Penrose drain are, respectively, kept until the fifth and sixth post–op day. The patient is then discharged.

The feasibility of the technique is hindered only by relative contraindications represented by huge pelvic dilatation, previous retroperitoneal surgery, previous renal trauma and infections (pyonephrosis).

15.3 Complications and Follow-Up

The complication rate is similar to the standard open approach. The principal complication is stenosis of the anastomosis. Fortunately, this is rare and 90–95% of cases are successful. In case of OTAP, recurrence could be due to fibrosis or ureter angles near the anastomosis; it is related to a difficult dissection that can cause tension and ischemia. Another rare complication is urinary leakage from the anastomosis determining a retroperitoneal urinoma (1–3%); however, leakage spontaneously resolves in the majority of cases and reintervention is extremely rare. Conversion to open surgery is necessary if the peritoneum is accidentally open because of the impossibility to create an adequate working chamber in the retroperitoneum.

Follow-up consists of repeated ultrasound at 3, 6, 12 months and then yearly. In our Centre, if pelvic dilation decreases over time and no further deterioration of the kidney echo-structure is seen, renography is not usually required [10]. If dilation does not improve and/or the echotexture worsens and/or symptoms appear, a renogram is performed.

15.4 Case Series

Since 2005, in our institution, the OTAP has been the preferred approach for hydronephrosis in children younger than 2 years of age [11]. Nevertheless, OTAP has also been used in children older than 2 years. In a range period of 15 years, we performed 156 OTAPs. Follow-up was available in 95.7% of all patients. We considered the minimum period of follow-up to be 1 year after surgery to define success. The mean operative time was 133 min and it was not influenced by crossing vessels. The mean hospitalization length was 6.71 days.

Conversion to open repair was required in seven cases (conversion to open surgery rate = 4.5%) with a mean age of 19 months: five accidental peritoneal opening that did not allow the retroperitoneoscopic phase and two technical difficulties, but these conversions occurred at the very beginning of our experience with OTAP (mostly in the first 8 years of experience with the technique).

Seven patients had complications due to recurrence of UPJ stenosis defined as a post–operative worsening of pelvic dilatation on ultrasound and persistence of impaired urinary flow pattern obstruction on dynamic MAG3 renography at 6 months after surgery (recurrence rate = 4.5%).

Regarding this complication, it is to say that these patients (4/7) mostly belong to the small group in which a stent was not used. This is the reason why we suggest the use of such stents, especially in very young patients.

At the beginning of our experience, we used an internal J-J ureteral stent; afterwards, as mentioned before, we tried not to use ureteral stents in a small series of patients, but this practice was abandoned due to increase in recurrence. At present, we are used to using external pyelo–ureteral stents that can be easily removed during hospitalization, with no sedation.

The postoperative course was characterized by urinary collection around the kidney (urinoma) in three patients (urinary leakage rate = 1.9%). One patient among these had a scarce urinary leakage and he was treated conservatively. In two cases, the urinary collection required a reintervention with the placement of a transanastomotic stent to replace the former one that was accidentally removed.

We have treated very young patients affected by severe forms of hydronephrosis for which an early surgical correction can be of some advantage. As a matter of fact, we demonstrated feasibility, in terms of efficacy and safety, of OTAP in the first 90 days of life in a case series of 23 patients [12].

All parents were satisfied with the aesthetical result.

Thus far, we have attempted a posterior muscle-sparing incision to approach the kidney in one patient, always through the retroperitoneal space (Posterior One Trocar Assisted Pyeloplasty, POTAP) [13].

Take-Home Points

- OTAP is a hybrid technique which combines the advantages of a minimally invasive retroperitoneoscopic approach with the high success rate of an open dismembered pyeloplasty.
- This technique consists of isolating the UPJ, thanks to a retroperitoneoscopic one-trocar approach and exteriorizing the UPJ through the lumbar incision, in order to perform an open dismembered pyeloplasty.
- OTAP is safe and feasible in very young patients.
- Complication and success rates are similar to those of the standard open technique.

References

1. Turner RM II, Fox JA, Tomaszewski JJ, Schneck FX, Docimo SG, Ost MC. Laparoscopic pyeloplasty for ureteropelvic junction obstruction in infants. J Urol. 2013;189(4):1503–7.
2. Peters CA, Schlussel RN, Retik AB. Pediatric laparoscopic dismembered pyeloplasty. J Urol. 1995;153(6):1962–5.
3. Yeung CK, Tam YH, Sihoe JD, Lee KH, Liu KW. Retroperitoneoscopic dismembered pyeloplasty for pelvi-ureteric junction obstruction in infants and children. BJU Int. 2001;87(6):509–13.
4. Hao G, Xiao J, Yang P, Shen H. Laparoscopic retroperitoneal dismembered pyeloplasty: single-center experience in China. J Laparoendosc Adv Surg Tech A. 2013;23(1):38–41.
5. El Gohary MA. Laparoscopic-assisted pyeloplasty in children. Pediatr Endosurg Innovative Tech. 2004;8:260–3.
6. Lima M, Tursini S, Ruggeri G, Gargano T, Libri M, Domini M. One trocar assisted pyeloplasty (OTAP): initial experience and codification of a technique. Pediatr Med Chir. 2007;29(2):108–11.
7. Marte A, Papparella A. One-trocar-assisted pyeloplasty: an attractive alternative to open pyeloplasty. Afr J Paediatr Surg. 2015;12(4):266–9.
8. Caione P, Lais A, Nappo SG. One-port retroperitoneoscopic assisted pyeloplasty versus open dismembered pyeloplasty in young children: preliminary experience. J Urol. 2010;184(5):2109–15.
9. Cobellis G, Nino F, Pierangeli F, Mariscoli F, Noviello C, Martino A. Retroperitoneoscopic one-trocar-assisted pyeloplasty in children: an age-related evaluation. J Laparoendosc Adv Surg Tech. 2017:651–4.
10. Almodhen F, Jednak R, Capolicchio JP, Eassa W, Brzezinski A, El-Sherbiny M. Is routine renography required after pyeloplasty? J Urol. 2010;184(3):1128–33.
11. Lima M, Ruggeri G, Messina P, Tursini S, Destro F, Mogiatti M. One-trocar–assisted pyeloplasty in children: an 8-year single institution experience. Eur J Pediatr Surg. 2015;25:262–8.
12. Lima M., Di Salvo N., Portoraro A., Catania VD, Maffi M., Ruggeri G. Feasibility, in terms of efficacy and safety, of video-assisted pyeloplasty (OTAP) in the first 90 days of life. J Ped Endosc Surg. https://doi.org/10.1007/s42804-019-00024-x.
13. Di Pace MR, Tripi F, Sergio M, Lima M, Cimador M. Posterior one-trocar-assisted pyeloplasty. J Ped Endosc Surg. 2019;1:33–6.

Laparoscopic Management of Extrinsic Uretero-Pelvic Junction Obstruction (UPJO) by Crossing Vessels

16

S. F. Chiarenza and C. Bleve

Learning Objectives

- To describe step by step the technique of laparoscopic polar vessel transposition (LPVT) in extrinsic uretero-pyelic junction obstruction (EUPJO).
- To present long-term outcomes of LPVH.
- To report the latest results of the major international papers about LPVH.
- To show a video with the technique of LPVH.
- To describe tips and tricks of LPVH.

16.1 Introduction

Dismembered Pyeloplasty (DP) was first described by Anderson and Hynes (AHDP) in 1949 [1]; this technique, both open and laparoscopic, remains, nowadays, the gold standard procedure to treat uretero-pyelic junction obstruction (UPJO). UPJO may be secondary to intrinsic muscle and collagen disorganization or to extrinsic compression due to crossing vessels (CV); the extrinsic obstruction is often present symptomatically in older children, frequently observed in adults and rarely in neonates. Von Rokitansky et al. in 1842 [2] first described the association between UPJ-obstruction and extrinsic etiology by lower pole CV. In case of pure extrinsic-UPJO, Hellström, also in 1949 [3], described an alternative approach to AHDP for the pure extrinsic-UPJO; it involved displacing the lower pole vessels cranially and then anchoring them to the anterior pelvic wall using vascular adventitial sutures. In order to prevent vascular damage to aberrant polar vessels, in 1959, Chapman [4] further modified this technique by securing a more superior position of the lower pole vessels within a wrap of the anterior redundant pelvic wall, without the need for vascular adventitial sutures. This technique has since been described in children in case of pure extrinsic-UPJO as an alternative to open dismembered pyeloplasty (DP). Pesce et al., in 1999 [5], reported the largest series of pediatric patients treated with vascular hitch (VH). Aberrant renal polar vessels usually can cause intermittent UPJO. These cases present a normal perinatal history, fol-

Supplementary Information The online version contains supplementary material available at [https://doi.org/10.1007/978-3-030-99280-4_16].

S. F. Chiarenza (✉) · C. Bleve
Department of Pediatric Surgery and Pediatric Minimally Invasive Surgery and New Technologies, San Bortolo Hospital, Vicenza, Italy
e-mail: fabio.chiarenza@aulss8.veneto.it; cosimo.bleve@aulss8.veneto.it

C. Esposito et al. (eds.), *Minimally Invasive Techniques in Pediatric Urology*,
https://doi.org/10.1007/978-3-030-99280-4_16

lowed by the subsequent onset of clinical signs and symptoms, often influenced by the child's hydration status, characterized by intermittent hydronephrosis on imaging and normal kidney function. The aberrant CV perfuses the lower pole of the kidney and typically cross over the UPJ. Currently, there are no definitive imaging techniques or intraoperative procedures available to confirm the etiology of UPJO. As noted by Schneider [6], one frequently encounters anatomic variability in the relationship between the renal pelvis and the lower pole vessels. Some authors have proposed DP to exclude intrinsic associated anomalies; others, in order to minimize technical difficulties and improve outcomes, have described simpler procedures that do not involve pyeloureteral anastomosis. In this chapter, we describe the minimally invasive approach to extrinsic-UPJO performed by laparoscopy. In order to reduce the risk of incomplete operation during laparoscopic vascular hitch (LVH), we suggest a simple and uncomplicated intraoperative test, diuretic test (DT), to confirm the relief of the obstruction. Since the renal pedicle and the position of obstructing polar vessels are anterior to renal pelvis and ureter, laparoscopic approach is the suitable technique to make easier the transposition of the aberrant pedicle. This technique gives excellent results in our hands.

16.2 Preoperative Preparation

A complete preoperative assessment is mandatory to make a correct diagnosis and to plan surgery. Complete medical history and a specific imaging examination are essential to confirm the diagnosis of extrinsic-UPJO. **The presence of extrinsic obstruction by CV must be suspected in case of:** absence/non significative renal pelvis dilation at prenatal or postnatal ultrasound; late presentation with intermittent symptoms (flank pain, or renal colic sometimes associated to vomit); marked hydronephrosis at the time of pain with primarily extrarenal dilatation.

All the patients with UPJO undergo ultrasonography/Doppler scan and MAG3 renogram,

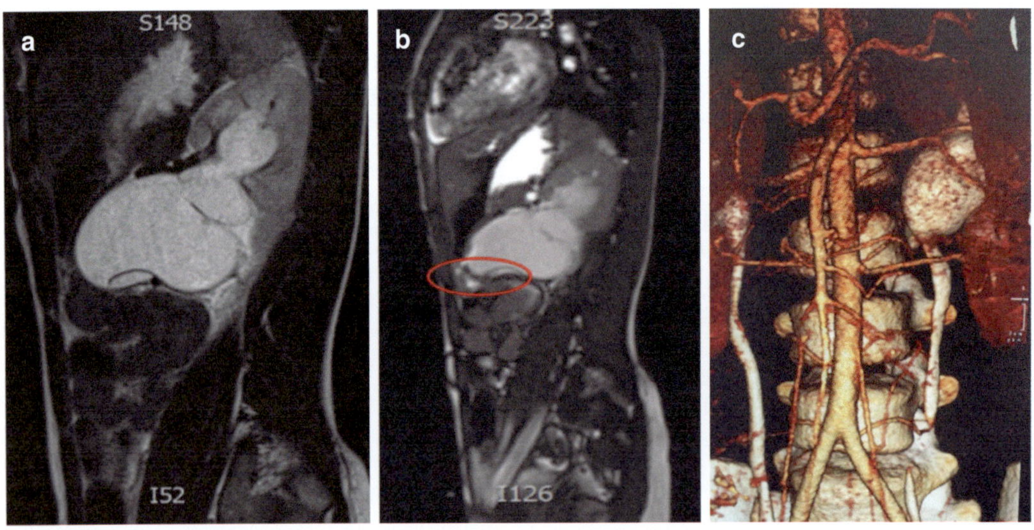

Fig. 16.1 A functional-magnetic-resonance-urography (fMRU) is reserved in case of doubtful suspected extrinsic obstruction. (**a**) Huge left pelvis distension; (**b**) Polar vessels compressing UPJ (red circle). (**c**) 3D RMN reconstruction

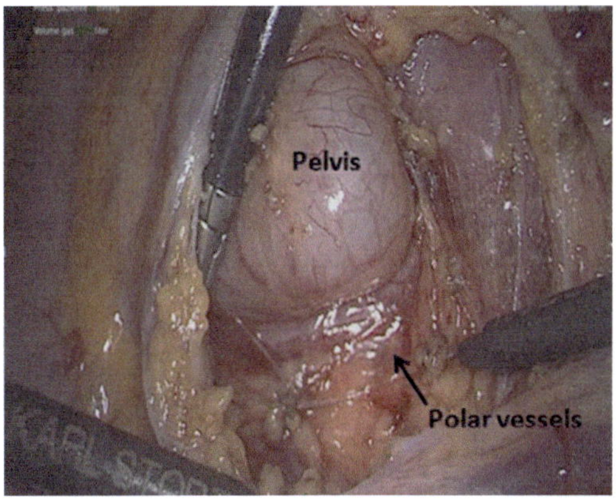

Fig. 16.2 Intraoperative corresponding view

respectively, with diuretic test confirming the obstructed patterns; in older patients, doppler scan can even detect obstructive extrinsic aberrant lower pole vessels. A functional-magnetic-resonance-urography (fMRU) is reserved in case of doubtful suspected extrinsic obstruction (Figs. 16.1a–c and 16.2) and or renal malformations such as horseshoe kidney.

Surgical indication is suggested in case of two or more of the following conditions: presence of clinical symptoms, obstruction on diuretic renogram (99mTc-MAG3); decrease in relative renal function; clear or suspected image of polar vessels on fMRU; worsening of intermittent hydronephrosis on follow-up.

The patients are hospitalized 24 h before surgery, starting with liquid diet, bowel cleansing with scheduled enemas and eventual laxative; these recommendations are suggested in order to obtain bowel deflation facilitating laparoscopic approach. All patients and their parents have to sign a specifically formulated informed consent before the procedure that must include not only the hitching procedure but also the possibility of a dismembered pyeloplasty also with "open" technique and potential intraoperative vascular complications. A general anesthesia and antibiotic prophylaxis with IV amoxicillin-clavulanic acid or cephalosporin is performed.

16.3 Positioning

Renal vascular pedicle and aberrant polar vessels are typically displaced anteriorly to the renal pelvis and UPJ, whereby a laparoscopic transperitoneal approach is advisable. In fact, the anterior access to the kidney ensures direct vision of the renal pedicle, aberrant vessel and renal pelvis and makes easier the anterior CV hitching. Just before the operation, a bladder catheter and nasogastric tube are positioned and the patient is placed in a semi-lateral supine position (45°) at the edge of surgical table to facilitate the instruments' movement. The surgeon's stand in front of the patient with the assistant to his left/right are trying to obtain for the surgical team the best possible ergonomics for the shoulders; scrub nurse is to the side of the surgeons (usually to the right) (Fig. 16.3a). The monitor is placed in front of the surgeon and at the back and toward the head of the patient.

16.4 Instrumentation

After a standard umbilical open approach, a 5 or 10 mm optical port is inserted; the trocar size depends on the weight and the age of the patient. Pneumoperitoneum is induced by insufflating CO_2 at the minimal pressure to obtain an acceptable operative space (pressure varies from 5 to 10 mmHg). An optical laparoscope is introduced to explore abdominal cavity; as in the majority of pediatric procedures, a 30° scope is

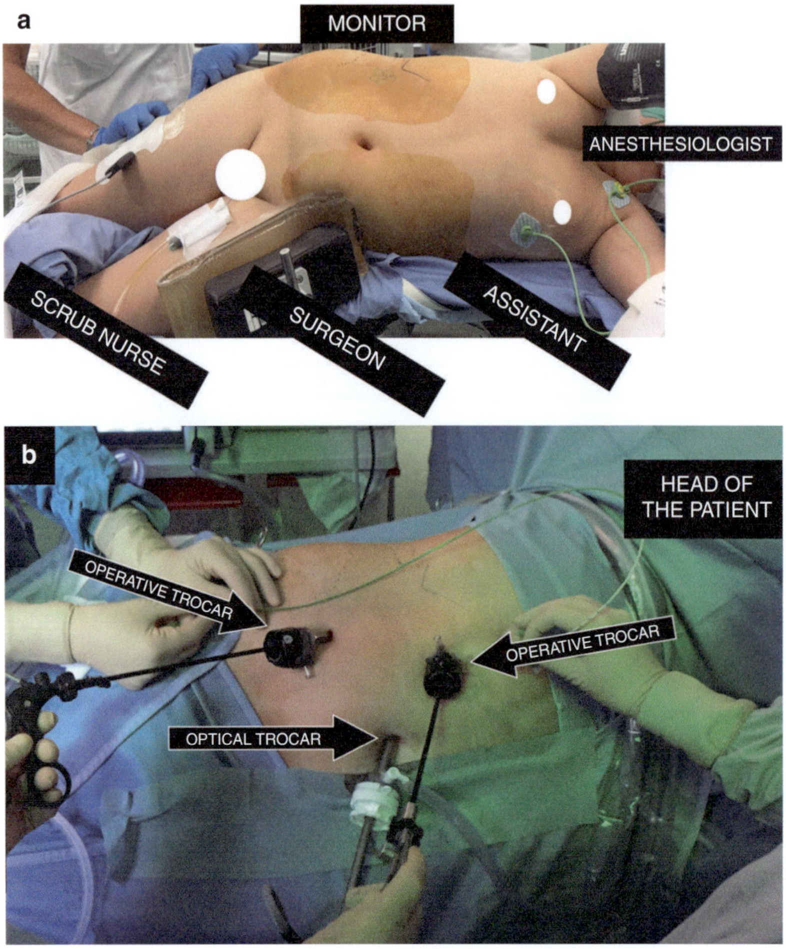

Fig. 16.3 (**a**) Patient position and team set-up. (**b**) Trocars' position

preferable to better visualize the different angulation of the operative field. Two other 3–5 mm working ports, according the weight of the patient and the surgeon's preference, are then placed, one in the epigastrium and one in the ipsilateral iliac fossa at the midclavicular line, to allow an ideal triangulation during the operation. Sometimes, it could be useful to use a third 3–5 mm lateral operative port to move the colon or to suspend the aberrant vessels during the UPJ dissection.

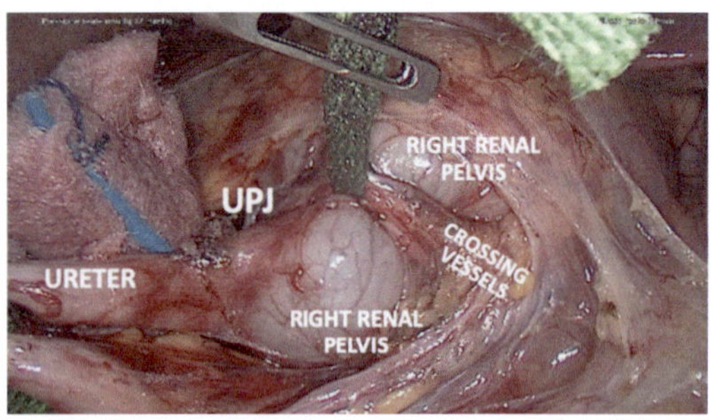

Fig. 16.4 Exposure of right dilated renal pelvis working just on the upper side of the colonic flexure that is freed. Suspension of CV

16.5 Technique

Once the operative trocar setting is obtained, the access to the retroperitoneal space is obtained on the left side, freeing the colonic flexure or usually through a window in the mesocolon, while on the right side, working just on the upper side of the colonic flexure that is freed (Fig. 16.4). Once the dilatated pelvis is identified, the obstructive CV must be visualized, dis-

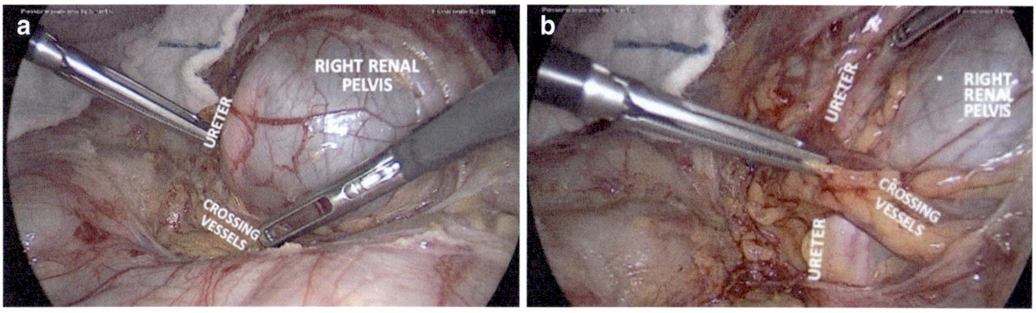

Fig. 16.5 (**a**) Dilated pelvis pre-diuretic test. (**b**) Empty pelvis after diuretic test and vessels mobilization

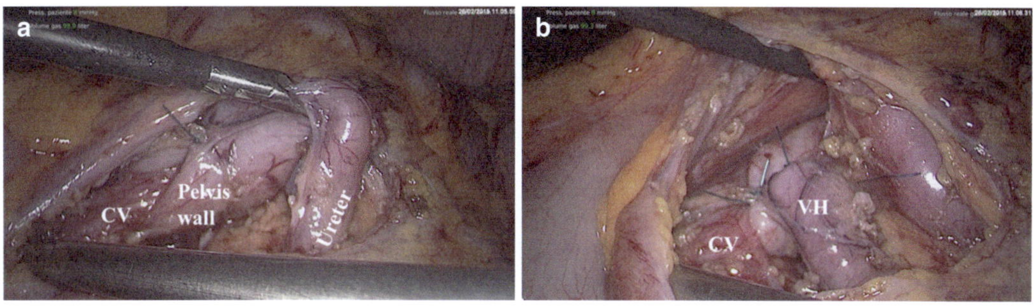

Fig. 16.6 (**a**) Loose wrap of the anterior pelvic wall around the aberrant polar vessels (pyelo-pyelic sleeve) (**b**). Vascular Hitch. To achieve and secure an adequate tunnel, the wrap with the anterior pelvic wall must be fixed with two/three interrupted stitches (3–4/0 non absorbable suture)

sected and mobilized off the UPJ and the proximal ureter. After complete mobilization of the CV pedicle, a diuretic test (DT) is then performed administering a bolus of normal saline (20 ml/kg IV before complete vessels mobilization), followed by furosemide (1 mg/kg IV). The success of the operation is obtained observing an easy urine passage through the junction (Fig. 16.5a, b). The UPJ is then carefully inspected for any ureter kinking and or intrinsic visible stenosis (significant narrowing). To be sure of a pure extrinsic obstruction, the CV must be temporarily transposed and the surgeon must observe: the peristalsis associated with the easy urine passage across the junction with satisfactory deflation of the renal pelvis. Once the test is successfully completed, the cranially displaced lower pole CV is then positioned away from the UPJ. Full mobility of the UPJ is confirmed by moving freely the upper and lower portions of the anterior pelvis wall just behind the CV as a shoeshine (shoeshine maneuver). At this point, a loose wrap of the anterior pelvic wall around the aberrant polar vessels (pyelo-pyelic sleeve) is prepared. To achieve and secure an adequate tunnel, the wrap with the anterior pelvic wall must be fixed with two/three interrupted stitches (3–4/0 non absorbable suture) (Fig. 16.6a, b). One possible tip is to pass the first suture transparietally, stabilizing and fixing the vascular bundle into the pelvic tunnel to assist the remaining suture. At the end of the procedure, it is very important to check the floppiness of the wrap and the absence of ischemia of the lower pole of the kidney. No double-J stent or abdominal drain is required.

16.6 Postoperative Care

In the postoperative period, the patients can start full oral feeding after few hours and according normal bowel movements. The analgesic requirement (Paracetamol every 6–8 h) is generally limited to the first 24 postoperative hours. All patients are discharged on the second or maximum on the third postoperative day.

16.7 Results and Personal Experience

In case of pure extrinsic-UPJO, the LVH success rate is almost 100% as reported in literature [7].

In our experience, median operative time was 95 min (range 45–125 min). Mean hospital stay was 2 days (range 2–4 days); these data are confirmed from recent literature that reports a median operative time of 105 min and a mean hospital stay of 1.8 days [7–9].

All patients treated underwent intraoperative-DT (furosemide) in the first stages of laparoscopy, which showed reduction of hydronephrosis after the complete mobilization of the vessels in 45 out of 48 children. A multicentric study by Chiarenza et al. reported similar results, in fact, after DT (furosemide), 51 out 54 patients were confirmed isolate extrinsic obstruction and underwent LCVT, while in three doubtful patients, dismember pyeloplasty was performed.

We did not report intraoperative or postoperative complications in our series of an 11 years-period. All patients had clinical evaluation and a renal-US at 1–6 months, and diuretic-renogram 6 months following surgery. Follow-up (range 12–132 months) showed complete resolution of symptoms (pain, hematuria) and decrease in hydronephrosis grade. Although none of the children displayed significant improvement in relative renal function, all of them showed improved drainage on 99mTc-MAG3-renogram and became unobstructed. One patient had recurrent symptoms of flank pain associated with recurrent pelvic dilatation 18 months after surgery. She underwent successful laparoscopic-AHDP 2 years after the original LVH-procedure. In our experience, long-term follow-up was very satisfactory; we followed at 5 years 37 patients. In all the patients, neither renal hypotrophy nor relapse and increase of renal blood pressure was recorded. At renal US, all the patients had complete resolution of the hydronephrosis, but four reported a mild hydronephrosis: three (SFU grade 1) and one (SFU grade 2) with occasional episodes of abdominal-flank pain. In the last patient, MAG3 renogram detected non obstructive pattern. Madec F. et al. reported similar results at long-term follow-up [7–11].

Tips and Tricks

- During laparoscopy, each case must be carefully evaluated regarding presence and position of CV, appearance of the UPJ, ureter course and DT-response of the dilated pelvis after vessels displacement. The main criteria to apply VH were the following: (I) hydronephrosis with presence of obstructing lower pole CV; (II) normal UPJ on inspection; (III) DT-response with emptying of the dilated pelvis after vessel displacement in order to confirm release of the obstruction and to exclude intrinsic-UPJ anomalies. We divided our patients with a suspicion of extrinsic UPJO by CV into two groups on the basis of anatomical relationships between CV, renal pelvis, UPJ and the ureter according Schneider's classification [6].
- In total, we treated 48 patients that we can divided into two groups.The AHDP group with the vessels placed in front of the UPJ, which present a really intrinsic stenosis (Schneider's second type): only three patients; the LVH group (45 patients), in which the vessels cross inferiorly the UPJ, resulting in variable ureteral kinking (defined as a ureteral curl or bend around the polar vessels similar to a swan-neck ureter), observing intraoperatively peristalsis and demonstrating the absence of intrinsic-UPJO (Schneider's third type). In particular, the very low incidence of relapse suggests that intraoperative-DT must be done and correctly in every suspect of extrinsic-UPJO (after CV transposition) to exclude associated intrinsic obstruction.

16.8 Discussion

UPJO is usually due to the presence of an aperistaltic-dysplastic narrow segment of the UPJ. It is often diagnosed with prenatal ultrasound, when a dilated pelvis is seen. The UPJ narrowing is caused by an incomplete recanalization process in utero at the cranial end of the ureter. The obstruction can result from an irregular arrangement (hypertrophied or virtually absent) of smooth muscle cells, causing a dysfunction of peristalsis. Besides this intrinsic etiology, crossing vessels (CV), as aberrant lower pole CV, represent the more frequent cause among extrinsic factors, above all in older children. CV are thought to cause from 40% to over 50% of extrinsic-UPJO in adults; they are more often ventrally located than dorsally to the UPJ; In the last case they are usually not obstructive. The arterial supply of accessory polar vessels usually arise directly from the aorta, while the venous supply arises from cava or iliac veins. The functional significance of vessels crossing the UPJ, causing the UPJ obstruction, is controversial and not a new one, but recently, thanks to the advent of advanced imaging techniques such as CT-scan and fMRU, the debate has been resurrected because of improved vessels detection.

The incidence of CV causing obstruction of the UPJ in children increases with age. CVs are very rarely noticed in newborns and infants. The CV incidence in children has been reported to range from 11 to 15%, but was as high as 58% in a series of older children with symptomatic UPJO and a history of normal antenatal renal ultrasonography. According to the literature, the average age of patients with a CV is between 7 and 11 years and is statistically higher than in patients with pure intrinsic obstruction. Open AHDP represents the gold standard procedure to treat UPJO in children, but the laparoscopic approach, developed in the last few decades, shows similar or even better outcomes. Laparoscopic pyeloureteral anastomosis in small children remains challenging, while robotic pyeloplasty in the last year has been felt to be technically easier. During the operation, in case of extrinsic polar CV, some authors have proposed AHDP to exclude intrinsic associated anomalies with the presence of CV. Nowadays, in case of pure extrinsic UPJO, valid minimally invasive alternative to AHDP can be considered laparoscopic vascular transposition. In the last years, we have assisted to an increasing number of papers regarding the treatment of pure extrinsic-UPJO by the relocation of lower pole CV in children The most recent series are reported by Schneider [6] and Miranda [12], with a successful outcome in up to 95% [13]; Polok, with a success rate of 93% [11] and by Chiarenza–Bleve, successful in 97% of patients, with a careful selection of candidates [14]. Meng and Stoller (in 2003) first reported laparoscopic vascular relocation using the Hellström technique in nine adults, with success in all cases. They observed that the herniation and subsequent ureteral kinking caused the obstruction and stated that changing the geometry may be enough to alleviate the obstacle [15]. Other important factors to consider are the numerous anatomical variants as described by Sampaio [16]. The double vascular bundles create a vascular window, facilitating the UPJ prolapse increasing obstruction. Vascular compression in these cases is in the proximal ureter. In these cases, the junction is certainly healthy, and the correction of the herniation is resolutive [6, 13]. This observation is supported histologically by the UPJ and CV analysis with the presence of normal muscle density, suggesting a different UPJ configuration between intrinsic and extrinsic obstruction. In this clinical condition, only patients with pure extrinsic-UPJO can be treated with this procedure, while any associated intrinsic UPJ abnormality must be ruled out. Janetschek has recommended always an UPJ exploration by a longitudinal incision in order to rule out the associated intrinsic anomalies, reported in up to 33% of their patients [17]. By histological analysis of resected UPJ tissue, some authors have showed evidence of intrinsic fibrosis and inflammation in cases where CV was thought to be the cause of obstruction. Some authors suggested that aberrant vessels may predispose the UPJ to the stenosis, favoring inflammatory episodes, infection; they could cause tension and ischemia, producing an urothelium fibrosis and stenosis, which could be one cause of the hypothetical failure of the VH-procedure [6, 12–18]. However, there is no evidence that the fibrosis can be progressive. Moreover, electron microscopy studies of extrinsic UPJ obstruction described immunohistochemically no significant structural changes in muscle or collagen content, in nerve distribution compared to normal controls, while intrinsically obstructed junction showed thinning of muscle fascicles with dense collagenous deposits when compared with controls. According to our experience, a careful patient selection is essential to obtain a high success rate performing LVH procedure. We usually consider three criteria: (1) preoperative patient selection; (2) accurate diagnostic studies; (3) performance of intraoperative-DT to confirm extrinsic obstruction. Among different imaging methods, preoperatory, none presents an accuracy of 100% in diagnosis of pure extrinsic-UPJO by CV. Indeed, we believe that an accurate clinical history remains the basis for correct selection of the patients affected from pure extrinsic-UPJO. In fact, it is mandatory to consider that these patients had usually no prenatal history of hydronephrosis; further, the majority presents intermittent colicky flank pain, sometimes associated with vomiting or hematuria. All patients show when symptomatic, marked hydronephrosis with a dilated pelvis associated to a mild calyceal dilatation that resolved shortly. Polok [11] reported success in 29/31 patients (93.54%); Godbole [18] in 12/13 patients with a median age of 10 years; Esposito C, Chiarenza S.F., Bleve C. et al. were successful in all 51 [8]. According to us, a success rate >90% with LVH procedure could be reached with close cooperation between surgeon and anesthesiologists to perform the intraoperative diuretic test correctly. The saline bolus needs to be timed so that the renal pelvis is well dilated prior to vessel dissection and mobilization. Once the aberrant pedicle is dissected away from the UPJ and after IV furosemide administration, a decreasing or emptying renal pelvis and a clear, visible peristalsis of UPJ usually confirm the extrinsic obstruction. If UPJ has intrinsic abnormalities associated, pelvic dilatation remains even after furosemide administration. The test is crucial because it allows to discriminate a variability in cases related to different factors: to the location of the abnormal vessels and their relations with the ureter and UPJ; the size of the vessels; the presence of hydronephrosis with sufficient tissue to allow the VH (index of the presence of an obstruction); the junction size and the presence of ureteral peristalsis. Miranda et al. performed laparoscopic vascular hitch with modified Whitaker test in 4 of 11 children. A fine needle was inserted percutaneously into the renal pelvis and the ureteral opening pressure was evaluated three times using a water column device. They assumed that if the opening pressure was lower than 14 cm of water, then the junction was considered to be unobstructed [6, 12]. VH procedure allows to preserve the UPJ integrity, eliminating the risk of leakage or urinoma and preserving the physiologic pyelo-ureteral motility and ureteral peristalsis; in addition, operative time is shorter. In our opinion, there is no need for invasive procedures like the Whitaker test. The puncture of the pelvis causes the risk of complications.

LVH is also particularly indicated and recommended in patients with symptomatic hydronephrosis due to CV in particular anatomic condition such as horseshoe kidney. In these cases, the UPJ anatomy is not favorable to a resection/re-anastomosis between ureter and renal pelvis [10]. As for the technical point of view, in our mind, laparoscopic vascular hitch seems to be effective and safe as procedure, but can only be performed on carefully selected patients (based on preoperative clinical and radiologic findings that are diagnostic of extrinsic-UPJO). The classical intraoperative, diuretic test with furosemide is simple to perform, does not extend the surgical time and maybe could reduce the risk of misdiagnosis.

References

1. Anderson JC, Hynes W. Retrocaval ureter; a case diagnosed pre-operatively and treated successfully by a plastic operation. Br J Urol. 1949;21:209–14.
2. Von Rokitansky CF. Handbuch der Pathologischen Anatomie. Vienna, Austria: Braumüller und Seidel; 1842.

3. Hellström J, Giertz G, Lindblom K. Pathogenesis and treatment of hydronephrosis. In: Presentedat VIII Congreso de la Sociedad International de Urologia, Paris, France. 1949.
4. Chapman TL. Urology in outline, vol. 82. Edinburgh, London: Churchill Livingstone; 1959.
5. Pesce C, Campobasso P, Costa L, Battaglino F, Musi L. Ureterovascular hydronephrosis in children: is pyeloplasty always necessary? Eur Urol. 1999;36:71–4.
6. Schneider A, Gomes FC, Delay C, Lacreuse I, Moog R, Becmeur F. Lower pole vessels in children with pelviureteric junction obstruction: laparoscopic vascular hitch or dismembered pyeloplasty? J Pediatr Urol. 2013;9:419–23.
7. Madec FX, Faraj S, Villemagne T, Fourcade L, Lardy H, Leclair MD. Laparoscopic transposition of lower-pole crossing vessels: long-term follow-up of 33 patients at puberty. J Pediatr Urol. 2016;12(4):226.e1–6.
8. Esposito C, Bleve C, Escolino M, Caione P, Gerocarni NS, Farina A, Caprio MG, Cerulo M, La Manna A, Chiarenza SF. Laparoscopic transposition of lower pole crossing vessels (vascular hitch) in children with pelviureteric junction obstruction. Transl Pediatr. 2016;5(4):256–61.
9. Chiarenza SF, Bleve C, Caione P, Escolino M, Gerocarni NS, Perretta R, La Manna A, Esposito C. Minimally invasive treatment of pediatric extrinsic ureteropelvic junction obstruction by crossing polar vessels: is vascular hitching a definitive solution? Report of a multicenter survey. J Laparoendosc Adv Surg Tech. 2017;27(9):965–71.
10. Bleve C, Bucci V, Conighi ML, Battaglino F, Costa L, Fasoli L, Zolpi E, Chiarenza SF. Horseshoe kidney and uretero-pelvic-junction obstruction in a pediatric patient. Laparoscopic vascular hitch: a valid alternative to dismembered pyeloplasty? Pediatr Med Chir. 2017;39(4):178. https://doi.org/10.4081/pmc.2017.178.
11. Polok M, Toczewski K, Borselle D, Apoznański W, Jędrzejuk D, Patkowski D. Hydronephrosis in children caused by lower pole crossing vessels-how to choose the proper method of treatment? Front Pediatr. 2019;7:83. https://doi.org/10.3389/fped.2019.00083. eCollection 2019.
12. Miranda ML, Pereira LH, Cavalaro MA, Carvalho Pegolo P, De Oliveira-Filho AG, Murray Bustorff-Silva J. Laparoscopic transposition of lower pole crossing vessels (vascular hitch) in children with pelviureteric junction obstruction: how to be sure of the success of the procedure? J Laparoendosc Adv Surg Tech. 2015;25(10):847–51.
13. Gundeti MS, Reynolds WS, Duffy PG, et al. Further experience with the vascular hitch (laparoscopic transposition of lower pole crossing vessels): an alternate treatment for pediatric ureterovascular ureteropelvic junction obstruction. J Urol. 2008;180:1832–6; discussion 1836.
14. Chiarenza SF, Bleve C, Fasoli L, et al. Ureteropelvic junction obstruction in children by polar vessels. Is laparoscopic vascular hitching procedure a good solution? Single center experience on 35 consecutive patients. J Pediatr Surg. 2016;51:310–4.
15. Meng MV, Stoller ML. Hellström technique revisited: laparoscopic management of ureteropelvic junction obstruction. Urology. 2003;62:404–8; discussion 408–9.
16. Sampaio FJ. The dilemma of the crossing vessel at the ureteropelvic junction: precise anatomic study. J Endourol. 1996;10:411–5.
17. Janetschek G, Peschel R, Franscher F. Laparoscopic pyeloplasty. Urol Clin North Am. 2000;27:695–704.
18. Godbole P, Mushtaq I, Wilcox DT, et al. Laparoscopic transposition of lower pole vessels e the 'vascular hitch': an alternative to dismembered pyeloplasty for pelvi-ureteric junction obstruction in children. J Pediatr Urol. 2006;2:285–9.

17 Minimally Invasive Redo-Pyeloplasty

Holger Till, Maria Escolino, and Ciro Esposito

Learning Objectives
- To describe step by step the technique of laparoscopic redo AHP.
- To describe the major aspects of robot-assisted redo AHP.
- To show a video of robot-assisted redo AHP.
- To present the latest results of international papers about redo AHP.

17.1 Introduction

Laparoscopic Anderson–Hynes pyeloplasty (AHP) has already been described in a previous chapter. In summary, it gained rapid acceptance among pediatric urologists once it had been technically refined and granted similar success rates like open AHP [1, 2]. Nevertheless, recurrences occur either by extrinsic causes like perirenal fibrosis, malposition of the primary AHP, kinking of the ureter or intrinsic scarring of the anastomosis. Besides endourological salvage maneuvers, redo pyeloplasty has been established for such cases with good functional results in experienced hands [3, 4]. The cornerstones for redo AHP remain the same as for primary pyeloplasty such as lateral spatulation of the ureter and tension free, water-tight anastomosis at the most dependent part of the renal pelvis. When robotic surgery was introduced, it became obvious that this technology can provide major advantages in both primary and redo AHP during dissection and suturing in restricted spaces [5–8].

The following manuscript elucidates the cornerstones of transperitoneal redo pyeloplasty with special attention to technical details of laparoscopic and robot-assisted approaches.

17.2 Preoperative Preparation

Patients for surgery must have proven secondary functional UPJO. Documentation include ultrasonography, holdup or significant delay in drainage on MAG3 diuretic renal renography and, in special cases, even radiologic demonstration of obstruction in an excretory urography. Preoperative retrograde pyelogram can also be performed so as to ascertain the anatomy of the

Supplementary Information The online version contains supplementary material available at [https://doi.org/10.1007/978-3-030-99280-4_17].

H. Till (✉)
Department of Paediatric and Adolescent Surgery, Medical University of Graz, Graz, Austria
e-mail: holger.till@medunigraz.at

M. Escolino · C. Esposito
Department of Pediatric Surgery, Federico II University of Naples, Naples, Italy
e-mail: maria.escolino@unina.it; ciroespo@unina.it

C. Esposito et al. (eds.), *Minimally Invasive Techniques in Pediatric Urology*,
https://doi.org/10.1007/978-3-030-99280-4_17

ureter and pelvis. Associated abnormalities like pelvic kidney or horseshoe kidney must be evident prior to surgery.

The child is given a preoperative enema the night before surgery. Preoperative antibiotic prophylaxis should be administered either with a broad spectrum medication or according to the child's specific urine testing.

Before surgery, parents are counselled for the minimal invasive procedure and the option for open surgery.

17.3 Positioning

17.3.1 For Conventional Laparoscopy

Positioning of the patient for redo AHP follows the same rules as for primary surgery. Before positioning the patient, most pediatric urologists would place a transurethral foley bladder catheter and connect it to a drainage bag as well as to a saline infusion bag for later "blue test" of the transanastomotic stent. Then the patient is placed in a semi-lateral position close to the edge of the operating table, with the ipsilateral side elevated. The patient is stabilized using adhesive bandage strapping to the operating table to allow rotation if deemed necessary.

17.3.2 For Robot-Assisted Approach

The patient is placed supine, and the affected side is elevated approximately 30° by placing a wedge cushion or jelly-roll under the patient's back. The patient is padded and secured firmly to the table. With tilting of the table, the intestines and colon fall away from the renal fossa. A sterile Foley catheter is inserted into the bladder.

17.4 Instrumentation for Conventional Laparoscopy

Essential

- 5 mm 30° laparoscope
- 2 × 3–5 mm working ports
- 3–5 mm atraumatic grasping forceps and scissors with fine tips
- 3–5 mm diathermy hook
- 3–5 mm needle holder
- Gauge 18 venous cannula.
- Fr 4 or Fr 5 double pigtail stent over guidewire.

Sutures

- 6–0 Vicryl sutures for infants
- 5–0 Vicryl sutures for children/adolescents
- 4- Prolene suture, straight needle to elevate the renal pelvis ("hitch-stitch")

17.5 Instrumentation for Robot-Assisted Approach

Essential

- 8 mm 30° robotic optic
- 2 × 8 mm robotic ports
- 1 × 5 mm conventional laparoscopic port
- Double pigtail stent over Terumo guidewire.
- 8 mm robotic monopolar curved scissors
- 8 mm robotic Cadiere grasper
- 8 mm robotic Maryland bipolar forceps
- 8 mm robotic needle driver
- 5 mm laparoscopic instruments (scissors, grasper, irrigation/suction device) to be used through the 5 mm assistant port.

Sutures

- 6–0 polydiaxone sutures
- 5–0 polydiaxone sutures

17.6 Technical Details of Laparoscopic Redo AHP

If the primary surgery had used a transperitoneal access and the original trocar positions seem to ergonomically fit the present procedure, the old scars should be used. For placement of the optic trocar, a 5–7 mm Hasson technique is used at the umbilicus. Two additional 3–5 mm instrument ports are introduced under direct vision. Redo surgery on the right side may require a liver retractor, which can easily be employed by a simple grasper crossing the entire upper abdomen underneath the liver and anchoring in the diaphragm.

Access to the UPJO does not differ from primary AHP except that the "heritage" of the previous surgery must be handled, i.e., adhesions of the colon to the kidney of peripelvic fibrosis requiring blunt and sharp dissection. Care must be taken in preserving the peri-ureteric vasculature. Any fibrotic band kinking the ureter is divided.

A hitch stitch to elevate the renal pelvis may make the procedure much easier, e.g., a 4/0 Prolene suture over a straight needle is passed percutaneously through the abdominal wall to the upper pole of the renal pelvis and passed back through the abdominal wall at the same entry point. This stitch serves to mark the upper limit of the line of the pyeloplasty during pelvic-ureteric anastomosis. More importantly, it also serves as a hitch stitch to stabilize and present the pelvis to facilitate intracorporeal suturing during the anastomosis. The renal pelvis is dismembered above the area of the pathology. Some authors recommend additional excision of redundant renal pelvis. If a concomitant intrarenal stone is present, at this point it is ideal using a flexible scope. If crossing vessels are still present, the ureter and renal pelvis are transposed to the opposite side. Finally, the proximal ureter is disconnected distal to the fibrotic segment and adequately spatulated on the lateral aspect.

Reconstruction starts with suturing the most dependent part of the renal pelvis to the apex of the spatulated ureter and continued at the posterior wall of the reduced renal pelvis (continuous or interrupted sutures). A stent is being placed transanastomotic and into the bladder. Its correct position may be confirmed by Methylen blue test.

Thereafter the anterior layer of the pelviureteric anastomosis is completed with continuous sutures and tied intracorporeally at the upper corner with the suture from the posterior anastomotic sutures.

The hitch stitch is released and the UPJ and the upper ureter are inspected to ensure a good, tension-free anastomosis and that no kinking has occurred.

17.7 Technical Details of Robot-Assisted Redo AHP

Peritoneal access is gained transumbilically using open technique with an 8 mm robotic port. A pneumoperitoneum of 12–15 mmHg is created and the robotic optic is introduced. Two additional 8 mm robotic ports are placed under direct vision, one in the midline between the umbilicus and the xyphoid, and the second in the mid-clavicular line 2 cm below the umbilicus. Finally, the fourth 5 mm assistant port is positioned on the pararectal line, mean 7-cm caudal to the robotic camera port. The table is tilted to raise the affected side. The DaVinci robot system (Intuitive Surgical, Sunnyvale, CA) is brought over the ipsilateral shoulder and is docked, using a three-arm configuration. Patient, trocars and robotic team positioning is represented in Fig. 17.1.

Adhesions with ipsilateral gut and omentum are first identified and adhesiolysis is performed releasing the gut and omentum (Fig. 17.2a). Then, the ipsilateral gut is mobilized in order to expose the retroperitoneal area. The ureter is identified in the virgin field, significantly below the UPJ (Fig. 17.2b). Careful dissection is then performed upward to expose the renal pelvis using blunt and sharp dissection with Maryland bipolar forceps and monopolar scissors that release the surrounding fibrosed tissue (Fig. 17.3a). Thereafter, the ureter and the pelvis are transected with excision of the fibrosed segment (Fig. 17.3b). The spatulation of the ureter on the lateral side and transection of the redundant renal pelvis is carried out (Fig. 17.3c). Identification of any crossing vessels, dismissed in the previous surgery, and their transposition behind the UPJ are performed. The AHP is carried out with 6–0 or 5–0 polydiaxone interrupted or running sutures, according to the surgeon's preference.

Once the posterior wall of pelvi-ureteric anastomosis is completed (Fig. 17.4a), a double-J stent is placed into the ureter in an anterograde fashion through the assistant port over a Terumo guidewire (Fig. 17.4b). Finally, the anterior wall of anastomosis is completed as

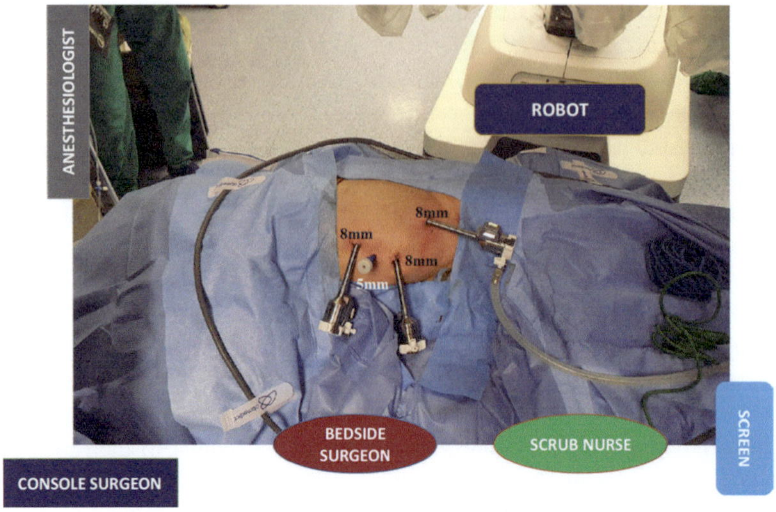

Fig. 17.1 Patient, trocars and robotic team positioning in robot-assisted redo AHP

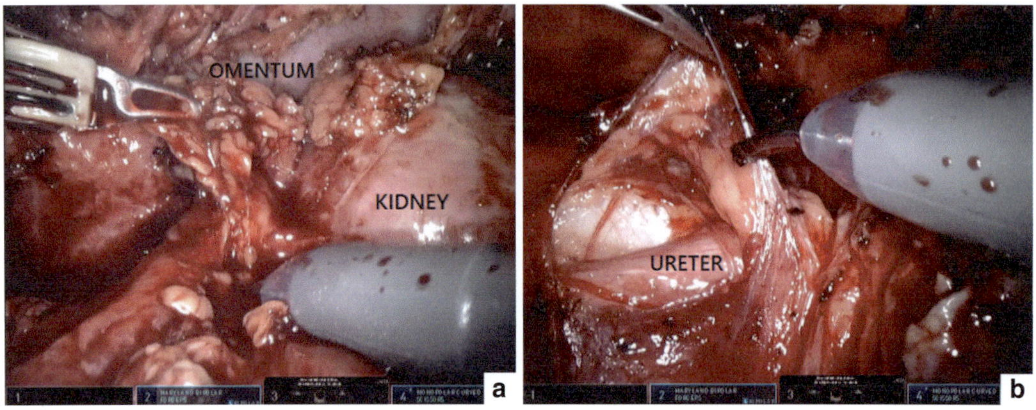

Fig. 17.2 Redo robot-assisted AHP technique: the adhesions with omentum are released and the ureter is isolated in a virgin field

well (Fig. 17.4c). An abdominal drain is placed through the 5-mm assistant port (Fig. 17.5). Trocars' orifices are closed using resorbable sutures.

17.8 Postoperative Care

Redo AHP usually requires no different postoperative care compared with primary surgery. Depending on the intraoperative findings, hospital setting and healthcare system, the patient is started on normal diet as tolerated on day 1 post-operatively and progressed accordingly. Postoperative analgesia is given until discharge. The Foley catheter and abdominal drain are usually removed after 2–3 days. The antibiotic prophylaxis is administered until the double pigtail stent is removed which is around 3–4 weeks after surgery. Unlike primary AHP, MAG3 diuretic renal renography may be advisable 3 months after removal of the stent.

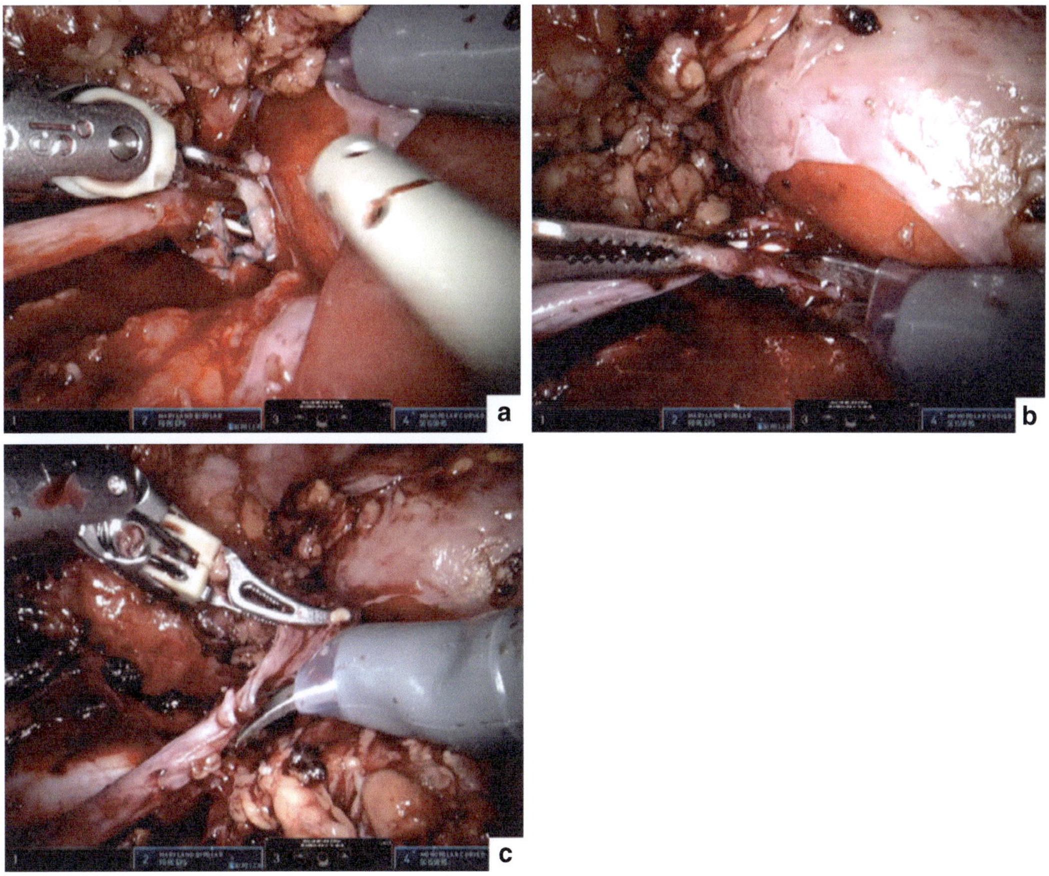

Fig. 17.3 Redo robot-assisted AHP technique: the previous AHP is identified (**a**), it is sectioned (**b**) and the ureter is spatulated laterally (**c**)

Tips and Tricks

- A hitch-stitch to elevate the renal pelvis may make several steps much easier.
- Avoid devascularization of the ureter.
- Avoid a secondary anastomosis under tension.
- Avoid urine leak and urinoma, as it translates into peripelvic fibrosis.
- Ensure adequate placement of stent intraoperatively.
- Identify and uncross any crossing vessels missed in the previous surgery.

17.9 Discussion

Recurrent UPJO is mostly the result of technical issues such as urinary extravasation leading to peripelvic fibrosis, ischemic injury to the ureter by excessive use of thermal energy or anastomosis under tension, which can cause more tissue reaction and fibrosis [9]. Once secondary UPJO has been confirmed by ultrasonography, MAG3 diuretic renal renography and, in special cases, even radiologic demonstration of obstruction in an excretory urography, drainage procedures may not be delayed. An attempt can be made to sal-

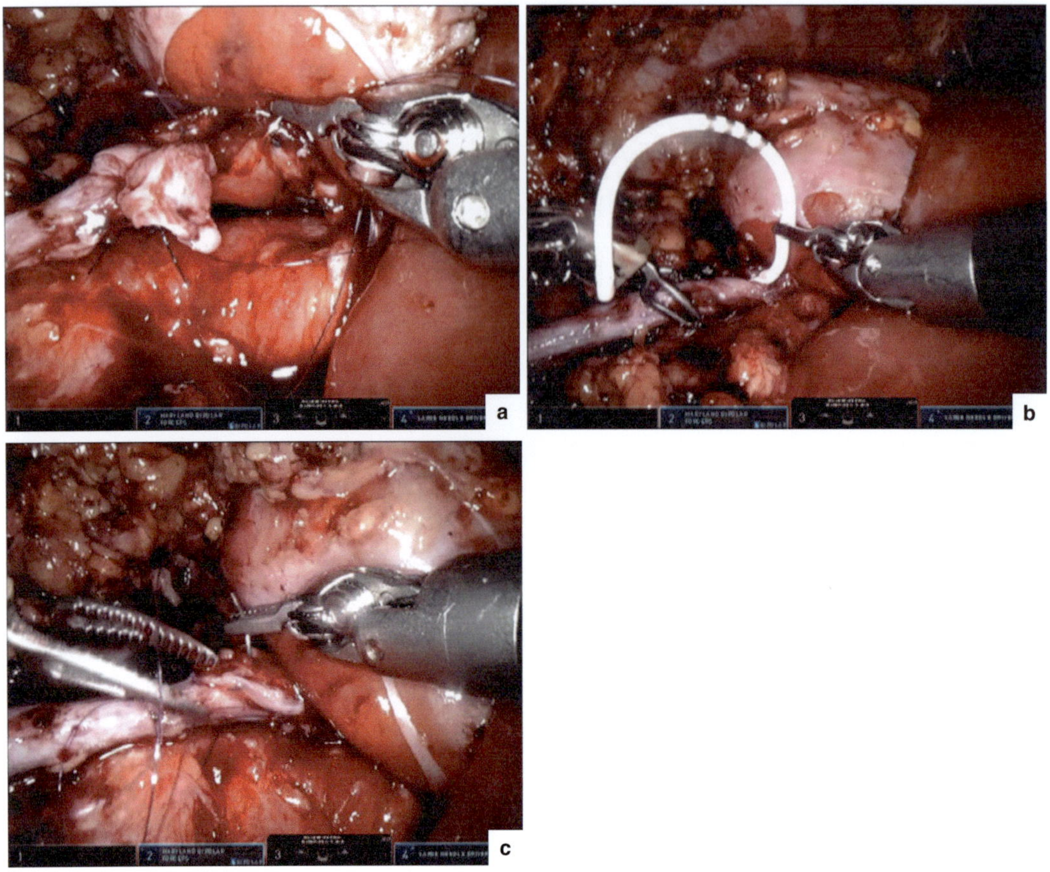

Fig. 17.4 Redo robot-assisted AHP technique: the posterior wall of new AHP is reconstructed (**a**), a double-J stent is inserted (**b**) and the anterior wall of new AHP is completed (**c**)

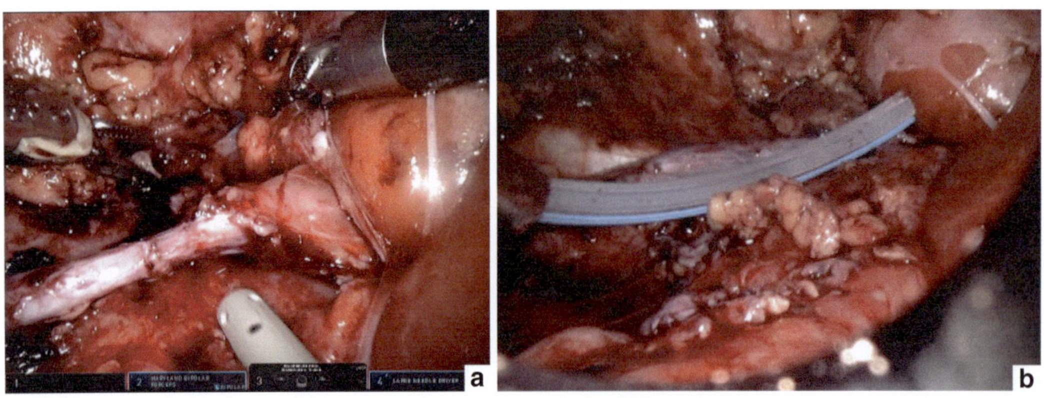

Fig. 17.5 Redo robot-assisted AHP technique: final result of redo AHP (**a**), an indwelling abdominal drain is finally placed (**b**)

vage the primary surgery by repetitive stenting, balloon dilatation or even endopyelotomy [10]. However, if the child remains symptomatic and renal function decreases, redo surgery is needed. Basically, redo surgery should aim to replace the primary pyeloplasty by a "better one." Care must be taken to preserve adequate blood supply to the upper ureter and renal pelvis and to create a tension free anastomosis at the most dependent part of the renal pelvis.

The access for redo pyeloplasty remains a matter of discussion. One basic consideration could be to avoid the primary access if possible, i.e., to choose the transperitoneal route in cases that had primarily been operated retroperitoneally and vice versa. On the other hand, the surgeon's experience with the "alternative route" should be excellent, because redo surgery will most likely be more demanding. In cases of long segment strictures of the ureter, a transperitoneal approach for redo pyeloplasty could be advisable because, unlike a retroperitoneal access laparoscopy, it allows for careful mobilization of the ureter all the way down to the bladder.

Laparoscopic redo pyeloplasty has gained increasing acceptance because it achieves almost comparable results like open redo pyeloplasty while providing the advantages of minimally invasive surgery. In a comparative study of open versus laparoscopic redo pyeloplasty in children [4], the authors found a 91.7% success rate of laparoscopic redo pyeloplasty vs. 100% in open redo pyeloplasty. Compared with redo open pyeloplasty, the mean operative time was longer (211.4 ± 32.2 vs. 148.8 ± 16.6, $P = 0.002$), estimated blood loss was higher (102 vs. 75 ml, $P = 0.06$), while hospital stay was shorter and pain score was lower in the laparoscopy group ($P = 0.02$). There were no intraoperative complications, while the postoperative complication rate was similar in the two groups (20.8 vs. 20.0%).

Although the laparoscopic technique mimics open surgery, it is not as versatile; however, it becomes technically more challenging in case of failed pyeloplasty.

More recently, the introduction of robotic system has reported additional advantages over conventional laparoscopy as it offers three-dimensional vision with increased magnification and depth of perception; it filters tremor and it provides an excellent surgeon's ergonomics [11, 12]. The dynamic versatility of EndoWrist Instrumentation allows easy intracorporeal suturing in a magnified 3-D environment. All these features result in an easier reconstructive procedure compared with laparoscopy and are useful especially in challenging scenarios such as recurrent UPJO [13].

In recent years, redo robot-assisted laparoscopic pyeloplasty (RALP) has gained wider acceptance because of the excellent exposure, delicate maneuvering of the instrument to facilitate fine dissection and the superb wrist-movement to re-establish the anastomosis [14–16]. This growing evidence reported very good outcomes of redo RALP in terms of feasibility, efficacy, safety and durability of the procedure [14–16]. Further studies and long-term follow-up evaluation should be awaited to confirm this evidence.

Take-Home Points

- Laparoscopic redo AHP can be safely and effectively performed in infants and children.
- The robot technology adds technical advantages such as the magnification of the view to identify peripelvic fibrosis and the "wrist-movement" for easy suturing.
- Larger series comparing "conventional laparoscopic" versus "robot-assisted" redo pyeloplasty are limited.
- Redo pyeloplasty requires advanced skills and should be reserved for experts in pediatric urology and specialized centers offering a variety of techniques and alternatives for management of secondary UPJO.

References

1. Wu Y, Dong Q, Han P, Liu L, Wang L, Wei Q. Meta-analysis of transperitoneal versus retroperitoneal approaches of laparoscopic pyeloplasty for uretero-pelvic junction obstruction. J Laparoendosc Adv Surg Tech A. 2012;22(7):658–62.
2. Huang Y, Wu Y, Shan W, Zeng L, Huang L. An updated meta-analysis of laparoscopic versus open pyeloplasty for ureteropelvic junction obstruction in children. Int J Clin Exp Med. 2015;8(4):4922–31.
3. Alhazmi HH. Redo laparoscopic pyeloplasty among children: a systematic review and meta-analysis. Urol Ann. 2018;10(4):347–53.
4. Abdel-Karim AM, Fahmy A, Moussa A, et al. Laparoscopic pyeloplasty versus open pyeloplasty for recurrent ureteropelvic junction obstruction in children. J Pediatr Urol. 2016;12(6):401.e1–6.
5. Esposito C, Masieri L, Castagnetti M, et al. Robot-assisted vs laparoscopic pyeloplasty in children with uretero-pelvic junction obstruction (UPJO): technical considerations and results. J Pediatr Urol. 2019;15(6):667.e1–8.
6. Salö M, Sjöberg Altemani T, Anderberg M. Pyeloplasty in children: perioperative results and long-term outcomes of robotic-assisted laparoscopic surgery compared to open surgery. Pediatr Surg Int. 2016;32(6):599–607.
7. Tam YH, Pang KKY, Wong YS, Chan KW, Lee KH. From laparoscopic pyeloplasty to robot-assisted laparoscopic pyeloplasty in primary and reoperative repairs for ureteropelvic junction obstruction in children. J Laparoendosc Adv Surg Tech A. 2018;28(8):1012–8.
8. Davis TD, Burns AS, Corbett ST, Peters CA. Reoperative robotic pyeloplasty in children. J Pediatr Urol. 2016;12(6):394.e1–7.
9. Persky L, McDougal WS, Kedia K. Management of initial pyeloplasty failure. J Urol. 1981;125:695–7.
10. Abdrabuh AM, Salih EM, Aboelnasr M, Galal H, El-Emam A, El-Zayat T. Endopyelotomy versus redo pyeloplasty for management of failed pyeloplasty in children: a single center experience. J Pediatr Surg. 2018;53(11):2250–5.
11. Spinoit AF, Nguyen H, Subramaniam R. Role of robotics in children: a brave New World! Eur Urol Focus. 2017;3(2–3):172–80.
12. Tasian GE, Casale P. The robotic-assisted laparoscopic pyeloplasty: gateway to advanced reconstruction. Urol Clin North Am. 2015;42(1):89–97.
13. Atug F, Burgess SV, Castle EP, Thomas R. Role of robotics in the management of secondary ureteropelvic junction obstruction. Int J Clin Pract. 2006;60(1):9–11.
14. Asensio M, Gander R, Royo GF, Lloret J. Failed pyeloplasty in children: is robot-assisted laparoscopic reoperative repair feasible? J Pediatr Urol. 2015;11(2):69.e1–69.e696.
15. Hemal AK, Mishra S, Mukharjee S, Suryavanshi M. Robot assisted laparoscopic pyeloplasty in patients of ureteropelvic junction obstruction with previously failed open surgical repair. Int J Urol. 2008;15(8):744–6.
16. Jacobson DL, Shannon R, Johnson EK, et al. Robot-assisted laparoscopic reoperative repair for failed pyeloplasty in children: an updated series. J Urol. 2019;201(5):1005–11.

18 Nephrectomy: Robotic Approach

Lorenzo Masieri, Giulia Bortot, Chiara Cini, Simone Sforza, and Alberto Mantovani

Learning Objectives
- To describe surgical steps of Robot-Assisted Radical Nephrectomy (RARN).
- To report the updates about the indications for RARN in Pediatric Urology.
- To describe tips and tricks of RARN in pediatric urology.
- To show a video of RARN technique.

18.1 Introduction

Radical nephrectomy (RN) is the recommended surgical approach in several diseases, in both adults and children.

In pediatric age, the indications for RN include benign diseases such as:

- Multicystic or dysplastic kidneys with or without renal hypertension.
- Non-functioning kidneys associated with reflux nephropathy.
- Non-functioning hydronephrotic kidney/infected kidney.
- Kidney-mediated hypertension not responding to pharmacological therapy.
- Xanthogranulomatous pyelonephritis.
- Protein-losing nephropathy (pre-transplantation nephrectomy).

And malignant diseases:

- Wilms tumor.
- Other renal tumors (renal cells carcinoma, RCC…) [1].

Currently, nephrectomy can be performed by different surgical approaches such as open surgery or mini-invasive surgery.

Open RN can be performed via retroperitoneal access (posterior or lateral) or with an anterolateral transperitoneal approach.

Regarding mini-invasive surgery, laparoscopic trans-peritoneal nephrectomy is a well-standardized procedure; more recently, robotic approach has also gained popularity in the pediatric field [2].

This chapter is focused on the operative technique of robot-assisted laparoscopic radical nephrectomy (RALN).

Supplementary Information The online version contains supplementary material available at [https://doi.org/10.1007/978-3-030-99280-4_18].

L. Masieri · G. Bortot (✉) · C. Cini · S. Sforza (✉)
A. Mantovani
Pediatric Urology Department, Meyer's Children Hospital, Florence, Italy
e-mail: lorenzo.masieri@meyer.it; giulia.bortot@meyer.it; chiara.cini@meyer.it; simone.sforza@unifi.it; alberto.mantovani@meyer.it

C. Esposito et al. (eds.), *Minimally Invasive Techniques in Pediatric Urology*,
https://doi.org/10.1007/978-3-030-99280-4_18

18.2 Preoperative Assessment

Preoperative examination should focus on clinical evaluation and patient's history. Anatomic characteristics of kidney and urinary tract, renal vessels and loco-regional nodes are defined with radiological investigations: renal ultrasonography (US), abdominal MRI scan or CT scan. Renal scintigraphy is used to evaluate residual renal function and the contralateral kidney.

It is important to emphasize that every patient is evaluated by a multidisciplinary team with pediatric nephrologists, radiologists, oncologists, in addition to urologists, in order to define the appropriate pathway.

Surgical procedure is discussed and described to parents and patients during the outpatient evaluation. A specifically formulated informed consent is administered during the last visit and has to be signed before the procedure. We endorse and apply, before, during and after any surgery, the WHO Surgical Safety Checklist. We check using a validated Italian translation of the original version [3].

Children are hospitalized the day before surgery. Regarding the prompt preoperative management, we usually do not prescribe intestinal preparation, but fasting from food or artificial milk is needed for at least 6 h, from breastfeeding for at least 4 h, from clear liquids for 1 h [4].

Patients receive a general anesthesia with orotracheal intubation, myorelaxation and transversus abdominis plane (TAP) block.

A Foley catheter is positioned into the bladder using sterile precautions just before surgery and is usually removed on first—second postop day, after complete mobilization of the patient. A nasogastric tube is placed in order to keep empty the stomach during the procedure and removed at the end of the surgery.

All patients receive antibiotic prophylaxis at the induction of anesthesia with broad-spectrum antibiotic (usually third generation cephalosporin).

18.3 Patient Positioning

The patient is placed in a semi-lateral decubitus close to the edge of the table, rotating the operative side up by 45° axially with the help of silicone pads underneath (Figs. 18.1 and 18.2). This position, allowing the retraction of the colon, provides a clear dissection of the ureter and a safe access to the renal pedicle.

Both the robotic console DaVinci® Xi and Si (Intuitive Surgery, Sunnyvale, CA) are available in our center. The surgeon sits at the console and the assistant stands at the operative table facing the monitor for laparoscopic assistance.

Three-arm configuration is usually set for a simple nephrectomy with a 5 mm port for the assistant. An additional trocar, if needed, can be placed more often on the right side, to retract the liver or on the left side to retract the spleen.

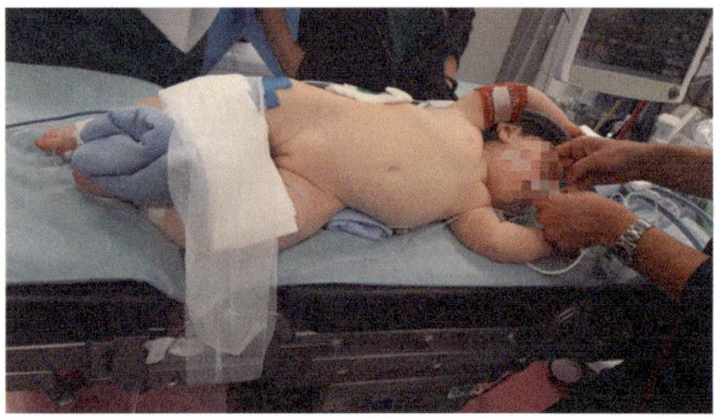

Fig. 18.1 Left flank position

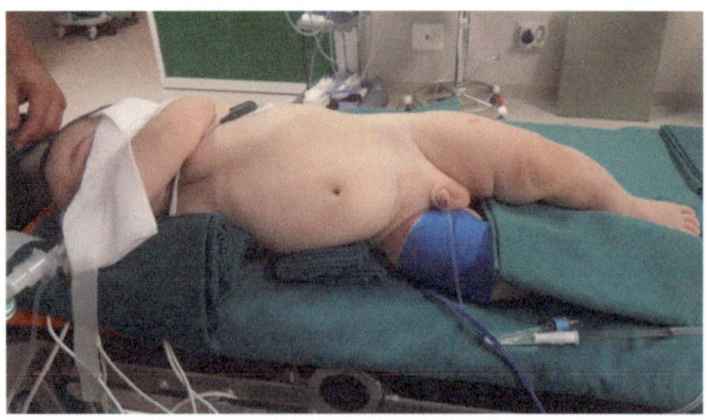

Fig. 18.2 Right flank position

18.4 Trocars and Instruments

We adopt an 8/10-mm trocar for 30-degree camera and 8 mm-robotic ports, while the assistant usually has a 5-mm trocar. We use monopolar curved scissors for the right robotic arm and Maryland fenestrated bipolar forceps for the left robotic arm. A robotic needle driver is rarely adopted for this procedure. The assistant may use laparoscopic Johann atraumatic fenestrated grasping forceps, suction device, clip applier, curved Metzenbaum scissors, endo clinch or needle holder, Hem-o-lok applier.

The hilar vessel control is usually performed using 5-mm titanium clips, or alternatively, using hemostatic devices such as Hem-o-lok, depending on vessels' size. An endo-bag is needed to remove the kidney, that is usually exteriorized through a mini-Pfannenstiel incision or through the umbilical port, depending on the dimension of the kidney.

18.5 Technique

RARN can be carried out through either a retroperitoneal or transperitoneal approach.

18.5.1 Transperitoneal Approach

We first place the 8/10 mm camera trocar infraumbilically: after the induction of pneumoperitoneum (8–10 mmHg), we insert the two 8-mm robotic trocars under vision. Robotic ports are placed on the emiclavear line, one 2 cm under the subcostal arch and the other 3 cm above the inguinal ligament. The 5-mm assistant port is positioned on the pararectal line, mean 6-cm caudal to the robotic camera port.

The ports are positioned in a sort of 'kite-like' appearance and as far apart as possible to reduce collisions (Fig. 18.3). Moreover, a slight traction of trocars, tenting the abdominal wall, appears to us useful to create some extra room and have adequate working space [5].

The da Vinci Xi or Si robot is then docked.

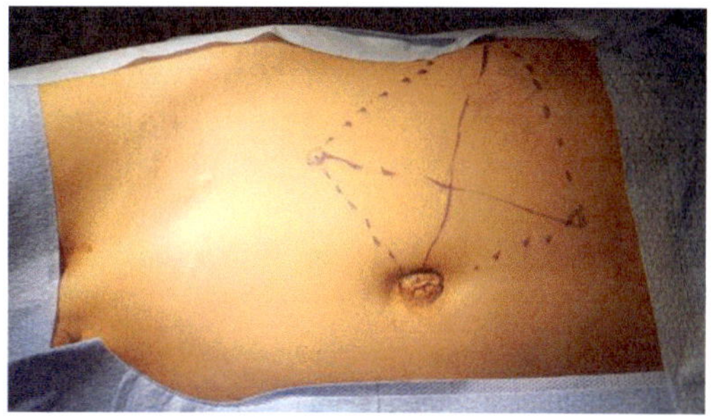

Fig. 18.3 Kite-like positioning of trocars

The colon is detached in correspondence of the Toldt's line and lowered. We then open the Gerota's fascia in order to have access to the kidney. The ureter is identified, isolated and clipped. The next step is to identify and isolate hilar vessels and possible accessory vessels. In dysplastic kidneys, aberrant arterial supply is common.

After the kidney is completely isolated, hilar vessels are clipped with titanium clip or Hem-o-lock and divided. Another option to manage the vessels is to seal them using sealing device, but we usually prefer the first technique.

Once resected, the kidney is placed into an endo-bag and then removed through a mini-Pfannenstiel incision, or through the umbilical port, depending on the size. An abdominal drainage can be left to check postoperative leakage, even if usually it is not necessary. Urethral catheter is usually removed on first—second postop day, after complete mobilization of the patient.

18.5.2 Retroperitoneal Approach

The 11th and 12th ribs, the iliac crest and the lumbar muscles are identified (Fig. 18.4).

An incision (1–1.5 cm) at the tip of the 12th rib following the anterior margin of the rib itself is performed, and the posterior fascia is opened to access the retroperitoneum. The retroperitoneal space is created performing a blunt dissection with gauzes, a dissection balloon or finger-guided maneuvers. These maneuvers have to be extremely delicate to avoid accidental lesions to the peritoneum that would allow the passage of

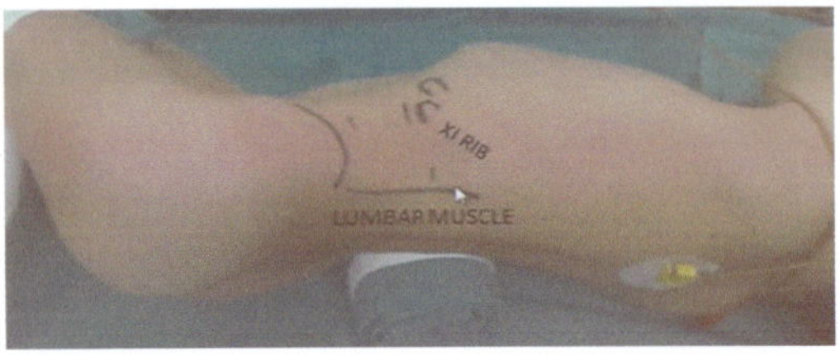

Fig. 18.4 Landmarks for retroperitoneal approach

gas in the abdomen, consequently losing the retroperitoneal space. An 8 mm trocar is positioned.

An 8–10 mm trocar for the camera is positioned on the iliac crest along the mid-axillary line. An 8 mm robotic trocar is then positioned along the psoas muscle below the 12th rib-vertebra angle.

Once all the trocars are positioned, pneumoperitoneum is induced and the da Vinci Si® or Xi® robotic surgical system (Intuitive Surgical, Sunnyvale, CA) is positioned and docked [6].

The kidney is retracted anteriorly and the dissection proceeds along the psoas muscle until the underlying renal vessels are identified. The renal hilum is then dissected and ligated using suture ligation, clips and/or robotic Hem-o-lok clips. The resected kidney is placed in an endo-bag and then removed through a mini incision, or through the camera port, depending on the size. An abdominal drainage can be left to check postoperative leakage. Urethral catheter is usually removed on first—second postop day, after complete mobilization of the patient.

We used to perform both techniques, despite the transperitoneal approach being preferred for simple nephrectomy, especially with lymphadenectomy, as it offers a wider working space compared to the retroperitoneal one.

18.6 Postoperative Care

Patients start liquid intake few hours postoperatively and following oral feeding. Analgesic therapy is prescribed by the Anesthesiologist according to our internal pain management protocol: Paracetamol (dosage 15 mg/kg at 6 to 8-h intervals) and Tramadol (dosage 1 mg/kg at 8-h intervals) are administered in the first 24–48 h postoperatively.

A short-term antibiotic therapy is performed for 48–72 h postoperatively.

Patients are usually discharged on second or third postoperative day (POD). An early postoperative outpatient control is scheduled on seventh–tenth POD to evaluate the surgical wound.

The subsequent follow-up depends on the underlying pathology that led to surgery, a multidisciplinary follow-up being preferred for all patients (urologists, nephrologists, oncologists, radiologists).

18.7 Results

Even if the robotics learning curve is flatter than the laparoscopic one, it is important to underline that the surgeon needs a significative robotic experience before performing a robot-assisted nephrectomy, especially for vessels management. Due to this, literature is still poor regarding robotic radical nephrectomy in pediatric patients.

In literature, robotic RN are performed especially and almost exclusively for Wilms tumors (small ones) and non-functioning atrophic kidneys [7–12].

Regarding the age of patients, in our center, we perform RARN and robot-assisted urological surgery preferably in children over 1 year of age, due to logistic (DaVinci® Robot is located in another pavilion), anesthesiologist's and surgeon's comfort.

However, in literature, many articles are emerging describing robot-assisted urological procedures even in children younger than 1 year of age [13, 14].

18.8 Complications and Management

Main complications in a mini-invasive RN are represented by: bleeding (immediate for intraoperative vessel damage or in the postoperative period for clips dislodgment) or damage to abdominal structure such as bowel, liver, spleen, or wound infection [1].

Complications could be managed, depending on which occurs, by redo surgery or explorative laparotomic surgery.

In our experience, to date, we have not experienced any intraoperative and postoperative complications, nor particular difficulties in performing the surgical technique described above.

Tips and Tricks

- Semi-lateral decubitus, with the operative side up by 45° with pads underneath, is crucial to optimize the surgery: the intestinal loops slide down and allows to have an excellent exposure of the renal lodge. Detaching the colon is important to easily expose the kidney and to isolate the ureter. At the end of the procedure, it is not necessary to reattach the colon to the abdominal wall.
- Ports positioned in a sort of 'kite-like' appearance, as far apart as possible, help to reduce robotic arms' collisions. Moreover, a slight traction of trocars, tenting the abdominal wall, appears to us useful to create some extra room and have adequate working space.
- An additional trocar may be useful especially when working on the right side to retract the liver, but sometimes it can be needed also on the left side, depending on the spleen's size and on the surgeon's preference.
- The use of sealing devices for tissue dissection makes the procedure bloodless, faster and safer.
- Regarding the management of hilar vessels, despite sealing devices having the FDA approval to seal vessels of 5–7 mm in diameter, we believe that it is safer to ligate separately hilar vessels with endoscopic clips (titanium or Hem-o-lok). If titanium clips are applied on vessels, it is forbidden to use monopolar energy or sealing devices to seal the vessels, in order to avoid the risk of clips' dislodgement.

18.9 Discussion

Advanced robotic procedures in Pediatric Urology field are now promoted by the use of new technologies available such as HD optics, miniaturized instruments, sealing devices, etc. and thanks to the robot-assisted surgical experience of adult Urologists.

However, to date, robot-assisted radical nephrectomy is not the Gold Standard in pediatric patients.

Indications for robotic approach in pediatric renal surgery are limited to clinical cases requiring nephrectomy with associated lymphadenectomy, partial nephrectomy or heminephrectomy/nephroureterectomy in duplication of the renal system; also, anatomical situations for which the robotic approach is more comfortable for the surgeon.

This procedure has not gained wider acceptance compared to the laparoscopic or the open approach, due to the high costs related to robotic surgery and because it is mostly indicated for reconstructive procedures. Da Vinci robotic system, moreover, is not available in all centers and only few pediatric surgeons and urologists have experience with robotic surgery.

The advantages of the robotic approach are the 3D vision with a complete and clear view of the entire urinary tract and the robotic arms' seven degrees of freedom allowing for more fine movements, especially in more challenging passages such as the exposure of renal hilar vessels.

Robotic nephrectomy is, anyway, a challenging procedure that can be performed only in pediatric centers with a very strong experience in minimally invasive surgery.

Take-Home Points

- Literature is still poor regarding robotic radical nephrectomy in pediatric patients.
- The learning curve for robotic nephrectomy is flatter than for the laparoscopic technique.

- The surgeon needs significative robotic experience before performing a robot-assisted nephrectomy, especially for vessels management.
- The advantages of the robotic approach are the 3D vision with a complete and clear view of the entire urinary tract and the robotic arms' seven degrees of freedom allowing for more fine movements, especially in more challenging passages such as the exposure of renal hilar vessels.
- The correct positioning of the patient and the robotic ports is already half the work done.

References

1. Guidelines of the Italian Society of Videosurgery in Infancy for the minimally invasive treatment of pediatric nephrectomy and partial nephrectomy. Videosurgery, Italian Society of. https://doi.org/10.4081/pmc.2019.231.
2. Cerulo M, Escolino M, Turrà F, et al. Benefits of retroperitoneoscopic surgery in pediatric urology. Pediatr Urol. 2018;19(5):33. (D Weiss, Section Editor).
3. WHO. www.who.int/patientsafety/topics/safe-surgery/checklist/en/.
4. Anderssona H, Schmitzb A, Frykholm P, et al. Preoperative fasting guidelines in pediatric anesthesia: are we ready for a change? Curr Opin Anaesthesiol. 2018;3:342–8.
5. Masieri L, Sforza S, Grosso AA, et al. Does the body weight influence the outcome in children treated with robotic pyeloplasty? J Pediatr Urol. 2020;16(1):109.e1–6.
6. Rogers C, Laungani R, Krane LS, et al. Robotic nephrectomy for the treatment of benign and malignant disease. BJU Int. 2008;102(11):1660–5.
7. Vardaa BK, Choa P, Wagnerb AA, Lee RS. Collaborating with our adult colleagues: a case series of robotic surgery for suspicious and cancerous lesions in children and young adults performed in a free-standing children's hospital. J Pediatr Urol. 2018;14, 182.e1(2):–182.e8.
8. Andolfi C, Kumar R, Boysen WR, et al. Current status of robotic surgery in pediatric urology. J Laparoendosc Adv Surg Tech. 2019;29(2):159–66.
9. Kibar Y, Yalçın S, Kaya E, et al. Our experiences with robot- assisted laparoscopic surgery in pediatric patients: the first case series from Turkey. Turk J Urol. 2017;43(3):355–60.
10. Cost NG, Liss ZJ, Bean CM, et al. Prechemotherapy robotic-assisted laparoscopic radical nephrectomy for an adolescent with Wilms tumor. J Pediatr Hematol Oncol. 2015;37(2):e125–7.
11. Waterloos M, Ploumidis A, Pappas A, et al. Robot-assisted resection of ectopic kidney in children: anatomical illustration. J Pediatr Urol. 2019;15(1):87–8.
12. Blanc T, Pio L, Clermidi P, et al. Robotic-assisted laparoscopic management of renal tumors in children: preliminary results. Pediatr Blood Cancer. 2019;66(Suppl 3):e27867.
13. Avery DI, Herbst KW, Lendvay TS, et al. Robot-assisted laparoscopic pyeloplasty: multi-institutional experience in infants. J Pediatr Urol. 2015;11(3):139.e1–5.
14. Finkelstein JB, Levy AC, Silva MV, et al. How to decide which infant can have robotic surgery? Just do the math. J Pediatr Urol. 2015;11(4):170.e1–4.

Laparoscopic Nephrectomy in Pediatric Patients

19

Susana Rivas Vila, Pedro López Pereira,
María José Martínez Urrutia,
Roberto Lobato Romera, Virginia Amesty Morello,
and Alfredo Aguilera Bazan

Learning Objectives

- To describe the technique of laparoscopic nephrectomy (LN), including positioning, instrumentation and surgical steps.
- To present the outcomes of LN.
- To compare the results of LN with other techniques such as open nephrectomy and retroperitoneal nephrectomy (RPN).
- To describe some tips and tricks for LN and the use of other available new technologies.
- To show images and video with the technique.

Supplementary Information The online version contains supplementary material available at [https://doi.org/10.1007/978-3-030-99280-4_19].

S. Rivas Vila (✉) · P. López Pereira
M. J. Martínez Urrutia · R. Lobato Romera
V. Amesty Morello
Pediatric Urology Unit, Hospital Universitario La Paz, Madrid, Spain
e-mail: susana.rivas@salud.madrid.org; pedroc.lopez@salud.madrid.org; mmartinezu@salud.madrid.org; Roberto.lobato@salud.madrid.org; mvirginia.amesty@salud.madrid.org

A. Aguilera Bazan
Adult Urology Unit, Hospital Universitario La Paz, Madrid, Spain
e-mail: alfredo.aguilera@salud.madrid.org

19.1 Introduction

At the beginning of the 1990's, Clayman described the first laparoscopic nephrectomy in adults [1]. Koyle et al. described the technique in children in 1993 [2]. Currently, nephrectomy is the most common urological indication for video-assisted surgical procedures in children. Over the years, LN has shown itself to be safe and effective, with additional benefits in so far as postoperative morbidity, hospital stay and cosmetic results when compared with open nephrectomy [3].

The most common indication for LN is the removal of non-functioning renal units that are secondary to VUR, MCK, UPJ obstruction or have an ectopic ureter [4]. Although results of LN in adult oncology patients are comparable to those of open surgery when the tumors are localized, few groups have recommended this technique to treat malign kidney processes in children [5–8].

With regard to other minimally invasive techniques like retroperitoneoscopic nephrectomy (RPN) in lateral decubitus or a pronus position, laparoscopy offers the advantages of a larger working space that allows the placement of more easily manipulated trocars and better orientation in the surgical field, resulting in a shorter learning curve than RPN. Also, this technique allows better access to ectopic pelvic kidneys and the more distal sections of the ureter, which makes it the

C. Esposito et al. (eds.), *Minimally Invasive Techniques in Pediatric Urology*,
https://doi.org/10.1007/978-3-030-99280-4_19

technique of choice for many authors when treating a *non-functioning* VUR kidney, since it avoids creating a long ureteral stump that might motivate new interventions [9, 10].

19.2 Preoperative Preparation

The patient's preoperatory evaluation includes a complete clinical history and physical exploration. The kidney and urinary tract should undergo an anatomical and functional study that includes ultrasound, DMSA scan and voiding cystography for those with suspected VUR or other anatomic anomalies.

Blood laboratory analyses should include biochemistry, coagulation time and blood count.

The patient will be evaluated by an anesthetist as part of the pre-surgical work-up and both, the parents as well as the child, if he/she is old enough, will be informed of the proposed procedure and should sign an informed consent form.

An intestinal preparation in the preparative period consisting of a liquid diet and enema should facilitate intestinal management during the procedure, particularly in the smallest patients.

Antibiotic prophylaxis is administered prior to surgery with a wide spectrum antibiotic. Surgery takes place under general anesthesia, muscular relaxation and orotracheal intubation.

Just before the procedure, a Foley catheter is placed in the bladder and a nasogastric tube inserted to relieve any stomach distension that may make the procedure more difficult.

19.3 Positioning

19.3.1 Patient's Position

The patient is placed in semi-lateral decubitus. To facilitate the surgeon's movements, it is best to place the patient close to the edge of the table and strap them into place to maintain their position. A pillow is placed below the axilla and also under the knees to avoid pressure lesions.

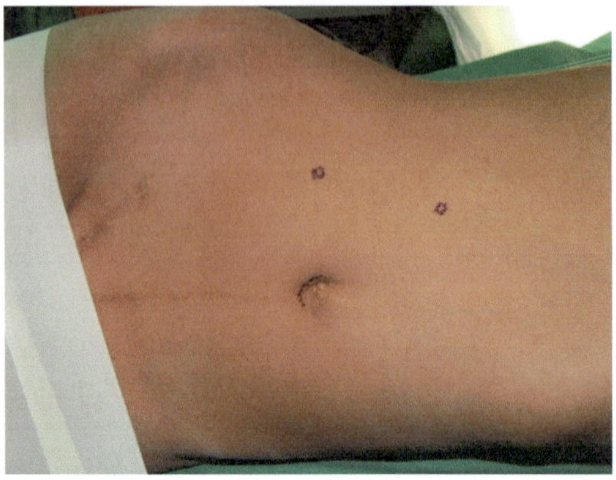

Fig. 19.1 Patient positioning and working ports for a right nephrectomy

This position causes gravity to shift the intestine outside the surgical field, facilitating colon detachment, and makes it possible to desiccate the entire length of the ureter and access the renal hilum (Fig. 19.1).

19.3.2 Positioning of Surgeons and Trocars

The surgeon and assistant will stand on the side contralateral to the kidney to be removed so that the kidney and the screen are in a straight line. If it is a nephrectomy of the left kidney, the surgeon will place themselves towards the patient's head and the assistant in the most caudal position; if it is a right kidney, the positions are reversed, with the assistant towards the patient's head and the surgeon in the caudal position. In both cases, the nurse in charge of the instruments will place themselves facing the surgeons and leave space for the laparoscopy tower.

The trocars will be placed forming a triangle such that the camera can be introduced through the umbilicus and the working ports placed in the ipsilateral upper and lower quadrants relative to the non-functional kidney. The umbilical port through which the 30° camera is introduced is 10 mm wide and will be used to extract the surgical piece. The use of Hasson-fixing trocars will facilitate the procedure. In older and/or obese patients, it may be necessary to displace incision

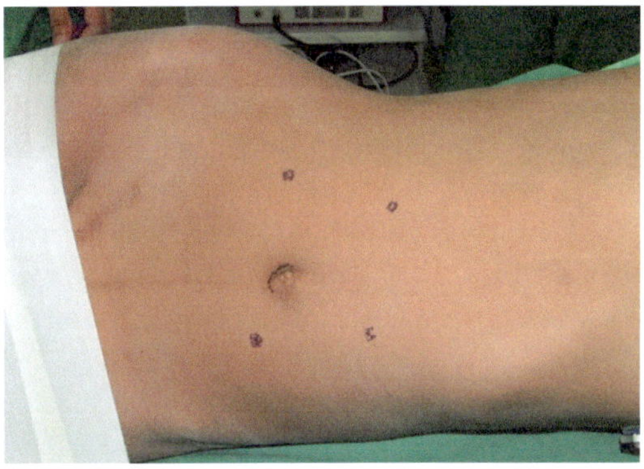

Fig. 19.2 Patient positioning for a nephrotic syndrome requiring bilateral nephrectomy

for the optic trocar port laterally towards the pararectal position.

Initially, three trocars will be placed, although it may become necessary to place a fourth trocar to retract the liver on the right side or the spleen to the left. The instrument ports will be 5 mm wide to allow the introduction of endoclips or a sealing device to control the hilar vessels. If a trocar is needed to lift the liver, it will be placed in a subxiphoid position, taking care to not damage the liver or the round ligament (Fig. 19.2).

19.3.3 Pneumoperitoneum

The umbilical trocar will be placed using an open procedure once the optic lens has been introduced and, once it has been confirmed that there is no visceral lesion or adherences, pneumoperitoneum will be produced by injecting sufficient CO_2 to achieve a minimum pressure that will allow us to work easily without surpassing 12–14 mmHg. The other trocars will be placed under direct vision.

19.4 Instruments

19.4.1 Equipment

You will require a laparoscopy tower that includes an optic lens, a camera, a xenon light source, screen, video recorder and CO_2 *pump* with a heating system. In addition to a 10 mm 30° optic lens, you will need two atraumatic forceps to manipulate the intestine and tissues, a curve dissector to individualize the renal hilum vessels, a dissection and cauterization hook, scissors, a 5 mm titanium clip applier, peanuts for drying and dissection and a sucker-rinser that should be ready in case of bleeding. If there is a Ligasure®, Utracison® or Starion MLS3® vessel-sealing device, the procedure can go faster. Except in cases in which nephrectomy is motivated due to infection or suspicion of a tumor, it is not necessary to introduce the piece in an endo-bag for extraction.

19.5 Technique

After achieving pneumoperitoneum and as a result of the patient's semi lateral decubitus position, gravity will cause the handles of the small intestine to drop, permitting access to the retroperitoneal space after detaching the colon (following the avascular line of Toldt). On the left side, colon detachment should go higher, sectioning the splenorenal ligaments, if necessary, to allow the descending colon to fall medially and have a more complete access to the renal hilum from the front. One must be especially careful with cauterization on this side since the pancreatic tail is quite close to the renal hilum and might be damaged.

Once colon detachment is achieved – either with electrocauterization or with a sealing device – the fascia of Gerota is opened to approach the kidney. Access to the kidney can also be made without detaching the colon, opening the mesocolon; however, this maneuver can be complicated in older children and those with more fatty tissue, and also it may cause damage in the colic vessels, motivating most authors to avoid it.

The psoas muscle serves as an anatomic guide for the entire intervention. The ureter and gonadal vein are found lying over the psoas and can be followed cranially to the renal hilum. Locating the ureter is easier in the most caudal position, since, in older patients, the fat of the Zuckerkandl cone may make it difficult in the area closest to the lower renal pole.

Excessive dissection of the posterior face of the kidney while accessing the renal hilum is not advisable since this may make it difficult to see the hilum (Figs. 19.3 and 19.4).

The following are the anatomic landmarks that identify the hilar vessels:

- *On the left,* the aorta crosses the field horizontally, the gonadal vein will guide us to the main renal vein and dissecting behind that vein will reveal the renal artery. A lumbar vein that reaches the main renal vein is quite common on the left side and it should be ligated before dissecting the renal artery. Once the artery is dissected, it is ligated with 5 mm titanium clips and sectioned. Last, we dissect and clip the renal vein.
- *On the right side*, the vena cava lies in a horizontal position, covered by the second duodenal portion on the anterior face, making it necessary to perform a Kocher maneuver to have easy access to the renal vein, behind which lies the renal artery. The same as on the left side, the first step is to dissect, ligate and section the renal artery before finally doing the same with the renal vein.

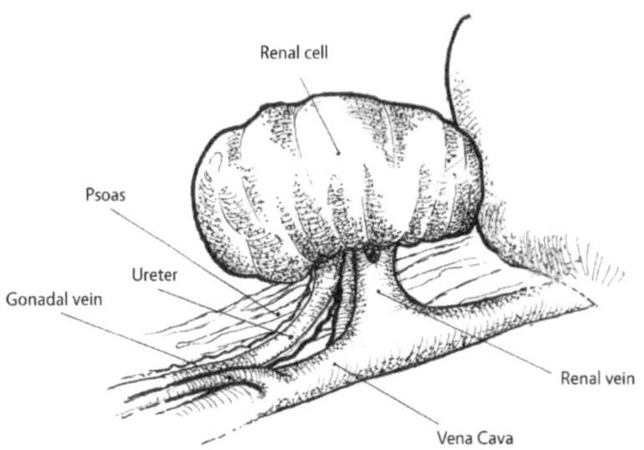

Fig. 19.3 Positions of the renal hilum vessels on the right side. Illustration by A. Aguilera

When the hilar vessels are less than 5 mm in diameter they can be closed with sealing devices without using clips.

After sectioning the renal hilum, we separate the kidney from its posterior adherences and continue caudally along the ureter as close as possible to the bladder. If the nephrectomy is motivated by a VUR, we must be especially careful when dissecting to leave the shortest possible ureteral stump and to ligate the ureter with an endoloop. We do not advise sealing devices to ligate the ureter. In cases without VUR, the ureter can be left open.

Before extracting the piece, we revise the hemostasis of the surgical field and reduce the pneumoperitoneum pressure for a few minutes.

The piece is extracted through the umbilicus, usually without a need for an endo-bag.

The trocars are removed under direct visual supervision to control any bleeding.

Fig. 19.4 Positions of the renal hilum vessels on the left side. Illustration by A. Aguilera

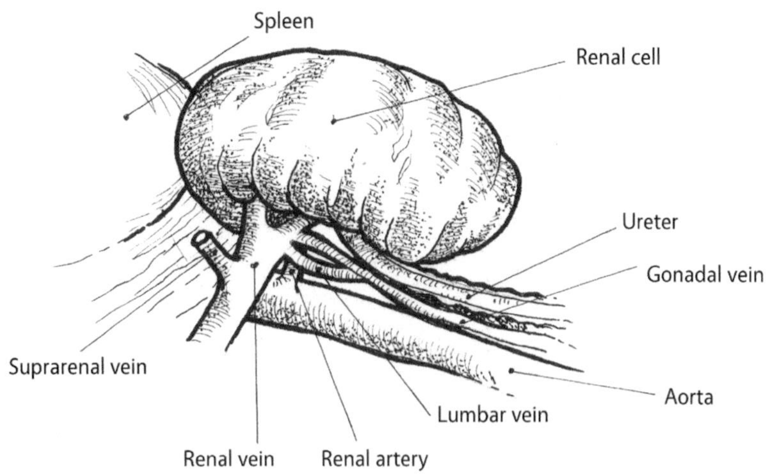

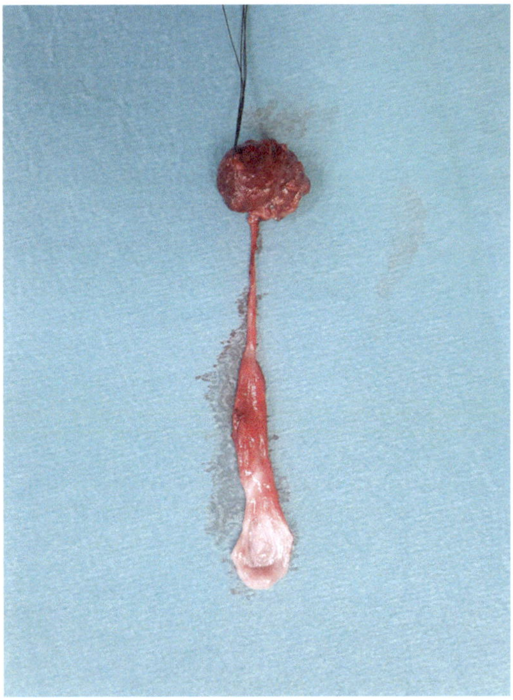

Fig. 19.5 Surgical piece (VUR non-functional kidney) removed through the umbilical port

Drainage is not necessary unless the patients have some infection.

In recent years, many papers have been published on single-port laparoscopic surgery to treat different urological pathologies in children, including some that require nephrectomy. These articles report a clinical result similar to that obtained with conventional laparoscopy, but better cosmetic results and less preoperatory morbidity (Fig. 19.5).

19.6 Postoperative Care

The patient regains oral tolerance within a few hours. Infusing the ports with local anesthesia before leaving the surgical theater will decrease the need for analgesia in the immediate postoperative period. Opioids are not necessary and generally the regular administration of paracetamol over the first 24 h after surgery will be enough to maintain the patient's comfort.

Antibiotic prophylaxis is maintained 24–48 h after surgery and, in our case, Ceftriaxona is usually administered in one daily intravenous dose during the hospital stay.

The patient is released 48 h after surgery and can renew daily activities progressively.

The first revision is done 1 week after surgery to control the surgical wounds and 1–3 months later a control ultrasound is performed.

19.7 Results

Few complications have been reported after LN, with a frequency of about 5% and the need to convert to open surgery quite rare. The infrequent complications include renal hilum vessel bleeding and port infection, which almost always only occur when an infected kidney is extirpated (*pyelonephritis xantogranulomatosa*). Reports of intestinal complications like perforation or ischemic damage secondary to mesocolon vessel lesion are extremely rare [11].

Surgical duration has decreased with the increase in experience of the groups with the surgery and the use of sealing devices and is now comparable with the open technique and less than with an RPN.

Most published series report that hospital stay is less than for open surgery and comparable to that of the RPN.

Less analgesia is needed than with the open technique and the amount needed is comparable to that required with patients recovering from RPN.

Laparoscopy allows complete dissection of the ureter up to the detrusor with a clear advantage over the open technique and RPN, thus avoiding the creation of a long ureteral stump that may necessitate the need for new interventions if it becomes infected [4, 10, 12, 13].

Single port LN has similar results to those of a conventional laparoscopic approach without increasing complications and also provides better cosmetic results [14].

Tips and Tricks

- Placing the patient in semi-lateral decubitus allows gravity to cause the intestines to drop, giving easier access to the renal area. Placing the patient on the edge of the operating table from which the surgeons work facilitates ergonomics and helps to make it easier to maneuver the instruments.
- When detaching the colon, one should follow the avascular line and coagulation and sealing devices can speed the maneuver and decrease surgical time. We do not advise a transmesocolon approach, particularly in older and/or obese patients. On the left side, it is necessary to disconnect the colon up to a higher level, even dissecting the splenorenal ligaments to be able to expose the renal hilum clearly. On the right side, it is necessary to perform a Kocher maneuver to move the second part of the duodenum so as to expose the anterior face of the vena cava and the entrance of the renal vein in the cava. Working on this *right* side, it may also be necessary to place a fourth trocar to shift the liver from the subxiphoid.
- The position of the psoas muscle is a reference point throughout the entire intervention. Identifying and following the ureter and gonadal vein cranially help to locate the renal hilum. It should be remembered that these structures might be found more medially than expected due to the patient's position and one should not try to locate the ureter very close to the inferior renal pole because the fat there will make it difficult to see.
- Sealing devices are helpful in detaching the colon, dissecting the renal hilum, sealing vessels less than 5 mm in diameter and freeing the posterior face of the kidney. They decrease surgical time and hemorrhagic complications. We recommend using 5 mm titanium endoclips on larger vessels. It is necessary to be especially careful when using the monopolar coagulating electrode near the clips since the current may provoke a burn that could cause the clip to come lose in the postoperative period.
- It is absolutely necessary to dissect the ureter caudally as far as possible in patients undergoing nephrectomy due to VUR. Also, in these cases, the distal portion of the ureter should be ligated with an endoloop.
- No advantages have been reported from repositioning and fixing the colon after detaching it.
- The kidney can be extracted through the umbilical port without using an endo-bag, unless the nephrectomy is due to an infection or tumor, in which case an endo-bag should be employed.

19.8 Discussion

At present, minimally invasive techniques are considered the gold standard in the treatment of non-malign pathologies that produce non-function of the renal union and necessitate nephrectomy in children [15].

Compared to the open technique, minimally invasive techniques for nephrectomy, known as MIS Nephrectomy, have been shown to provide advantages in so far as postoperative morbidity, hospital stay and cosmetic results are concerned without increasing the complication rate. In addition to these benefits, the laparoscopic approach makes it possible to remove the ureter much more distally than when using an open technique approach via a lumbotomy, and it decreases the need for later interventions to remove the ureteral stump if there is pyoureter or infection [4]. By allowing simultaneous access to the renal space and pelvis, laparoscopy makes it possible to perform the nephrectomy and procedures affecting the most distal part of the upper urinary tract without making new incisions.

There is a consensus among pediatric urologists and surgeons regarding their preference for MIS techniques when performing nephrectomy, although the debate on the advantages and inconveniences of the transperitoneal approach versus the retroperitoneal one continues [9, 12, 13, 16–19].

The most obvious advantage of the transperitoneal approach is the existence of a larger working space that allows easy trocar placement and the use of a larger number of trocars. Also, the peritoneal space facilitates kidney access in patients with prior pyelonephritis, massive hydronephrosis, ectopic kidneys, horseshoe kidneys or when a bilateral nephrectomy is required.

On the other hand, a retroperitoneal approach reproduces the steps of the classic open technique, avoids entering the peritoneum and colon detachment, easing direct access to the kidney and renal hilum without risk of damaging intrabdominal organs. By avoiding the peritoneum, it decreases the risk of intestinal adherences and postoperative eviscerations, as well as confining possible complications like hematomas and urinomas to the retroperitoneal space, thus producing less damage to the patient.

However, the retroperitoneal space is small and must be created for the surgery, trocar placement is more difficult and, as the kidney is above the instruments, they must be directed upwards at an acute angle, making triangulation with the camera more difficult. In patients with recurrent pyelonephritis, prior renal surgeries or xanthogranulomatous pyelonephritis, it can be nearly impossible to create sufficient working space in the retroperitoneal area.

Accidental lesion of the peritoneum during surgery may decrease the already scarce working space and might force the conversion of the RPN into an LN or even an open nephrectomy.

Given these drawbacks, the learning curve is quicker for transperitoneal procedures and many authors consider an LN to be easier and quicker than an RPN, with no differences between the techniques in so far as postoperative stay and morbidity.

Certain pathologies as well as the patient's age may favor the choice of one approach or the other. In nephropathies secondary to reflux, in which as much ureter as possible must be removed, LN offers better results since the resulting ureteral stump is less than 5 mm in length, in comparison to the up to 5 cm resulting from the retroperitoneal approach on a patient in pronus position, the position that gives the worst access to the distal ureter.

Castellan et al. advise a transperitoneal approach for small patients with large kidneys and for those in whom a complete ureterectomy is necessary. In patients over 12 months of age who do not require the ureterectomy, they recommend RPN [19].

Esposito et al. state that LN is mandatory in cases undergoing nephrectomy due to VUR, in pelvic ectopic kidneys and preferable in nearly all the indications, reserving RPN almost exclusively for the infrequent cases that require nephrectomy due to MCK [15].

Most authors do not report significant differences in surgical time, complications, postoperative morbidity or hospital stay between LN and RPN; thus the indication of one or the other should be made on an individual basis in function of the patient's pathology and the surgeon's preferences and experience. It is advisable to have experience with both techniques so that the surgeon can offer the one that is best for each patient [13, 17, 18].

Another controversy that has arisen recently is whether LN, commonly accepted to treat localized malign pathologies in adults, can be used for this purpose in children. In 2017, Duarte et al. published their experience with LN to treat Wilms Tumor in children after neoadjuvant chemotherapy (the SIOP protocol). They propose its use only for patients with small tumors that have shrunk in response to chemotherapy. They argue that laparoscopy allows abdominal inspection in search of metastases, a radical nephrectomy and the extirpation of perihilar and para-aortic ganglia. Their results in a group of 24 patients aged 10–93 months who underwent LN show that the procedure could be done by laparoscopy in all cases and the hospital stay was 2–3 days. The authors did not report any intraoperative tumor spillage and after a follow-up of 6.65 years, two patients have had relapses, one in the lung and the other in the liver [6].

Varlet et al. published a retrospective multicentric study with 17 patients who underwent LN to treat malign renal tumors; 16 had neoadjuvant chemotherapy according to the SIOP protocol, and one (renal carcinoma) surgery alone. It was possible to complete the treatment laparoscopically without any tumor rupture in 16 patients, and the largest tumor was 8 cm. After a follow-up ranging from 11 to 77 months, 15 children were well, 1 had a local relapse and another, with a clear cell sarcoma, had died. The authors conclude that radical nephrectomy via a transperitoneal approach is a valid option to treat Wilms tumor and other malign renal tumors [8].

Take-Home Points

- LN is a safe and effective therapy that can be considered a gold standard procedure for kidney removal in children, particularly in cases with reflux nephropathy.
- We highly recommend LP in patients under the age of 12 months with large kidneys and in all cases requiring total ureterectomy.
- You need an optic lens of 10 mm and 30° and 2–3 5 mm trocars. It is quite easy to remove the kidney through the optic orifice. No endo-bag is required except in cases of kidney infection.
- The new hemostatic devices like *the* Starion MLS3R, UltracisionR or LigasureR are not strictly necessary, but they facilitate dissection, decrease the risk of bleeding and permit faster and safer surgery.
- The fixation of the colon is not strictly necessary. No drainage is needed except in some cases of kidney infection.

References

1. Clayman RV, Kavoussi LR, Soper NJ, Dierks SM, Merety KS, Darcy MD, Long SR, Roemer FD, Pingleton ED, Thomson PG. Laparoscopic nephrectomy. N Engl J Med. 1991;324(19):1370–1.
2. Koyle MA, Woo HH, Kavoussi LR. Laparoscopic nephrectomy in the first year of life. J Pediatr Surg. 1993;28(5):693–5.
3. You D, Hong S, Lee C, Kim KS. Feasibility and safety of laparoscopic ablative renal surgery in infants: comparative study with children. J Urol. 2012;188(4):1330–4.
4. Traxel EJ, Minevich EA, Noh PH. A review: the application of minimally invasive surgery to pediatric urology: lower urinary tract reconstructive procedures. Urology. 2010;76(1):115–20.
5. Cabezalí Barbancho D, Guerrero Ramos F, López Vázquez F, Aransay Bramtot A, Gómez FA. Laparoscopic approach for Wilms tumor. Surg Laparosc Endosc Percutan Tech. 2014;24(1):22–5.
6. Duarte RJ, Cristofani LM, Odone Filho V, Srougi M, Dénes FT. Videolaparoscopic radical nephrectomy after chemotherapy in the treatment of Wilms' tumor: long-term results of a pioneer group. J Pediatr Urol. 2017;13(1):50.e1–5.
7. Tolley DA, Esposito MP. Laparoscopic and renal sparing approaches to tumours of the ureter and kidney. Surg Oncol. 2002;11(1–2):47–54.
8. Varlet F, Petit T, Leclair MD, Lardy H, Geiss S, Becmeur F, Ravasse P, Rod J, de Lambert G, Braik K, Lardellier-Reynaud F, Lopez M. Laparoscopic treatment of renal cancer in children: a multicentric study and review of oncologic and surgical complications. J Pediatr Urol. 2014;10(3):500–5.
9. Esposito C, Valla JS, Yeung CK. Current indications for laparoscopy and retroperitoneoscopy in pediatric urology. Surg Endosc. 2004;18(11):1559–64.
10. Escolino M, Farina A, Turrà F, Cerulo M, Esposito R, Savanelli A, Settimi A, Esposito C. Evaluation and outcome of the distal ureteral stump after nephroureterectomy in children. A comparison between laparoscopy and retroperitoneoscopy. J Pediatr Urol. 2016;12(2):119.e1–8.
11. Aksenov LI, Granberg CF, Gargollo PC. A systematic review of complications of minimally invasive surgery in the pediatric urological literature. J Urol. 2020;203(5):1010–6.
12. Valla JS. Retroperitoneoscopic surgery in children. Semin Pediatr Surg. 2007;16(4):270–7.
13. Kim C, McKay K, Docimo SG. Laparoscopic nephrectomy in children: systematic review of transperitoneal and retroperitoneal approaches. Urology. 2009;73(2):280–4.
14. Soto-Aviles OE, Escudero-Chu K, Perez-Brayfield MR. Laparoscopic single-site surgery in pediatric urology: where do we stand today? Curr Urol Rep. 2015;16(10):68.
15. Esposito C, Becmeur F, Steyaert H, Szavay P. ESPES manual of pediatric minimally invasive surgery. Springer: Switzerland. 2019. ISBN 978-3-030-00963-2.
16. Esposito C, Escolino M, Corcione F, Draghici IM, Savanelli A, Castagnetti M, Turrà F, Cerulo M, Farina A, Settimi A. Twenty-year experience with laparoscopic and retroperitoneoscopic nephrectomy in children: considerations and details of technique. Surg Endosc. 2016;30(5):2114–8.

17. Lorenzo Gómez MF, González R. Laparoscopic nephrectomy in children: the transperitoneal vs the retroperitoneal approach. Arch Esp Urol. 2003;56(4):401–13.
18. Taue R, Izaki H, Koizumi T, Kishimoto T, Oka N, Fukumori T, Takahashi M, Kanayama HO. Transperitoneal versus retroperitoneal laparoscopic radical nephrectomy: a comparative study. Int J Urol. 2009;16(3):263–7.
19. Castellan M, Gosalbez R, Carmack AJ, Prieto JC, Perez-Brayfield M, Labbie A. Transperitoneal and retroperitoneal laparoscopic heminephrectomy--what approach for which patient? J Urol 2006;176(6 Pt 1): 2636–2639.

Retroperitoneal Laparoscopic Nephrectomy

20

Elie Farah, Aline Broch, Nathalie Botto, and Thomas Blanc

Learning Objectives
- To describe step by step the technique of retroperitoneal laparoscopic nephrectomy (RLN).
- To show a (Videos 20.1 and 20.2) with the technique of RLN.
- To describe tips and tricks of RLN and to show all the new technologies available in pediatric urology that can be adopted to perform an RLN.

20.1 Introduction

The standard therapeutic management of a poorly or nonfunctioning kidney in children connected to a refluxing, obstructed, or dysplastic ureter is nephrectomy with total or proximal ureterectomy. The aim of surgery is to prevent urinary tract infections or limit the risk of hypertension. In cases of reflux nephropathy with/without megaureter, it is essential to continue the resection all the way down to the vesico–ureteric junction.

Since the introduction of minimal invasive nephrectomy in 1991 by Clayman for adults, and only 2 years later by Koyle for children, the approach has quickly gained general acceptance among pediatric urologists [1, 2]. Report of minimally invasive nephrectomies in children was first published in 1998 for the retroperitoneal approach [3]. Laparoscopic nephrectomy has been shown to be a safe, viable alternative to traditional open surgery, with potential advantages of shorter hospital lengths of stay, decreased postoperative analgesic use, and improved cosmesis [4, 5].

Technically speaking, the surgical steps for pediatric nephroureterectomy follow the same principles independent of the surgical approach. Both, the transperitoneal as well as the retroperitoneal route have been established [6]. The retroperitoneoscopic approach has advantages of direct kidney visualization, decreased risk of intra-abdominal adhesions, and reduced in-patient stay, compared with open or transperitoneal laparoscopic surgery [7].

In this chapter, we report the technique of retroperitoneal laparoscopic nephrectomy in infants and children.

Supplementary Information The online version contains supplementary material available at [https://doi.org/10.1007/978-3-030-99280-4_20].

E. Farah · A. Broch · N. Botto · T. Blanc (✉)
Department of Paediatric Surgery and Urology, Necker-Enfants Malades University Children Hospital, Paris, France

AP-HP Centre – Université de Paris, Paris, France
e-mail: eliefarha@hotmail.com; aline.broch@aphp.fr; nathalie.botto@aphp.fr; thomas.blanc@aphp.fr

C. Esposito et al. (eds.), *Minimally Invasive Techniques in Pediatric Urology*,
https://doi.org/10.1007/978-3-030-99280-4_20

20.2 Preoperative Preparation

All the patients are operated under general anesthesia with orotracheal intubation and they received a nasogastric tube. Bladder catheter is not needed.

20.3 Positioning

The procedure starts with a crucial step to achieve a successful retroperitoneal access: proper positioning of the patient.

The surgeon and his team stay behind the patient (Fig. 20.1).

The child is placed in the lateral position close to the edge of the table, using lumbar padding to stretch the costo–iliac distance without flexing the operating table. Non-stretch adhesive banding secures this position and prevents displacement either forwards or backwards. The upper leg is stretched while the lower leg is flexed, with no contact between them to avoid compression.

The landmarks are the twelfth rib, the costovertebral angle, and the top of the iliac crest.

20.4 Initial Access, Insufflation, and Trocar Placement

Retroperitoneal access is achieved through the first access incision (15 mm), one finger width from lower border of the twelfth rib.

A perpendicular dissociation of the muscles will approach the Gerota's fascia under vision (Fig. 20.2). The Gerota's fascia is opened at its most posterior part under vision.

The first blunt trocar is introduced directly inside the opened Gerota's fascia.

A working space around the kidney is created directly by a 5 or 10 mm 0° laparoscope and by gas insufflation dissection, with no need for finger or balloon dissection.

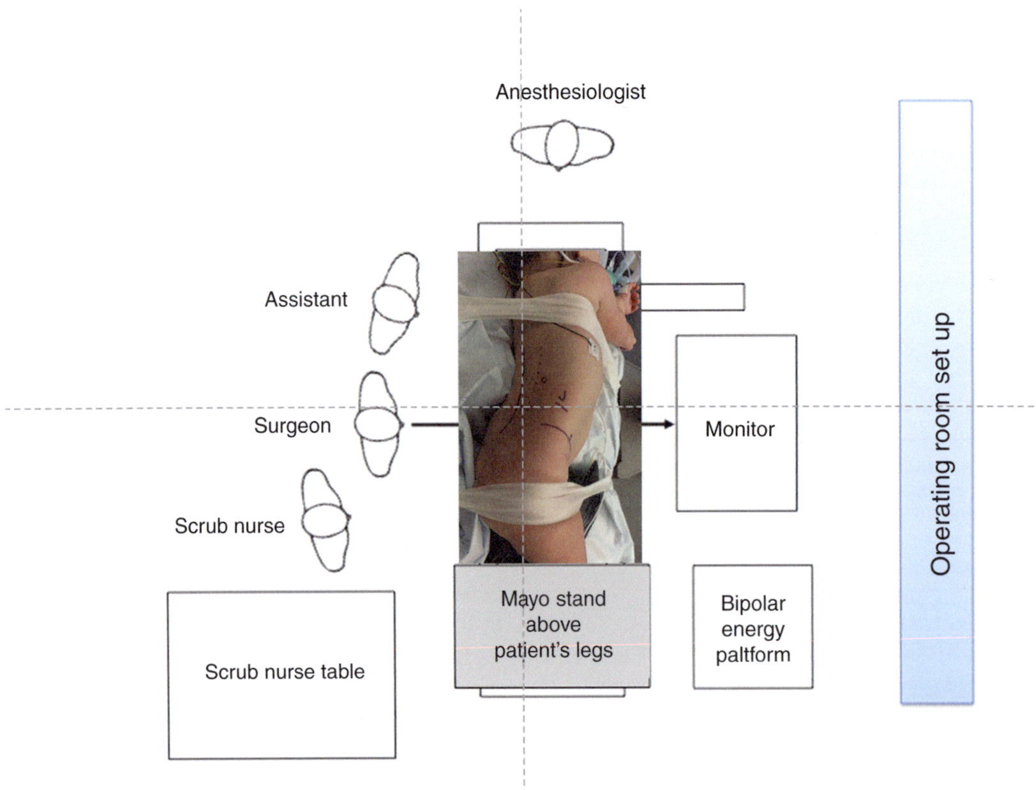

Fig. 20.1 Operating room set-up for right retroperitoneoscopy

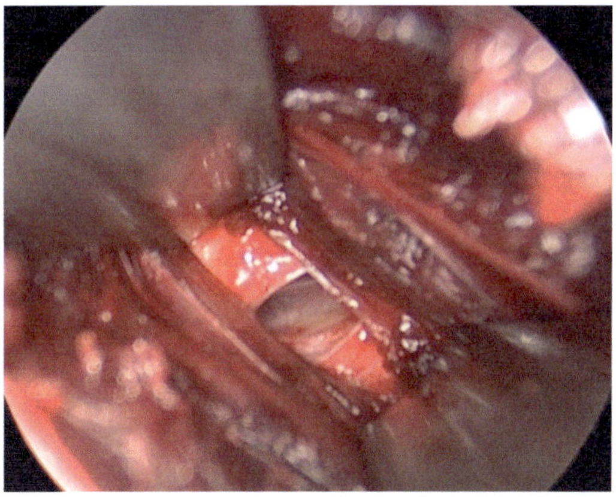

Fig. 20.2 Perpendicular dissociation of the muscles to approach the Gerota's fascia

This allows insufflation to push the kidney upscreen (medially) without the need for individual kidney retraction to expose the renal pedicle.

The space around the kidney is created.

The second trocar (5 mm-operative trocar) is inserted posteriorly under vision in the costovertebral angle, in front of the lumbosacral muscle.

Third trocar insertion is in the anterior axillary line, a finger width from the top of the.

iliac crest.

20.5 Instrumentation

- Three ports (5-5-5 mm or 10-5-5 mm).
- Atraumatic fenestrated grasping forceps to manage tissues.
- Clip applier for vessel control and scissors or sealing device.
- Suction and aspiration device in case of bleeding.
- Endo-bag to remove the kidney.
- Endoloop to ligate the distal ureter in case of refluxing ureter.

20.6 Surgical Technique

The kidney is approached posteriorly.

The psoas, the landmark during the whole procedure, is downscreen, the kidney is up screen.

The lower pole of the kidney and the ureter are identified.

The kidney remains attached anteriorly to the peritoneum and is lifted gently in order to identify and control the pedicle.

The renal artery and the renal vein are isolated separately.

Hilar vessels can be sealed and divided with a sealing device, either the 5-mm LigaSure® (Covidien US, MN) or harmonic scalpel, that allows a faster and safer surgery without bleeding, although hemoclips (Hem-o-lok®) can also be used, depending on the renal vessel size.

Other pedicles can be controlled with the same technique.

The ureter can be preserved for a future kidney transplantation and the ureter is then divided at the level of UPJ.

If VUR is present, the ureter should be isolated as far down as possible to the bladder base and ligated, using preferably an endoloop.

The kidney is freed from the peritoneum and placed in a laparoscopic retrieval bag and removed piecemeal so that the incision size does not need to be increased.

No drain is left in situ.

20.7 Results

From 2010 to 2020, 130 laparoscopic total nephrectomy were performed in the Department of Paediatric Surgery and Urology at Necker-Enfants Malades University Children Hospital, including 95 retroperitoneal laparoscopic total nephrectomies, performed by six surgeons. Transperitoneal laparoscopic nephrectomies were excluded from further analysis.

Mean age at surgery was 6.2 years (2 months–16 years).

Indication for surgery was

- Vesico–ureteric reflux ($n = 33$).
- Nephrotic syndrome ($n = 21$).
- PUJ obstruction ($n = 15$).
- VUJ obstruction ($n = 11$).
- Multicystic dysplastic kidney ($n = 6$) (Fig. 20.3).
- Simplex ureterocele ($n = 5$).

- Duplex kidney ($n = 2$).
- Renal artery stenosis ($n = 1$).
- Urolithiasis ($n = 1$).

Six bilateral nephrectomies were performed for nephrotic syndrome, including one HSK.

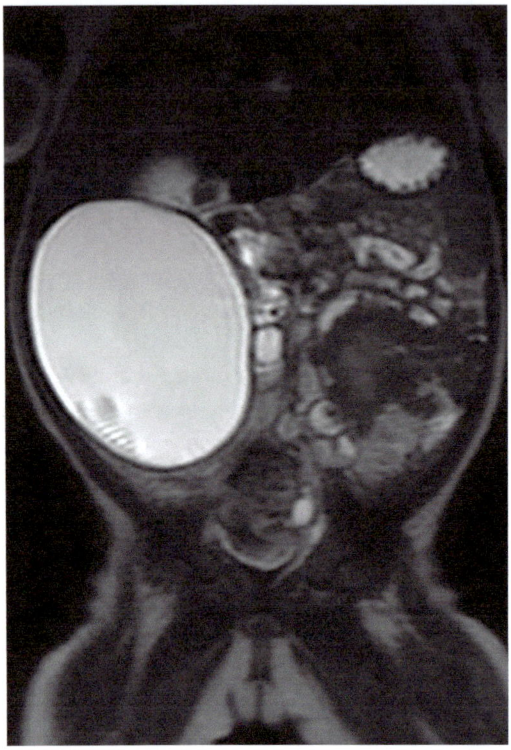

Fig. 20.3 Multicystic dysplastic kidney

Mean duration of surgery was 110 min (range 44–265 min).

Mean length of hospital stay was 3.5 days (range 1–16), with 45% of children discharged at day 1 postoperatively.

Three cases (3%), with previous kidney surgery for UPJ obstruction or partial nephrectomy, were converted to open surgery.

Four children were re-operated for recurrent UTIs due to refluxing ureteric stump (Fig. 20.4).

The median length of follow-up was 3.5 years (range 2 months–9 years).

Tips and Tricks

- Leave the kidney attached to the peritoneum.
- Landmark: psoas muscle.
- Use sealing devices for tissue dissection to make the procedure bloodless, faster, and safer.
- In case of peritoneum opening, insert a Veress needle in the peritoneum through the abdominal wall.

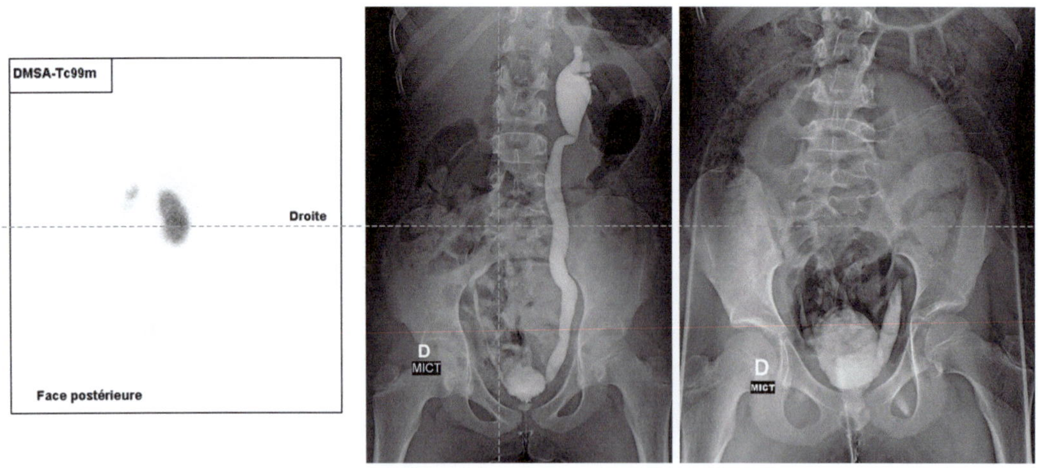

Fig. 20.4 Symptomatic refluxing ureteric stump

20.8 Discussion

Nephrectomy in pediatric patients is a treatment option for benign, nonfunctioning kidneys with a history of obstructive uropathy, vesico–ureteral reflux, multicystic dysplastic kidney, UPJ obstruction or stone disease [8, 9]. Nephrectomy before renal transplantation is indicated in children with ESRD who have severe proteinuria, polyuria, or hypertension [10].

Although open nephrectomy, either via an abdominal or flank incision, has long been considered the "gold standard," minimally invasive/laparoscopic nephrectomy has gained acceptance over the last two decades as a safe and effective surgical option in pediatric patients. It has been associated with shorter lengths of hospital stay, decreased pain medication use, earlier return to normal activities, and improved cosmetic results [11, 12].

Given the paucity of knowledge regarding use of pediatric nephrectomy in the United States, Sammon et al. explored the trends in incidence across age and gender [13]. While the annual incidence of nephrectomy is stable, the use of minimally invasive nephrectomy is expanding in the pediatric population. The median age of patients undergoing minimally invasive nephrectomy (MIN) was greater than those undergoing the open approach (7 vs. 3 years, $p < 0.001$). The majority of nephrectomies were for benign indications (73.8% vs. 26.2%), with only 2.2% of MIN procedures performed for malignancy. Median annual hospital volume for pediatric nephrectomy was 12 (IQR 6–23), with MIN more likely to be performed at institutions with greater annual volumes (median 15, IQR 7–26).

There is still some controversy concerning which approach to choose: transperitoneal or retroperitoneal. Arguments to advocate one approach are more theoretical than true objective criteria. The transperitoneal approach offers the advantages of a larger working space; however, it requires more dissection to reach the kidney and the colon must be reflected. Although there is a theoretical risk of intra-abdominal injury while performing a transabdominal technique, it remains rare. The retroperitoneal approach has the advantage of direct access to the urinary tract and an easier detection of crossing vessels. It also reduces manipulation and contact with the intraperitoneal organs. However, the longer time needed for the retroperitoneal approach is related to the limited working space. Shoma et al. published the first prospective randomized study that compared the transperitoneal approach and the RA in adults in 2007 [14]. Both approaches had satisfactory comparable outcomes without a significant difference in the success rate. The RA was associated with a longer operative time (189 vs. 149 min).

We routinely do all laparoscopic renal surgery through the RA, and we reserve the transperitoneal approach for selected indications. We believe that in experienced centers, the team should be familiar with both approaches and decide which is easier for the team to apply routinely, keeping the alternative approach for selected indications. The choice of performing a transperitoneal approach or the RA should be based mainly on the personal preference and experience of the individual surgeon.

Esposito et al. reported their 20 years of experience in laparoscopic and retroperitoneoscopic nephrectomy. All the removed kidneys were nonfunctioning because of benign diseases: VUR (84), UPJO (38), multicystic dysplastic kidney (20), xanthogranulomatosis pyelonephritis (4), nephropathy causing uncontrollable hypertension (2) and nephrolithiasis (1). Based on their experience, they concluded that LN is easier and faster to perform compared to RN. They consider xanthogranulomatous pyelonephritis or other kidney infections or in case of previous renal surgery as contraindication for retroperitoneoscopy. In case of VUR, they prefer LN because it is fundamental to remove all the ureter. Finally, this group clearly prefers to perform nephrectomy using laparoscopy rather than retroperitoneoscopy.

Interestingly, we have recently reported that the unilateral retroperitoneal approach allows total nephrectomy in horseshoe kidney for benign disease. Port placement was modified due to the anatomy of the HSK: one 5-mm port was, as usually, at the costo–vertebral angle, but the other

5-mm port was placed above the iliac crest at the external margin of the lumbosacral muscle. The dissection was safe with section of the vessels close to the HSK. Despite significant variation of the origin and distribution of the vessels, it was completed in excellent condition.

Retroperitoneal access preserves the abdominal cavity, which will remain intact for peritoneal dialysis if favored by the nephrology team. Szymanski et al. reported their experience with retroperitoneoscopic nephrectomy in children on peritoneal dialysis [15]. They performed three bilateral synchronous, one bilateral staged, and six unilateral RPNs 1in 0 children with a mean age of 12 years. Peritoneal dialysis was initiated at a median of 9 h postoperatively and dialysate volume was titrated to target within a median of 60 hours. One patient with a small peritoneotomy needed temporary hemodialysis despite intraoperative airtight repair. They conclude that retroperitoneoscopic nephrectomy for end stage renal disease is a safe, effective technique that preserves peritoneal integrity in children who require immediate postoperative peritoneal dialysis. Avoiding post-nephrectomy hemodialysis decreases patient morbidity, preserving vessels for future vascular access. Compared to the literature on laparoscopy in this setting, retroperitoneoscopic nephrectomy can be considered the ideal approach for minimally invasive nephrectomy in patients on peritoneal dialysis.

Nephroureterectomy, through retroperitoneoscopy, anterolateral abdominal incision, or through a lumbotomy does not allow excision of the entire ureter, even in very small children. In case of refluxing ureter, the ureter has to be divided as low as possible in the deep pelvis. A dual approach (retroperitoneal and inguinal approach) has been recommended when complete excision of the kidney and ureter is required [16]. The risk of recurrent urinary tract infections due to stasis of infected urine in the refluxing ureteric stumps has been described, with symptoms mimicking pyelonephritis, even though the kidney had been removed [17]. Controversy persists in regard to treatment of the lower defunctionalized segment of ureter and it has been recommended in such cases to divide the stump where it entered the bladder and to suture the bladder hiatus [18, 19].

Hence, the length of the remaining ureteric stump in reflux nephropathy is a key parameter of success. Escolino et al. published an evaluation of the distal ureteral stump after NU in children comparing the TPN versus RPN approach [20]. The authors included 21 consecutive patients (median age 3.5 years; range 1–10 years). They found a longer operating time for RPN versus TPN (80 vs. 50 min). The length of the distal ureteric stump was significantly shorter after TPN (range 3–7 mm) versus RPN (range 2–5 cm). In conclusion, the authors stated that TPN permits removal of all ureter near to the bladder dome. In children with non-functioning kidneys due to VUR, they recommend performing a laparoscopic rather than RPN nephrectomy.

Laparoendoscopic single-site surgery (LESS) means working through one access, most commonly the umbilicus. This technique challenges the paradigm of conventional laparoscopy to angulate the instruments for optimal working spaces. Instead, it introduces significant ergonomic difficulties such as clashing (of the ports outside), crowding (of the instruments within the single port), and, most important, crossing of the instruments [21, 22]. The latter means that all intuitive movements of conventional laparoscopy become counterintuitive.

Despite all euphoria for LESS, the surgical performance remains a matter for vivid discussions due to the different ergonomics. Tam from Hong Kong found that LESS nephrectomy took longer than conventional laparoscopy (mean 156 vs. 99 min) and no postoperative complications occurred [23]. The authors conclude that LESS nephrectomy is safe and effective with a minimal invasive nature comparable to conventional laparoscopy. However, they recommend further studies to investigate the implication of patient selection and the cosmetic benefits of LESS.

Cherian et al. reported the first single incision retroperitoneoscopic pediatric nephrectomy in two patients, including one child with bilateral synchronous nephrectomy, using an advanced access platform (GelPOINT Mini) [24].

Take-Home Points

- Ablative surgery, such as nephrectomy, is an excellent procedure to begin your experience in retroperitoneal approach.
- 0° laparoscope to create your working space.
- Only 3 trocars.
- Sealing devices are very helpful to perform a bloodless, safer, and faster procedure.
- In case of nephroureterectomy, perform distal ureterectomy to the level of the bladder hiatus and ligate the ureteric stump in patients with refluxing ureter in order to avoid postoperative symptoms associated with recurrent UTIs.
- Large multicystic dysplastic kidney is an excellent indication for retroperitoneal laparoscopic nephrectomy.

References

1. Clayman RV, et al. Laparoscopic nephrectomy: initial case report. J Urol. 2017;197(2S):S182–6. https://doi.org/10.1016/j.juro.2016.10.074.
2. Koyle MA, Woo HH, Kavoussi LR. Laparoscopic nephrectomy in the first year of life. J Pediatr Surg. 1993;28(5):693–5. https://doi.org/10.1016/0022-3468(93)90034-I.
3. El-Ghoneimi A, Valla JS, Steyaert H, Aigrain Y. Laparoscopic renal surgery via a retroperitoneal approach in children. J Urol. 1998;160(3 Pt 2):1138–41. https://doi.org/10.1097/00005392-199809020-00047.
4. Kim C, McKay K, Docimo SG. Laparoscopic nephrectomy in children: systematic review of transperitoneal and retroperitoneal approaches. Urology. 2009;73(2):280–4. https://doi.org/10.1016/j.urology.2008.08.471.
5. Ku JH, Yeo WG, Choi H, Kim HH. Comparison of retroperitoneal laparoscopic and open nephrectomy for benign renal diseases in children. Urology. 2004;63(3) https://doi.org/10.1016/j.urology.2003.11.040.
6. Esposito C, et al. Twenty-year experience with laparoscopic and retroperitoneoscopic nephrectomy in children: considerations and details of technique. Surg Endosc. 2016;30(5):2114–8. https://doi.org/10.1007/s00464-015-4472-7.
7. Leclair MD, Vidal I, Suply E, Podevin G, Héloury Y. Retroperitoneal laparoscopic heminephrectomy in duplex kidney in infants and children: a 15-year experience. Eur Urol. 2009;56(2):385–91. https://doi.org/10.1016/j.eururo.2008.07.015.
8. Yucel S, Brown B, Bush NC, Ahmad N, Baker LA. What to anticipate with experience in pediatric laparoscopic ablative renal surgery. J Urol. 2008;179(2):697–702. https://doi.org/10.1016/j.juro.2007.09.092.
9. The development of laparoscopic surgical skills in pediatric urologists: longterm outcome of a mentorship-training model. https://pubmed-ncbi-nlm-nih-gov.proxy.insermbiblio.inist.fr/16274518/. Accessed 17 August 2020.
10. Sheinfeld J, Linke CL, Talley TE, Linke CA. Selective pre-transplant nephrectomy: indications and perioperative management. J Urol. 1985;133(3):379–82. https://doi.org/10.1016/S0022-5347(17)48983-X.
11. Peters CA. Laparoscopy in pediatric urology. Curr Opin Urol. 2004;14(2). Curr Opin Urol:67–73. https://doi.org/10.1097/00042307-200403000-00004.
12. Lee RS, Retik AB, Borer JG, Diamond DA, Peters CA. Pediatric retroperitoneal laparoscopic partial nephrectomy: comparison with an age matched cohort of open surgery. J Urol. 2005;174(2):708–12. https://doi.org/10.1097/01.ju.0000164748.00339.4c.
13. Sammon JD, et al. Pediatric nephrectomy: incidence, indications and use of minimally invasive techniques. J Urol. 2014;191(3):764–70. https://doi.org/10.1016/j.juro.2013.09.063.
14. Shoma AM, El Nahas AR, Bazeed MA. Laparoscopic pyeloplasty: a prospective randomized comparison between the transperitoneal approach and retroperitoneoscopy. J Urol. 2007;178(5):2020–4. https://doi.org/10.1016/j.juro.2007.07.025.
15. Szymanski KM, Bitzan M, Capolicchio JP. Is retroperitoneoscopy the gold standard for endoscopic nephrectomy in children on peritoneal dialysis? J Urol. 2010;184(4 Suppl):1631–7. https://doi.org/10.1016/j.juro.2010.04.019.
16. Persad R, Kamineni S, Mouriquand PDE. Recurrent symptoms of urinary tract infection in eight patients with refluxing ureteric stumps. Br J Urol. 1994;74(6):720–2. https://doi.org/10.1111/j.1464-410X.1994.tb07113.x.
17. Malek RS, Moghaddam A, Furlow WL, Greene LF. Symptomatic ureteral stumps. J Urol. 1971;106(4):521–8. https://doi.org/10.1016/S0022-5347(17)61332-6.
18. Ade-Ajayi N, Wilcox DT, Duffy PG, Ransley PG. Upper pole heminephrectomy: is complete ureterectomy necessary? BJU Int. 2001;88(1):77–9. https://doi.org/10.1046/j.1464-410X.2001.02249.x.
19. Kim KS, Kim Y, Oh SJ. Natural history of refluxing distal ureteral stumps following upper tract surgery in children with ectopic ureter or ureterocele. Urol Int. 2001;67(2):142–6. https://doi.org/10.1159/000050970.
20. Escolino M, et al. Evaluation and outcome of the distal ureteral stump after nephro-ureterectomy in children. A comparison between lapa-

roscopy and retroperitoneoscopy. J Pediatr Urol. 2016;12(2):119.e1–8. https://doi.org/10.1016/j.jpurol.2015.10.007.
21. Soto-Aviles OE, Escudero-Chu K, Perez-Brayfield MR. Laparoscopic single-site surgery in pediatric urology: where do we stand today? Curr Urol Rep. 2015;16(10). Current Medicine Group LLC 1 https://doi.org/10.1007/s11934-015-0542-6.
22. Kim PH, et al. Early comparison of nephrectomy options in children (open, transperitoneal laparoscopic, laparo-endoscopic single site (LESS), and robotic surgery). BJU Int. 2012;109(6):910–5. https://doi.org/10.1111/j.1464-410X.2011.10524.x.
23. Tam YH, et al. Laparoendoscopic single-site nephrectomy and heminephroureterectomy in children using standard laparoscopic setup versus conventional laparoscopy. Urology. 2013;82(2):430–6. https://doi.org/10.1016/j.urology.2013.02.057.
24. Cherian A, De Win G. Single incision retroperitoneoscopic paediatric nephrectomy: early experience. J Pediatr Urol. 2014;10(3):564–6. https://doi.org/10.1016/j.jpurol.2013.12.018.

Posterior Prone Retroperitoneoscopic Nephrectomy

21

Naser Al-Soudan Al Anazi, Sara Lobo, and Imran Mushtaq

Learning Objectives

- To describe step by step the technique of posterior prone retroperitoneoscopic nephrectomy (PPRN).
- To present outcomes of retroperitoneoscopic versus transperitoneal nephrectomy.
- To show a video with the technique of PPRN.
- To describe tips and tricks of PPRN.

21.1 Introduction

Pediatric laparoscopic nephrectomy was first described in 1993 by Das et al. [1] Laparoscopic approaches to the kidney include transperitoneal (TP), posterior prone retroperitoneoscopic (PPR), and lateral retroperitoneoscopic (LRP) routes. Gaur initially described the retroperitoneal approach, which is now the approach of choice for most laparoscopic urological surgeons. However, the transperitoneal route still has a role when performing renal ablative surgery for tumors or when performing laparoendoscopic single site (LESS) surgery. Regardless of the approach utilized, the benefits to the child in terms of a faster postoperative recovery and improved cosmesis are without question.

This chapter is focused on the operative technique of posterior prone retroperitoneoscopic nephrectomy (PPRN).

21.2 Indications

A laparoscopic nephrectomy is indicated in the following cases:

- Poorly functioning or non-functioning kidney.
- Multicystic dysplastic kidney.
- Reflux-associated nephropathy.
- Congenital nephrotic syndrome.
- Pre-transplant native kidney nephrectomy.

Supplementary Information The online version contains supplementary material available at [https://doi.org/10.1007/978-3-030-99280-4_21].

N. A.-S. Al Anazi (✉) · S. Lobo · I. Mushtaq
Great Ormond Street Hospital, London, UK
e-mail: naser.alanazi@gosh.nhs.uk; naseralsoudan@gmail.com; sara.lobo@gosh.nhs.uk; mushti@gosh.nhs.uk

C. Esposito et al. (eds.), *Minimally Invasive Techniques in Pediatric Urology*,
https://doi.org/10.1007/978-3-030-99280-4_21

21.3 Contraindications

- Previous renal surgery.
- Renal malignancy.
- Xanthogranulomatous pyelonephritis.
- Coagulation disorders.

21.4 Pre-Operative Preparation

- Recent imaging in the form of a recent renal ultrasound scan and MAG3/DMSA scan must be available.
- In children with a history of vesicoureteric reflux, the micturating cystogram images must also be available for review.
- The renal ultrasound provides information about the size of the kidney, degree of hydronephrosis, and, in the case of a multicystic kidney, regarding the number and size of cysts. This allows for determining the approach for specimen removal: endopouch, cyst aspiration, port site extraction.
- Routine preoperative blood tests, which should include serum creatinine, hemoglobin level, and a group/save of serum. Clotting parameters do not need to be checked routinely unless there is a history of bleeding disorders.

21.5 Positioning

The patient is positioned fully prone under general anesthesia. The exposed dorsal and lateral aspects of the trunk are prepared and draped in a sterile manner. For more details, refer to the posterior prone retroperitoneoscopic access chapter.

21.6 Anesthesia

Anesthesia for MIS procedures in children requires endotracheal intubation and the use of volatile and/or intravenous anesthetic agents. Children are at significant risk of developing hypothermia during laparoscopic surgery, especially with prolonged operating times and a high gas flow. Therefore, the use of underbody/overbody warming mats is recommended for all cases. The current trend is to combine general anesthesia with caudal or local anesthesia.

21.7 Instrumentation

- Primary camera port—6 or 10 mm Hasson, 1–2 secondary 5 mm instrument ports.
- 30°- 5 mm laparoscope
- Kelly forceps (×2) for dissection.
- Metzanbeum scissors.
- Harmonic scalpel for coagulation/division of vessels or 5 mm endoclip applicator.
- Endoloop.
- Endopouch for specimen retrieval.

21.8 Technique

- A 5 mm transverse incision is made midway between the iliac crest and the tip of the 12th rib, just lateral to the outer border of the sacrospinalis muscle. This will be used as the camera port (CP) (Fig. 21.1). Through this incision, a small area of the retroperitoneum is dissected bluntly with artery forceps to allow the insertion and inflation of a balloon to create the retroperitoneal working space [2, 3].
- A Hasson cannula is inserted into the port site, followed by insufflation of the retroperitoneum with CO_2 to a pressure of 10–12 mmHg and a flow of 1–3 L/min.
- An instrument port is placed under direct vision below the tip of the 11th/12th ribs and above the iliac crest, and if required a second instrument port can be placed 2–3 cm medial to the camera port traversing the sacrospinalis muscles (Fig. 21.2).
- Gerota's fascia is incised in a cruciate manner to enter the perinephric space (Fig. 21.3) The kidney is dissected on its posteromedial aspect to expose the hilar vessels: these are individually displayed and divided between hemoclips or with a harmonic scalpel (Fig. 21.4).

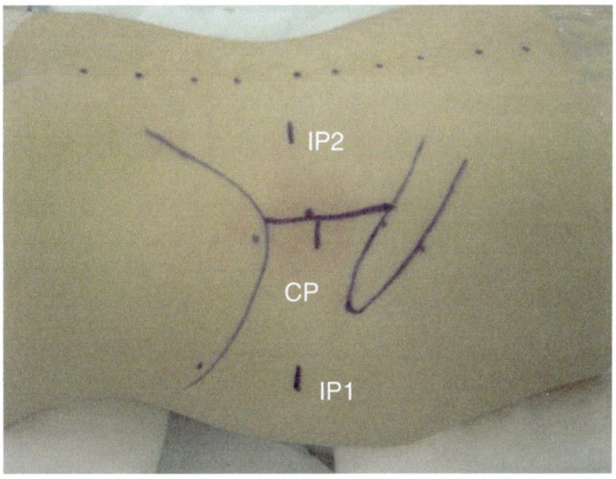

Fig. 21.1 Diagram showing surface landmarks and location of port sites (CP Camera Port, IP1 Instrument port 1, IP2 Instrument port 2)

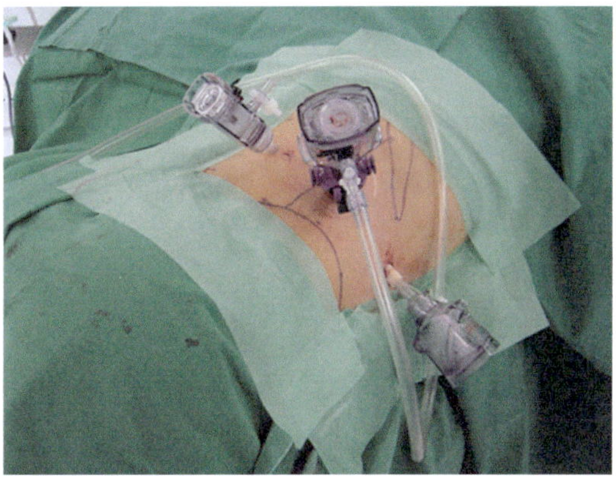

Fig. 21.2 Diagram showing the arrangement of the ports after insertion

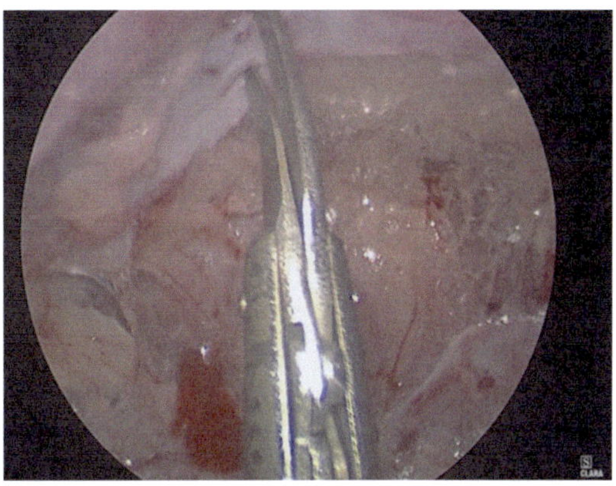

Fig. 21.3 Laparoscopic view of the Gerota's fascia which is incised in a cruciate manner to enter the perinephric space

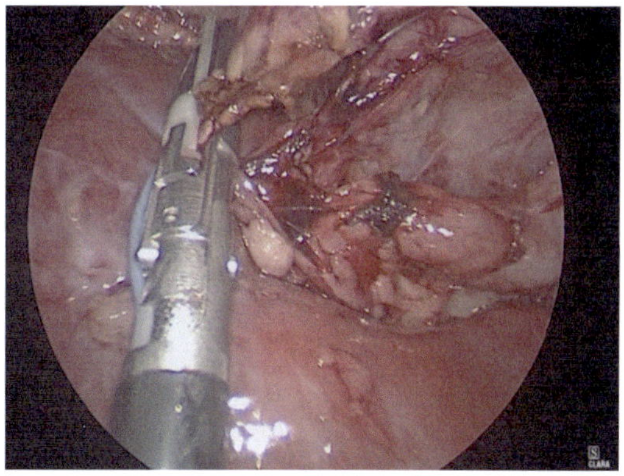

Fig. 21.4 Laparoscopic view of the renal hilar vessels and division using a Ligasure device

- The ureter should be traced inferiorly as far as necessary and divided. In children with ipsilateral vesicoureteric reflux, the ureter should be ligated or the bladder drained with a urethral catheter for 48 h.
- The kidney is then mobilized on all surfaces until it is completely free of all attachments. This can be accomplished with a single instrument but with exceptionally large or previously infected kidneys, it may require a second instrument to provide counter-traction.
- Small kidneys or those with minimum parenchyma can be removed directly via the camera port, whereas larger specimens may require entrapment in an Endopouch retrieval device and piecemeal removal.

21.9 Postoperative Care

- Can start fluids and diet on return to the ward.
- As bacteremia may occur during the procedure, oral antibiotics to cover the immediate postoperative period may be required in some cases.
- The patient is discharged when mobilizing with adequate control of pain with simple analgesia.

21.10 Complications

21.10.1 Peritoneal Tear

The posterior prone approach minimizes the risk of a peritoneal tear as compared to other approaches for retroperitoneoscopic surgery. It can occur in the following situations: dissecting balloon is inflated too rapidly; the balloon is too large for the size of the patient and in children on peritoneal dialysis, where the peritoneum is very delicate.

21.10.2 Balloon Rupture

Rupture of the dissecting balloon can occur when the balloon is inflated too rapidly, with overinflation of the balloon or when excessive external pressure is applied over the balloon. When it occurs, the ruptured balloon must be carefully examined for lost fragments, which should be sought and removed from the patient.

21.10.3 Intraoperative Bleeding

Intraoperative bleeding is most likely due to slipping of hemoclips from a renal vein or due to inadvertent damage to a renal vein or vena cava by a laparoscopic instrument. In most cases, hemorrhage can be controlled by the prompt application of hemoclips to the affected vessel. Uncontrollable hemorrhage will require conversion to an open approach to ligate or over sew the bleeding vessel.

21.10.4 Urine Leak

A retroperitoneal urinoma can occur from the reflux of urine from the distal ureteric stump or from the cut surface of the kidney following heminephrectomy. The risk can be kept to a minimum using an endoloop suture on the renal parenchyma and by endoloop ligation of refluxing ureters as opposed to the use of hemoclips or the harmonic scalpel to seal the ureter. Most urinomas will resolve with the placement of a urethral catheter for at least 48–72 h. A persistent urine leak or an infected urinoma may require the placement of a percutaneous wound drain.

21.11 Results

A recent study from Scotland compared the results of laparoscopic and open nephrectomy in children. It was found that a laparoscopic nephrectomy may take longer to perform but that the children suffer less postoperative pain and have a shorter duration of hospital stay. Furthermore, they found that those children who had a retroperitoneoscopic nephrectomy made an even faster recovery. The technique of retroperitoneoscopic nephrectomy is now well established and has been shown to be applicable to all age groups, with a low conversion (<3%) and complication rate. The technique has been adapted to the management of children who have end-stage renal disease and who require bilateral native kidney nephrectomy. As the peritoneum can be maintained intact, it allows for immediate postoperative peritoneal dialysis.

Tips and Tricks

- A visible lateral bulge during balloon inflation confirms an extraperitoneal location of the balloon.
- The aim should be to inflate the dissecting balloon outside Gerota's fascia, and then incise this under direct vision. This approach will minimize bleeding from the perinephric adipose tissue which bleeds easily.
- For rapid and optimum access to the renal hilum, dissection is started at the inferior pole of the kidney and continued superiorly along the medial aspect of the kidney pushing it laterally and downwards to expose the posteromedial surface and the renal hilum.

- The lateral and inferior attachments of the kidney are maintained intact to facilitate exposure of the renal pedicle by a natural retraction of the kidney.
- Ureterectomy and ureteric ligation can be done after the kidney is extracted out of the patient in an extracorporeal manner.
- With increasing experience, the procedure can be completed with a camera port and single instrument port (SIMPL nephrectomy).
- Bleeding points should be meticulously controlled throughout the procedure with monopolar diathermy.
- A multicystic dysplastic kidney or hydronephrotic kidney may be decompressed by aspiration and withdrawn directly via the camera port wound.

21.12 Discussion

The retroperitoneoscopic approach has several advantages over the transperitoneal laparoscopic approach to the kidney. It avoids the risk of injury to intra-abdominal organs and enables a quicker recovery. It also facilitates easy positioning of the patient and direct access to the kidney resulting in a decreased operative time.

Take-Home Points

- Minimally invasive alternatives to conventional open urological procedures are now practiced in major pediatric urology centers [4, 5].
- Both the transperitoneal and retroperitoneoscopic approaches are utilized in children, although the retroperitoneoscopic technique is favored for renal surgery in benign conditions [5].
- Posterior prone retroperitoneoscopic nephrectomy can be utilized for most of the renal surgeries with minimal complications [5, 6].

References

1. Das S, Keizur JJ, Tashima M. Laparoscopic nephroureterectomy for end-stage reflux nephropathy in a child. Surgical Laparoscopy & Endoscopy. 1993;3(6):462–5
2. Gill IS, Munch LC, Lucas BA, Das S. Initial experience with retroperitoneoscopic nephroureterectomy: use of a double-balloon technique. Urology. 1995;46(5):747–50.
3. Cho A, Asimakidou M, Mushtaq I. Access for retroperitoneoscopic surgery. J Pediatr Urol. 2019;15:287–8.
4. Lee RS, Retik AB, Borer JG, Diamond DA, Peters CA. Pediatric retroperitoneal laparoscopic partial nephrectomy: comparison with an age matched cohort of open surgery. J Urol. 2005;174(2):708–11.
5. Gundeti MS, Patel Y, Duffy PG, Cuckow PM, Wilcox DT. Imran Mushtaq an initial experience of 100 paediatric laparoscopic nephrectomies with transperitoneal or posterior prone retroperitoneoscopic approach. Pediatr Surg Int. 2007;23:795–9.
6. Cho A, Mushtaq I. Retroperitoneoscopic lower pole heminephrectomy. J Pediatr Urol. 2019;15:89–90.

22 Robot-Assisted Partial Nephrectomy in Children

Ibtissam Kassite, Aurélien Binet, Anne Letouze, Thierry Villemagne, Karim Braik, and Hubert Lardy

Learning Objectives
- To describe step by step the technique of robot-assisted partial nephrectomy (RAPN).
- To present long-term outcomes of RAPN.
- To report the latest results about RAPN published in the literature.
- To show a video with the technique of RAPN.
- To share tips and tricks of RAPN.

Supplementary Information The online version contains supplementary material available at [https://doi.org/10.1007/978-3-030-99280-4_22].

I. Kassite · A. Binet · A. Letouze · T. Villemagne
K. Braik · H. Lardy (✉)
Pediatric Surgery Department, Clocheville Hospital, Tours, France
e-mail: ibtissam.kassite@univ-tours.fr; aurelien.binet@univ-tours.fr; a.letouze@chu-tours.fr; t.villemagne@chu-tours.fr; k.braik@chu-tours.fr; hubert.lardy@univ-tours.fr

22.1 Introduction

The management of duplication anomalies of the upper urinary tract depends on many factors: the presence of an ureterocele, a vesico-ureteric reflux of the lower pole, symptoms … The aim of all treatment is to conserve as much normal renal parenchyma as possible.

Currently, different minimally invasive surgical approaches can be used: mostly, laparoscopy, retroperitoneoscopy, and robotic surgery.

Laparoscopic (transperitoneal or retroperitoneal) partial nephrectomy has been reported to be a technically challenging procedure, performed only in pediatric institutions with advanced experience in pediatric laparoscopy [1]. Robotic technology was introduced to ease laparoscopic surgery and to facilitate the expansion of minimally invasive surgery for more complicated procedures, with the added benefits of three-dimensional visualization of the operative environment, elimination of surgeon tremor, the dexterity afforded by instruments. Indeed, this can allow correct identification of anatomical variation and precise control of technically challenging tasks such as delicate dissection of renal hilum.

The aim of this chapter is to focus on the operative technique and the results of robot-assisted partial nephrectomy (RAPN).

C. Esposito et al. (eds.), *Minimally Invasive Techniques in Pediatric Urology*,
https://doi.org/10.1007/978-3-030-99280-4_22

22.2 Preoperative Preparation

Preoperative imaging is performed to specify duplication anatomy. Patients are primarily evaluated with cystography, renal ultrasonography, and scintigraphy scans. If anatomy remains unclear, magnetic resonance imaging can be performed. It provides comprehensive morphologic and functional information on duplicated renal collecting system, as well as demonstrating barely or nonfunctional renal pole. It helps surgical planning by delineating each renal moiety in complicated duplex systems.

Urine testing is performed preoperatively, and preoperative antibiotic prophylaxis is prescribed according to the results.

Surgery is carried out after obtaining parent's approval and after explaining in detail the known benefits, risks, and expectations of RAPN. All the procedures are performed in general anesthesia, and a single dose of antibiotic prophylaxis with cefazolin is administered according to local protocol. No caudal or epidural anesthesia is needed to help in pain control after surgery.

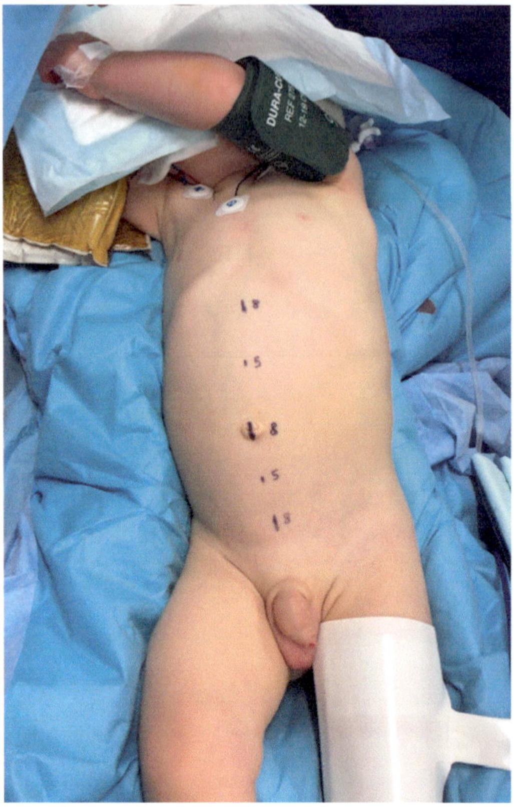

Fig. 22.1 The patient is lying in a vacuum mattress with padding at all pressure points

22.3 Positioning

Patients are positioned in a lateral decubitus position with the ipsilateral side raised using a vacuum mattress (shell mattress), so that they can lie more securely (Fig. 22.1). The patient is sufficiently padded at all pressure points to prevent injury. The robot is positioned over the ipsilateral flank. All procedures are carried out using three arms: one camera arm and two instrument arms (8 mm each). Two additional 5-mm non-robotic accessory ports are used for introducing sutures, suction, irrigation devices, and exposing the working space (Fig. 22.2).

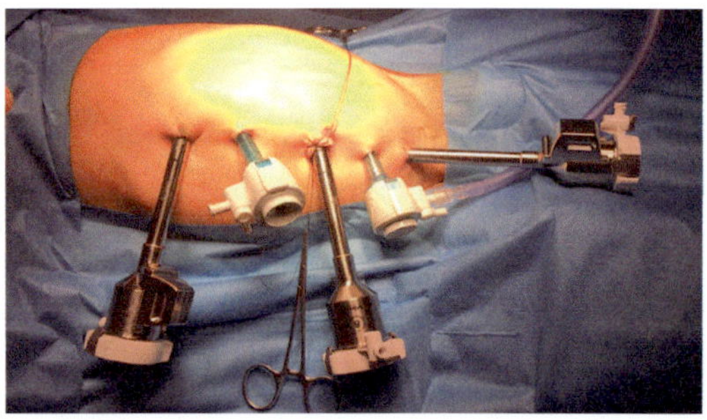

Fig. 22.2 Position of ports for a left partial nephrectomy: 3 robotic ports (8 mm) and 2 non-robotic accessory ports (5 mm)

22.4 Instrumentation

We used two atraumatic fenestrated forceps to handle and manipulate tissues. Monopolar scissors are used in the right-handed 8-mm port and a precise bipolar forceps in the left hand.

We used clips or Ligasure to control the hilar vessel.

We used endoloop (Vicryl Endoloop-0, Ethicon Endo-surgery, Cincinnati, Ohio, USA) or clips to ligate the distal ureter. A flexible silicone loop (Vesseloops®) is needed to retract and expose the nonfunctional moiety. A suction and irrigation device is needed to better expose the working space.

22.5 Technique

No cystoscopic evaluation is performed and no catheterization of the preserved ureter is realized.

The procedure is performed through a transperitoneal approach. The colon is mobilized to reach the kidney in the retroperitoneal space. Sometimes, a transmesocolic approach is performed without colon mobilization. During upper pole partial nephrectomy, the upper pole ureter is identified and freed from the lower ureter. It is then passed behind the lower pole vessels (uncrossing manoeuvre). The blood vessels to both moieties are then identified before carrying out ligation. The upper pole vessels are ligated with nonabsorbable clips or ligasure or absorbable 3-0 Vicryl sutures. A line of demarcation between vascularized and devascularized renal tissue appears clearly on the renal surface after vascular control. Monopolar electrocautery or Ligasure are used to transect the renal tissue.

For lower pole PN, the uncrossing manoeuvre is unnecessary. The equivalent surgical process is carried out after identifying the normal ureter and the functional moiety. The cut margin of the normal moiety is left open with no sutures. Sometimes sealants are used if hemostasis is required. During dissection, renal cavities may be opened in some cases of hugely dilated pelvis in order to help define anatomy and identify clearly the nonfunctional moiety, particularly in case of nondilated ureter. The ureter is then dissected as far as possible down to the bladder to allow a nearly complete ureterectomy, but extensive pelvic dissection of the distal ureter is avoided. Ureteral stump is systematically secured using endoloop and removed through the camera port. No peritoneal drainage is leaved. All of the ports are closed under direct visual control with absorbable 4-0 Vicryl sutures. No bladder catheter is left in place.

22.6 Postoperative Care

Postoperative analgesia typically includes alternating anti-inflammatory drugs and paracetamol (acetaminophen), with narcotics administered as needed. As for the immediate postoperative course, usually children start liquid diet within few hours after surgery. Patients are discharged from the hospital after adequate oral intake and good pain control.

At follow-up, some examinations are performed systematically: renal Doppler ultrasonography every 3 months postoperatively, to assess functionality of the remnant moiety. Poor parenchymal blood flow on Doppler study and/or significant reduction in volume of the remaining moiety during follow-up is considered as renal functional loss. It is not our current practice to perform postoperative renal scintigraphy, if the remaining moiety appears normal or unchanged with adequate decompression or significantly improved hydronephrosis on postoperative ultrasound. In case of functional loss of the remnant moiety in Doppler study and if the patient has clinical presentation (hypertension), a total nephrectomy can be proposed. Sometimes, there is a fluid collection surrounding the margin of the remnant moiety, which is usually asymptomatic.

Urinary tract infections (UTIs) are treated with antibiotics in hospitalization. In case of recurrent febrile UTIs, a cystography scan is then be performed to look for de novo vesico- ureteral reflux in the remaining ureteral stump or the remnant renal moiety.

22.7 Results

In our institution, 18 patients underwent RAPN between 2007 and 2020, performed by three pediatric surgeons (Table 22.1). The median age at surgery was 4.2 years (range 0.9–12) with a median weight of 13.5 kg (range 8.6–27). Averaged operating time was 160.3 min and ranged from 88 to 280 min. All 18 RAPNs were completed totally under robotic assistance without conversion to open surgery.

Intraoperative complications occurred in one patient: a vascular injury which was sutured robotically without need of conversion. Postoperatively, three patients had Clavien–Dindo grade II complications [2]:

- One thrombosis of renal vein and artery. This patient showed a renal (remnant moiety) functional loss, due to vascular injury during RAPN. This patient had clinical presentation (postoperative fever and abdominal pain) and showed poor parenchymal blood flow on Doppler study with thrombosis of the ipsilateral renal vein and artery.
- Two patients had one postoperative UTI.

The median postoperative stay was 3 days (range 2–10). The median time for need of analgesia was 2 days [1–4]. On follow-up (median 4.2 months range 2–49), in all other patients, the postoperative period was uneventful.

In the literature reporting the outcome of RAPN in children published over the last 20 years (Table 22.2), the conversion rate described in all papers ranged between 0% and 14% [3–6]. The median operating time varied between 90 min and 446 min depending on the indications [3, 5]. The complication rate varied between 9% and 21%. These were mainly recurring febrile UTI secondary to refluxing ureteral stump or fluid collections around the kidney. In some series, some patients needed further surgery to remove the distal remnant ureteral stump because of recurrent febrile UTIs [6, 7]. These procedures were done robotically

Table 22.1 Patients' characteristics

Number of patients	18
Age[a] (years) (range)	4.2 (0.9–12)
Weight[a] (kg) (range)	13.5 (8.6–27)
Indications for surgery	Recurrent urinary tract infections
	Incontinence
	Abdominal pain
	Unfunctional moeity
Operative time[a] (min) (range)	146 (88–280)
Conversion	0
Complications	3
Time to no need for analgesic[a] (days)	2 (1–4)
Length of stay[a] (days)	3 (2–10)
Follow-up[a] (months)	4.2 (2–49)

[a]Median

Tips and Tricks

- In partial nephrectomy, it is very helpful to use vessel loops to identify the right ureter and the right vessels to facilitate the dissection of the nonfunctional moiety.
- In case of hugely dilated renal cavities, a transparietal needle aspiration can be useful. Renal cavities can be opened to help to define anatomy and margin of resection, particularly in case of large cavities.
- To avoid injury of the normal moiety by extensive dissection, we suggest to do a nonanatomical resection of the nonfunctional moiety leaving the bottom of renal cavities.

22.8 Discussion

Over the last 20 years, robotic partial nephrectomy has been reported to be safe and feasible in paediatric population [8].

Table 22.2 Previous reports of robotic partial nephrectomy in children

Study	Number of cases	Age	Weight (kg)	Indication	Approach	Operating time (min)	Complications	LOS (days)	Follow-up (months)
Pedraza [3]	1	4 years		Bilateral duplicated systems	Transperitoneal	440	No	2	NM
Olsen [6]	14	4.9 (0.5–20.2) years		Unilateral duplicated system	Retroperitoneoscopy	176 (120–360)	2 conversions	1 (1–4)	8 (1–24)
Lee [21]	9	7.2 years		Unilateral duplicated system	Transperitoneal	275		2.9	6
Cost [10]	1	14 years		Renal cell carcinoma	Transperitoneal	180	NM	2	6
Mason [22]	21	4.1 (0.3–16.7) years		Unilateral duplicated system	Transperitoneal	301 (165–526)	1 iatrogenic forniceal rupture 1 incarcerated hernia at the umbilical port	1.6 (0.8–3.8)	24 (3–80)
Ballouhey [20]	15	20 (7–39) months	10.9 (8.2–14.9)	Unilateral duplicated system	Transperitoneal	201 (130–245)	1 Omentum hernia	3.4 (1–7)	46.4 (25–68)
Tostivint [23]	1	14 years		Unilateral duplicated system	Transperitoneal	235	NM	3	3
Kapoor [4]	3	32.9 (7–46) months	13.7 (10.4–13.6)	Bilateral duplicated systems		446 (356–503)	No	1.7	18.3 (7–36)
Malik [7]	16	37.5 (3–189) months	17.8 (8–73.5)	Unilateral duplicated system	Transperitoneal	135	2 secondary ureterectomy	2 (1–3)	22.1 (3–56)
Herz [14]	19	3.1 years (4 months–10.5 years)		Unilateral duplicated system	Transperitoneal	209 (169–330)	4 VUR (lower ureter)	NM	NM
Wiestma [24]	1	11 months	10.7	Unilateral duplicated system	Transperitoneal	NM	NM	1	1
Varda [13]	27	3.5 (0.6–31) years		Unilateral duplicated system		206 (147–391)	4UTIs 5 fluid collections	1 (1–12)	1.1 years (0–5.5)
Neheman [25]	18	43.9 (17–131) months	14.4 (9.9–32.8)	Unilateral duplicated system	Transperitoneal	256 (163–458)	4 UTIs	2 (1–4)	NM
Blanc [9]	3	7.3 (3.2–14.1) years		2 Wilm's tumor 1 tubulopapillary carcinoma	Retroperitoneoscopy	123 (110–140)	No	3.3 (2–4)	13 (12–14)
Sala [5]	1	3 years	14	Bilateral Wilm's tumor	Transperitoneal	90	No	2	NM

LOS length of stay, *NM* not mentioned, *VUR* vesicoureteral reflux, *UTI* urinary tract infections

The technical difficulty in pediatric partial nephrectomy relies on the delicacy of the renal vasculature of the remnant segment. Robotic assistance allows precise dissection of the moiety, limits mobilization of the remnant pole, and facilitates vessels' isolation.

In children, partial nephroureterectomy is indicated for treatment of patients with poorly functioning moiety and/or symptomatic duplicated systems (recurrent urinary tract infections [UTIs], incontinence, pain), and/or associated vesicoureteral reflux.

Some authors published their experience with robotic partial nephrectomy for oncological indications such as unilateral or bilateral Wilm's tumors, tubulopapillary, or renal cell carcinomas [5, 9, 10].

In partial nephrectomy, the main complications reported are recurrent febrile UTI secondary to refluxing ureteral stump and urine leakage at the resection area. According to some authors, the risk of damaging the lower pole ureter and bladder does not justify the routine excision of the ureteral stump, which is symptomatic (recurrent UTIs) in only 8–10% of cases [11, 12].

Therefore, if a surgical removal is necessary subsequently, it can be performed robotically. As to fluid collections or urinomas, in the majority of cases, they resolved spontaneously or remained stable and asymptomatic. In the series by Varda et al., in two cases, it was found to be associated with pain [13]. One patient was managed successfully with drainage and sclerotherapy, while another failed with this approach and needed open redo partial nephrectomy. In the existing robotic series, no loss of function of the remnant moiety was reported [7, 14]. In our series, one patient experienced renal atrophy. This is explained by vascular injury during the procedure. Particularly when mobilizing and controlling the upper pole as well as additional traction on the hilum when obtaining vascular control there is a greater risk of ischemia of the remnant moiety and therefore loss of renal function [7].

In 2004, Pedraza et al. reported the first case of robot-assisted partial nephrectomy for bilateral duplicated collecting systems in a 4-year-old girl [3]. Since then, many authors adopted robotic approach for this procedure (Table 22.2) since the robot offered advantages such as precise visualization of the moieties and precise vascular control [8].

Some authors reported their experience with robotic retroperitoneoscopy (RP) [6, 9], whereas others performed this procedure through a transperitoneal (TP) approach (Table 22.2). RP is reported to be technically more difficult due to the creation of a nonexisting operative working space [1, 15]. It's also difficult according to some authors to well position the trocars which may be difficult to move because the retroperitoneal space is too small [16]. Also, there is a risk to open the peritoneum during dissection. Specifically with the retroperitoneoscopic approach, Wallis et al. postulated that infants may be at higher risk for residual ischemia in the remaining moiety, given the smaller working space with the hemodynamic effects of CO_2 insufflation on renal blood flow [17].

Blanc et al. reported three cases of partial nephrectomy for oncological indications by adopting retroperitoneoscopic approach [9]. According to the author, this approach spares the peritoneal cavity in case of new developing lesions, and when radiotherapy is indicated (positive margins), it can be limited to retroperitoneal space avoiding *in to* irradiation of the abdomen.

Transperitoneal approach allows performing a complete ureterectomy near the bladder dome avoiding leaving a residual distal ureteral stump, which may cause recurrent febrile UTIs because of reflux on the residual ureteral stump, needing reoperation. In Esposito series, in RP, the ureter can be removed until it crosses the iliac vessels leaving in place the last 5–6 cm of the ureter, thus they recommend the transperitoneal approach when complete excision of the ureter is required like in reflux nephropathy [1].

Also, the TP approach is preferable to retroperitoneoscopy in case of ectopic pelvic kidneys [18, 19]. On the basis of their 20-year experience in pediatric minimally invasive nephrectomy, Esposito et al. preferred performing nephrectomy using the TP approach since it's easier, faster, and safer compared to RP [1]. Sala et al. recommend the use of a TP approach for bilateral nephrectomy for Wilm's tumor since it provides direct access to the kidneys and the renal hilum, and a very good view of the tumors [5]. Moreover, it allows operating on the contralateral side by reinserting the same ports after flipping the patient [5].

Laparoscopy is physically demanding whereas with the robotically assisted system, the surgeon sits relaxed at the console. Robotically assisted system is specifically useful in limiting traction on vasculature and reducing the risk of resultant ischemic damage [7].

In a series by Ballouhey et al., in comparison with the open approach, robotic system provided similar renal outcomes, lower hospital stay, and less postoperative pain, even in lower weight patients [20].

It combines the advantages of the precision of an open approach and the benefits in term of hospital stay, postoperative pain, complications, and cosmetic results of the laparoscopic approach [20]. They found also that infants undergoing RAPN used half the amount of morphine than those undergoing open partial nephrectomy. Robotic surgery with the small port incisions causes less pain than open surgery, and thus allows a shorter recovery [20].

Varda reported that robotic approach for partial nephrectomy was comparable to open approach regarding safety and operating time, with a shorter length of stay with robotic system [13].

In conclusion, we believe partial nephrectomy is a good application of robotic surgery since this device allows a safer dissection of renal hilum, a safer vascular control. Thus, it improves the feasibility and the quality of this procedure.

Take-Home Message

- The indications of partial nephrectomy in children must be selected carefully and good anatomical assessment must be performed preoperatively.
- Minimally invasive surgery is appropriate for this indication either in laparoscopy or robotic.
- Robotic technology allows better surgical ergonomics with fine and precise dissection.
- The main complication is loss of the remnant moiety principally due to vascular thrombosis or injury.
- This surgical treatment cure patients definitively with excellent results.

References

1. Esposito C, Escolino M, Corcione F, Draghici IM, Savanelli A, Castagnetti M, et al. Twenty-year experience with laparoscopic and retroperitoneoscopic nephrectomy in children: considerations and details of technique. Surg Endosc. 2016;30(5):2114–8.
2. Dindo D, Demartines N, Clavien P-A. Classification of surgical complications: a new proposal with evaluation in a cohort of 6336 patients and results of a survey. Ann Surg. 2004;240(2):205–13.
3. Pedraza R, Palmer L, Moss V, Franco I. Bilateral robotic assisted laparoscopic heminephroureterectomy. J Urol. 2004;171(6 Pt 1):2394–5.
4. Kapoor V, Elder JS. Simultaneous bilateral robotic-assisted laparoscopic procedures in children. J Robot Surg. 2015;9(4):285–90.
5. Sala LFM, Guglielmetti GB, Coelho RF. Bilateral nephrectomy robotic-assisted laparoscopic in children with bilateral Wilms' tumor. Urol Case Rep. 2020;31:101146.
6. Olsen LH, Jørgensen TM. Robotically assisted retroperitoneoscopic heminephrectomy in children: initial clinical results. J Pediatr Urol. 2005;1(2):101–4.
7. Malik RD, Pariser JJ, Gundeti MS. Outcomes in pediatric robot-assisted laparoscopic Heminephrectomy compared with contemporary open and laparoscopic series. J Endourol. 2015;29(12):1346–52.
8. Muneer A, Arya M, Shergill IS, Sharma D, Hammadeh MY, Mushtaq I. Current status of robotic surgery in pediatric urology. Pediatr Surg Int. 2008;24(9):973–7.

9. Blanc T, Pio L, Clermidi P, Muller C, Orbach D, Minard-Colin V, et al. Robotic-assisted laparoscopic management of renal tumors in children: preliminary results. Pediatr Blood Cancer. 2019;66(Suppl 3):e27867.
10. Cost NG, Geller JI, DeFoor WR, Wagner LM, Noh PH. A robotic-assisted laparoscopic approach for pediatric renal cell carcinoma allows for both nephron-sparing surgery and extended lymph node dissection. J Pediatr Surg. 2012;47(10):1946–50.
11. De Caluwé D, Chertin B, Puri P. Long-term outcome of the retained ureteral stump after lower pole heminephrectomy in duplex kidneys. Eur Urol. 2002;42(1):63–6.
12. Ade-Ajayi N, Wilcox DT, Duffy PG, Ransley PG. Upper pole heminephrectomy: is complete ureterectomy necessary? BJU Int. 2001;88(1):77–9.
13. Varda BK, Rajender A, Yu RN, Lee RS. A contemporary single-institution retrospective cohort study comparing perioperative outcomes between robotic and open partial nephrectomy for poorly functioning renal moieties in children with duplex collecting systems. J Pediatr Urol. 2018;14(6):549.e1–8.
14. Herz D, Smith J, McLeod D, Schober M, Preece J, Merguerian P. Robot-assisted laparoscopic management of duplex renal anomaly: comparison of surgical outcomes to traditional pure laparoscopic and open surgery. J Pediatr Urol. 2016;12(1):44.e1–7.
15. Borzi PA. A comparison of the lateral and posterior retroperitoneoscopic approach for complete and partial nephroureterectomy in children. BJU Int. 2001;87(6):517–20.
16. Valla J-S. Retroperitoneoscopic surgery in children. Semin Pediatr Surg. 2007;16(4):270–7.
17. Wallis MC, Khoury AE, Lorenzo AJ, Pippi-Salle JL, Bägli DJ, Farhat WA. Outcome analysis of retroperitoneal laparoscopic heminephrectomy in children. J Urol. 2006;175(6):2277–80. discussion 2280–2
18. Esposito C, Valla JS, Yeung CK. Current indications for laparoscopy and retroperitoneoscopy in pediatric urology. Surg Endosc. 2004;18(11):1559–64.
19. Hammad FT, Upadhyay V. Indications for nephrectomy in children: what has changed? J Pediatr Urol. 2006;2(5):430–5.
20. Ballouhey Q, Villemagne T, Cros J, Szwarc C, Braik K, Longis B, et al. A comparison of robotic surgery in children weighing above and below 15.0 kg: size does not affect surgery success. Surg Endosc. 2015;29(9):2643–50.
21. Lee RS, Sethi AS, Passerotti CC, Retik AB, Borer JG, Nguyen HT, et al. Robot assisted laparoscopic partial nephrectomy: a viable and safe option in children. J Urol. 2009;181(2):823–8. discussion 828–9
22. Mason MD, Anthony Herndon CD, Smith-Harrison LI, Peters CA, Corbett ST. Robotic-assisted partial nephrectomy in duplicated collecting systems in the pediatric population: techniques and outcomes. J Pediatr Urol. 2014;10(2):374–9.
23. Tostivint V, Doumerc N, Roumiguie M, Beauval J-B, Rischmann P, Soulie M, et al. Laparoscopic robot-assisted partial nephrectomy with total ureterectomy in a symptomatic complete duplicated system: advantages of transperitoneal approach. Prog Urol. 2014;24(12):738–43.
24. Wiestma AC, Cho PS, Hollis MV, Badway J, Yu RN. Robot-assisted laparoscopic lower pole partial nephrectomy in the pediatric patient. J Pediatr Urol. 2016;12(6):428–9.
25. Neheman A, Kord E, Strine AC, VanderBrink BA, Minevich EA, DeFoor WR, et al. Pediatric partial nephrectomy for upper urinary tract duplication anomalies: a comparison between different surgical approaches and techniques. Urology. 2019;125:196–201.

23 Laparoscopic Partial Nephrectomy in Pediatric Patients

Ciro Esposito, Maria Escolino, Alessandra Farina, Fulvia Del Conte, Vincenzo Coppola, Mariapina Cerulo, Giuseppe Autorino, and Alessandro Settimi

Learning Objectives

- To describe step by step the technique of laparoscopic partial nephrectomy (LPN).
- To present long-term outcomes of LPN.
- To report the latest results of the major international papers about LPN.
- To show with a video the technique of LPN.
- To describe tips and tricks of LPN and to show all the new technologies available in pediatric urology that can be adopted to perform a LPN.

Supplementary Information The online version contains supplementary material available at [https://doi.org/10.1007/978-3-030-99280-4_23].

C. Esposito (✉) · M. Escolino · A. Farina
F. Del Conte · V. Coppola · M. Cerulo · G. Autorino
A. Settimi
Pediatric Surgery Unit, Federico II University of Naples, Naples, Italy
e-mail: ciroespo@unina.it; maria.escolino@unina.it; alessandra.farina@unina.it; fulvia.delconte@unina.it; vincenzocoppola1992@gmail.com; mariapina.cerulo@unina.it; autorino.giuseppe@gmail.com; settimi@unina.it

23.1 Introduction

Duplication of the renal system is one of the most common congenital anomalies of the urinary tract. The majority of these anomalies remain clinically silent. A smaller number of them becomes evident as a consequence of hydronephrosis, vesicoureteral reflux (VUR), or incontinence [1]. Recently, antenatal diagnosis permits to identify many urologic anomalies, including different variants of ureteral duplications, which are clinically asymptomatic.

A duplex renal system often has one moiety that is either poor or nonfunctioning. In such cases, there is indication to remove surgically the nonfunctioning moiety [2]. The surgical management of children with renal duplication depends on a variety of factors such as parenchymal function of each unit and presence or absence of concomitant anatomic anomalies and pathologies, such as ectopic ureterocele or VUR [3–5]. Currently, different surgical approaches can be used to perform partial nephrectomy such as posterior retroperitoneal, lateral retroperitoneal, laparoscopic trans-peritoneal, and more recently robotic approach [6–8].

In case of duplex system with nonfunctioning moiety and a huge refluxing megaureter, laparoscopy is the approach of choice.

This chapter is focused on the operative technique of laparoscopic partial nephrectomy (LPN).

C. Esposito et al. (eds.), *Minimally Invasive Techniques in Pediatric Urology*,
https://doi.org/10.1007/978-3-030-99280-4_23

23.2 Preoperative Preparation

Preoperative examinations should focus on the anatomical malformations of the entire urinary tract and their functional implications. Investigations have to include renal ultrasonography and DMSA renal scintigraphy or a magnetic resonance (MR) urogram. In some cases, cystoscopy may help to understand the anatomy. An intestinal preparation with simethicone, enema, and liquid diet is desirable, especially in young children.

Preoperative antibiotic prophylaxis should be administered either with a broad-spectrum medication or according to the child's specific urine testing.

All patients and their parents have to sign a specifically formulated informed consent before the procedure. Patients receive a general anesthesia with oro-tracheal intubation and myorelaxation. A Foley catheter is positioned into the bladder using sterile precautions just before surgery and a nasogastric tube is placed in order to keep empty the stomach during the procedure.

23.3 Positioning

In case of laparoscopic partial nephrectomy (LPN), the patient should be placed in a semilateral decubitus position, close to the edge of the operating table, with the ipsilateral side elevated using a pad underneath. The surgeon and the assistant stand on the contralateral side, facing the pathology and the monitor in a straight line on the patient's back (Fig. 23.1). This approach uses the gravity for the retraction of the colon, allows clear dissection of the ureter till down to the bladder level, and provides a safe access to the renal pedicle. We always adopt a 10-mm 30° optic since we usually remove the kidney moiety through the optic orifice. In laparoscopy, we start the procedure using three trocars, even if we sometimes need an additional fourth trocar, more often on the right side, in order to retract the liver or alternatively on the left side in order to retract the spleen or the loops. In general, we prefer to adopt 5-mm working trocars so as to use intraoperatively a clip applier for vessel control, a sealing device, or a peanut, that have 5-mm diameter. The trocars are positioned in triangulation with the optic in order to achieve a better ergonomics (Fig. 23.2): one port for the optic in the umbilicus and two working ports in the upper and lower quadrant (always ipsilateral to the diseased kidney) for the instruments.

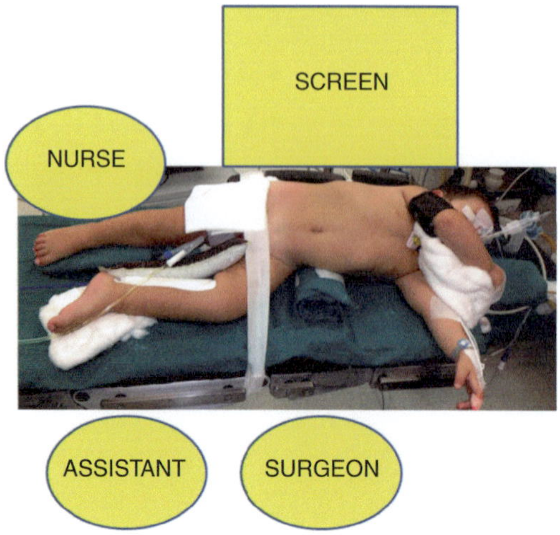

Fig. 23.1 The patient is positioned in semilateral decubitus on the operative table with the screen on his back, and the surgeon and the assistant in front of him

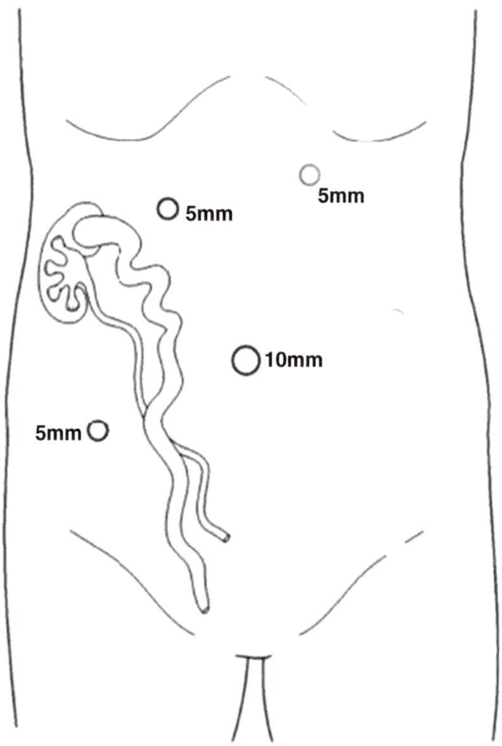

Fig. 23.2 We prefer to use 4 trocars: one 10-mm optic trocar in the umbilicus and two 5-mm working trocars and a fourth 5-mm trocar to retract the liver or the spleen

23.4 Instrumentation

Before starting laparoscopy, we usually perform a cystoscopy, and we place a stent into the normal moiety ureter. In this step, we adopt an 9.5 Fr operative cystoscope. Regarding the laparoscopic procedure, we adopt a 10-mm 30° optic and all 5-mm instruments. We use two atraumatic fenestrated grasping forceps to manage tissues, one curved dissector to isolate vessels, a hook cautery to perform dissection, and scissors to cut. We usually adopt an endoloop to ligate the distal ureter. A needle holder is rarely adopted for this procedure. The hilar vessel control is usually performed using 5-mm titanium clips, or alternatively, using hemostatic devices such as Starion MLS3 or Ligasure, that may be useful to perform a faster and safer dissection. A peanut may be helpful during the dissection. It is safe to prepare a suction and aspiration device and put it on the bench because it may be useful in case of bleeding. No endo-bag is needed to remove the kidney moiety that is usually exteriorized through the umbilical trocar orifice, except for cases of infected kidney. In the last 3 years, we adopted indocyanine green (ICG)-enhanced fluorescence technology in order to easily identify the vascularization and to guide the parenchymal resection of the nonfunctioning moiety. To use ICG technology, you need a special equipment represented by a special camera system and a special laparoscope equipped with a specific filter for near-infrared (NIR) light detection and obviously a vial of ICG dye (5 mg/mL) to be injected intravenously during the procedure.

23.5 Technique

The technique is divided in two phases: cystoscopy and laparoscopy. Cystoscopy is performed as the first step of the procedure with the aim to place a stent into the ureter of the normal functioning pole to be adopted intraoperatively as a guide to avoid injury to the normal ureter during the dissection of the nonfunctioning moiety ureter.

In the laparoscopy phase, as the loops slide down due to the semilateral decubitus, the colon is detached and lowered before opening the Gerota's fascia and access to the kidney. An alternative could be to pass through a trans-mesocolic window, but it may be challenging especially in older children due to abundant fatty tissue in the meso and a considerable risk of vascular injury. For this reason, most authors prefer to detach the colon. This step can be performed using hook cautery or a sealing device that allows a faster and safer surgery without bleeding. After opening the Gerota's fascia, the ureter of the affected moiety is identified and isolated, and it is dissected upward to the kidney. Thereafter, hilar vessels of the affected moiety are identified, isolated separately, and finally clipped and divided. Another option to manage the vessel is to seal them using sealing device. After vessels ligation, a demarcation line shows the dissection plane between the normal and the ischemic moiety that can be easily sectioned using sealing device. Thereafter, the affected pole is separated from the posterior attachment, and the ureter is isolated downward, up to the bladder dome. If VUR is present into the affected kidney moiety, the ureter should be isolated far down as possible to the bladder base and ligated, using preferably an endoloop. If VUR is not present, the ureter can be left open.

In the last 3 years, we adopted ICG-enhanced fluorescence in order to better identify the vessels of the nonfunctioning moiety and to guide the surgeon during the parenchymal resection.

ICG is injected intravenously, using a dosage of 0.3 mg/mL/kg, just after the division of the Gerota's fascia and ICG-guided NIRF allows to visualize the vascularization of the kidney within 2 min. ICG-enhanced fluorescence is very useful to identify the main hilar vessels and the vessels supplying the upper/lower moiety (Figs. 23.3 and 23.4). After

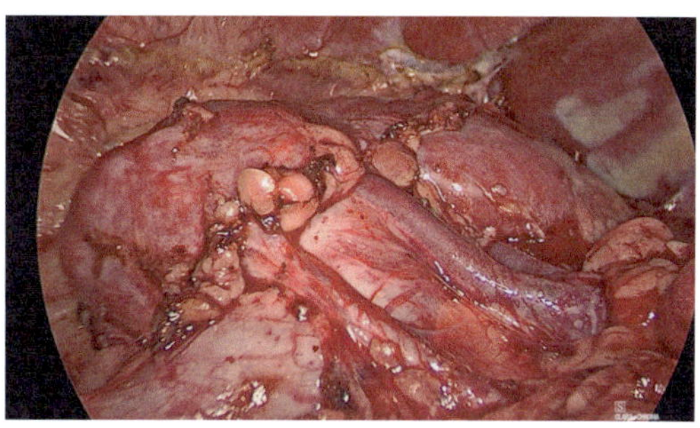

Fig. 23.3 View of the main renal vessels and two lower pole vessels at standard white light imaging in a lower pole partial nephrectomy

division of supplying vessels, ICG-enhanced fluorescence is useful to delineate the anatomical boundary or dissection plane between the two moieties and finally check the perfusion of the normal moiety following the parenchymal resection of the nonfunctioning one (Figs. 23.5 and 23.6).

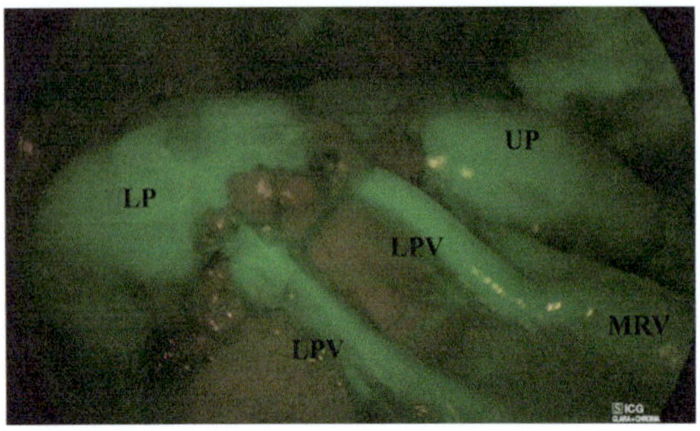

Fig. 23.4 Using ICG-enhanced fluorescence, the renal vessels and renal parenchyma appear green colored. (LP) lower pole; (UP) upper pole; (MRV) main renal vessels; (LPV) lower pole vessels

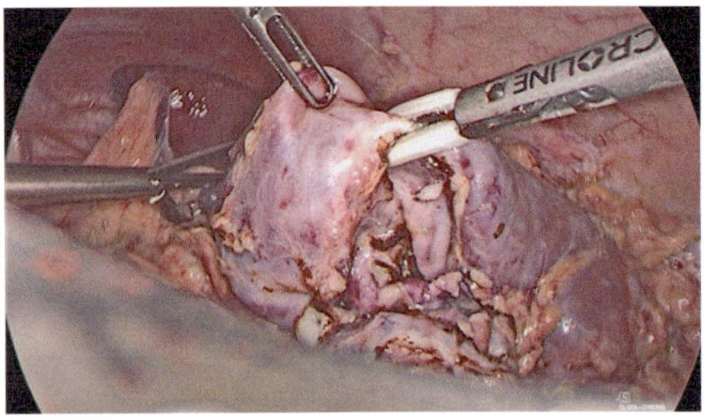

Fig. 23.5 After vessel ligation, the nonfunctioning upper pole moiety is resected using sealing device

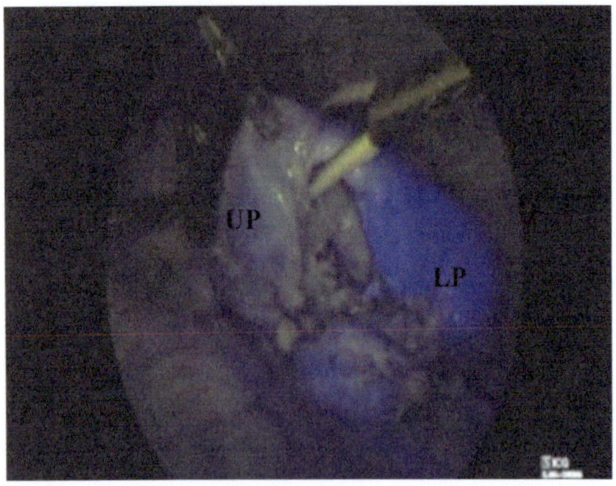

Fig. 23.6 ICG-enhanced fluorescence allowed to identify the demarcation line between the normal lower pole and the ischemic upper pole

In laparoscopy, the resected moiety and the ureter are removed through the umbilical orifice. An indwelling abdominal drain can be left to check postoperative urinary leakage.

23.6 Postoperative Care

Patients start oral feeding few hours postoperatively. Analgesic therapy is rarely necessary; paracetamol (dosage 15 mg/kg at 8-h interval) is usually administered in the first 12–24 h postoperatively. A short-term antibiotic therapy is performed for 48–72 h postoperatively. Patients are discharged from hospital on second or third postoperative day (POD). Postoperative clinical controls are scheduled on 7th and 30th POD and thereafter annually. A renal Doppler ultrasonography is performed 1 month and 1 year postoperatively to check the vascularization of the remaining moiety (Fig. 23.7). Finally, a renal scintigraphy is performed 1 year postoperatively to assess the function of the remaining moiety.

23.7 Results

The median duration of surgery in our experience is 95 min (range 80–125). The conversion rate of laparoscopic partial nephrectomy, when performed by experienced surgeons, is near 0% [9–

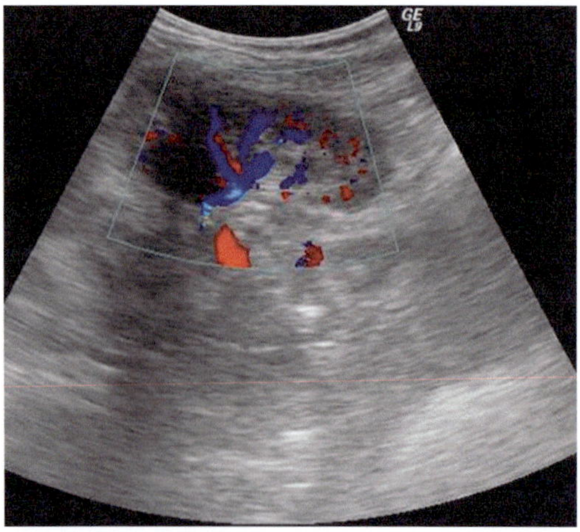

Fig. 23.7 At 1-month follow-up, a Doppler renal ultrasonography is performed to check the vascularization of the remaining renal moiety

11]. It is important to underline that you should accomplish this procedure only after a robust experience with total nephrectomy.

The indications for surgery include recurrent urinary tract infections (UTIs), secondary to VUR and/or obstructive ureterocele, loss of kidney moiety function, and ectopic ureter causing (pseudo) incontinence [12, 13].

A recent multicenter study by Esposito et al. [2] reported 10/52 (19.2%) complications (4 urinomas, 2 recurrent UTIs in symptomatic ureteral stumps, 4 prolonged urinary leakages), classified as grade II according to Clavien–Dindo grading system [14], but no conversions to open surgery or intraoperative complications were recorded. The patients with prolonged urinary leakage were managed conservatively, leaving the bladder catheter and the drainage in situ until the complete resolution of the leakage (max 10 days) [2, 9]. In the same study, in one patient, who underwent upper partial-nephrectomy, the urinary leakage was discovered intraoperatively, and methylene blue dye was injected into the stent, previously introduced into the normal ureter via cystoscopy, in order to identify the leakage point and close it with interrupted stitches [2].

In the study by Esposito et al. [2], the remaining complications (four urinomas and two recurrent UTIs in symptomatic refluxing ureteral stumps) are resolved spontaneously or after antibiotic therapy, without the need of a new surgical procedure [2, 9]. Renal Doppler ultrasound was normal in all patients, either 1 month or 1 year after surgery. Postoperative DMSA scan demonstrated no loss of function of the residual kidney moiety (mean 37.8%) compared with preoperative value (mean 38.1%) in all operated children [2, 9].

Analyzing the literature reporting the outcome of LPN in children published over the last 10 years [6–8], a 0% conversion rate was described in all papers. The median operative time varied between 90 min and 198 min. The complications rate varied between 7.4% and 52.9% [14–16].

Tips and Tricks

- In case of partial nephrectomy, it is very useful to perform a cystoscopy before starting laparoscopy in order to place a stent in the normal ureter to avoid damaging it during the procedure. Regarding the laparoscopic phase, the patient's position in semilateral decubitus is a crucial point for the success of the procedure; in fact, using this patient's positioning, the loops slide down and you have an excellent exposure of the renal lodge. It is fundamental to detach the colon when you have to perform a partial nephro-ureterectomy; in this way, you can easily expose the kidney and isolate the entire ureter up to the bladder dome. An additional fourth trocar may be useful especially on the right side to retract the liver but sometimes also on the left side; in such case, the need of a fourth trocar depends on the spleen's size and on the surgeon's preference. Probably at the beginning of experience, it is better to use always four trocars, independently from the affected side, in order to have an adequate exposure of the operative field.
- A very useful expedient in our experience is to check the integrity of the parenchymal resection edge by injection of methylene blue dye into the ureteral catheter positioned preoperatively into the ureter of the normal functioning moiety. In this way, we can see that the normal functioning of kidney moiety has not been opened during the resection of the nonfunctioning moiety. We also suggest to leave an indwelling abdominal drain for at least 24–48 h postoperatively to check an eventual urinary leakage.
- Finally, another important recommendation is to always perform distal ureterectomy to the level of the bladder hiatus and to ligate the ureteric stump in patients with refluxing ureter in order to avoid postoperative symptoms associated with recurrent UTIs.

- Another useful expedient is to use sealing devices for tissue dissection that make the procedure bloodless, faster, and safer.
- Regarding the management of hilar vessels also if sealing devices have the FDA approval to seal vessels of 5–7 mm in diameter, we believe that it is safer to ligate hilar vessels using endoscopic clips. It is also important to remember that if you use clips to close vessels, it is forbidden to use monopolar energy or sealing devices to seal the vessels between clips, in order to avoid the risk of clips dislodgement that may occur immediately or later in the postoperative period.
- At the end of the procedure, it is not necessary to re-attach the colon to the abdominal wall.
- ICG technology may be useful to identify kidney vascularization and to guide the surgeon during the parenchymal resection, allowing a clear identification of the demarcation line between the ischemic and the perfused moiety.

23.8 Discussion

Laparoscopic partial nephrectomy has gained widespread acceptance for benign kidney pathologies in pediatric patients over the last two decades [9, 10, 17].

Advanced laparoscopic procedures in pediatric urology field are now facilitated by the use of the advanced technologies available on the market as HD cameras, miniaturized instruments, and special sealing devices [11]. Furthermore, new imaging technologies such as ICG-enhanced fluorescence allow easier intraoperative visualization of the kidney anatomy and its vasculature and subsequently safer dissection of the anatomic structures [7, 18]. Excluding oncological indications, the main indication for partial nephrectomy in children is to remove a nonfunctioning upper or lower pole secondary to complicated duplex anomalies of the kidney [7].

Laparoscopic partial nephrectomy is technically more demanding than laparoscopic nephrectomy [12]. In particular, during the resection of the nonfunctioning moiety, there is the risk to damage the vascularization of the residual kidney and also the risk of urine leakage at the level of the parenchymal resection or at the level of the residual ureteral stump [7].

After the first description of laparoscopic partial nephrectomy in children by Jordan and Winslow more than 25 years ago in 1993 [19], this procedure has gained wider acceptance compared to the open approach, thanks to the reported advantages of decreased hospital stay, lower analgesic requirements, and better cosmesis [14].

This procedure can be carried out through either a retroperitoneal or transperitoneal approach [10].

Although there is no evidence in the international literature about which technique between laparoscopy and retroperitoneoscopy is the best to adopt to perform LPN, analyzing the international literature, it seems that retroperitoneoscopy has a higher rate of conversion and a higher number of major complications compared to LPN [15].

The most frequent complications occurred in our experience in LPN were urinomas and prolonged leakages that are related to urine leakage at the level of the parenchymal resection or of the residual ureteral stump [2]. This leakage could be due to residual excretive structures of an incompletely resected kidney moiety or to the opening of the normal functioning kidney moiety.

Based upon our experience, it seems that the prolonged leakage can be due also to an excessive peritoneal secretion due to the fact that the colon is mobilized to better expose the kidney and ureter. We also recorded two cases of recurrent UTIs due to symptomatic residual ureteric stumps [2, 9].

The use of laparoscopy to perform partial nephrectomy has the main benefit of a good overall exposure of the anatomy of the kidney and its vasculature; in particular, it is extremely easy to identify the vascularization of the nonfunctioning kidney, thanks to the use of a 30° optic. Furthermore, during the dissection of the dilated ureter, it is very important to identify and save the gonadal vessels, that cross the ureter on the left side, in male patients.

In conclusion, we believe that laparoscopic partial nephrectomy is easier compared to the other approaches adopted to perform partial nephrectomy in MIS (retroperitoneoscopy, prone position), but it still remains a challenging procedure performed only in pediatric centers with a strong experience in minimally invasive surgery. In our experience, the principal advantages of the laparoscopic approach include the complete and clear view of all urinary tract, the excellent exposure of renal hilar vessels, and the possibility to remove the entire ureter up to the bladder dome.

Take-Home Points

- You've to start to perform LPN only after a strong experience in total nephrectomy.
- Before starting LPN it's preferable to perform a cystoscopy and to position a catheter in the ureter of the normal moiety in order to avoid injuries during the dissection.
- You need 3/4 trocars with an optic of 10-mm 30°, because you have to remove the specimen thorough the umbilicus.
- New technologies as sealing devices and ICG-enhanced fluorescence imaging may be helpful to perform a bloodless, safer, and faster procedure.
- A long-term outcome is crucial to check the complications and the status of the remaining moiety.

References

1. Jiang D, Wang Q, Shi Z, Sun J. Congenital anomalies of the kidney and urinary tract in children with congenital heart defects. Kidney Blood Press Res. 2020;45(2):307–13.
2. Esposito C, Varlet F, Patkowski D, Castagnetti M, Escolino M, Draghici IM, Settimi A, Savanelli A, Till H. Laparoscopic partial nephrectomy in duplex kidneys in infants and children: results of an European multicentric survey. Surg Endosc. 2015;29(12):3469–76.
3. Borzi PA, Yeung CK. Selective approach for transperitoneal and extraperitoneal endoscopic nephrectomy in children. J Urol. 2004;171:814–6.
4. Wang DS, Bird VG, Cooper CS, et al. Laparoscopic upper pole heminephrectomy for ectopic ureter: initial experience. Can J Urol. 2004;11:2141–5.
5. Piaggio L, Franc-Guimond J, Figueroa TE, Barthold JS, Gonzalez J. Comparison of laparoscopic and open partial nephrectomy for duplication anomalies in children. J Urol. 2006;175:2269–73.
6. Esposito C, Miyano G, Caione P, Escolino M, Chiarenza F, Riccipetitoni G, Yamataka A, Cerulo M, Savanelli A, Settimi A, Valla JS. Retroperitoneoscopic heminephrectomy in duplex kidney in infants and children: results of a multicentric survey. J Laparoendosc Adv Surg Tech A. 2015;25(10):864–9.
7. Neheman A, Kord E, Strine AC, Vander Brink BA, Minevich EA, DeFoor WR, Reddy PP, Noh PH. Pediatric partial nephrectomy for upper urinary tract duplication anomalies: a comparison between different surgical approaches and techniques. Urology. 2019;125:196–201.
8. Polok M, Dzielendziak A, Apoznanski W, Patkowski D. Laparoscopic heminephrectomy for duplex kidney in children-the learning curve. Front Pediatr. 2019;7:117.
9. Esposito C, Escolino M, Miyano G, Caione P, Chiarenza F, Riccipetitoni G, Yamataka A, Savanelli A, Settimi A, Varlet F, Patkowski D, Cerulo M, Castagnetti M, Till H, Marotta R, La Manna A, Valla JS. A comparison between laparoscopic and retroperitoneoscopic approach for partial nephrectomy in children with duplex kidney: a multicentric survey. World J Urol. 2016;34(7):939–48.
10. Yao D, Poppas DP. A clinical series of laparoscopic nephrectomy, nephro-ureterectomy and heminephroureterectomy in the pediatric population. J Urol. 2000;163:1531–5.
11. Robinson BC, Snow BW, Cartwright PC, DeVries CR, Hamilton BD, Anderson JB. Comparison of laparoscopic versus open partial nephrectomy in a pediatric series. J Urol. 2003;169:638–40.
12. Elashry OM, Wolf JS Jr, Rayala HJ, McDougall EM, Clayman RV. Recent advances in laparoscopic partial nephrectomy: comparative study of electrosurgicals electrode and ultrasound dissection. J Endourol. 1997;11:15–22.
13. El-Ghoneimi A, Valla JS, Steyaert H, Aigrain Y. Laparoscopic renal surgery via a retroperitoneal approach in children. J Urol. 1998;160:1138–41.
14. Dindo D, Demartines N, Clavien PA. Classification of surgical complications. A new proposal with evaluation in a cohort of 6336 patients and results of a survey. Ann Surg. 2004;240:205–13.
15. Singh R, Wagener S, Chandran H. Laparoscopic management and outcomes in non-functioning moi-

eties of duplex kidneys in children. J Pediatr Urol. 2010;6:66–9.
16. Schneider A, Ripepi M, Geiss S. Laparoscopic transperitoneal partial nephrectomy in children under 2 years old: a single-centre experience. J Pediatr Urol. 2010;6(2):166–70.
17. Janetschek G, Seibold J, Radmayr C, Bartsch G. Laparoscopic heminephro-ureterectomy in pediatric patients. J Urol. 1997;158:1928–30.
18. Esposito C, Del Conte F, Cerulo M, Gargiulo F, Izzo S, Esposito G, Spagnuolo MI, Escolino M. Clinical application and tecnica standardization of indocyanine green (ICG) fluorescence imaging in pediatric minimally invasive surgery. Pediatr Surg Int. 2019;35(10):1043–50.
19. Jordan GH, Winslow DH. Laparoendoscopic upper pole partial nephrectomy with ureterectomy. J Urol. 1993;150:940–3.

Partial Nephrectomy Using Retroperitoneoscopy

24

Matthieu Peycelon, Valeska Bidault, Annabel Paye-Jaouen, and Alaa El-Ghoneimi

Learning Objectives

- To describe step by step how to perform a laparoscopic retroperitoneal partial nephrectomy.
- To present long-term outcomes of laparoscopic retroperitoneal partial nephrectomy.
- To report the latest results of the major international articles about laparoscopic retroperitoneal partial nephrectomy.
- To show a video with a laparoscopic retroperitoneal partial nephrectomy procedure.
- To describe tips and tricks of laparoscopic retroperitoneal partial nephrectomy.
- To discuss the management of complications.

24.1 Introduction

Laparoscopic procedures in pediatric urology are gaining popularity with an increasing number of centers performing advanced surgery due to improvements in equipment and expertise. Currently, nephrectomy is an accepted laparoscopic procedure in children and is included in the routine practice of many centers [1] Partial nephrectomy is technically more demanding than total nephrectomy and needs more laparoscopic experience showed by higher conversion rate and possible renal and extrarenal complications [2] Since the first description of partial nephrectomy in children by Jordan et al., the procedure has been reported either through transperitoneal or retroperitoneal approaches and more recently the surgery is also feasible by robotic assisted technique [3–8]. Partial nephrectomy is a well-established option for the treatment of nonfunctioning renal moieties in duplex kidneys. Most indications are represented by high-grade reflux in lower moieties and nonfunctioning upper moieties caused by ureterocele or ectopic distal implantation of the ureter [4]. Retroperitoneal approach is preferable for partial nephrectomy as it resembles more closely the approach used in open surgery [9]. Due to the limited indications of partial nephrectomy in children, the number of patients in most reported series to date remains small [9]. The emergence of alternative procedures to partial nephrectomy had also

M. Peycelon · V. Bidault · A. Paye-Jaouen
A. El-Ghoneimi (✉)
Department of Pediatric Urology, Robert-Debré University Hospital, APHP, Paris, France

National Reference Center of Rare Urinary Tract Malformations (MARVU), Paris, France

Université de Paris, Paris, France
e-mail: matthieu.peycelon@aphp.fr; valeska.bidault@aphp.fr; annabel.paye-jaouen@aphp.fr; alaa.elghoneimi@aphp.fr

C. Esposito et al. (eds.), *Minimally Invasive Techniques in Pediatric Urology*,
https://doi.org/10.1007/978-3-030-99280-4_24

reduced significantly the number of these procedures (ureterocele incision, low transureteroureterostomy for duplex system).

24.2 Preoperative Preparation

A duplex renal system often has one moiety that is either poor or nonfunctioning. Excluding oncological indications, partial nephrectomy is usually done in children to remove surgically a nonfunctioning upper or lower pole secondary to complicated duplex anomalies of the kidney. The usual pathology of the upper pole is recurrent urinary tract infections (UTIs), persistent obstruction associated with an ureterocele after endoscopic incision or incontinence secondary to an ectopic ureter [1, 8, 10–12]. The usual pathology in the lower pole is UTIs and vesicoureteric reflux (VUR) [13, 14].

Patient preparation is not different from the conventional pediatric urology preparation. Any specific diet measures are prescribed before surgery. Usual recommendations for general anesthesia preparations are followed. All patients are screened for blood type. Serum electrolytes, creatinine, and coagulation studies are performed, and all patients should have preoperative sterile urine cultures. The child is on strict diet depending on his/her age, according to international pediatric anesthesia guidelines (usually between 4 h and 8 h), and premedicated before going to the operating room. Some surgeons recommend fluid diet and enema on the night preceding surgery [10]. Cystoscopy, ureteral stent insertion, and indwelling bladder catheter are recommended to facilitate the identification of one of the poles. A nasogastric tube may be placed after the endotracheal general anesthesia. Noninvasive hemodynamic and ventilatory monitoring is needed during the laparoscopic polar nephrectomy in either trans- or retroperitoneal approach. Cephalosporin is administered intravenously at the induction time.

24.3 Positioning

The retroperitoneal access is done by a lateral approach. The patient is placed lateral, with a lumber padding to laterally flex the patient to expose the area of trocars placement, between the last rib and the ileac crest. Yeung et al. used different positioning according to the side of the kidney: semi-prone for the right side and semi-lateral for the left side [15].

24.4 Instrumentation

Regarding the laparoscopic retroperitoneal procedure, we adopt a10-mm 0° optic and two 5 mm working trocars. We use one atraumatic fenestrated grasping forceps, one 5-mm scissors, one 5-mm bipolar, and sealing devices.

24.5 Technique

24.5.1 Retroperitoneal Access

24.5.1.1 Lateral Approach

The patient is placed lateral, with enough flexion of the operating table so as to expose the area of trocar placement, between the last rib and the iliac crest. In infants and young children (under 6 years), our preference is to use lumber padding to laterally flex the patient without flexing the operating table. Retroperitoneal access is achieved through the first incision, 10–15 mm in length, and one finger width from the lower border of the tip of the 12th rib. The use of narrow retractors with long blades allows a deep dissection despite a short incision. Gerota's fascia is approached by a muscle splitting blunt dissection, then it is opened under direct vision and the first blunt trocar (10 mm, 0° lens) is introduced directly inside the opened Gerota's fascia. A working space is created by gas insufflation's dissection, and the first trocar is fixed with a purse-string suture that is applied around the deep fascia to ensure an air-tight seal and to allow traction on the main trocar if needed to increase the working space. This suture is preferably done before putting the trocar as the small incision is too tight around the trocar. We prefer this type of fixation to the disposable self-retaining trocar, as we find that this type of trocar is relatively large and interferes with the mobility of instruments. A second trocar (5 mm) is inserted posteriorly in the costovertebral angle, in front of the lumbosacral muscle. A third trocar (5 mm) is inserted in the anterior axillary line, a finger width from the top of the iliac crest. To avoid transperitoneal insertion of this trocar, the working space is fully developed, and the deep surface of the anterior wall muscles is identified before trocar insertion. Insufflation pressure does not exceed 12 mm, and the CO_2 flow rate is progressively increased from 1 L to 3 L/min. Access to the retroperitoneum and creation of the working space are the keys to success in retroperitoneal renal surgery. Age and weight are not limiting factors for this approach [14]. Young children have less fat and the access is easier. The authors' preference is for the lateral approach; it allows any type of renal surgery at any age with good exposure to the distal ureter.

24.5.1.2 Other Techniques to Access the Retroperitoneal Space

Since the description by Gaur, balloon dissection has been the method applied by most urologists [16]. Disadvantages of the balloon are the cost of the disposable material and the possible complications related to rupture of the balloon [17]. On the other hand, balloon dissection allows creating a working space without opening Gerota's fascia, which is important for radical removal of malignant tumors in adults. Capolicchio et al. [26] described a modification of lateral access [18]. They recommend the insertion of the first trocar through the costovertebral angle. This modification helped the authors to avoid an accidental peritoneal tear during access through the first lateral incision and allowed a smaller incision for the laparoscope. One of the possible disadvantages of the use of this device is that the placement of the device can be badly inserted and the Gerota's fascia would be approached more anteriorly. This common mistake may lead to the drop down of the kidney and makes more difficult the retroperitoneal approach with the need to retract the kidney upward. Micali et al. reported the use of the Visiport visual trocar to access directly to the retroperitoneal space, which was originally described by Cadeddu et al. [19, 20]. The advantage of this method is the possibility to use a small incision for the first trocar, which is helpful in reconstructive surgery but not in ablative surgery as the first incision is needed for organ retrieval.

24.5.2 Retroperitoneal Laparoscopic Upper Pole Partial Nephroureterectomy

Cystoscopy at the beginning of the procedure is advised to confirm and define the underlying pathology, and in our last decade practice, we insert routinely a ureteral catheter to the remaining moiety ureter. This step will allow to connect methylene blue to the ureteral catheter and to inject the dye just before the parenchyma transection. The advantage of this step is to easily find the healthy ureter to remain (especially if the pathologic ureter is not significantly dilated) and to confirm after the parenchymal transection that no leak from the remaining collecting system is identified.

As previously described, the kidney is approached posteriorly [1]. The upper pole ureter is identified at the lower pole of the kidney and dissected very close to its wall not to injure the vascularization of the lower pole ureter. We found it helpful to ligate the proximal ureter before cutting it, so the proximal ureter remains dilated facilitating the dissection of the upper pole. The upper pole ureter is lifted off the vessels by blunt dissection superiorly. The upper pole ureter is used as a handle to facilitate this part of dissection. The plan between the dilated upper pole pelvis and the lower pole parenchyma is easily identifiable by blunt dissection until the edges of the thin parenchyma of the upper moiety are recognized. At this step, the upper pole vessels are identified running from the aorta or the renal vessels to the upper pole parenchyma. They are either clipped or coagulated depending on their size. The upper pole is identified by color changes after vessel ligature and mostly by the difference in aspect between normal lower pole and dilated dysplastic upper pole. In cases of having difficulty to individualize upper pole vessels, the parenchymal transection is started before the vascular control of the upper pole. Sometimes, it is safer to go through the dilated cavity of the upper pole to identify the limit of parenchymal transection. Many options are available to transect the parenchyma. Surgeons must choose the device that they are most familiar with. The device can be monopolar hook, bipolar energy, sealing devices, or harmonic scalpel. We have been using the harmonic scalpel with the curved jaws, as it provides a clean cut at the junction between upper and lower poles. To minimize mobilization of the lower pole and consequently the risk of indirect vascular trauma of the renal pedicle, the lower pole remains attached to the peritoneum during all the steps of the procedure. The upper pole is freed completely from peritoneal attachments before transecting the parenchyma to avoid any transperitoneal bowel injury. The distal part of the upper ureter is left opened and suction of its contents is done to decompress the ureterocele. If it is a refluxing ectopic ureter, the distal ureter is dissected as far as possible and is ligated by endocorporeal knots or endoloop. Drain is not routinely used except in specific cases of severe adhesions secondary to repeated infections or any doubt of opening the collecting system.

24.5.3 Retroperitoneal Laparoscopic Lower Pole Partial Nephrectomy

The access is the same as for the upper pole. The lower pole ureter is identified and followed till the lower pole pelvis to be sure of its identification. Contrary to the upper pole nephrectomy, full dissection of the lower pole vessels is necessary before transecting the parenchyma. As the main pathology is a VUR with repeated UTIs, the lower pole is usually retracted and easily identified from the healthy upper pole parenchyma. The ureter is ligated near to the bladder to avoid postoperative reflux in a long ureteral stump.

24.5.4 Robot-Assisted Laparoscopic Partial Nephrectomy (RALPN)

Described by Lee et al. in 2009, RALPN could be performed using the Vinci Surgical System [5]. The affected side is elevated by a 30° wedge and the patient is secured carefully to the operating table. With the abdomen flat, transperitoneal port access is gained either using a Veress needle or via the modified Hasson technique. A camera port (12 mm) is placed at the umbilicus. A second port is placed superior to the umbilicus in the midline approximately 10 cm from the umbilical port. A third working port (5 or 8 mm) is positioned at the ipsilateral anterosuperior iliac spine laterally at a 45° offset and 10 cm from the umbilical port. A fourth 5-mm port is placed if necessary, particularly in right cases to lift the liver edge and expose the upper pole of the kidney. The table is angled to raise the affected side to a 60° flank position. The robot is positioned on the ipsilateral side of the patient and angled over the shoulder. The three robotic arms are then engaged to the laparoscopic ports. A 30° lens is used in the down position. In patients undergoing lower pole nephrectomy, the inferior port may need to be placed more inferior and medial to avoid being too close to the working area and limiting mobility. In the sole patient undergoing concomitant antireflux surgery, the robot is repositioned to the foot of the patient and the camera port remains in the umbilicus [21, 22]. The ipsilateral lower working port is used along with a contralateral mid clavicular port at the level of the umbilicus. This arrangement would be similar if removal of the distal ureter into the deep pelvis is desired. The kidney is exposed by reflecting the colon medially. The ureter from the nonfunctioning moiety is identified and mobilized as distally as the iliac vessels. The ureter is then divided if there is no vesicoureteral reflux and ligated if there is a refluxing moiety. The affected pole is manipulated using the divided ureter as a handle. The vessels to the moiety are identified and briefly compressed with a dissecting tool if there was any uncertainty as to their association. Vessels are divided in the standard fashion using either suture or titanium clips. The renal pelvis of the nonfunctioning pole is separated from the normal pole parenchyma using blunt dissection to identify better the demarcation between the functioning and nonfunctioning pole. The nonfunctioning pole is excised using electrocautery or harmonic scalpel along the line of vascular demarcation.

Perirenal fat is used as a bolster before closing the cut surface of the remaining pole with 4/0 absorbable monofilament sutures. Some authors advise closing the cut surface of the remaining pole with 4/0 absorbable sutures [22]. After inspection for hemostasis, a retroperitoneal drain is placed if there is concern about remnant pole collecting system injury. The specimen is removed through the camera port. Local anesthetic could be injected into the trocar site wounds. The bladder catheter is usually removed on postoperative day 1 or 2.

The retroperitoneal approach is also feasible and have been reported by few centers who already use the retroperitoneal approach for robotic pyeloplasty [23, 24].

24.6 Postoperative Care

Bladder drainage is not mandatory. The postoperative care is mainly analgesics and standard recommended postoperative surveillance for hemodynamic and urine output. The current hospital stay in the recent series is between 1 and 2 days. With the progress of anesthesia and analgesic management, most of children recover with excellent pain control, and they return to activity early. Recently in some highly experienced centers, day-care partial nephrectomy has been applied without major complications [1, 8, 13, 25–28]. Postoperative fever or uncontrolled pain should be the alarming signs for complications on the remaining moiety or ureter. Leak should be excluded and managed promptly.

To achieve the best outcomes on mid-term and long-term follow up, it is mandatory to exclude any damage of the remaining moiety. Monitoring renal function following heminephrectomy merits special attention. We routinely performed a renal Doppler ultrasonography (US) at 1 and 6 months postoperatively. The follow-up in our series was reported up to 12 years postoperatively. We find that dimercaptosuccinic acid (DMSA) scintigraphy is not mandatory if no abnormality is detected on US such as cortical thinning, large hydronephrosis, or poor Doppler flow. In our practice, we complete an abnormal US by a functional imaging. However, Wallis et al. insisted on the importance of DMSA renal scan and not only Doppler studies even if it shows a normal hilar blood flow [9].

A multicentre French retrospective cohort study of 9 years included 30 patients all undergoing laparoscopic partial nephrectomy (LPN) evaluated by renal US and DMSA scintigraphy pre- and postoperatively [14]. Long-term follow-up with US and DMSA showed that none of this cohort had complete loss of lower pole renal function. Mean lower pole renal function directly related to LPN was not significantly different after versus before surgery for the entire cohort, for the <12-month group and for the >12-month group. Partial loss of function was identified in 17% of the patients (mean function loss, 9.3 ± 6% at a median age of 13 months). They concluded that systematic postoperative DMSA was not mandatory if US remains normal.

24.7 Results and Discussion

Though laparoscopic retroperitoneal partial nephrectomy is a challenging procedure, early publications have shown that it can be performed in a comparable operative time to that of an open procedure [1]. The mean (range) operative time was 146 min (50–180) and 152 min (75–240) for the open surgery and the laparoscopic groups, respectively. The main advantage to the laparoscopic approach is that it shortens significantly the length of hospital stay. The mean (range) hospital stay was 1.4 days (1–3) and 3.9 days (3–5) for the laparoscopic and open surgery groups, respectively ($p < 0.0001$). Eight of 13 children were discharged the day after the laparoscopic procedure.

Robinson et al. compared, in a prospective nonrandomized study, costs and outcome of LPN to open surgery in children [29]. Mean operative time in the laparoscopic and open groups was 200.4 and 113.5 min, mean hospital stay was 25.5 h and 32.6 h, respectively ($p < 0.0005$). Patients in the laparoscopic group required lower doses of analgesics than those who had open surgery. The main disadvantage reported in this series was a longer operative time in case of LPN. The operative time in this series was relatively longer than in other pediatric series, and probably it will be shortened with experience.

Valla et al. have reported 37% of intraoperative complications, mainly residual perirenal collections at the transection line [12]. The major complication is, however, the loss of function of the remaining moiety. We have lost one kidney early in our experience in a 7-year-old child after upper pole nephrectomy. We believe that the main surgical mistake was to free the remaining moiety from the peritoneum which increased the risk of twisting the main renal pedicle. Wallis et al. have reported functional loss of the remaining moiety in two children who were 6- and 7-month-old, respectively [9]. They insisted on the importance of following these children by DMSA renal scan and not only with a Doppler US, which may show normal hilar blood flow. They concluded that in children under 1 year, there was a higher risk for complications. Leclair et al. have also reported higher conversion and complication rates in children under 1 year [4].

Castellan et al. compared the transperitoneal with the retroperitoneal approach [30]. Four of the five complications (80%) were reported in patients younger than 1 year and the authors concluded that the complication rate does not depend on the surgical approach but rather on the age of the patient. Conversion to open surgery was relatively high in this series, which reported the early experience of advanced laparoscopic surgery (retroperitoneal or transperitoneal approaches), but recent published series are more encouraging on the feasibility and the safety of the procedure, as Dénes et al. have reported no conversion in a series of 18 LPN [31].

We have reviewed our experience with retroperitoneal partial nephrectomy in a series of 58 consecutive cases with special interest in our group of patients under 1 year [21, 32]. Among the tenlaparoscopic retroperitoneal upper partial nephrectomies performed in children under 1 year, only one had a complication in our first year of experience which required conversion to identify the line of parenchymal section. Others had no complications nor required conversion, even for a 60-mm dilated upper pelvis in a 1-month old child. Mean (range) operative time was 150 min (75–180). One child had an asymptomatic urinoma at 2 years of age. All children had a well-vascularized remaining moiety after a mean follow-up of 36 months (6–60) [21].

Ballouhey et al. have compared retrospectively perioperative outcomes between robotic and open partial nephrectomy in a multicenter study [33]. The study was focused on young children weighting less than 15 kg. The robotic group has shorter hospital stay and less postoperative analgesics than the open surgery group. They found no difference in operative time. None of their cohort had a loss of function of remaining moiety [33].

To investigate the natural history of cystic lesions following LPN in children, Esposito et al. reviewed the US imaging reports performed during the follow-up of 125 children (transperitoneal approach in 83 children and a retroperitoneal approach in 42 children) [34]. The mean follow-up was 4.2 years. At US, an avascular cyst related to the operative site was found after 61/125 procedures (48.8%). A total of 13 on 61 cysts (21.3%) disappeared after a mean of 4 years, 26/61 (42.6%) did not significantly change in dimension, 17/61 (27.8%) decreased in size, and only 5 of the 61 cysts (8.3%) enlarged. The cysts were asymptomatic in 51 children (83.6%), while they were associated with UTIs and abdominal pain in the remaining 10; none required a reintervention. They concluded that US finding of a simple cyst at the operative site after LPN can be common during the follow-up, with an incidence of nearly 50%. No correlation between cyst formation and type of surgical technique was found. As there was no association between cysts and clinical outcomes, renal cysts after LPN can be managed conservatively, with periodic US evaluations.

Tips and Tricks

The major complication, even rare, is the loss of function of the remaining moiety. We learned from our early complications that some aspects are necessary to make the retroperitoneal approach easier and safer:

- Excellent comprehension and anatomical definition of the duplex anomaly before surgery.
- The technique should be standardized to reduce complications.
- The remaining moiety should be kept attached to peritoneum, if the retroperitoneal approach is chosen.
- The pathological ureter should be kept dilated by ligature at the beginning of surgery.
- Retrograde insertion of ureteral catheter to allow methylene blue injection is recommended when possible and necessary in cases of lower pole nephrectomy or atypical upper pole nephrectomy.

Take-Home Points

- Laparoscopic retroperitoneal partial nephrectomy remains a challenging laparoscopic procedure. The main limiting factor is the learning curve and not the age at surgery or the degree of dilatation. Nevertheless, in children under 1 year of age, surgery should be done with great care and by the most experienced surgeon of the team. We believe that both retroperitoneal and transperitoneal approaches are now safely feasible with comparable results and recommend that the surgical teams concentrate on and improve the technique of their choice, instead of trying to compare approaches. It is clear from the published reports that the main objective is to avoid the high complication rate in the beginning of the experience. Mentored learning of the procedure is recommended before starting to proceed on one's own [35].

References

1. El-Ghoneimi A, Farhat W, Bolduc S, Bagli D, McLorie G, Khoury A. Retroperitoneal laparoscopic vs open partial nephroureterectomy in children. BJU Int. 2003;91(6):532–5.
2. El-Ghoneimi A, Valla JS, Steyaert H, Aigrain Y. Laparoscopic renal surgery via a retroperitoneal approach in children. J Urol. 1998;160(3 Pt 2):1138–41.
3. Jordan GH, Winslow BH. Laparoendoscopic upper pole partial nephrectomy with ureterectomy. J Urol. 1993;150(3):940–3.
4. Leclair M-D, Vidal I, Suply E, Podevin G, Héloury Y. Retroperitoneal laparoscopic heminephrectomy in duplex kidney in infants and children: a 15-year experience. Eur Urol. 2009;56(2):385–9.
5. Lee RS, Sethi AS, Passerotti CC, Retik AB, Borer JG, Nguyen HT, et al. Robot assisted laparoscopic partial nephrectomy: a viable and safe option in children. J Urol. 2009;181(2):823–8. discussion 828–9
6. Miyano G, Takahashi T, Nakamura H, Doi T, Okawada M, Koga H, et al. Retroperitoneoscopic nephrectomy/heminephrectomy in children planned, performed, and managed by supervised senior pediatric surgical trainees. J Laparoendosc Adv Surg Tech A. 2013;23(8):723–7.
7. Bansal D, Cost NG, Bean CM, Noh PH. Pediatric laparo-endoscopic single site partial nephrectomy: feasibility in infants and small children for upper urinary tract duplication anomalies. J Pediatr Urol. 2014;10(5):859–63.
8. Esposito C, Varlet F, Patkowski D, Castagnetti M, Escolino M, Draghici IM, et al. Laparoscopic partial nephrectomy in duplex kidneys in infants and children: results of an European multicentric survey. Surg Endosc. 2015;29(12):3469–76.
9. Wallis MC, Khoury AE, Lorenzo AJ, Pippi-Salle JL, Bägli DJ, Farhat WA. Outcome analysis of retroperitoneal laparoscopic heminephrectomy in children. J Urol. 2006;175(6):2277–80. discussion 2280–2
10. Peters CA. Laparoendoscopic renal surgery in children. J Endourol. 2000;14(10):841–7. discussion 847–8

11. El-Ghoneimi A. Paediatric laparoscopic surgery. Curr Opin Urol. 2003;13(4):329–35.
12. Valla J-S, Breaud J, Carfagna L, Tursini S, Steyaert H. Treatment of ureterocele on duplex ureter: upper pole nephrectomy by retroperitoneoscopy in children based on a series of 24 cases. Eur Urol. 2003;43(4):426–9.
13. Nerli RB, Vernekar R, Guntaka AK, Patil SM, Jali SM, Hiremath MB. Laparoscopic hemi/partial nephrectomy in children with ureteral duplication anomalies. Pediatr Surg Int. 2011;27(7):769–74.
14. Joyeux L, Lacreuse I, Schneider A, Moog R, Borgnon J, Lopez M, et al. Long-term functional renal outcomes after retroperitoneoscopic upper pole heminephrectomy for duplex kidney in children: a multicenter cohort study. Surg Endosc. 2017;31(3):1241–9.
15. Yeung CK, Tam YH, Sihoe JD, Lee KH, Liu KW. Retroperitoneoscopic dismembered pyeloplasty for pelvi-ureteric junction obstruction in infants and children. BJU Int. 2001;87(6):509–13.
16. Gaur DD. Laparoscopic operative retroperitoneoscopy: use of a new device. J Urol. 1992;148(4):1137–9.
17. Adams JB, Micali S, Moore RG, Babayan RK, Kavoussi LR. Complications of extraperitoneal balloon dilation. J Endourol. 1996;10(4):375–8.
18. Capolicchio J-P, Jednak R, Anidjar M, Pippi-Salle JL. A modified access technique for retroperitoneoscopic renal surgery in children. J Urol. 2003;170(1):204–6.
19. Micali S, Caione P, Virgili G, Capozza N, Scarfini M, Micali F. Retroperitoneal laparoscopic access in children using a direct vision technique. J Urol. 2001;165(4):1229–32.
20. Cadeddu JA, Chan DY, Hedican SP, Lee BR, Moore RG, Kavoussi LR, et al. Retroperitoneal access for transperitoneal laparoscopy in patients at high risk for intra-abdominal scarring. J Endourol. 1999;13(8):567–70.
21. Peycelon M, El-Ghoneimi A. Heminephrectomy for duplex kidneys. In: Gundeti MS, editor. Surgical Techniques in Pediatric and Adolescent Urology. Jaypee Brothers Medical Publishers (P) Ltd; 2020. https://emedicine360.com/surgical-techniques-in-pediatric-and-adolescent-urology.
22. Malik RD, Pariser JJ, Gundeti MS. Outcomes in pediatric robot-assisted laparoscopic heminephrectomy compared with contemporary open and laparoscopic series. J Endourol. 2015;29(12):1346–52.
23. Olsen LH, Jorgensen TM. Computer assisted pyeloplasty in children: the retroperitoneal approach. J Urol. 2004;171(6 Part 2):2629–31.
24. Olsen LH, Rawashdeh YF, Jorgensen TM. Pediatric robot assisted retroperitoneoscopic pyeloplasty: a 5-year experience. J Urol. 2007;178(5):2137–41. discussion 2141
25. Schneider A, Ripepi M, Henry-Florence C, Geiss S. Laparoscopic transperitoneal partial nephrectomy in children under 2 years old: a single-centre experience. J Pediatr Urol. 2010;6(2):166–70.
26. Pearce R, Subramaniam R. Minimally invasive partial or total nephrectomy in children: a comparison between transperitoneal and retroperitoneal approaches. Pediatr Surg Int. 2011;27(11):1233–7.
27. Esposito C, Miyano G, Caione P, Escolino M, Chiarenza F, Riccipetitoni G, et al. Retroperitoneoscopic heminephrectomy in duplex kidney in infants and children: results of a multicentric survey. J Laparoendosc Adv Surg Tech A. 2015;25(10):864–9.
28. Suson KD, Wolfe-Christensen C, Elder JS, Lakshmanan Y. Practice patterns and outcomes of pediatric partial nephrectomy in the United States: Comparison between pediatric urology and general pediatric surgery. J Pediatr Urol. 2015;11(4):171.e1–5.
29. Robinson BC, Snow BW, Cartwright PC, De Vries CR, Hamilton BD, Anderson JB. Comparison of laparoscopic versus open partial nephrectomy in a pediatric series. J Urol. 2003;169(2):638–40.
30. Castellan M, Gosalbez R, Carmack AJ, Prieto JC, Perez-Brayfield M, Labbie A. Transperitoneal and retroperitoneal laparoscopic heminephrectomy--what approach for which patient? J Urol. 2006;176(6 Pt 1):2636–9. discussion 2639
31. Dénes FT, Danilovic A, Srougi M. Outcome of laparoscopic upper-pole nephrectomy in children with duplex systems. J Endourol. 2007;21(2):162–8.
32. Matta R, Paye-Jaouen A, Peycelon M, Badawy H, Al Hazmi H, Carricaburu E, et al. Laparoscopic retroperitoneal partial nephrectomy in children; standardized technique can make it safe even in infants. 27th Congress of the ESPU; 2016; Harrogate, Yorkshire (United Kingdom).
33. Ballouhey Q, Binet A, Clermidi P, Braik K, Villemagne T, Cros J, et al. Partial nephrectomy for small children: robot-assisted versus open surgery. Int J Urol. 2017;24(12):855–60.
34. Esposito C, Escolino M, Troncoso Solar B, Iacona R, Esposito R, Settimi A, et al. Diagnosis and long-term outcome of renal cysts after laparoscopic partial nephrectomy in children. BJU Int. 2017;119(5):761–6.
35. Cook A, Khoury A, Bagli D, McLorie GA, El-Ghoneimi A, Farhat WA. The development of laparoscopic surgical skills in pediatric urologists: long-term outcome of a mentorship training model. Can J Urol. 2005;12(5):2824–8.

25 Retroperitoneoscopic Prone Partial Nephrectomies

Marc-David Leclair

> **Learning Objectives**
> - Understand specific advantages of prone position for retroperitoneoscopy.
> - Learn surgical steps of partial nephrectomy.

25.1 Introduction to Retroperitoneoscopic Partial Nephrectomies

The first cases of laparoscopic total and partial nephrectomies have been reported in the early 1990s in adult and children. Most total and partial nephrectomies in children are performed for non-functioning symptomatic kidneys or moieties, secondary to renal dysplasia, obstructive uropathy, or vesico-ureteric reflux. Symptoms warranting the indication include infections, hypertension, stones, and loin pain.

Whether the kidney should be approached by transperitoneal or retroperitoneal laparoscopy has been an endless debate among pediatric urologists, although both approaches have specific advantages and drawbacks.

It is generally accepted that total nephrectomy is the procedure of choice to acquire and develop experience with retroperitoneoscopy, although indications remain rare. Laparoscopic partial nephrectomy is technically more demanding than total nephrectomy. Main indications are represented by nonfunctioning upper moieties secondary to obstructive uropathy (ureterocele, ectopic ureter), or lower moieties destructed by reflux or PUJ obstruction.

Upper-pole nephrectomy usually represents the majority of indications. The main technical difficulty for retroperitoneoscopy may be the limited working space in small infants with massively dilated upper tract [1, 2]. Lower-pole nephrectomies are usually performed in older children and involve less dilated upper tract. The procedure, however, may remain difficult due to the size of the moiety to resect and deep involvement of the lower calyces in the upper moiety. The main difficulty of both procedures relies on a clear and undoubtable identification of the vascular anatomy and requires meticulous dissection before any definitive vessels ligation be performed.

Supplementary Information The online version contains supplementary material available at [https://doi.org/10.1007/978-3-030-99280-4_25].

M.-D. Leclair (✉)
Pediatric Surgery, Department of Pediatric Surgery and Urology, Hôpital Mère-Enfant, Nantes Hospital, University of Nantes, Nantes, France
e-mail: mdleclair@chu-nantes.fr

C. Esposito et al. (eds.), *Minimally Invasive Techniques in Pediatric Urology*,
https://doi.org/10.1007/978-3-030-99280-4_25

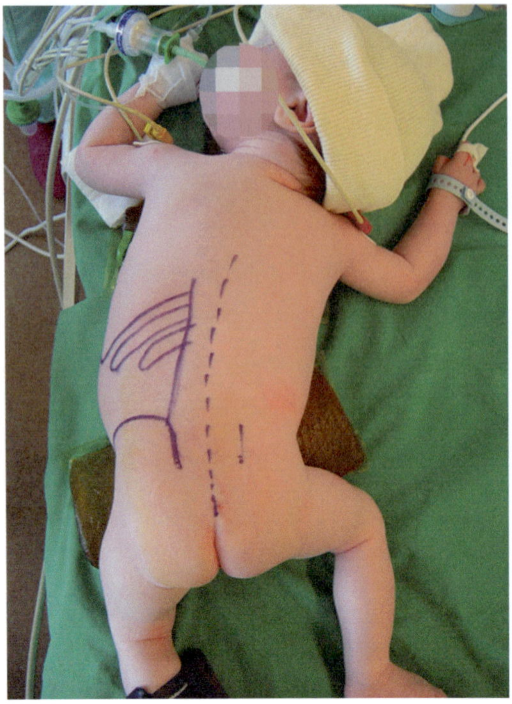

Fig. 25.1 Prone installation for a left retroperitoneoscopic approach. Note that the infant is placed along the edge of the operating table to facilitate the movements of the most lateral and dependent trocar. Note also the slightly curved installation of the patient, to enlarge the space between the 12th rib and the iliac crest

25.2 Patient Positioning

The lateral position has been the historical route for retroperitoneal access; however, the prone position for posterior retroperitoneoscopic approach [3] has raised recent interest among pediatric urologists. The patient is placed in a fully prone position, with rolls placed under the chest and the pelvis to allow the abdominal contents to fall away in a dependent position [4]. The indicated side of the child is brought close to the edge of the table to allow maximum freedom of mobility for the most dependent operating port. The patient should also be positioned such as to enlarge the space between the iliac crest and the 12th rib (Fig. 25.1).

25.3 Instrumentation

Limited working space of the retroperitoneum translates externally in a very limited skin area to insert trocars. It is mandatory to use at least 5 mm instrumentation, or smaller when available. We use very few different instruments, mainly atraumatic grasper (Babcock-type or windowed grasper), a fine curved bipolar used both as a fine tip dissector and for elective coagulation of small vessels, and scissors. Any sealing device in 5 mm or 3 mm diameter is useful, especially for the step of parenchyma division. Specimen is extracted directly through the posterior/medial wound, usually the largest, without the need for a specimen bag (which is anyway difficult to deploy in the retroperitoneal space).

25.4 Trocars Placement and Working Space Creation (Video 25.1)

A transverse skin incision is made along the lateral edge of the sacro-lumbar muscle, and a home-made balloon is introduced percutaneously in the retroperitoneum after the fascias have been punctured. The retroperioneal working space is then fully developed by insufflation of the balloon, posterior and lateral to the kidney, outside of the Gerota's fascia. In a striking contrast with the technique used by most experts in lateral position retroperitoneoscopy (which implies opening and insufflating within the Gerota's fascia at the very beginning of the procedure), it is important to stress the fact that in prone position, most of the working space is developed outside of the Gerota fascia, before it is ultimately incised. A 5-mm trocar is placed through the incision, and the retroperitoneum is insufflated. Additional ports (Fig. 25.2) will be inserted under direct vision, at the tip of the 12th rib for the laparoscope, and a lateral operating port as lateral and anterior as possible, taking great care not to insert it through the peritoneum.

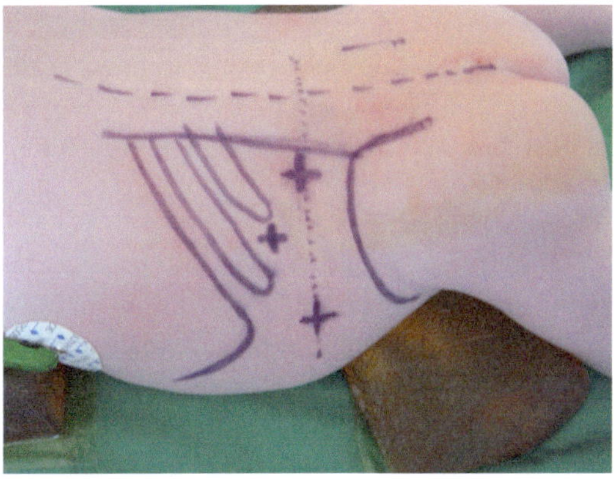

Fig. 25.2 Prone left retroperitoneoscopy. Ports are inserted along the sacrospinalis musculature at mid-distance between the iliac crest and the last rib, at the tip of the last rib, and laterally as low and lateral as possible

25.5 Technique

It can be of great help to perform a cystoscopy at the beginning of the procedure, especially if both ureters are small or have no major diameter discrepancy. A ureteral stent can be inserted especially in the moiety that is planned to be left intact. It allows easier identification of both ureters during the dissection. During parenchymal division, methylene blue injection in the "remaining moiety" may help to detect any calyceal beach. Some experienced teams advocate early ligation of the pathological ureter at the beginning of the procedure that will remain dilated and facilitate further dissection of the moiety [5].

After insufflation of the retroperitoneal space at 8 mmHg to 10 mmHg pressure, 3 mm to 5 mm-0° laparoscope is inserted in the first incision trocar (most medial) to allow direct vision for the introduction of the two other 3 mm or 5 mm ports. The laparoscope will then switch position to be used through the middle-trocar at the tip of the 12th rib.

The Gerota fascia is incised horizontally, and the posterior aspect of the kidney and the renal hilum is exposed.

25.5.1 Upper-Pole Nephrectomy (Video 25.2)

The dissection starts at the upper pole of the kidney and usually easily identifies the upper ureter emerging from the renal sinus. It is generally unnecessary to dissect at the lower pole of the kidney and look for renal main pelvis and lower ureter; upper-moiety vascular branches will be electively identified and divided along the upper pole. A posterior upper-pole artery is usually very easy to identify and divide. In case of any doubt on the vascular territory of any vessels, a clamp and release test can be performed by gentle occlusion of the arterial branch with an atraumatic grasper. The next step is to perform division of the upper-pole ureter; the ligation should be performed 2–3 cm from the renal sinus, allowing to use the proximal stump as a handle and expose the anterior aspect of the renal sinus. Following the contact of the anterior surface of the proximal ureter, the dissection should identify the main upper-pole vessels, with an anterior artery emerging from the main renal artery. After clear identification of the vascular anatomy is ascertained, vessels can be safely divided, using clips (Hemolock® 5 mm clips for example) or sealing devices.

After vessels control, the step of parenchymal section is now greatly facilitated by the use of modern sealing devices (Harmonic® scalpel, Ligasure®). It is important that the remaining moiety is kept attached to the peritoneum and mobilized as little as possible all along the procedure, to avoid vascular injury caused by intraoperative traction and accidental postoperative torsion. Any doubt on accidental calyceal breach of the remaining moiety should drive thorough evaluation, intracorporeal suturing repair, or open conversion if necessary.

After parenchymal division, a supplementary ureterectomy can be performed, starting from the distal stump of the previously divided ureter. It usually needs to be uncrossed from the main renal pedicle and carefully dissected away, as distal as possible, from the intact ureter paying great attention not to jeopardize the common vascularization.

25.5.2 Lower-Pole Nephrectomy (Video 25.3)

Technical steps are similar, but some important differences must be stressed. The dissection starts below the lower pole of the kidney, and in the absence of major dilatation difference between both moieties, it can sometimes be difficult to ascertain which ureter is which. The dissection then proceeds directly along the main renal pedicle, to determine where vessel division will preserve upper-moiety vascularization. The artery is dissected and ligated first, which is a significant advantage of the prone posterior approach. It usually helps to underline clear demarcation on the parenchyma surface to assist later parenchymal division. Surgical steps then follow open-surgery guidelines, and after division of the most posterior vascular branches of the lower pole, it is often helpful to divide the pelvi-ureteric junction and proceed to further dissection along the anterior aspect of the pelvis, to electively identify small lower-pole anterior vessels.

Parenchyma division may be a challenging step; In contrast to the upper-pole nephrectomy, it may sometimes be safer to proceed to parenchyma division directly through the median calyceal cavities, leaving a small rim of ischemic lower-moiety parenchyma.

25.6 Postoperative Course

The minimally invasive retroperitoneal access allows very short hospital stay. We observed steady decrease of length of hospitalization in our experience, and hospital stay is now routinely limited to one postoperative night and discharge the next morning. The antalgic requirements are usually very limited, and return to normal feeding is allowed in the next hours after the end of the procedure.

The partial nephrectomy in prone position is even feasible as day-case surgery, as in our experience (Fig. 25.3).

Working space suction drain placement or bladder drainage are unnecessary in typical cases of partial nephrectomy.

Of note, postoperative fever (38° or above) is frequently observed at day 2 or 3 postoperatively, and very likely related to parenchymal ischemia if a small rim of renal tissue has been left in place to allow safe bloodless parenchymal division. Obviously, prolonged postoperative fever should drive adequate blood and urine sampling to rule out any postoperative complications.

25.7 Discussion

The retroperitoneal area is a virtual space, thus the creation of an adequate working volume is an essential phase of every retroperitoneoscopic procedures. This first step, potentially problematic for beginners in terms of orientation and adequation of the space created to the size of the child, may have slowed down the diffusion of the technique as it requires significant learning curve to be mastered.

The creation of the working space can be achieved either under direct control vision with repeated movements of the laparoscope or blindly with the insufflation of a balloon of appropriate size percutaneously inserted (a home-made balloon can easily be manufactured using one finger of a surgical glove secured at the tip of a large catheter). When using a balloon, the ideal site for percutaneous insertion may not be at the tip of the 12th rib, but more along the lateral edge of the sacrolumbar muscles, due to the high risk of transperitoneal insertion and subsequent pneumoperitoneum (Fig. 25.4). This site will eventually be the location of the most medial operative port.

A thoughtful positioning of the child is also of outstanding importance, considering the limited space between the iliac crest and the 12th rib in young children. Every effort should be made to

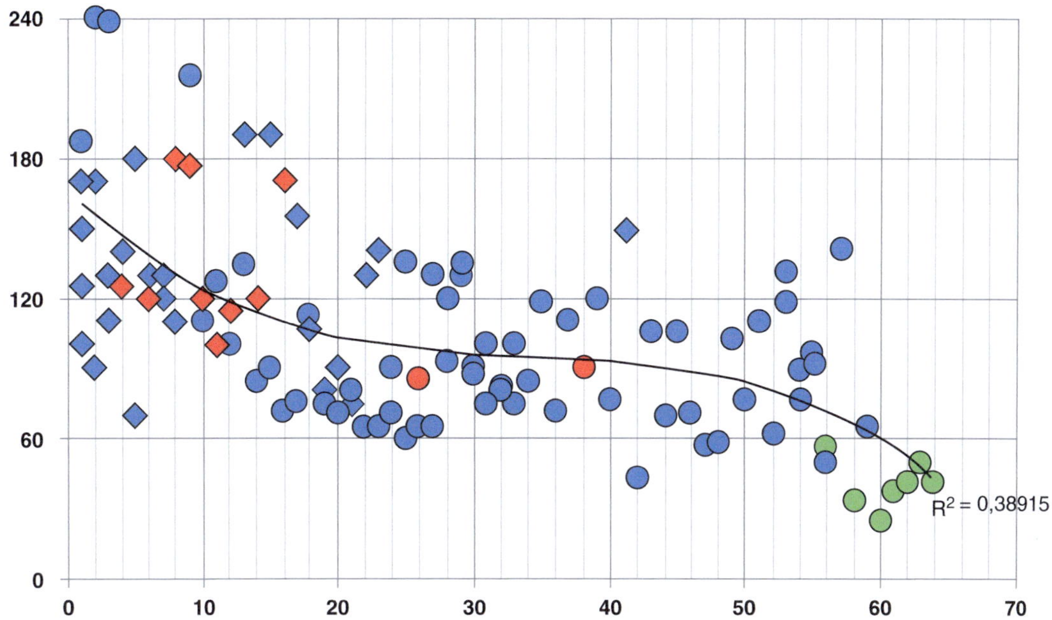

Fig. 25.3 Example of learning curve for partial nephrectomies (single institution experience, 1993–2016, unpublished data). Vertical axis: duration of procedure in minutes. Horizontal axis: ranking order of cases. Total number of procedures: 110 (one surgeon: 65; one surgeon: 35; 4 surgeons: 1–5 procedures) Squares: lateral position retroperitoneoscopy; Circles: prone position. Red: conversion to open surgery; Green: day-case procedure

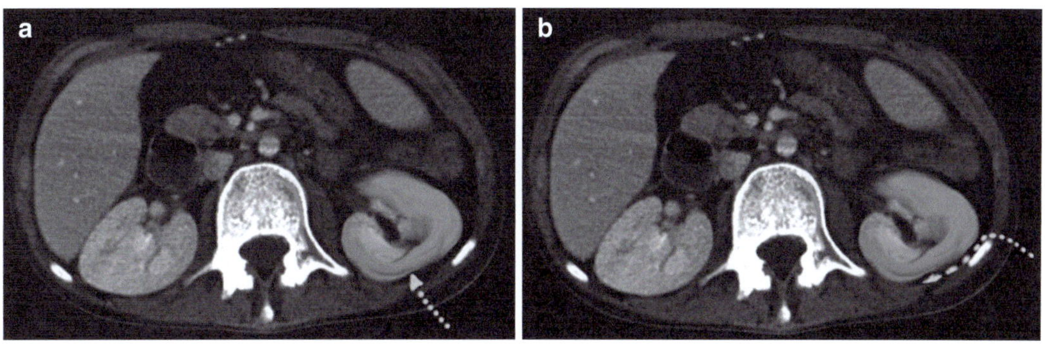

Fig. 25.4 Schematic view of abdominal CT scan, showing point of entry of the first trocar. (**a**) Arrow shows the path of a balloon inserted along the lateral edge of the sacrospinalis muscle. (**b**) Arrow shows the path of the approach at the tip of the 12th rib. Note the presence of the peritoneal lateral cul-de-sac

enlarge this space, by using flexible operative table or bolsters while installing the patient.

In retroperitoneoscopy, the orientation of the surgeon in such an unusual space may be confusing, and actually relies on one major landmark: the psoas muscle, which should be constantly kept in a fixed position, usually at the bottom of the field of view in lateral position or at the ceiling in prone.

An important point is the necessity of mobilizing the kidney itself as less as possible until complete control of the vascular structures. Indeed, the natural peritoneal attachments of the kidney will help the exposure, avoiding the need for additional ports, sometimes difficult to introduce considering the limited space.

25.8 Prone Vs Lateral Approach

The kidney can be approached retroperitoneoscopically with both approaches, with comparable difficulties and similar learning curves. The lateral approach has been the historical and logical route for retroperitoneoscopy, in analogy with the conventional access for open renal surgery. However, the prone posterior approach offers undeniable advantages, like a direct and early access to the renal pedicle. In lateral position, it is often necessary to retract and hold the kidney at the "ceiling" of the working space to maintain access to the renal vessels, whereas the prone position allows direct access to the vessels, without the need for an instrument to maintain this space opened. The benefit of gravity permitted by prone installation also provides a larger working space, without the need for excessive CO_2 insufflation. The posterior route is a very versatile approach, especially in small infants in whom the limited working space may be critical. In our opinion, this approach is superior to the conventional lateral route when meticulous and prolonged dissection of the renal hilum is necessary (partial nephrectomies), and for bilateral cases as it avoids the need for changing the installation. Another advantage of the prone position is that any accidental peritoneal opening will have very limited impact on the working space and will be barely recognized intraoperatively. The main drawbacks are the time needed for urgent open conversion, if major vascular injury occurs, and a somewhat limited access to the deep pelvis in older children after 5–7 years of age [3]. When complete resection of the lower ureter is mandatory in old patients, the lateral approach may allow to extend the ureterectomy lower in the deep pelvis, beyond the division of the iliac vessels.

25.9 Retroperitoneoscopy: Pros and Cons

The choice for transperitoneal or retroperitonal laparoscopy for renal access is an on-going debate among pediatric urologists [6–9].

One of the major arguments for the retroperitoneal access is that it reproduces exactly what had been previously performed and advocated for decades for renal surgery. The risk of bowel adhesions is not theoretical and may have been underestimated, especially in the procedures that will involve some urine leakage. One has to keep in mind this hazard when planning a laparoscopic procedure, considering the long life span of the pediatric patients.

In children with ESRF already under peritoneal dialysis, the retroperitoneoscopic approach is certainly superior to transperitoneal laparoscopy, as it has been clearly shown that it allows faster return to dialysis. Bilateral procedures, although uncommon, will be best approached through prone posterior access without the need for changing the installation.

The small working volume and the difficulties of orientation of the surgeon's mind in this unusual volume represent significant limitations that have hindered the widespread adoption of the technique. Mentored learning is especially recommended, and standardization of the procedures helps to reduce complications. It is obvious in the pediatric literature that, with the development of minimally invasive techniques, a shift can be observed from retroperitoneal open surgery toward transperitoneal laparoscopic procedures, especially for the most technically challenging indications (heminephrectomies, pyeloplasties, adrenalectomies). However, this trend may be viewed as a devious effect, as experienced groups have extensively shown the feasibility of all these procedures through retroperitoneoscopy, after adequate teaching and safe learning curve.

Take-Home Messages

- Retroperitoneoscopic partial nephrectomy is a challenging procedure, in relatively rare indications.
- Creation of the working space is the most important step.
- It is mandatory to clearly expose vascular anatomy before any vessels ligation.
- Leaving all peritoneal attachments of the kidney intact allows easier exposition of the renal hilum and vessels.

References

1. Leclair MD, et al. Retroperitoneal laparoscopic heminephrectomy in duplex kidney in infants and children: a 15-year experience. Eur Urol. 2009;56(2):385–9.
2. Wallis MC, et al. Outcome analysis of retroperitoneal laparoscopic heminephrectomy in children. J Urol. 2006;175(6):2277–80. discussion 2280–2
3. Borzi PA. A comparison of the lateral and posterior retroperitoneoscopic approach for complete and partial nephroureterectomy in children. BJU Int. 2001;87(6):517–20.
4. Mushtaq I, Haleblian G. Laparoscopic heminephrectomy in infants and children: first 54 cases. J Pediatr Urol. 2007;3(2):100–3.
5. El-Ghoneimi A. Laparoscopic partial nephrectomy in children. Dialogues in pediatric. Urology. 2008;30(1):2–3.
6. El-Ghoneimi A, et al. Retroperitoneal laparoscopic nephrectomy in children: at last the gold standard? J Pediatr Urol. 2006;2(4):357–63.
7. El-Ghoneimi A, et al. Laparoscopic renal surgery via a retroperitoneal approach in children. J Urol. 1998;160(3 Pt 2):1138–41.
8. Gundeti MS, et al. An initial experience of 100 paediatric laparoscopic nephrectomies with transperitoneal or posterior prone retroperitoneoscopic approach. Pediatr Surg Int. 2007;23(8):795–9.
9. Jayram G, et al. Outcomes and fate of the remnant moiety following laparoscopic heminephrectomy for duplex kidney: a multicenter review. J Pediatr Urol. 2011;7(3):272–5.

Management of Kidney Stones Using RIRS

26

Lorenzo Masieri, Alfonso Crisci, Alberto Mantovani, Chiara Cini, and Simone Sforza

Learning Objectives

- To describe step by step the technique of retrograde intrarenal surgery in children (RIRS).
- To report the latest results of the major international papers about pediatric RIRS.
- To show a video with the technique of RIRS.
- To describe tips and tricks of RIRS and to show all the new technologies available in
- pediatric urology that can be adopted to perform this technique.

Supplementary Information The online version contains supplementary material available at [https://doi.org/10.1007/978-3-030-99280-4_26].

L. Masieri (✉) · A. Crisci · A. Mantovani · C. Cini
S. Sforza
Pediatric Urology Department, Meyer's Children Hospital, Florence, Italy
e-mail: lorenzo.masieri@meyer.it; alfonso.crisci@unifi.it; alberto.mantovani@meyer.it; chiara.cini@meyer.it; simone.sforza@unifi.it

26.1 Introduction

RIRS stands for retrograde intrarenal surgery, a minimally invasive surgical strategy that respects the natural anatomy of the urinary tract. It is the endoscopic evaluation of the upper urinary tract in a retrograde fashion with rigid or flexible instruments and represents a milestone of the modern treatment of urinary stones.

Indeed, stone disease is an important increasing clinical problem in pediatric urology practice. As per the European Urology Association (EAU) guidelines, RIRS represents one of the primary treatment choices for renal stones up to 2 cm [1, 2] EAU–European Society of Pediatric Urology (ESPU) guidelines suggest RIRS as a valid alternative option for stones up to 2 cm.

Moreover, as recently reported, there is an increasing demand of RIRS for pediatric stones with a growing number of surgeons using this technique [3, 4]. Different articles reported shorter hospital stay, lower radiation exposure, and lower complication rate related to RIRS when compared to PCNL, especially for stones between 10 and 20 mm. Furthermore, evidences suggest that, although urinary lithiasis is less prevalent in children than in adults, it is associated with significant morbidity and incidence is increasing [5]. Indeed, refinements in endoscopic instrumentations, the widespread popularization of endourology, and the recognition of minimal invasiveness of endo-

C. Esposito et al. (eds.), *Minimally Invasive Techniques in Pediatric Urology*,
https://doi.org/10.1007/978-3-030-99280-4_26

scopic approach, with powerful lasers and new instruments, have led to evolving interest in adopting the technique not only in adults but also in the pediatric patients [6].

In this light, our chapter is focused on the preoperative and perioperative details, on practical tips and tricks, on the outcomes and on a brief reporting of the literature of RIRS in children.

26.2 Preoperative Preparation

To approach pediatric RIRS, you need to gain endourological experience on adults or in one of the few large caseload pediatric centers in endourology to not only improvise but also be familiar with different endoscopic instruments and disposables.

Pre-operative diagnostic assessment usually requires abdominal ultrasonography and plain filming of the abdomen (KUB). This will give us information on the number of the stones, their location in the kidney, their size and their radiopacity. To plan how to better tackle the stone, you will need to add an intraoperative retrograde pyelogram that will paint our path to the stone, highlighting the upper urinary tract details and congenital malformations or narrowings. This, together with the direct visualization of the urinary tract, can provide the surgeon with sufficient anatomical data.

Optional low-dose protocol non-contrast computed tomography (NCCT) scan (standard in adults) could give us critical preoperative information on the stone hardness measured in Hounsfield units (HU) and on the pelvicalyceal anatomy, especially in a dilated system.

Clarify parents the concept of single procedure/single RIRS: every "single" RIRS could be a staged procedure (presenting–surgery–stent removal) requiring up to three general anesthesia.

Inform parents of the real chance/risk of staged procedures/repeated RIRS to obtain stone-free status (SFS). Primary SFR is 80% for less than 1.5 cm stones. Parents should be aware of nature, risks, and possible therapeutical alternatives of the RIRS.

You must have perfect knowledge of your instruments and be aware of the compatibility of your flex scopes with your UAS (ureteral access sheath).

Always culture urine preoperatively and administer proper antibiotic treatment until the urine becomes sterile. In non-toilet-trained patients, use urine collection pads.

Administer prophylactic perioperative wide-spectrum antibiotics to patients before surgery and continue for 48 postoperative hours. In non-toilet-trained children, continuous antibiotic prophylaxis should be given until stent removal.

We believe that passive dilation of the ureter with a double-J stent kept in place 1–2 weeks before RIRS is the way to dramatically decrease the risk of potential complications of active dilation of the ureter in younger children, whether or not you will use an UAS. Primary URS/RIRS can be performed safely in older children. Pre-stenting protects against possible severe UAS-induced ureteral injury. Keep in mind that most children with an obstructive/symptomatic stone require a double-J stent, so these patients arrive already pre-stented at RIRS.

26.3 Positioning

The procedure is performed under general anesthesia in dorsal lithotomy position, or frog leg position, (Fig. 26.1) with X-ray image intensifier screening. Positioning an infant on the surgical table in the lithotomy position is always a moment of concern for anesthetist and surgeon. While the standard stirrups can be used to hold the legs for lithotomy position in adolescents, they are impossible to use in neonates and infants because of the greater discrepancy in size, with the legs often left dangling and insufficiently secure. Furthermore, stirrups are cumbersome for C arm positioning. Taking advantage of the anatomy of the hip joint of the infants that allow the flexed hip to be abducted to 90° the perineum is brought to the edge of the operation table, both hip joints are symmetrically flexed, abducted, and externally rotated, and also a towel roll of appropriate size is placed on either side below the flexed

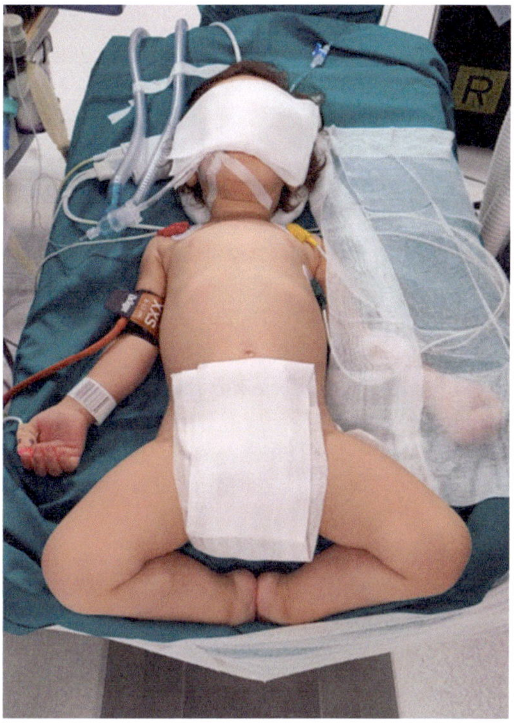

Fig. 26.1 Frog leg position

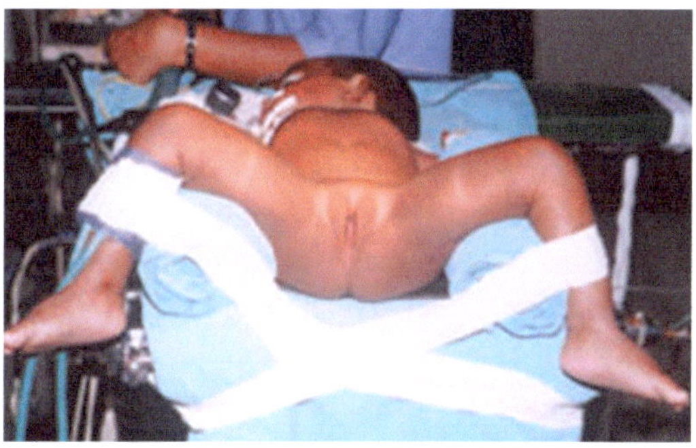

Fig. 26.2 Dorsal lithotomy position

knees (Fig. 26.2). As the towel rolls are soft, neurological complications from compression are unlikely. Radiolucent cloth rolls also permit on-table radiography.

26.4 Instrumentation

One unique aspect of URS in children is the smaller ureteral diameter compared to adults, which more often results in failure to access the ureter. The goal is to remove all the stones in order to reduce the high incidence of recurrence, keeping safety at first place and respecting the anatomy. We need to use smaller instruments. RIRS could not exist as we know it today without the development of miniaturized, actively deflectable (dual 270° deflection) flexible ureterorenoscope with excellent optical properties. These instruments are expensive and delicate; they need a structured maintenance plan to be cost-effectively used. In fiberoptic scopes, light and image are transmitted in analog format through optic fibers, whereas illumination in digital scopes is made by optic fibers or by a diode, and image capture is charged by a digital sensor located at the distal end of the endoscope.

The 7.5-Fr fiberoptic flexible ureterorenoscope Flex X^{2S} (Karl Storz, Germany) is the thinnest on the market. Olympus fiberoptic URF-P7 has a diameter of 7.95 Fr, with a 4.5 Fr evolution tip.

Reusable Digital flexible scopes in adults showed improved visual quality compared to fiberoptic counterparts and consequently achieved 20% shorter operative laser time. The thinnest currently in market are 8.5 Fr wide (Storz Flex XC and Olympus URF-V3). They better fit into 11/13 or 12/14 Fr UAS. They are more expensive and larger in diameter, but they are lighter, and they are becoming the standard of care for RIRS in the adult. They should be part of the armamentarium of the pediatric endourologist being aware that they could be used only in the compliant ureter of an older child. Both fiberoptic and digital instruments have a 3.6 Fr working channel, 67–69 cm shaft length and 6–8 cm flexible tip length.

Recently, disposable single-use digital flexible ureteroscopes have been released in the market to eliminate the inconsistent performance and maintenance hassles associated with reusable scopes. They provide no sterilization and maintenance costs and eliminate the risk of cross infection. Being very light, their ergonomics design brings good manipulation experience to doctors. Their goal is also to give high cost performance benefits to both patients and hospitals. The LithoView from Boston Scientific is currently the most used with a 7.7 Fr tip diameter and 9.5 Fr outer diameter. Pusen Uscope UE3022 has 9.5 Fr outer diameter. OTU WeScope has a 7.4 Fr tip and a 8.6 Fr outer diameter.

RIRS era started with development of the Holmium-Yag pulsated Laser. There are various generations of laser machines ranging from low power (≤20 W) to high power (120 W). High power machines allow for much more setting (PE pulse energy, Fr pulse frequency, PD pulse duration) adjustment, thus allowing the stone to be disintegrated into fragments *Fragmentation: high PE, low Fr, short PD) or converted into dust/powder (Dusting: low PE, high Fr, long PD) (Popcorning: higher Fr, small calix, fiber in contact with the stone)* (Fig. 26.3).

The fragments can be removed by nitinol tipless baskets <=1.9 Fr/120 cm advanced in the working channel of the scope, and dust/powder exits with the irrigation fluid without the need for retrieval devices. Baskets and laser fibers inserted in the working channel decrease significantly the irrigation flow.

Thulium fiber laser technology has evolved and is gaining attention now that it is capable of pulsed emission. In comparison to Ho-YAG lithotripsy, it is two to four times faster for dusting, generates finer particulate and produces minimal or no retropulsion without any significant heat production. Thullium fiber laser has recently been launched in the market for endourological use.

The Tuohy Borst adapter/port seal connector is a small but pivotal accessory for RIRS. It allows controlled access to the working channel of the flexible ureteroscope, preventing the backflow of fluid around the laser fiber/basket introduced through the working channel, improving irrigation and visibility, and blocking the laser fiber at the right distance from the tip of the scope.

A good irrigation is important in endourology. Warm normal saline is used. Gravity irrigation at 80 cm height is preferred to limit pressure build up in the collecting system but combined with a hand- assisted irrigation system providing on-demand forced irrigation to provide proper visibility. Modulation of irrigation is essential. Manual pumps are the best system. These handheld devices should be used carefully because it can generate dangerous high pressure picks especially when the working channel is empty.

UAS are used to establish a conduit during endoscopic urological procedures in the upper urinary tract. They are essential as RIRS facilitators. Most UAS have a hydrophilic coating, radio-opaque markings, and a tapered tip with a smooth transition between dilator and outer sheath. UAS improve visualization, reduce intrarenal pressure, decrease surgery time and complications, increase SFR, and preserve endoscope life allowing multiple passes of instruments. UAS are manufactured at lengths from 13 to 55 cm and inner diameters from 9.5 Fr to 16 Fr.

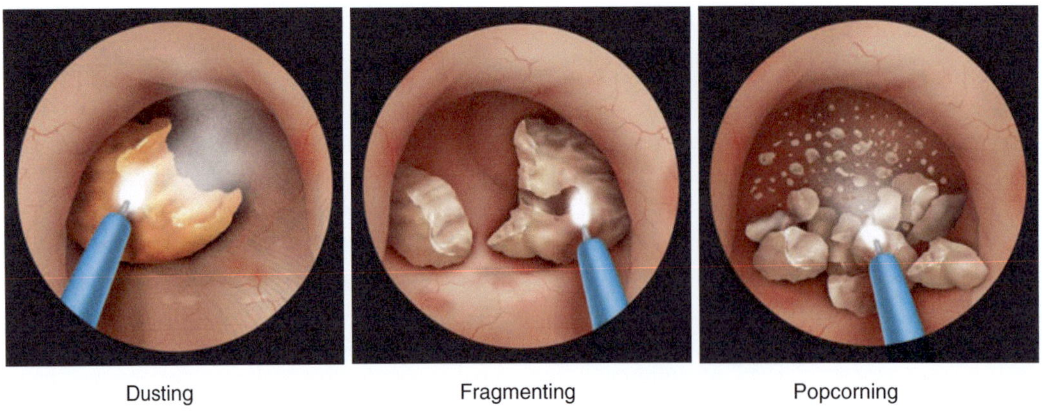

Fig. 26.3 Different setting of holmium laser lithotripsy (Desai and Ganpule; *BJUI Surgical Atlas*, 2011)

The 13 cm long/9.5–11.5-Fr Flexor UAS (Cook Medical, USA) is the shortest and the thinnest in the market, but it can barely accommodate the thinnest flexible scope. Always ensure to have a good backflow of irrigation out of the UAS and also consider the 10/12 Fr or 11/13 Fr UAS (Cook, Boston Scientific, Olympus, Rocamed, Applied Medical, Richard Wolf, etc.). Neither the most used disposable (LithoView-Uscope) nor the reusable digital flexible scopes fits in the 9.5–11 Fr UAS. You must have perfect knowledge of your instruments and be aware of the compatibility of your flex scopes with your UASs.

Semirigid ureteroscopes for diagnostic or therapeutic purpose are an essential part of RIRS. A 4.5 to 6.5 Fr, 31 or 43 cm long, 3.3 Fr wc, semi-rigid ureteroscope (Needle Ureteroscope, Richard Wolf, USA) or a 7.3 Fr, 25 cm long, 3.6 Fr wc, semirigid pediatric ureterorenoscope (Karl Storz, Germany) or a 6.5 to 7 to 9.9 Fr, 34 or 43 cm long, 4.8 Fr wc, semirigid adult ureterorenoscope (Karl Storz, Germany), or a 6.4 to 7.8 Fr, 33 or 43 cm, 4.2 Fr wc, semirigid adult ureteroscope (Olympus, Japan) are the smallest instruments available.

Every surgeon uses his favorite guidewire for RIRS, but the leading principle is that we want a stiff radiopaque wire with a flexible tip to advance the flexible scope and/or the UAS. Metallic-Polytetrafluoroethylene (PTFE) wires are more stable but kinkable, however, nitinol hydrophilic wires have a tendency to slip out but are not kinkable and are more likely to slide past an obstruction. Hybrid guidewires are a good option. We prefer nitinol stiff hydrophilic guidewires (150 cm length/0.035 in.) with flexible straight tip either as working or as safety wire.

26.5 Technique

RIRS endourological technique must be standardized and reproducible. You need to have and to be familiar with different endoscopic instruments and disposables. You need to gain endourological experience on adults or in one of the existing large case-load pediatric centers in endourology. Pediatric RIRS is technically identical to adult RIRS. It can be performed with semirigid or flexible ureteroscope. One unique aspect of RIRS in children is the smaller ureteral diameter compared to adults, which more often results in failure to access the ureter. Operating on a 2 yo child is different than treating a 12 yo, and we need to adjust to the anatomical features encountered and not the contrary (Fig. 26.4).

Fig. 26.4 Mean ureteral diameter according to the age of the children

	Mean ureteral diameter (mm)	
Age	CUSSEN 1967	HELLSTROM 1985
0–3 m	3.5	3.0
3–12 m	3.6	3.1
1–3 y	3.5	3.6
3–6 y	4.1	4.3
6–9 y	4.6	4.6
9–12 y	4.9	4.8

26.5.1 Our Procedure Step by Step

- The procedure is performed under general anesthesia in lithotomy position, or frog leg position, with X-ray image intensifier screening usually located on the left of the patient and with the endoscopic tower usually placed on the right.
- Surgeon and first assistant/scrub nurse is the best team composition.
- Cystoscopy with a 11 Fr instrument before puberty.
- Double-J stent removal if in place (we believe in passive dilation of the ureter in younger children especially under 3–4 yo).
- Insert nitinol stiff hydrophilic guidewire (0.035 in. 150 cm length) with a straight flexible tip into the renal pelvis under fluoroscopy guidance. Always keep an eye on the tip of the guidewire since rarely it can perforate the kidney and give hemorrhagic complications.
- Retrograde pyelogram with contrast medium with a 5–6 Fr ureteral catheter (serves as a road map for the endoscopic procedure and tests the compliance of the upper urinary tract and confirms the location of the stone).
- Diagnostic or therapeutic semirigid ureteroscopy. Instrument size must be decided according to the compliance of the urinary system. Remember to carefully introduce ureteroscope with a railway/two guidewires technique and to leave one stiff guidewire as safety wire secured to the surgical drape. The safety guidewire is the one that saves from the sins committed inside the ureter.
- Semirigid ureteroscopy provides a gentle active dilation of the already passively dilated ureter, treats simultaneous ureteral stones, detects ureteral stenosis. Longer semirigid ureteroscope can be passed inside a 35–36 cm UAS.
- Semirigid laser ureteroscopy can also effectively treat renal pelvis or upper caliceal stones in compliant systems.
- If you plan or need to use a flexible ureteroscope, whenever you can smoothly advance an UAS, go and do it! In the adult, it has demonstrated to decrease surgery time and complications, increase SFR, preserve endoscope life. It will make the difference!
- Advance under continuous fluoroscopy UAS over a stiff working guidewire up to the proximal ureter. UAS size must be adapted to anatomical specificity.
- Flexible ureteroscopy and direct visualization of the stones: Make sure to always have a good backflow of irrigation out of the UAS.
- Gravity irrigation of warm normal saline at 80 cm height combined with a hand-assisted irrigation system provides on-demand forced irrigation for proper visibility.
- For small (less than 1 cm) and soft (less than 1000 HU) stones, when you foresee effective dusting and no need for repeated extraction of the flexible scope, you could guide directly the flexible scope over a working wire without the UAS and proceed with holmium laser vaporization.
- Keep surgery time under 60′–90′ and keep intrarenal pressure low to decrease pyelovenous backflow and risk of urosepsis.
- Stones are vaporized or fragmented using 200–275 μm holmium laser fiber. Small fibers have same efficacy, more flexibility, more irrigation, less retropulsion and allow better scope deflection compared to larger ones.
- The holmium laser generator can be set to dusting (e.g., 0.2–0.5 J; 20–80 Hz; LP), fragmenting (e.g., 0.8–1.2 J; 6–10 Hz; SP) or popcorning (e.g., 0.5 J; 80 Hz; SP) parameters. When treating renal stones, a complete dusting technique consists of two phases: contact laser lithotripsy (painting, chipping), followed by noncontact laser lithotripsy (popcorning).
- The goal is a stone-free status. At the end of the stone laser treatment, all visible fragments other than dust are carefully removed with the help of a basket (a 1.9 Fr/120 cm nitinol tipless stone retrieval basket is a good compromise between endurance and size) and sent for analysis.
- After completion of the procedure, UAS is removed under visual control, to assess eventual ureteral injury and stones.
- Remember to decrease as much as possible child radiation exposure.

- Always put up a double-J ureteral stent (depending on the age and the height of the patient, 3–6 Fr, 10–28 cm) at the end of the surgery whenever you use an UAS or when you feel the procedure was even mildly complicated or based on the length of the case. A mono-J ureteral catheter left in place 24 h could be used after a short and straightforward procedure.
- Place Foley urethral catheter.

26.6 Postoperative Care

Stone free is defined using a combination of being endoscopically stone-free immediately after URSL and radiologically stone-free on follow-up imaging. Stone-free status is particularly critical in pediatric patients because of the higher risk of recurrence.

Keep child hydrated with e.v. fluids. Keep urethral catheter for 12–24 h in uncomplicated cases.

Physical examination to check for hematuria and fever. Discharge 24–48 h after the procedure in uncomplicated cases.

Send stone fragments for physical analysis with X-ray diffraction crystallography or infrared spectroscopy.

Double-J removal can be done 10–15 days after RIRS usually under general anesthesia.

If a second RIRS is needed to ensure complete SF status, this must be planned accordingly after 2–3 weeks (at the time when usually double-J stent is removed).

Follow-up child at 1–3 and 6 months, and then yearly with abdominal ultrasound, urine analysis, and urine culture.

Refer child to pediatric nephrologist for a full biochemical metabolic analysis.

26.7 Results

A recent well-written non-systematic review by Silay et al. analyzed the status of surgical treatment of stones in pediatric urology and SWL; in their analysis, they also reported four studies on RIRS. They concluded that success rates between 80% and 100% are achieved with RIRS for kidney stones <2 cm but may require pre-stenting in smaller children [7]. SWL usually requires multiple sessions under general anesthesia in younger children.

When compared to others techniques, retrospective comparative reports have indicated that RIRS provides at least similar stone-free rate as mini PCNL in pediatric patients with intermediate-sized renal stones. Resorlu et el., in the larger multicenter study on RIRS, discuss the outcomes of mini PCNL and RIRS in children for 10–30 mm renal calculi. They recorded 201 pediatric patients who underwent mini PCNL (n = 106) or RIRS (n = 95). Primary SFR was 84.2% for the RIRS group and 85.8% for the mini PCNL group ($p = 0.745$). These percentages increased to 92.6% and 94.3% with adjunctive therapies for RIRS and mini PCNL, respectively. Minor complications classified as Clavien I or II occurred in 17% and 8.4% in mini-perc and RIRS, respectively. Seven patients in the mini PCNL group received blood transfusions, whereas none of the children in the RIRS group were transfused ($p = 0.015$) [8].

Indeed, Wang et al. compared micro PCNL (group 1) and RIRS (group 2) in treating 1 and 2 cm solitary renal stones in pediatric patients aged less than 3 years [9]. There were 27 patients in group 1 and 30 patients in group 2, and the patients mean ages were 19 ± 9.9 months and 21 ± 7.8 months, respectively ($p = 0.462$). The stone size was 1.60 ± 3 cm in group 1 and 1.7 ± 0.2 cm in group 2 ($p = 0.217$); the mean surgical time was 52 ± 7 min in group 1 and 48 ± 9 min in group 2 ($p = 0.163$) while the SFR at 1 month after surgery was 88.9% in group 1 and 86.7% in group 2 ($p = 0.799$). The complication rate was similar with 14.8% and 16.7% in group 1 and group 2, respectively ($p = 0.714$).

A large recent experience is reported by Suliman et al. (56 stone episodes in 36 patients) with a favorable outcome. Primary RIRS was successful in 42/56 (75%) with a second FURS performed in 11 cases, bringing the cumulative clearance to 89%; clearance rates of more than 70% after first RIRS were achieved with stones up to 17 mm. The authors described excellent results similar to the adult population, they treated also small infants as young as 17 months and showed how even multiple stones may be treated in one session. Importantly, there were neither immediate ureteric complications nor long-term problems such as ureteric strictures, with no evidence of dilation on follow-up control [3].

Another large series is described by Erkurt et al.. They evaluated the efficacy and safety of RIRS to treat renal stones in preschool age (<7 years) in a total of 65 children with a mean stone size that was 14.66 ± 6.12 mm (7–30 mm) and a relative low operative time (mean 46.47 ± 18.27 min). The authors reported that in five (7.69%) patients, the initial procedure failed to reach the renal collecting system and ended with the insertion of a pigtail stent. The stone-free rates were 83% and 92.3% after the first and second procedure, respectively. They reported post-operative hematuria (Clavien I) in six (9.2%) patients, urinary tract infection with fever (Clavien II) was observed in 10 (15.4%) patients while an ureteral wall injury (Clavien III) was noted in two (3%) patients [10].

A large cohort study was recently published by Li et al. on 45 patients that presented upper urinary stones treated using RIRS combined with holmium laser lithotripsy. The size of the calculi was 1.7 cm (0.8–3.3) with 11 stones over 2 cm. The overall operative success rate was 97.8% (44/45); 1 patient (2.2%) was complicated by intraoperative ureteric laceration and was converted to laparoscopic pyelolithotomy and ureter-bladder reimplantation. After the first RIRS, there was stone clearance in 38 patients (84.4%), and second or third phase lithotripsy were needed for six patients (13.3%). Severe postoperative gross hematuria occurred in one patient and high fever occurred in two patients [11].

These large series demonstrated the safety and efficacy of RIRS in the pediatric population despite the fear that instrument size might limit the application of FURS to children.

Most of the pediatric literature on RIRS is about adolescents. Regarding children of low weight and younger age, Berrettini et al. assessed the safety of RIRS with UAS focusing on patients under 20 kg. They analyzed 13 patients with a median age of 3.91 ± 1.8 years (mean ± SD) who underwent 16 RIRS. Mean patient weight and stone burden were 14.88 ± 3.81 kg (range 10–20 kg) and 15.5 ± 3.8 mm (median 16 mm), respectively. All patients were pre-stented, a UAS was used in 15 out of 16 (93.8%) procedures and SFS was reached in 81.3% of cases after the first surgery with 100% after auxiliary procedures. Postoperative hematuria (Clavien I) occurred in three (18.8%) children and was resolved with hydration and clot removal, postoperative urinary tract infections with fever (Clavien II) were observed in two (12.5%) patients while hydrocalyx (Clavien IIIb) was noted in one (6.3%) patient. Patients with stones located in the lower pole calices ($p = 0.024$) and with mixed composition ($p = 0.036$) had a greater prevalence of complications than those with calculi of other compositions located in other sites. The authors demonstrated that RIRS with UAS is feasible, safe, and effective in very young children under 20 kg, with no ureteral stenosis or vescicoureteral reflux or late UTI or hydronephrosis at 22.4 months follow-up. As reported in this chapter, younger children could evocate an higher incidence of complications [12].

Indeed, another important issue, when the surgeon approaches kidney stones, is the nature of the stones themselves. Cystine calculi are resistant to SWL and are one of the most challenging types in the pediatric setting because of their high risk of rapid recurrence especially in the presence of residual fragments. Even if patients with cystine stones may present in older ages, the majority of patients are diagnosed during childhood and require multiple invasive treatment. Yuruk et al. described the largest consecutive series of 14 children with this type of stones treated with RIRS, the mean age was 10.9 ± 2.2 years (range: 7–15) and mean stone size was 13.6 ± 2.4 mm (range: 10–18); UAS was used in 12 (85.7%) patients. At 4 weeks follow-up, SFR was 100%. The authors report of a quite short mean operation time (38.2 ± 7.2 min, range: 30–50) underlines how cystine stones are sensitive to holmium laser treatment. Mild ureteral laceration was observed in one case during the procedure and another case developed fever on the second postoperative day. During a mean follow-up period of 25.7 ± 5.2 months, stone recurrence was noted in one patient. The authors concluded that RIRS is the surgical treatment of choice to manage cystine stone [13].

In conclusion, we recently reported a comparison between a pediatric (group A) and an adult cohort (group B) to assess the learning curve of an adult endourologist. There was no statistically significant difference between RIRS in group A and group B regarding gender, laterality, size of the stone, length of stay (p = 1.000), and operative time (group A: mean = 70, IQR 60–80; group B: mean = 80, IQR 63–105; p = 0.466). While the mean size for stone surface area in group A was 90 (IQR 80–144) mm^2 and for group B it was 100 (IQR 90–165) mm^2; there was no statistically significant difference between the two groups (p = 0.137). Moreover, no statistically significant difference was found regarding stone-free rate (p = 0.624). In facts, 13 out of 15 patients in group A (86.7%) and 12 patients in group B (80%) were stone-free after the procedure. All the patients, two (13.3%) in the pediatric and three (20%) in the adult group, respectively, who had not achieved SFS after the first procedure, were submitted to a second RIRS who gained SFS without need of ulterior treatment. Hematuria and fever were noticed in one patient for both groups requiring antibiotic treatment (Clavien II) and a longer period of stay [4].

Tip and Tricks

- The laser fiber should be advanced in the flexible scope only when the instrument is straight, better if inside the UAS.
- When you tackle a stone with holmium laser lithotripsy remember to adjust to the characteristics of the stone. Start with low power and low frequency settings and check how the stone respond. The darker stone is harder than the lighter stone. If the stone is very hard and less than 1 cm size, a winning strategy is to set the laser for fragmentation and obtain few fragments to basket out. You should be very careful to mold reasonable size fragments that fit into your UAS and into the ureter without getting stuck.
- A 2 cm stone produces at least sixty-four 0.5 mm fragments that need to be extracted, making the procedure time-consuming and hazardous. With such a stone, a better strategy is extreme and patient dusting. Laser Popcorn is useful for residual fragments.
- When snow-effect of prolonged dusting impairs your visibility, take your time to flush progressively out the dust with irrigation.
- Whenever possible relocate a lower pole stone in the renal pelvis or in an upper calix to preserve the instrument life and increase the SFR.
- Cleave laser fiber every 10–15 min with metallic scissor to reduce fiber tip degradation. To avoid repeated and potentially harmful laser fiber insertions, cleave it without retrieving it from the scope.
- Remember to check for bladder fullness during surgery and either empty it with a small tube advanced alongside the scope/UAS or with a small suprapubic percutaneous drainage to be removed at the end of the procedure.
- Since reusable flexible scopes are fragile, in tough cases where the risk of scope damage is high it could be wise to use a disposable instrument.
- During RIRS make sure that you do not move/advance with UAS. To avoid damage to the ureter, you can move UAS only over a wire and with the obturator inserted.
- If UAS doesn't fit in smoothly, you can try to remove the safety guidewire to facilitate the insertion.
- If wide-breathing excursions of the patient impair the precision of your lithotripsy increasing the risks of bleeding complications, remember to ask anesthetist to modulate respiration of the patient decreasing the extent of breathing excursion or providing short periods of apnea.
- Try to always perform endourological procedures with your skilled assistant/team.

26.8 Discussion

Since the first paper on the use of URS for stone treatment in children have been published by Ritchey et al. in 1988, ureteroscopy management has become increasingly common in pediatric stone patients [14, 15]. Recently, RIRS has gained attention as an effective method for stone lithotripsy in the proximal ureter, in the renal collecting system, especially in the lower calyx, providing less invasiveness compared to PCNL [16]. Indeed, RIRS allows lithotripsy and removal of the stones through a natural channel of the human body. Surgical urinary tract trauma, bleeding, and other complications are significantly reduced in comparison to PCNL, laparoscopic, and open approaches. RIRS minimizes operative time and hospital stay and has an acceptable reproducibility and a shorter learning curve [11].

RIRS is less invasive than PCNL and is therefore the most preferred approach to treat renal calculi in patients with a bleeding diathesis and in recurrent cystine stone formers. This method has the advantages of high efficiency, minimal invasiveness, and repeatability.

Other indications are SWL-resistant stones, multiple kidney stones, simultaneous ureteric and kidney stones, and also lower pole stones <1.5 cm.

RIRS can be used to minimize morbidity of the percutaneous access of PCNL by Endovision puncture of the renal papilla of the targeted calix or be constituent part of the ECIRS (endoscopic combined intrarenal surgery) approach.

RIRS has also been compared with PCNL for large stone over 2 cm, concluding that RIRS has the advantages of decreased radiation exposure, fewer complications, and shorter hospital although PCNL maintains a better stone-free rates [17]. Moreover, RIRS can be performed safely in children, even in infants younger than 1 yo and has become a popular modality to treat upper ureteric and renal stones ≤2 cm [12].

Patients with bilateral renal stones, although simultaneous RIRS is technically feasible, should be managed in two separate sessions for safety reasons.

A recent systematic review of children undergoing RIRS for both kidney and upper ureter stones reported an aggregate success rate of 87.5% and a complication rate of 10.5%. When outcomes are limited to intrarenal stones in children, FURS can achieve stone-free rates of 58–91% after a single treatment. The authors data show how both stone location and stone burden are important factors for treatment success [18].

Whatley et al. wrote the most recent systematic review searching for all English language articles in patients ≤18 years from 1990 to 2018 who underwent FURS. They found 11 studies on 431 patients, with a mean age of 8.5 years; mean stone size was 13 mm (range, 1.5–30 mm). SFR was 87% (58–100%) with a mean complication rate of 12.6% ($n = 55$) (range, 0–31.3%) and 76% needing a post-operative ureteric stent insertion. Five articles were from Turkey, two from the United States, two from the United Kingdom, and one each from France and Australia. Although there are still only a few studies on FURS for pediatric stone disease, RIRS is growing in numbers and appears safe and effective [19]. The most frequent complications are fever and urinary tract infection, hematuria, and post-operative pain, including stent discomfort. No Clavien V complication (ureteral avulsion) is mentioned in this series, but Li et al. in 2019 reported on a ureteral laceration requiring ureter-bladder reimplantation [11, 19]. There was no data found in the literature on the development of ureteric strictures following URS in the pediatric population.

Complications increase with length of the procedure, stone burden, and younger age. This indicates that RIRS is particularly delicate and should be recommended with caution in younger children. Never force the boundaries of primary RIRS for a higher SFR but plan a second look procedure. Prolonged surgery comes with prolonged high intrarenal pressure and high risk of sepsis.

Most of the literature on pediatric RIRS includes adolescents. SFR decrease with stone burden, younger age, and for lower pole stones in case of acute infundibulopelvic angle. Stones

>2 cm and staghorn stones confer a high risk for treatment failure [12, 20].

Although EAU/ESPU guidelines consider SWL the first option of treatment for kidney stones, a critical view of SWL outcomes coupled with improved instrumentation for RIRS has resulted in a shift in practice across the United States and Europe, with lower rates of SWL compared to RIRS. The long-term effects of SWL are not clear. In a prospective series comparing SWL with RIRS for renal stones under 2 cm, Ibrahim A. et al. showed stone-free rate of single session RIRS higher than that of SWL (86.6% vs. 70%) but the difference was not statistically significant, probably because of the small number of cases. In a retrospective analysis, Freton L et al. showed better single-session SFR for FURS vs. SWL, despite more complex urinary stones (multiple, lower pole, etc.) and without increasing morbidity. In single stones less than 2 cm size, SRF was 78.6% vs. 50%; $p = 0.06$ [7]. This SFR difference is especially wide in case of lower pole stones [20].

Another issue is to pre-stent children before surgery and the use of UAS.

Primary URS/RIRS can be performed safely in older children as in the adults. Passive dilation of the ureter with a double-J stent kept in place 1–2 weeks before RIRS is the way to dramatically decrease the risk of potential complications of active dilation of the ureter in younger children according to the small caliber of the ureter, whether or not you will use an UAS. Pre-stenting does allow for more reliable access to the ureter (almost 100% UAS smooth insertion vs. around 50% success without pre-stenting in preschool children [11]) and has been associated with shorter operative time and better stone clearance rates in retrospective studies in adults. Deciding a sharp age threshold to pre-stent children is not possible because other factors need to be taken into account like body weight and physical body development, but considering ureteric diameters (Fig. 26.4), one could suggest to pre-stent patients under 3–4 yo age. The risk-benefit ratio for additional anesthetic compared to potentially improved outcomes with pre-stenting deserves anyway further investigation [3].

The use of UAS in children is still under debate because of the potential risk of ureteral injury and vesicoureteral reflux related to the relatively large caliber of the instruments. Pre-stenting protects against possible severe UAS-induced ureteral injury. Recent data demonstrate the safety of UAS in the pediatric population and even in children under 20 kg [11, 12, 21].

As on today, the final decision whether to proceed with a primary or secondary (with pre-stenting) RIRS and whether to use UAS or not depends to a great extent on the endourological experience of the surgeon and the type of endoscopic instrumentation available.

We should inform parents of our personal results and complications with RIRS and discuss with them other possible alternatives.

To overcome his boundaries, RIRS in the future will need further downsizing of the instruments to improve the safety profile, but this will come with more time-consuming procedures. Extraction of fragments can't be mechanical but should be hydrodynamic to reduce surgery time. The dusting technique will have to be maximized acting on different laser setting or thanks to Thulium fiber laser.

Last but not the least, as we previously reported, another interesting topic is the learning curve of this procedure. It is commonly thought that RIRS is relatively more difficult to perform in children due to the narrower space that makes it more challenging to maneuver the instrument.

Moreover, usually preoperative anatomical and stone data are lacking in the children because diagnostic assessment is done with US scan before the surgery instead of CT scan.

Despite these limitations, the increasing demand for pediatric stone management in daily clinical practice in tertiary referral center leads adult's surgeons to perform RIRS in this subset of patients without a high expertise in children. We assessed that surgeons who have achieved high expertise in adult's field could confidently approach pediatric age population with efficacy and safety comparable with adults, even in his first series, as seen for other surgical procedures as a robotic procedure.

A twin surgeon approach with a pediatric urologist and an experienced adult endourologist has also been recommended for achieving good results in pediatric patients. The results also seem to be equally good in medium and high volume centers.

In conclusion, the use of ureteroscopy for the treatment of pediatric kidney stones has increased, and RIRS represents a safe and effective option with high SFR and low complication rate. Pediatric population is surgically and technically more challenging than adults and must be addressed with great attention and preparation.

Take-Home Points

- RIRS can be performed safely with high SFR in children, even in infants younger than 1 yo, and has become a popular modality to treat upper ureteric and renal stones ≤2 cm.
- RIRS can be performed by a pediatric urologist/surgeon only after a good experience with URS in children better if mentored by a skilled adult endourologist or can be performed by an adult endourologist better if mentored by a pediatric urologist/surgeon.
- Standardize your technique, make it reproducible. You must have perfect knowledge of your instruments and be aware of the compatibility of your flex scopes with your UASs.
- Inform parents of your results with RIRS and of possible alternatives for kidney stones.
- Clarify parents the concept of single procedure/single RIRS: every "single" RIRS could be a staged procedure (pre-stenting–surgery–stent removal) with up to three general anesthesia.
- Adapt the instruments to the ureter and Never Force the progression or the extraction of your instruments. Use the smallest equipment available.
- Always use a safety guidewire to be on the safer side.
- Care should be taken to ensure that the radiation exposure to the child during the procedure is minimized as there is now a well-documented relationship of radiation dosimetry and the development of secondary malignancies.

References

1. Van Cleynenbreugel B, Kılıç Ö, Akand M. Retrograde intrarenal surgery for renal stones—part 1. Turk J Urol. 2017;43(2):112–21.
2. Tekgül S, Stein R, Bogaert G, Nijman RJM, Quaedackers J, 't Hoen L, et al. European Association of Urology and European Society for Paediatric Urology Guidelines on Paediatric Urinary Stone Disease. Eur Urol Focus. 2021:S2405–4569(21)00158–9. https://doi.org/10.1016/j.euf.2021.05.006.
3. Suliman A, Burki T, Garriboli M, Glass J, Taghizadeh A. Flexible ureterorenoscopy to treat upper urinary tract stones in children. Urolithiasis. 2020;48(1):57–61. https://doi.org/10.1007/s00240-018-1083-5.
4. Sforza S, Tuccio A, Grosso AA, Crisci A, Cini C, Masieri L. Could surgical experience of adult endourologist overcome the learning curve of retrograde intrarenal surgery in children? Urolithiasis. 2020;48(5):459–64. https://doi.org/10.1007/s00240-019-01161-x.
5. Clayton DB, Pope JC. The increasing pediatric stone disease problem. Ther Adv Urol. 2011;3(1):3–12.
6. Faure A, Boissier R. Optimal settings for the holmium: YAG laser in pediatric endourology: tips and tricks. J Pediatr Urol. 2020;16(2):244–50. https://doi.org/10.1016/j.jpurol.2020.03.002.
7. Selcuk M, Ellison JS, Tailly T, Caione P, Catto J. Update on urinary stones in children: current and future concepts in surgical treatment and shockwave lithotripsy. Eur Urol Focus. 2017;3(2–3):164–71. https://doi.org/10.1016/j.euf.2017.07.005.
8. Resorlu B, Unsal A, Tepeler A, Atis G, Tokatli Z, Oztuna D, et al. Comparison of retrograde intrarenal surgery and mini-percutaneous nephrolithotomy in children with moderate-size kidney stones: results of multi-institutional analysis. Urology. 2012;80(3):519–23.
9. Wang W, Ge Y, Wang Z, Wang L, Li J, Tian Y. Comparing micropercutaneous nephrolithotomy and retrograde intrarenal surgery in treating 1-2 cm solitary renal stones in pediatric patients younger than 3 years. J Pediatr Urol. 2019;15(5):517.e1–6.
10. Erkurt B, Caskurlu T, Atis G, Gurbuz C, Arikan O, Pelit ES, et al. Treatment of renal stones with flexible ureteroscopy in preschool age children. Urolithiasis. 2014;42(3):241–5.

11. Li J, Yu H, Zhou P, Pan H, Li R, Wang Y, et al. Application of flexible ureteroscopy combined with holmium laser lithotripsy and their therapeutic efficacy in the treatment of upper urinary stones in children and infants. Urol J. 2019;16(38):343–6.
12. Berrettini A, Boeri L, Montanari E, Mogiatti M, Acquati P, De Lorenzis E, et al. Retrograde intrarenal surgery using ureteral access sheaths is a safe and effective treatment for renal stones in children weighing < 20 kg. J Pediatr Urol. 2018;14(1):59.e1–6. https://doi.org/10.1016/j.jpurol.2017.09.011.
13. Yuruk E, Tuken M, Gonultas S, Colakerol A, Cakir OO, Binbay M, et al. Retrograde intrarenal surgery in the management of pediatric cystine stones. J Pediatr Urol. 2017;13(5):487.e1–5. https://doi.org/10.1016/j.jpurol.2017.01.015.
14. Esposito C, Masieri L, Bagnara V, Tokar B, Golebiewski A, Escolino M. Ureteroscopic lithotripsy for ureteral stones in children using holmium: yag laser energy: results of a multicentric survey. J Pediatr Urol. 2019;15(4):391.e1–7. https://doi.org/10.1016/j.jpurol.2019.05.004.
15. Ritchey M, Patterson DE, Kelalis PPSJ. A case of pediatric ureteroscopic lasertripsy. J Urol. 1988;139:1272–4.
16. Mandeville JA, Caleb P. Pediatric urolithiasis. Curr Opin Urol. 2009;19(4):419–23.
17. Saad KSM, Youssif ME, Hamdy SAIN, Fahmy A, El Din Hanno AG, El-Nahas AR. Percutaneous nephrolithotomy vs retrograde intrarenal surgery for large renal stones in pediatric patients: a randomized controlled trial. J Urol. 2015;194(6):1716–20.
18. Ishii H, Griffin S, Somani BK. Review ureteroscopy for stone disease in the paediatric population: a systematic review. BJU Int. 2015;115(6):867–73.
19. Whatley A, Jones P, Aboumarzouk O, Somani BK. Safety and efficacy of ureteroscopy and stone fragmentation for pediatric renal stones: a systematic review. Transl Androl Urol. 2019;8(Suppl 4):S442–7.
20. Featherstone NC, Somani BK, Griffin SJ. Ureteroscopy and laser stone fragmentation (URSL) for large (≥1 cm) paediatric stones: outcomes from a university teaching hospital. J Pediatr Urol. 2017;13(2):202.e1–7.
21. Traxer O, Thomas A. Prospective evaluation and classification of ureteral wall injuries resulting from insertion of a ureteral access sheath during retrograde intrarenal surgery. J Urol. 2013;189(2):580–4.

Management of Kidney Stones Using Perc/Micro-perc as Minimally Invasive Percutaneous Procedures

27

Paolo Caione, Giuseppe Collura, Michele Innocenzi, Mauro De Dominicis, Laura Del Prete, Ermelinda Mele, and Nicola Capozza

Learning Objectives

- To update on percutaneous treatment of stone disease in pediatric age and discuss the minimally invasive different options
- To describe step by step the technique of mini-perc by ClearPetra equipment
- To describe step by step the technique of micro-perc by a 4.8 gauge stylet
- To show mini-perc and micro-perc procedures by two videoclips
- To describe tips and tricks of PCNL, mini- and micro-perc in pediatric age, to optimize results and reduce the complication rates

Supplementary Information The online version contains supplementary material available at [https://doi.org/10.1007/978-3-030-99280-4_27].

P. Caione (✉) · G. Collura · M. Innocenzi
L. Del Prete · E. Mele · N. Capozza
Division of Pediatric Urology, "Bambino Gesù" Children's Hospital, Rome, Italy
e-mail: caionep.urologiaped@gmail.com; giuseppe.collura@opbg.net; michele.innocenzi@opbg.net; laura.delprete@opbg.net; ermelinda.mele@opbg.net; nicola.capozza@opbg.net

M. De Dominicis
Division of Urology, "Cristo Re" Hospital, Rome, Italy
e-mail: mauro.dedominicis@ospedalecristore.it

27.1 Introduction

Renal stone disease in pediatric age is a significant problem to treat even today, and there is a need to optimize diagnostic and surgical approach [1]. The incidence of upper tract urinary stones in children is reported as representing 0.1– 5% of urolithiasis in adult age [2], but it seems to have increased in Western countries in recent decades, due to metabolic disorders and due to modified alimentary habits from the first period of life [1, 3]. Moreover, urolithiasis in children is associated with considerable morbidity and presents higher recurrent rate than in adults [4].

Thus, the goal to achieve stone-free status is paramount in pediatric age patients. Improvements in new technologies and devices for the urological treatment of pediatric nephrolithiasis have been borrowed from adult experience and adopted to the smaller anatomical features of children, especially in pre-school age [5]. According to the European Association of Urology (EAU) and European Society for Pediatric Urology (ESPU) guidelines, shock wave lithotripsy (SWL) is still the initial option in pediatric renal stones [6] but continuous advances in endoscopic and percutaneous technology and equipment have obtained to reach recently higher success rates with low complication and reduced morbidity. Endoscopic uretero-

C. Esposito et al. (eds.), *Minimally Invasive Techniques in Pediatric Urology*, https://doi.org/10.1007/978-3-030-99280-4_27

lithotripsy (ULT), retrograde intra-renal surgery (RIRS), percutaneous nephrolithotomy (PCNL) with its mini-invasive variants as mini-percutaneous lithotripsy (Mini-PCNL) and micro-percutaneous access to calyceal system (micro-perc) are offered and adopted in pediatric renal stone disease [7].

We will focus on technical refinements in recent percutaneous procedures for renal stones in pediatric age, with special attention to new technologies and perspectives in discussion.

27.2 Preoperative Preparation

A rigorous workup is mandatory prior to proceeding with any urological treatment [8]. Accurate familial and personal medical history, repeated urinalysis, and urine culture are the first steps. Blood laboratory investigations, including blood cells count, coagulation profile, serum creatinine, protein, and electrolytes, are needed before any surgical approach. Blood group must be determined with availability of erythrocyte transfusion if needed. High-quality imaging is paramount to address properly the stone disease treatment: renal ultrasonography (US) and plain abdomen X-ray after adequate bowel preparation are the required traditional imaging tests (Fig. 27.1a).

Nowadays, X-ray is commonly replaced by low-dose non-contrast computerized tomography (CT) scan of the abdomen, for quantitative assessment of the stone burden and for better definition of the stone number and localization within the renal calyceal, pyelic, and ureteral system (Fig. 27.1b). Pretreatment determination of Hounsfield Units density by CT can be used to distinguish the harder stones, commonly when composed by cysteine or struvite, from other types of calculi [9]. This information is useful to address the urologist to the most appropriate lithotripsy treatment. Renal scintigraphy (DMSA or MAG3) can be required to assess relative kidney function and any urinary outflow obstruction before lithotripsy.

Finally, the percutaneous treatment, with its variants mini-perc and micro-perc, must be selected individually for any patient, choosing between the different available options that include SWL, ULT, RIRS, PCNL, and its variants or open surgical approach [8].

27.3 Positioning

Classically, percutaneous renal approaches are carried out on patient in prone position, as for any nephrostomy positioning [10]. The prone

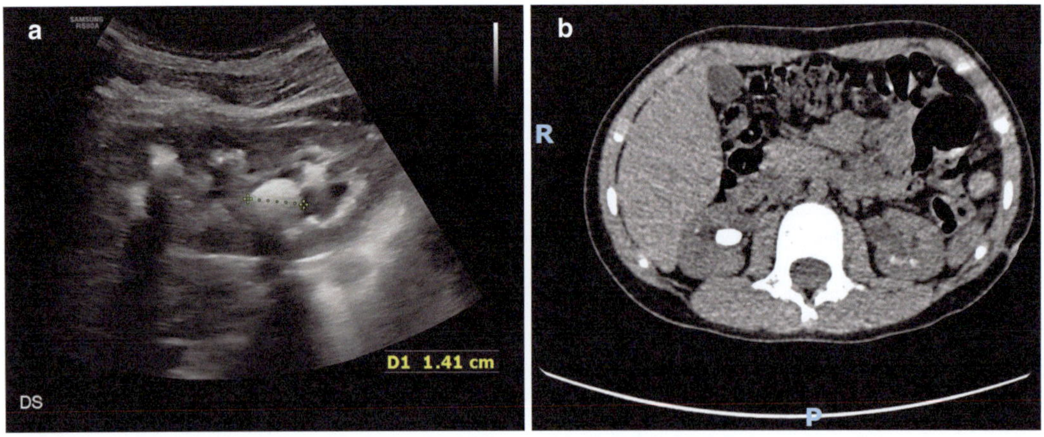

Fig. 27.1 (**a** and **b**): stone imaging. (**a**) US picture of a 14 mm stone in lower portion of right kidney pelvis in a 7-year boy. (**b**) CT abdominal scan, better defining the endopyelic stone (1150 Hounsfield Units density) in the same boy

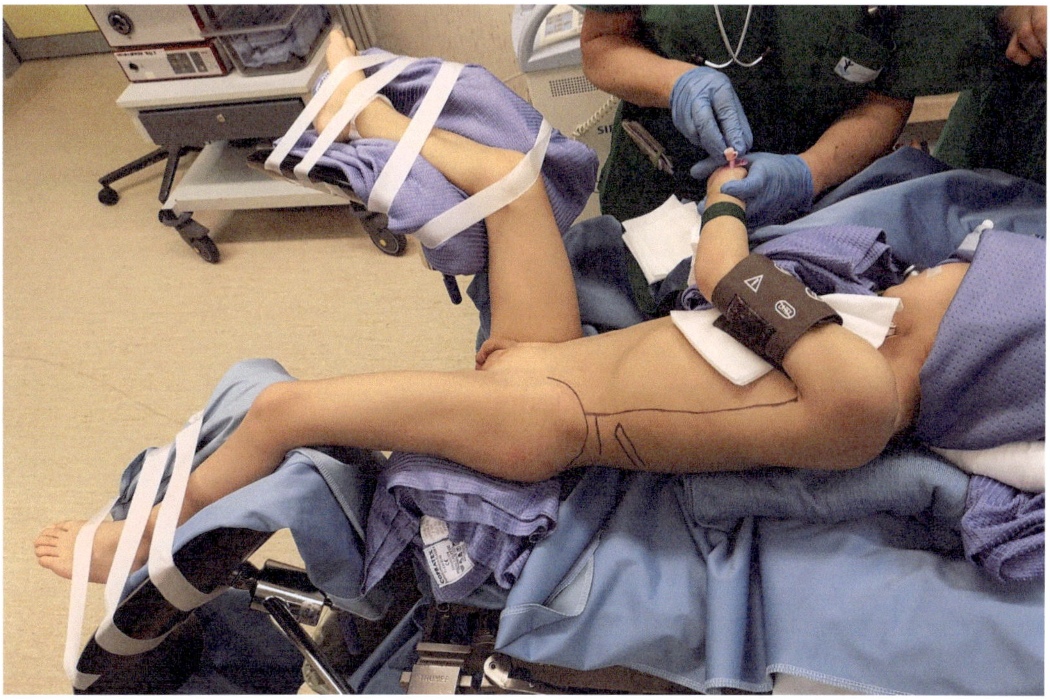

Fig. 27.2 The Valdivia Urìa modified Galdakao position of the pediatric patient during the percutaneous procedures for renal lithotripsy

position is still the most commonly utilized approach in adult patients. Recently, the supine position of the patient gained popularity, with several variants, although multiple renal accesses could be more difficult to perform. In particular, the Valdivia Urìa modified Galdakao position is preferred for several advantages [11, 12]: shorter time and easier positioning of the patient on the surgical table, easier fragments clearing, reduced risk of colonic lesion, and better anesthesiologist respiratory control [13].

In our institution, we adopt only the Valdivia Urìa modified Galdakao position (Fig. 27.2): the patient lays supine on the urological table, with two small pillows under the ipsilateral shoulder and buttock. The ipsilateral arm is flexed on the opposite side over the chest and the contralateral leg is placed in flexed and abducted position (Fig. 27.2). The posterior axillary line and the 12th rib are marked. The position guarantees simultaneously retrograde uretero-renoscopy and antegrade percutaneous access to the kidney [11].

27.4 Instrumentation

PCNL is still considered the gold standard treatment for large renal calculi (diameter > 2 cm) even in pediatric age, mimicking from adult urological procedures. Although the use of adult size instruments is referred to be safe [13], miniaturization of instrumentation is able to reduce significantly invasiveness in the pediatric population, especially in very young children who undergo renal percutaneous approaches [7, 8].

The instrumentation, mainly borrowed from adult urology, includes availability in the operating room of high-definition ultrasonographic device. A portable X-ray machine with the "C-arch" must be kept beside the operating table,

Table 27.1 Equipment required in the operating room for PCNL-miniperc-microperc procedures

Disposable	Not disposable
Pollack ureteral catheter (4–5 °F)	Portable US machine
Ciba needle 18 G	Portable X-ray machine with "C arch"
Standard guide wire (0.025–0.035 in.)	Pediatric operative cystoscopy set (8–9.8; 12; 14 °F)
Sensor hybrid guide wire with hydrophilic 5 cm tip and nitinol+PTFE core 140 cm	Semirigid ureteroscopes 5° optic (6.5–7.5 F 60 cm; 4.5–6.5 F 57 cm)
Amplatz guide wire 145 cm 0.035 inch (super-stiff; extra-stiff)	Flexible nephroscope (7.5 F 67 cm Flexion 270° vision 88°)
Amplatz dilatator up to 24 °F	Nephroscope 12 F (mini-PCNL)
High-pressure balloon dilatator (17 cm 24 °F; 16 cm 18 °F) with Amplatz sheath	Nephroscope 24 F (PCNL)
Basket 1.9–2.2 °F	Holmium-YAG laser 30 W
Clear Petra sheath (16 °F 13 cm) With aspiration system (mini-PCNL)	Trilogy combinate energy machine (US+ ballistic)
Open tip occluding catheter (10 °F 50 cm)	Microperc set
Dual-lumen catheter (10 °F 50 cm)	Optic fibers 200–550 μm for Holmium YAG laser
Probe for combinate energy machine 340 mm 10.3 °F (PCNL) 341 mm 5.7 °F (mini-PCNL)	
Optic fibers 200–550 μm for Holmium YAG laser	
Double-J ureteral stent 4.5–6 °F (14–24 cm)	
Contrast media solution	

with contrast media for pyelogram to allow precise pointing of the stone within the renal pelvis and calyx. Both ultrasonography and retrograde pyelogram can be used to guide properly the percutaneous access to the collecting system by means of a delicate navigation maneuver [14].

Percutaneous access to kidney requires a Ciba needle for the kidney sting and a series of different tools to perform the dilatation of the percutaneous way through the flank abdominal wall. The polyurethane Amplatz dilators in ascending order up to 24 °F or the metallic telescopic dilators, proposed by Alken, have been widely used from the 1980s [15]. Usually, we adopt the high-pressure "balloon" dilatation system that allows quicker dilatation in a single passage through the abdominal wall and the kidney, reducing the risk of parenchymal trauma and bleeding due to vascular injury [16]. Different caliber Amplatz sheath cannulas (14–24 °F) are required to adopt to the nephroscope and several 0.0035 to 0.0018 metallic or hydrophilic guide wires are used (Table 27.1).

A 22 F nephroscope (Karl Storz, Tubingen, Germany) is used for classic PCNL in older children and adolescents. In order to reduce invasiveness and bleeding complications, we adopt the mini-perc procedure, with smaller percutaneous access (16–18 F Amplatz cannulas) and 12 F nephroscope (Karl Storz). Flexible nephroscope or flexible ureteroscope (Karl Storz, Wolf, Girus Acmi) may be ready for residual stone fragments extraction by basket or laser tripsy. Fragmentation is carried out by different sources of energy: ballistic and pneumatic energy by 1.9 (0.8–2.5) mm probe (Swiss Lithoclast), ultrasound energy, Holmium:YAG laser by 200–500 micron fibers (Sphinx 30 W laser machine, LISA Laser, Pleasanton, California, United States) (Table 27.1). The micro-perc uses a special kit, with a 4.85 °F needle containing a 0.9 mm optic fiber and a 200 micron laser fiber (Figs. 27.3 and 27.4).

For any percutaneous procedure, complete setup for pediatric cystoscopy, ureteral catheterization, retrograde pyelogram, with 4–5 °F Pollak, and occluding catheters are needed. Semirigid and flexible ureteroscopes, caliber 6 °F–8 °F, must be available if a retrograde procedure (ULT or RIRS) should be associated combined with the percutaneous antegrade approach [11]. As final remark, it must be

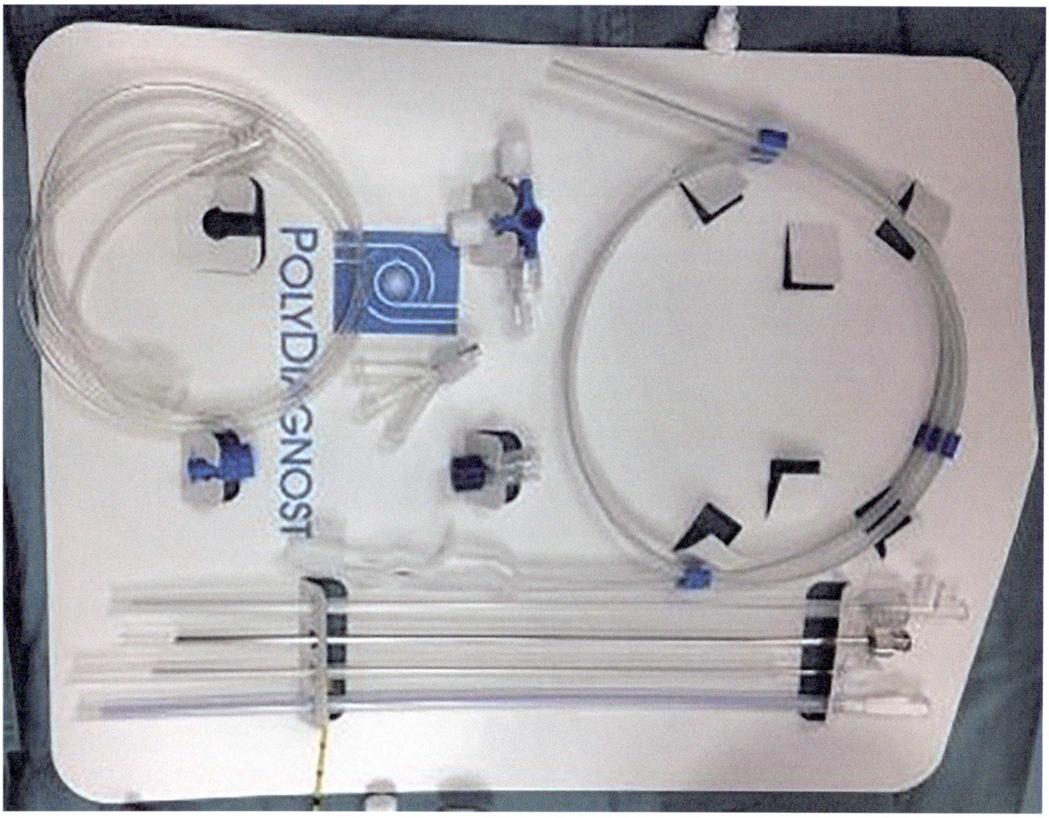

Fig. 27.3 The micro-perc setting with the 4.85 °F needle and the three-way connector and optic fiber for laser-tripsy

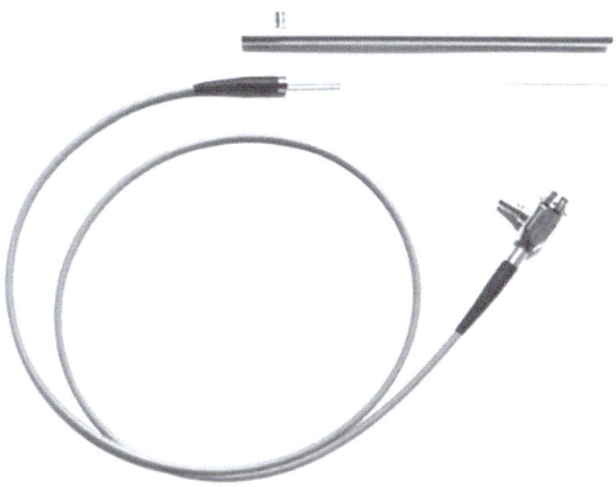

Fig. 27.4 The 272 micron laser fiber inserted in the central port of the three-way connector and the syringe for manual controlled, low pressure, irrigation

stressed that complete endourological equipment suitable for pediatric patients must be available in the operating room, before starting any percutaneous procedure.

27.5 Technique

27.5.1 Perc/Mini-perc Procedure

The patient is put on the urological table in supine Valdivia Urìa modified Galdakao position [10] under general anesthesia by tracheal intubation. Posterior axillary line, 12th rib, and iliac crest are marked. Transurethral cystoscopy allows retrograde catheterization of the affected ureter and contrast media is injected carefully through an occluding open tip catheter positioned at the pyelo-ureteral junction. Opacification of the pyelo-calyceal system is obtained using the "C-arch" fluoroscopic X-ray machine combined with US to guide the selected calyx. If possible, only US can be used for stone pointing guidance.

As the selected calyx has been reached by the tip of the Ciba needle, a guide wire is inserted

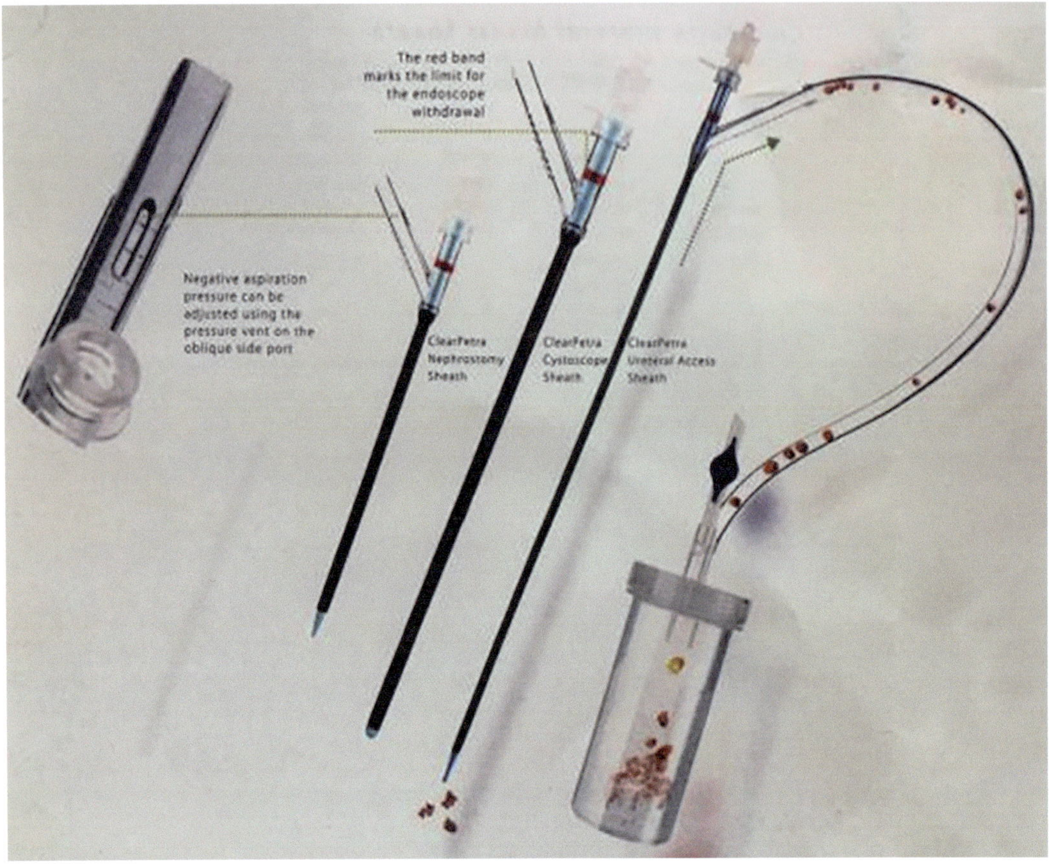

Fig. 27.5 The ClearPetra System with the aspiration channel that can be manually controlled

into the pelvis under X-ray control, and dilatation of the nephrostomy access is obtained by high-pressure balloon or by progressive Amplatz dilators, up to 26 °F for classic **PCNL**, 16 °F for the **mini-perc**, or finally 12 °F for the so-called **"ultra-mini-perc" (UMP)**. Amplatz sheath of 24 or 16–14 or 12 °F is positioned, according to the chosen caliber of the procedure. A second "safety" guide wire is passed through the sheath. The nephroscope caliber should be 3–4 °F smaller than the sheath to allow good saline irrigation and easy fragments outflow. We prefer the mini-perc procedure with 12 °F pediatric nephroscope through a 16 °F sheath that guarantees good endoscopic visual, efficient irrigation, and reduces the invasiveness of the standard PCNL. Recently, a new device has been introduced in our institution, the **"ClearPetra System."** It is a new single-use 14 °F–16 °F sheath that allows direct calyx access with continuous aspiration and irrigation flow (Fig. 27.5). The continuous irrigation (60–80 mL/min) is performed through the nephroscope channel, whereas the negative aspiration pressure (150–200 mmHg) is manually controlled through a lateral channel with multiple orifices (Fig. 27.5). Stones and fragments are attracted at the sheath opening and laser lithotripsy is carried out without risk of stone retropulsion. As lithotripsy source of energy, Holmium YAG laser passes through a 272 micron fiber, with low energy and high frequency (30 W, 0.6 J, 8 Hz). Stone fragments pass easier between sheath and nephroscope and are extracted through the lateral slanting tube into a bottle. Larger fragments are aspirated into the Clear-Petra sheath when the nephroscope is partially extracted. At the end of the procedure, a 10 °F nephrostomy tube is positioned and a 4.5 °F double-J is often left postoperatively, with transurethral Foley catheter.

27.5.2 Micro-perc Procedure

Micro-perc procedure has been recently offered to treat lower pole stones, small diameter (less than 20 mm) with a really minimally invasive procedure. The patient is in supine Valdivia modified position; open tip occluding catheter is positioned at the pyelo-ureteral junction. The procedure adopts a single-step percutaneous calyceal puncture using a single 4.85-°F needle. When the collecting system access is achieved, the inner stylet is removed and a three-way connector is attached to the sheath. A 0.9 mm high-resolution (10,000 pixels) optic flexible wire connected with the telescope is passed through the sheath. The other side port is used for intermittent saline irrigation by manual control (Figs. 27.3 and 27.4). A 200 micron laser fiber is passed through the connector central port and stone fragmentation is performed under direct vision using high frequency and low energy (0.6–0.8 J). Complete fragmentation and stone clearance is checked by direct vision and fluoroscopic control before needle removal. No nephrostomy tube is left. The transurethral catheter and bladder Foley are removed at 18–24 h from surgery.

27.6 Postoperative Care

Children who undergo mini-perc procedure receive wide-spectrum antimicrobial treatment and fluid overload during the three postoperative days. Postoperative pain assessment is detected by the "face-legs-activity-cry-consolability" (FLACC) scale in children younger than 4 years or the "visual analogic scale" (VAS) in older patients. Paracetamol requirement (15 mg/kg body weight at 6 h intervals, if needed) is fulfilled. Hemoglobin decrease and complications are detected. Nephrostomic tube is closed at day 2 and removed at day 3 if hematuria is controlled and transurethral catheter is removed at hospital discharge. Renal US and abdominal X-ray are performed at 1 month and 3 months postoperatively. Stone clearance is defined as achieved if no residual calculi or asymptomatic fragments less than 4 mm diameter are detected. Metabolic disorders (mainly idiopathic hypercalciuria and cystinuria) are monitored for the required nephrological treatment and long-term prevention of stone recurrence is needed.

The postoperative care after micro-perc procedure is really simple: very little postoperative pain is usually observed, with minimal requirement of paracetamol. The transurethral bladder catheter is removed simultaneously within 18–24 h. The patient is discharged consequently, continuing antimicrobial prophylaxis in the subsequent 2 weeks. US and, if required, X-ray check, as well as long-term patient monitoring, are similar to the PCNL procedure.

27.7 Results

The stone composition in our experience is summarized in Table 27.2. The youngest children treated with micro-perc and mini-perc were 13 and 18 months old, respectively. The mean operative time ranged from 58 to 150 min (mean 88 min), shorter in micro-perc procedures. Stone-free rate was achieved in 83% of our patients after a single mini-perc procedure. Non-significant asymptomatic residual fragments were observed in 5% of children and observed at long-time follow-up. A secondary procedure was required in 12% of children who underwent mini-perc: usually, we adopted retrograde access to renal pelvis and calyx by RIRS with laser lithotripsy, usually at the time of double-J removal.

Table 27.2 Stone composition in pediatric age

Dihydrate calcium oxalate	39.5%
Monohydrate calcium	16.2%
Struvite	23.5%
Cystine	10.4%
Uric acid	2.3%
Other or not detected	8.1%

(From Salerno et al. [1])

Postoperative pain was very limited, especially after the micro-perc procedure, with the FLACC/VAS scale <3 often also in the mini-perc patients. The Paracetamol requirement was limited to the first or second postoperative day. The blood loss was insignificant in the micro-perc and limited to the first 3–5 postoperative days in the mini-perc, with 0.5 to 2.1 gr% hemoglobin decrease. No gross hematuria was observed, but two patients required limited blood transfusion in mini-perc procedures.

In 1 out of the eleven child patients who received micro-perc procedure, we observed stone migration into the pelvis that required conversion to RIRS. No other significant complications were observed, unless transient febrile urinary tract infection in one patient.

Tip and Tricks

- The percutaneous procedures for renal stone disease in pediatric age are not easy to perform and it is necessary to be confident with common urological endoscopy before approaching it with safety and efficacy. We recommend to start any percutaneous procedure with the support of an experienced endourologist, as mentor. It seems realistic that at least 20 procedures should be performed with mentoring protection before becoming independent in PCNL and its variants.
- The supine position of the patient, according to Valdivia Urìa modified Galdakao, is very useful to allow retrograde access combined with the percutaneous antegrade approach. The positioning at the pyelo-ureteral junction of the open tip occluding catheter as preliminary act is a very effective advice, avoiding stones or fragments migrating into the ureter during the percutaneous lithotripsy maneuvers.
- As soon as the access into the selected calyx is reached and the sheath is positioned, a crucial point is to put a second "safety" guide wire into the renal pelvis and proximal ureter. At the end of the procedure, we suggest to leave a small caliber nephrostomy tube (10 °F caliber) in mini-perc procedures. No nephrostomy but transurethral pyelo-ureteral catheter fixed to a Foley bladder catheter is adopted in micro-perc.
- It must be stressed that no force should be applied during any endourological procedure. Renal parenchyma injury, urinary tract wall perforation, and significant bleeding are the possible complications, if the endoscopic maneuvers are not appropriate. The hemorrhage risk is always possible and it is reported up to 8%, but sometimes it could be a severe complication [7, 13].

27.8 Discussion

Renal stone disease causes significant morbidity in pediatric age population, for the reported increased incidence worldwide in developed countries, for the symptomatic involvement of the affected kidneys and urinary tract, and lastly for the difficult treatment, both medical and surgical, especially in younger children [1, 7]. Therefore, every effort should be made to achieve stone-free status in pediatric population. The smaller anatomical characteristics of the urinary tract in younger children may challenge any urological treatment. There is no complete agreement that really does exists at the moment on the most efficacious and most safe modality for treatment of renal stone disease in children [5].

Medical management, as adequate fluid intake, restricted dietary salt, and metabolic disorders treatment have demonstrated to be useful in prevention of recurrence, whereas alpha-blockers drug administration is given for stimulating small ureteral stones expulsion. Although it is still reported to be the first line of treatment even in pediatrics [6], the use of SWL in children has often been unpredictable or shown partial results, general anesthesia is needed and it can require pre-stenting the urinary tract by double-J positioning. Moreover, repeated sessions may be necessary [7, 8].

In the last few decades, innovative endourological procedures have been introduced progressively in children affected by urolithiasis, borrowed from the experience of adult urology. Retrograde endoscopic procedures, as ULT or RIRS, have good results for ureteral or limited burden pyelo-calyceal stones (<20 mm), but it presents high costs and poor durability of the small flexible instrumentation, and could be difficult to perform if the ureter caliber is very small, requiring pre-stenting [5, 17].

Percutaneous procedures to reach renal stones for lithotripsy have been demonstrated as highly effective, especially to treat large or staghorn pyelo-caliceal stones, with stone-free rate up to 90–95%, but the risk of major complication, namely bleeding, is reported to be 6–8% [8, 13, 17]. Recently, less invasive percutaneous techniques have been extended in pediatric age, due to the advent of miniaturized endourological instrumentation, such as mini-perc, UMP, and micro-perc.

For renal pyelic calculi, mini-perc has been demonstrated to have significantly higher stone clearance rate than PCNL ($p < 0.001$) with minor complication rate (5.1%) in a group of 129 children compared with 115 pediatric patients who received standard PCNL [17]. In our experience, mini-perc has evolved as the main technique adopted for pyelo-caliceal stones, with high stone-free rate and minor complication rate if compared with standard PCNL and retrograde procedures as RIRS. The ClearPetra System is a special 14 °F or 16 °F single-use sheath that improves the efficacy of the mini-perc in our recent experience. It allows continuous irrigation, performed through the 12 °F nephroscope, and negative aspiration pressure, manually controlled through a lateral channel of the device with multiple orifices (Fig. 27.5). The stones and fragments are attracted at the ClearPetra sheath opening, reducing the risk of retropulsion and allowing easier lithotripsy. Fragments are aspirated between sheath and nephroscope, if smaller, or into the sheath in case of bigger burden stone residual. The continuous negative aspiration through the side port on the ClearPetra System presents several advantages, also in our recent experience: it reduces the intraluminal pressure in the urinary tract, improves the visual field from bleeding and stones powder, prevents stone retropulsion during lithotripsy, reduces the operative time, and increases efficacy and safety.

A further miniaturization, the UMP, has been described by Desay et al. [18] utilizing a 11 °F instrument through a 13 °F Amplatz sheath, with a reported stone-free rate of 86.6% and few complications, including conversion to mini-perc in two cases on 62 patients included in the study. The real advantage of UMP compared to mini-perc is still not demonstrated in our opinion. Ureteroscopic lithotripsy has been established as the standard treatment for small ureteric calculi and for residual stone fragments inside pelvis or intra-calyceal [19]. No more indications should be given for open surgical or laparoscopic approaches to stone disease in pediatrics, except in cases of severe skeletal abnormalities, associated urinary tract obstruction, or failed endoscopic treatments [1, 7].

The micro-perc device is a recent novel instrument proposed by Desay MR et al. in 2011 [20] that really carries to extreme the miniaturization of percutaneous procedures, adopting a single-step calyceal puncture using a 4.85 °F needle (Figs. 27.3 and 27.4). The laser-tripsy is carried out by a 272 micron fiber inserted in the central port of a three-way connector and passing inside the 4.85 °F lumen needle, with 10,000 pixel optic wire and low-pressure irrigation from the lateral ports of the connector. The micro-perc has been demonstrated really to be a minimally invasive procedure, allowing lithotripsy under direct vision with a scarless access to lower calyx and pelvis. The procedure requires short operative time and short hospitalization, with minimal analgesic support, and could be considered as a new frontier for treatment of selected renal calculi in lower pole, but it presents several significant in contra's. It needs experienced hands, with very precise selection of indications: small diameter stones in lower pole calyx or pelvis and limited number (1 or 2) of stones. The endoscopic vision is reduced and needs no endoluminal bleeding. The percutaneous maneuver is delicate and it is performed as single short access by the almost large needle present in the set, having 4.85 °F caliber, without safety guide wire. Thus, we consider the access to the selected calyx more challenging and the hemorrhagic risk higher than in the mini-perc procedure. For these reasons, recently, we prefer mini-perc with ClearPetra system as first choice percutaneous approach for renal stones treatment.

In conclusion, significant technical improvements have been reached in recent years also in pediatric stone disease, modifying our approach towards mini-invasive video-surgical procedures and increasing safety and efficiency. Future advancements are on the horizon that offers the promise of further increasing the efficiency and safety of current procedures, minimizing complications and invasiveness [6].

Take-Home Messages

- The percutaneous procedures need mentoring at beginning and achievement of experience but have very high success rate (up to 95% stone-free rate).
- Availability of full endourological equipment is required in the operating room.
- Attention must be paid to never force the maneuver; safety guide wire is strongly advised.
- If there is difficulty in progression of the procedure or poor visual, do not hesitate to stop the procedure and drain the urinary tract.

References

1. Salerno A, Gerocarni Nappo S, Matarazzo E, De Dominicis M, Caione P. Treatment of pediatric renal stones in a Western Country: a changing pattern. J Pediatr Surg. 2013;48(4):835–9.
2. D'Addessi A, Bongiovanni L, Sasso F, Gulino F, Falabella R, Bassi P. Extracorporeal shockwave lithotripsy in pediatrics. J Endourol. 2008;22:1–11.
3. Novak TE, Lakshmanan Y, Trock BJ, Gearhart JP, Matlanga BR. Sex prevalence of pediatric kidney disease in the United States: an epidemiological investigation. Urology. 2009;74:104–7.
4. Noe HN, Stapleton FB, Jerkins GR. Clinical experience with pediatric urolithiasis. J Urol. 1983;129:1166–8.
5. Caione P, Matarazzo E, Battaglia S. Stone treatment in children: where are we today? Arch It Urol Androl. 2010;82(1):45–8.
6. Radmayr C, Bogaert G, Burgu B Radmayr C, Bogaert G, Burgu B, Dogan HS, Nijman JM, Rawashdeh YFH, et al. EAU Guidelines on Paediatric Urology. 2022;74–81.
7. Silay MS, Ellison JS, Tailly T, Caione P. Update on urinary stones in children: current and future concepts in surgical treatment and shockwave lithotripsy. Eur Urol Focus. 2017;9(Aug):465–9.
8. Caione P, Collura G, Innocenzi M, De Dominicis M, Gerocarni Nappo S, Capozza N. Percutaneous endoscopic treatment for urinary stones in pediatric patients: were we are now. Transl Pediatr. 2016;5:266–74.
9. Roy OP, Angle JF, Jenkins AD, Schenkman NS. Cone beam computed tomography for percutaneous nephrolithotomy: initial evaluation of a new technology. J Endourol. 2012;26:814–8.
10. Valdivia Urìa JC, Valle Gerhold J, Lòpez Lòpez JA, et al. Technique and complications of percutaneous nephroscopy: experience with 557 patients in the supine position. J Urol. 1998;160(6 pt 1):1975–8.
11. Ibarluzea G, Scoffone CM, Cracco CM, et al. Supine Valdivia and modified lithotomy position for simultaneous anterograde and retrograde endourological access. BJU Int. 2007;100(1):233–6.
12. De SM, Autorino R. Quarto g et al: supine versus prone position in percutaneous nephrolithotomy for renal stones treatable with a single percutaneous access: a prospective randomized trial. Eur Urol. 2008;54:196–202.
13. Goyal NK, Goel A, Sankhwar SN. A critical appraisal of complications of percutaneous nephrolithotomy in paediatric patients using adult instruments. BJU Int. 2014;113:801–10.
14. Bianchi G, Rosa M. PCNL: cosa è cambiato. Urologia. 2014;81(2):108–14.
15. Alken P. The telescope dilators. World J Urol. 1985;3:7–10.
16. AJ LR. Percutaneous access. In: Smith AD, Badlani GH, Kavoussi LR, editors. Smith's Textbook of Endourology. St Louis: Quality Medical; 1996. p. 199–210.
17. Yadav P, Madhavan K, Syal S, Farooq A, Srivastava A, Ansari MS. Technique, complications and outcomes of pediatric urolithiasis management in a tertiary care hospital: evolving paradigms over the last 15 years. J Pediatr Urol. 2019;15(6):665–9.
18. Desai J, Solanki R. Ultra-mini percutaneous nephrolithotomy (UMP): one more armamentarium. BJU Int. 2013;112:1046–9.

19. Tsai SH, Chung HJ, Tseng PT, Wu YC, Tu YK, Hsu CW, Lei WT. Comparison of the efficacy and safety of shockwave lithotripsy, retrograde intrarenal surgery, percutaneous nephrolithotomy and minimally invasive percutaneous nephrolithotomy for lower pole renal stones: a systematic review and network meta-analysis. Medicine. 2020;99(10):e19403.
20. Desai M, Mishra S. "Microperc" micro percutaneous nephrolithotomy: evidence to practice. Curr Opin Urol. 2012;22(2):134–8.

Place of Laparoscopic and Robotic Surgery in the Management of Kidney Urolithiasis

28

H. Steyaert and S. Luycks

28.1 Introduction

Stone disease is uncommon in developed countries [1]. Since years, non-surgical options are used in the treatment of the majority of cases of kidney (and ureteral) stones disease in children.

Medical expulsion therapy (MET) is the first-line treatment for most stones <10 mm encountered in children. But alternative techniques are also described [2].

For renal stones <20 mm having failed MET, EAU/ESPU and AUA guidelines still recommend extracorporeal shock wave lithotripsy (ESWL) as first-line treatment [3]. ESWL is effective and harmless [4].

However, recent development of paediatric flexible ureteroscopes, PCNL in children, and laser lithotripsy allow to attain better stone-free rates with less procedures (Fig. 28.1). Finally, less than 5% of the cases still need a real surgical approach [5].

When surgery is scheduled, again a minimal invasive approach (laparoscopic or retroperitoneoscopic, eventually robotically assisted) is the rule. Indications for open surgery are exceptional nowadays but still more frequent in paediatric surgery [6, 7].

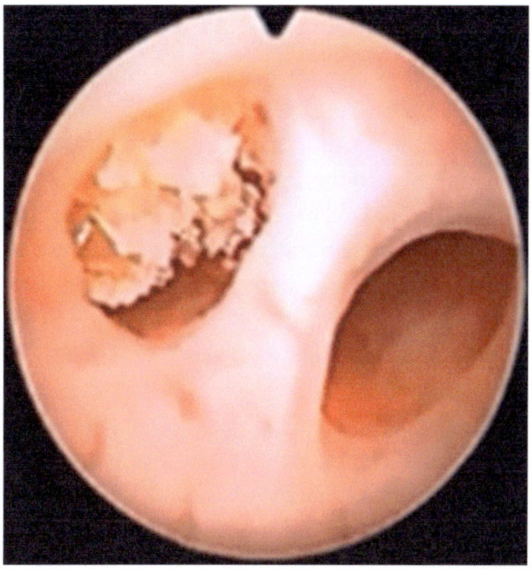

Fig. 28.1 Little stone accessible for several endourologic techniques

28.2 Indications

The contemporary indications for laparoscopic kidney stone management are well-defined [8]. They may be divided into five categories:

1. anatomical abnormalities of the kidney, for example, pelvic or horseshoe kidney but also some cases of malrotated kidney,

H. Steyaert (✉) · S. Luycks
Departement of Pediatric Surgery, Université Libre de Bruxelles (ULB), Hôpital Universitaire des Enfants Reine Fabiola (HUDERF), Brussels, Belgium
e-mail: henri.steyaert@huderf.be; stephane.luyckx@huderf.be

C. Esposito et al. (eds.), *Minimally Invasive Techniques in Pediatric Urology*, https://doi.org/10.1007/978-3-030-99280-4_28

2. the presence of a congenital anomaly such as a PUJ obstruction that could be treated in the same time,
3. symptomatic stones present in calicle diverticula not easily amenable to an endourological approach,
4. large impacted renal calculi (with eventual kidney loss),
5. renal pelvic stones >1 cm diameter or smaller refractive for ESWL or recurrent after first ESWL approach.

Even in those cases (e.g., malrotated or horseshoe kidney), the combination of a surgical approach and the use of PCNL that is guided under laparoscopic control may be an option [9].

Eventually, the choice of the best approach will depend on the available material and the experience of the surgical team. For those two reasons, urological management of stones in children should be concentrated in high-volume centres where expertise with updated material is at disposal.

When a surgical approach is decided, we know that a minimal invasive approach decreases the morbidity of an open one but at the price of a mostly challenging renal reconstruction, in particular, in anatomically abnormal kidneys. For that reason, more and more teams advocate the use of robotic assistance [10].

More reports, at least in adults, show that the use of a robot may increase stone clearance with fewer auxiliary procedures in most difficult cases [11].

28.3 Pre-Operative Preparation

A pre-operative evaluation should first include ultrasonography and isotope scanning. The high rate of metabolic abnormalities in children with urinary stones suggests that all should undergo nephron-metabolic evaluation. Such evaluation can be performed before or after stone management. Magnetic resonance (MR) urogram or a contrast-enhanced CT are mandatory in order to know exactly how the anatomy of the urinary tract is delineated, but also to be aware of the anatomy of the blood vessels in those cases were the kidney is abnormally positioned.

This may help in the decision to choose between a retro or trans-peritoneal approach even in cases of horseshoe and malrotated kidneys for which the transperitoneal way seems best adapted.

Pre-operative antibiotic prophylaxis should be administered either with a broad-spectrum medication or according to the child's specific urine testing.

All parents and patients (depending on their age) have to sign an informed consent before the procedure.

Patients receive a general anaesthesia with oro-tracheal intubation and myorelaxation.

Before positioning the patient in the laparoscopic suite, a cystoscopy with placement of a JJ stent is undertaken. This JJ stent can also be pushed percutaneously through the kidney pelvis, once opened and stones extracted, depending on surgeon's preference and anatomy of the patient's urinary tract. After positioning the patient, room has to be made for fluoroscopic material. For that reason, the use of an "integrated operating room" where the screens are fixed on arms coming from above facilitates the management.

28.4 Positioning

28.4.1 Non-robotic Minimal Invasive Surgery

28.4.1.1 Transperitoneal

The patient is placed with a 60° lateral tilt (operated kidney up). All the pressure points are consciously padded.

The surgeon and the assistant stand on the contralateral side of the operated kidney in front of the patient. The idea is always the same: having everything in line: the surgeon, the target, and the screen (in the back of the patient).

Care must be taken with the arms. Mostly, the ipsilateral one is placed near the head to avoid elongation of the brachial plexus. Patient will be secured to the bed with two bands across the chest and legs.

In children, an open approach is essential for the first trocar that is inserted through the umbilicus. A 5 mm optical system is mostly used but a 10 mm gives a better view and may be a good option in case large stones are to be removed.

All optical systems are 30° ones because they give the opportunity to look over the colon and may help to minimize colon dissection or need for positioning of the optical trocar outside the umbilicus in older children.

Working trocars are placed around the optical one; generally one in the epigastrium and one in the ipsilateral fossa iliaca some cm from the iliac crest. In case of horseshoe kidney, the position of the working trocars will be adapted under direct view depending on the position of the kidney that is mostly closer to the pelvis and to the midline. Two working trocars are mostly enough. Size of those trocars (3 mm or 5 mm) will depend on the surgeon's experience, the age of the child, and the eventually planned auxiliary percutaneous procedures. In case exposure is not optimal, an accessory trocar in the epigastric area could be useful in particular in order to retract the liver on the right side.

28.4.1.2 Retroperitoneal

Patient will be positioned in a strict lateral position with a bag under the limb in order to allow maximal opening of the space between the tip of the 11th rib and the iliac crest. In an older child, flexion of the operating table can be used in order to increase that effect.

Then again care must be taken with the arms. Mostly the ipsilateral one is placed near the head. Patient will be secured to the bed with two bands across the chest and legs.

Surgeon and assistant stand in the back of the patient. Nurse may stand in the front if she has her own screen.

28.4.2 Robotic Minimal Invasive Surgery

Since the authors only have the experience of a transperitoneal approach with the robot, they will only describe this approach.

Placement of the trocars can differ depending on the used robotic system. Since authors do not use the last generation of the Da Vinci robot (Intuitive*), the position of the trocars is quite the same for a laparoscopic approach. With the last generation robot, all the trocars are to be placed in line with the optical trocar positioned in the umbilicus. Use of single port system is also possible but authors are yet to gain experience in this. Authors fix all their trocars to the skin, even for robotic surgery. The muscular wall is indeed thin in children.

The main concern is to be sure that the trocars are separated at least for 5–8 cm, what is sometimes difficult to obtain in little children. That's why there is mostly a limitation in patients weighing less than 20 kg. In case the surgeon is willing to use such robotic assistance for little children, it's mandatory to elevate the child from the table with a thick mattress in order to gain few cm of movements for the robotic arms outside the area of the mattress.

Another concern in robotic surgery is the need for an accessory trocar. This trocar has to be placed in such a manner that the assistant can use the instruments in good fashion in line with a screen but also outside the area of robotic arms movements.

This trocar will mostly be placed in the opposite lateral fossa iliaca. Long instruments are needed if the child is over 10 years of age.

If fluoroscopy is needed, dedocking of the robot is advised using the trocars laparoscopically, in order to help the percutaneous manoeuvres.

Docking and dedocking takes few seconds in experienced hands.

28.5 Instrumentation

Cystoscopes and JJ stents from different sizes (depending on the age of the patient) are needed. All materials have to be checked before the beginning of the procedure.

Regarding the laparoscopic procedure, a 5 or eventually a 10 mm 30° optic is used. Two atraumatic fenestrated grasping forceps are used in order to manage tissues and other things. A fine curved dissector is used in order to obtain fine dissection (around vessels, ureter, etc.). Authors prefer to use bipolar cautery systems even if a monopolar hook can do the job. A hook is always good to have, for example, for faster dissection. Alternatively, other electrocautery systems may be used such as harmonic scalpel (for dissection of colon attachments) or Ligasure* depending on the availability and surgeon's habits.

Other needed instruments are a suction-irrigation system, a pair of scissors, 1 or 2 curved needle holders, endobags, and sometimes clip appliers.

Depending on the age of the child, 3 mm or 5 mm sets will be used with a preference for the 5 mm ones in particular when accessory manoeuvres are scheduled.

Intraoperative US devices are also a +.

Even if most papers report the use of 8 mm instruments when robotic surgery is used, authors are using the 5 mm Da Vinci (Intuitive*) set. This set has three main disadvantages:

1. Not a complete 360° movement.
2. A longer working part of the instruments necessitating more space inside the abdomen.
3. A much less number of instruments at disposal.

If these limitations are really obvious in little children, they are not so in older ones.

Not to forget: due to the fact that a lot of instruments will be introduced through the accessory trocar, for example, aspiration-irrigation, endobag, clips, the accurate positioning of this trocar is of main concern.

Depending on the pre-operatively decided strategy, a flexible cystoscope with a variety of flat-wire baskets could be useful. Small calibre dye or holmium: YAG laser may be necessary for fragmentation or vaporization of large stones.

In case of concomitant cystoscopy, use of two cameras is the best option.

28.6 Technique (Transperitoneal)

28.6.1 Pelvic and Calyceal Stones

First step is to reflect the colon along the white line of Told. Harmonic scalpel makes this part easier. Once the pelvis of the kidney is freed, its ureter (by the indwelling stent) and main vessels recognized, the stone is identified by the bulge, by touching it with a forceps or, if needed, using intraoperative US.

Once the stone is found, an inverted V-shaped incision is made on the pelvis paying attention not to incise too close to the PUJ, avoiding the use of electrocautery in this area, after introduction of the dissector in order to get around the stone. The stone is extracted using a large forceps and put in an endobag. It is important to avoid fragmentation of the stone if possible (Fig. 28.2). A finger tip of a glove (latex-free) can also be used and is perhaps easier to manipulate. Once the stone is delivered, the pyelolithotomy is closed using either a 4 or 5-0 absorbable suture. Knots are to be made outside the lumen.

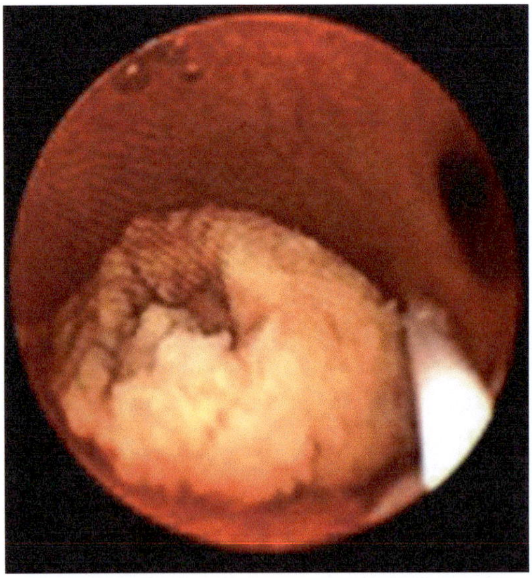

Fig. 28.2 Large pelvic stone (PUJ obstruction) ideally extracted in one piece

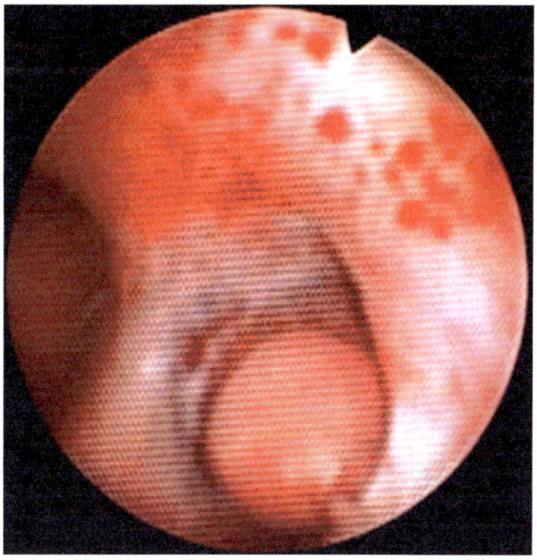

Fig. 28.3 Renal papilla stone: good indication for a combined procedure

In case stones are located in a distant calyx, a flexible instrument is useful (Fig. 28.3). This instrument will be pushed through the trocar most in line with the calyx to be treated. Authors suggest not to hesitate to put an accessory trocar if the working ones are not correctly in line for an easy removal.

28.6.2 Pelvic Stone and UPJ Obstruction

In case of concomitant stone and PUJ obstruction, the operation begins exactly in the same manner as above but the V-shaped incision is made closer to the PUJ. Once the surgeon has dealt with the stones, a transcutaneous thread will secure the pelvis to the anterior abdominal wall before beginning with the ureteral incision and spatulation. Further step depends on surgeon's preference. Best option is mostly not to separate completely the ureter from the pelvis before beginning the first running suture. Some teams put a second transcutaneous thread on the ureter. This can be specifically useful in the beginning because things are better stabilized. Generally only two running sutures are required if the incision of the pelvis was not too far from the PUJ. This will also depend on the size of the delivered stone. In case of larger pelvic resection, a third running suture is conducted in order to close the pelvis. Some authors use interrupted sutures for the anastomosis part.

It's in this indication that robotic assistance is of great interest due to the enhanced movements permitted by the robotic arms.

28.6.3 Nephrectomy for Calculus Disease

In very exceptional cases, a nephrectomy is indicated for xantogranulomatous pyelonephritis. Those nephrectomies are challenging due to adhesions and distorted anatomy.

The operation begins again by largely reflecting the colon. Second step is to recognize both the ureter and the pelvis. An ureteral stent helps to do this. Third step is to recognize and dissect the vessels of the renal hilum. Hem-o-Lock clips are very useful in this part of the surgery because once fixed they will not slip away during the sometimes very difficult dissection of the rest of the kidney. Use of the harmonic scalpel may facilitate the dissection of the adhesions to surrounding tissues. Care must be taken not to enter the infected kidney, reason why it is wise to dissect outside the Gerota's area in case of necessity. On the upper pole, a more subcapsular dissection is performed in order to avoid an unnecessary adrenalectomy. Finally, the ureter is double clipped and cut in between in order to avoid spillage of pus. An endobag is mandatory in order to extract the infected kidney.

28.7 Technique (Retroperitoneal)

28.7.1 Diverticula

Trocars are classically placed with the optical one under the tip of the 11th rib and the two operating ones a little bit more caudally, above the iliac crest (one more anterior and the other one more posterior).

After open access to Gerota's fascia through incision of the muscle layers, a working space is created with the help of the scope and insufflation. Then, under visual control, the two operating trocars are inserted. Landmarks are visualized: the psoas muscle, the ureter, and the kidney that is located in the upper part of the field.

Depending on the site of the diverticulum, part of the kidney is freed from the peritoneum. It is sometime interesting to put a sling around the vessels in order to help to control bleeding during opening of very large diverticula. An ultrasonic probe is useful to localize the stones. If not available, stones can be identified by direct puncture. The thinnest part of the cortex is incised and diverticulum partially removed (marsupialization) if necessary with the help of the harmonic scalpel in order to get access to the stones. Once the stone(s) have been removed, a stitch will close the communication with the calyces. The renal parenchyma is to be closed using gross stitches (ideally with patches) in case of bleeding that can't be controlled by monopolar cautery. Haemostatic meshes are also useful.

A JJ stent will drain the urinary tract.

28.7.2 Nephrectomy

Nephrectomy for xantogranulomatous pyelonephritis can also be performed by retroperitoneoscopy.

Introduction of trocars is the same as described above.

After recognition of the three landmarks (psoas, ureter, pelvis), the hilum is dissected. Advantage here is that the vessels are just in front of the surgeon. After clipping and severing the renal vessels, dissection of the kidney can be started. Adhesions make it also not an easy task with the risk of opening the peritoneum with gas "leakage" and reduced space available.

Several options are to be considered in that case:

1. Inserting a Veress needle through the umbilicus increases gas flow (deflates the abdomen and inflates the retroperitoneal space).
2. Using a stitch in order to close the hole if not too big.
3. Putting a more anterior accessory trocar in order to close the hole in between the two jaws of a forceps
4. Widely opening the hole, transferring surgeon and the assistant to the front of the patient and continuing the procedure transperitoneally.

28.8 Post-Operative Care

At the end of the operation, all trocar sites are closed, even the 3 mm ones in little children, at the level of the fascia.

Patients start oral feeding once they are discharged from the recovery room, beginning mostly with liquids. Pain medication is given according to hospital protocols. Most of the time, there is no need for level 2 or 3 analgesics after the first night.

Antibiotics are usually given for 48–72 h. The urine catheter is removed in the first or second postoperative day. Antibioprophylaxis during JJ stenting is not recommended. Patients are discharged 2 or 3 days after operation. JJ stent is mostly removed between 2 weeks and 1 month postoperatively. Follow-up will depend on the type of surgery and the chemical analysis of the calculus.

28.9 Results

Series are scarce even in adults.

Case reports about stone removal in horseshoe kidneys using combined techniques (laparoscopy and endourology) are described [8, 9]. Most of the series don't comprise more than 15 to 30 cases [11].

Some papers show good results of concomitant treatment of urolithiasis and UPJ obstruction [12].

There are more and more reports about a robotic approach for stones [10, 11, 13–15].

In children, series are very scarce [16, 17]. Results are globally good except in one paper describing staghorn stone management in adolescents [18, 19].Robot-assisted surgery has a good stone-free rate after a single procedure [6]. Because stones in the paediatric population have a high recurrence rate, it is especially important to prevent stone recurrence by ensuring complete stone clearance.

Tips and Tricks

- Well-defined pre-operative strategy is a key point for success in stone management.
- Having all needed material and positioning accurately the patient is of main concern before beginning MIS for stone disease.
- Having a good flushing system is important (suction/irrigation).
- Blue dye may be useful to check for leakage after suturing.
- Ureteral stenting prior to surgery helps during dissection and in order to find the stone (opacification just before beginning surgery).
- Don't hesitate to put accessory trocars (eventually 3 mm ones) if exposure is not optimal.

28.10 Discussion

Indications for a laparoscopic or retroperitoneoscopic approach in the management of upper urinary stones in children are decreasing with the development of modern and miniaturized endourologic treatments [4].

In guidelines, ESWL remains the gold standard for first-line treatment even in staghorn calculus. Relative contraindications are the stones from infective origin. They are bulky and have a soft matrix not really suitable for ESWL [16].

In case of large stone, repeated ESWL may be necessary raising the question of several general anaesthesia where a surgical approach can solve the problem at once [18]. Percutaneous techniques are actually treating the vast majority of the cases. In toddlers, the flexible ureteroscopes will mostly do the job, and in little children, where there may raise a concern about damaging the urethra (especially in boys), percutaneous nephrotomy techniques (PERC and micro PERC) are becoming gold standards. Nevertheless, those techniques are not without potential complications such as bleeding, sepsis, and radiation exposure [19]. Finally, recurrence of stone disease is frequent, making it necessary knowing all the armamentarium of techniques [20].

Furthermore, those endourologic techniques are difficult to use in anatomical abnormal kidneys and may raise the risk of spreading stone fragments. In such cases, minimal invasive surgery eventually combined with endourologic techniques may be an option [21]. MIS can also be considered as a salvage procedure when the less invasive once failed [19]. In case of UPJ associated with stones, first MIS approach is an excellent option in order to treat the stones and the UPJ obstruction during the same operation [22]. Robot is a perfect tool in this situation [12].

When nephrectomy is indicated, MIS is also the ideal treatment in particular through a retroperitoneal approach [23]. But retroperitoneal approach will essentially be used for a stone in a diverticula (Nephrolithotomy) even if this is the most logical for general kidney access (Pyelolithotomy). Nevertheless, authors have to admit that the retroperitoneal way is certainly not the first choice for the majority of the surgical teams dealing with renal diseases.

In conclusion, even if some papers still describe high percentage of open approach (up to 20%) for kidney stones in children in comparison with adult series, authors think there is, in fully equipped countries, no indication any more for an open approach [5]. Discussion between a fully endourologic, a laparoscopic endourologic, or a complete MIS surgical approach (trans or retroperitoneal) will depend on several factors such as size, type, and position of the stones in the kidney, anatomy of the kidney, material at disposal, age of the patient, and experience of the team. Options are to be discussed with the parents and the child after thorough explanation and a collegial decision taken by surgeon and parents. In case of MIS, the help of the robot will make this surgery much easier.

Take-Home Messages

- Stone disease in children is rare, in particular in developed countries.
- More and more endourologic or percutaneous techniques exist.
- Need for expensive material and experience are in high demand for concentration in high volume centres.
- Minimal invasive surgical approach has the advantage to treat mostly stones and eventual associated congenital abnormalities in one time whereas other strategies may need several general anaesthesia.
- Normally, there is no place anymore for open surgery in the management of kidney stones in children.

Acknowledgments Authors would like to thank Adam Halinski (see ref. 20) for provision of some images.

References

1. Lopez M, Hoppe B. History, epidemiology and regional diversities of urolithiasis. Pediatr Nephrol. 2010;25(1):49–59.
2. Faure A, Dicrocco E, Hery G, Boissier R, Bienvenu L, Thirakul S, Maffei P, Panait N, Karsenty G, Merrot T, Alessandrini P, Guys J-M, Lechevallier E. Postural therapy for renal stones in children: a rolling stones procedure. J Pediatr Urol. 2016;12(4):252.e1–6. https://doi.org/10.1016/j.jpurol.2016.02.019.
3. EAU Guidelines. Edn. presented at the EAU Annual Congress Amsterdam 2020. ISBN 978-94-92671-07-3.
4. Tejwani R, Wang H-HS, Wolf S, Wiener JS, Routh JC. Outcomes of shock wave lithotripsy and ureteroscopy for treatment of pediatric urolithiasis. J Urol. 2016;196:196–201. https://doi.org/10.1016/j.juro.2016.02.2975.
5. Paik ML, Wainstein MA, Spirnak JP, Hampel N, Resnick MI. Current indications of open surgery in treatment of renal and ureteral calculi. J Urol. 1998;159:374–9.
6. Lee RS, Passerotti CC, Cendron M, Estrada CR, Borer JG, Peters CA. Early results of robot assisted laparoscopic lithotomy in adolescents. J Urol. 2007;177:2306–10.
7. Simforoosh N, Aminsharifi A. Laparoscopic management in stone disease. Curr Opin Urol. 2013;23:169–74.
8. Ganpule AP, Preshant J, Desai MR. Laparoscopic and robot-assisted surgery in the management of urinary lithiasis. Arab J Urol. 2012;10(32):32–9.
9. Maheshwari PN, Bhandarkar DS, Shah RS, Andankar MG, Saple AL. Laparoscopy-assisted transperitoneal percutaneous nephrolithotomy for recurrent calculus in isthmic calix of horseshoe kidney. J Endourol. 2004;18:858–61.
10. Suntharasivam T, Mukherjee A, Luk A, Aboumarzouk O, Somani B, Prasad RB. The role of robotic surgery in the management of renal tract calculi. Transl Androl Urol. 2019;8(Suppl 4):S457–60.
11. Hemal AK, Nayyar R, Gupta NP, et al. Experience with robotic assisted laparoscopic surgery in upper tract urolithiasis. Can J Urol. 2010;17:5299–305.
12. Jensen PH, Berg KD, Azawi NH. Robot-assisted pyeloplasty and pyelolithotomy in patients with ureteropelvic junction stenosis. Scand J Urol. 2017;51:323–8.
13. Müller PF, Schlager D, Hein S, et al. Robotic stone surgery—current state and future prospects: a systematic review. Arab J Urol. 2017;16:357–64.
14. Swearingen R, Sood A, Madi R, et al. Zero-fragment nephrolithotomy: a multi-center evaluation of robotic pyelolithotomy and nephrolithotomy for treating renal stones. Eur Urol. 2017;72:1014–21.
15. Badalato GM, Hemal AK, Menon M, Badani KK. Current role of robot assisted pyelolithotomy. For the management of large renal calculi: a contemporary analysis. J Endourol. 2009;23:1719–22.
16. Valla JS, Yeung CK, Steyaert H. Minimally invasive surgery and management of urinary tract stone in children. In: Bax K, Georgeson K, Rothenberg S, Valla JS, Yeung CK, editors. Endoscopic surgery in infants and children. Springer, Berlin; 2008. p. 681–8.
17. Soltani MH, Simforoosh N, Nouralizadeh A, Sotoudeh M, Mollakoochakian MJ, Shemshald HR. Laparoscopic pyelolithotomy in children less than two years old with large renal stones: initial series. Urol J. 2016;13(5):2837–40.
18. Casale P, Grady RW, Joyner BD, Zeltser IS, Kuo RL, Mitchell ME. Transperitoneal laparoscopie pyelolithotomy after failed percutaneous access in the pediatric patient. J Urol. 2004;172(2):680–3. discussion 683
19. Agrawal V, Bajaj J, Acharya H, Chanchalani R, Raina VK, Sharma D. Laparoscopic management of pediatric renal and ureteric stones. J Pediatr Urol. 2013;9(2):230–3.

20. Halinski A, Halinski AN, Zaniew M, Bartosz Kudlinski B, Soltysiak J, Sobolewski B, Steyaert H. Interest of URS-L in the treatment of ureterolithiasis in preschool children. Front Pediatr. 2019;7:324. https://doi.org/10.3389/fped.2019.00324.
21. Masieri L. Laparoscopic approach to urinary stones. In: Esposito C, Becmeur F, Steyaert H, Szavay P, editors. ESPES manual of pediatric minimally invasive surgery. Springer, Berlin; 2019. p. 389–92.
22. Stein RJ, Turna B, Nguyen MM, Aron M, Hafron JM, Gill IS, et al. Laparoscopie pyeloplasty with concomitant pyelolithotomy. Technique and outcomes. J Endourol. 2008;22:1251–5.
23. Merrot T, Ordorica-Flores R, Steyeart H, Ginier C, Valla JS, Merrot T. Is diffuse xanthogranulomatous pyelonephritis a contraindication to retroperitoneoscopic nephroureterectomy? A case report. Surg Laparosc Endosc. 1998;8(5):366–9.

29 MIS Management of Symptomatic Simple Renal Cysts

Maria Escolino, Fulvia Del Conte, Vincenzo Coppola, Mariapina Cerulo, and Ciro Esposito

Learning Objectives

- To describe step-by-step laparoscopic and robot-assisted approach to simple renal cysts.
- To present long-term outcome of the technique.
- To report the available evidence in the current pediatric literature about MIS management of simple renal cysts.
- To show a video tape of robot-assisted treatment of simple renal cysts.
- To describe tips and tricks of the technique and all innovative technologies available to improve surgical treatment of simple renal cysts.

Supplementary Information The online version contains supplementary material available at [https://doi.org/10.1007/978-3-030-99280-4_29].

M. Escolino (✉) · F. Del Conte · V. Coppola
M. Cerulo · C. Esposito
Pediatric Surgery Unit, Federico II University of Naples, Naples, Italy
e-mail: maria.escolino@unina.it; fulvia.delconte@unina.it; vincenzocoppola1992@gmail.com; mariapina.cerulo@unina.it; ciroespo@unina.it

29.1 Introduction

Simple renal cysts (SRC) are benign, unilateral, and solitary lesions arising outside the renal parenchyma with no communication with the collecting system [1]. SRC are rare in childhood and increase in frequency during adulthood [2]. Renal cysts can be classified as being either simple or complex [3]. The criteria to define renal cysts as "simple" include (a) absence of internal echoes; (b) posterior enhancement; (c) a round/oval shape; (d) sharp/thin posterior walls [3, 4]. They are commonly asymptomatic and are incidentally diagnosed. A small number of patients (5%) may become symptomatic and present with abdominal or flank pain and less frequently hypertension, hematuria, recurrent urinary tract infections, cyst rupture, and pelvicalyceal obstruction [1, 5].

To date, there is no consensus about the optimal protocol for the surveillance, imaging, or treatment of renal cysts in children [6]. Surgical treatment is commonly indicated in patients with symptomatic or rapidly enlarged cysts (>6 cm) and complex renal cysts with malignancy risk [7]. Different treatment options for symptomatic cysts have been described and include aspiration with or without instillation of sclerosing agents,

C. Esposito et al. (eds.), *Minimally Invasive Techniques in Pediatric Urology*,
https://doi.org/10.1007/978-3-030-99280-4_29

percutaneous resection, and open or laparoscopic decortication [7]. Percutaneous techniques are not easy to apply in children and have been associated with high recurrence rate and need for repeat procedure [8, 9]. Laparoscopic management has become a valid alternative because it is minimally invasive and has a high success rate in terms of cyst recurrence [7, 10]. More recently, robotic surgery has also been reported as a viable treatment option for SRC [11, 12]. However, there is very limited evidence in the current pediatric literature about MIS management of SRC. In this chapter, we described the laparoscopic and robot-assisted approach for treatment of simple renal cysts in pediatric patients.

29.2 Pre-Operative Preparation

Pre-operative work-up includes renal ultrasonography, DMSA renal scintigraphy, and magnetic resonance imaging (MRI) or computed tomography (CT) (Fig. 29.1). SRC are classified into stages I-IV, according to the Bosniak classification upon CT or MRI findings [13]. Stages I–II represent 95% of SRC and are considered as simple or benign, whereas stages III–IV demonstrate high vascularity and are considered as complex or potentially malignant. The recently revised Bosniak classification considers SRC bigger than 3 cm automatically as stage IIF (F for follow-up) and recommends serial follow-up studies to prove benignity [4]. An accurate pre-operative imaging study is crucial to exclude cyst communication with the collecting system and to plan the surgical strategy (Fig. 29.2). Urine analysis with culture and sensitivity is obtained in all patients. A bowel preparation with simethicone, enema, and liquid diet may be useful, especially in younger children. All patients should receive intra-operative antibiotic prophylaxis.

After the induction of general anesthesia with oro-tracheal intubation, a Foley bladder catheter

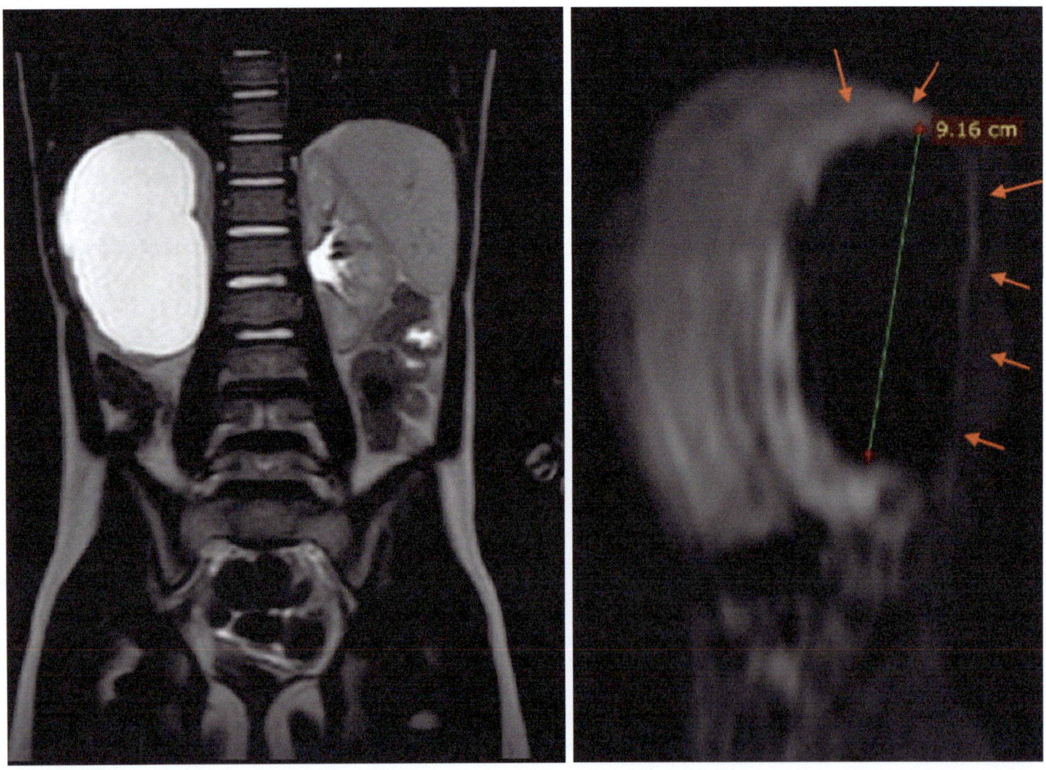

Fig. 29.1 Pre-operative CT of a giant renal cyst: arrows indicate the thin renal parenchyma compressed by the cyst

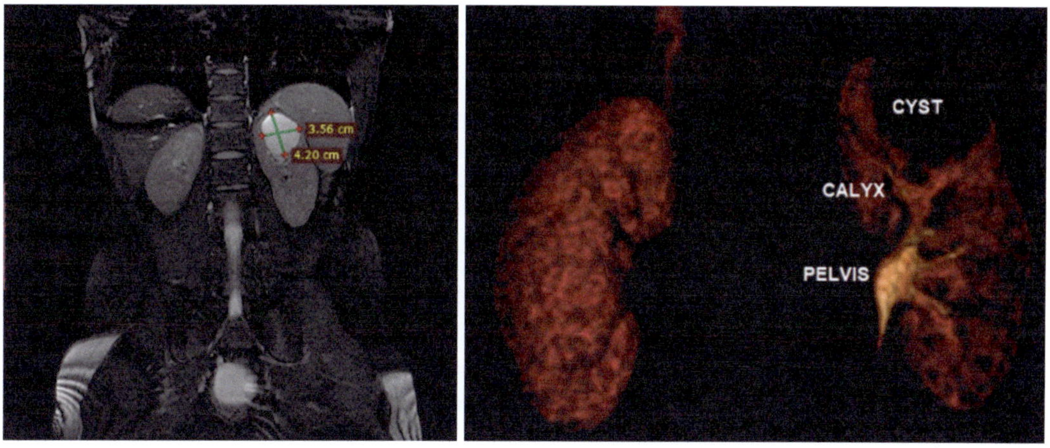

Fig. 29.2 Pre-operative CT imaging showed size and location of the renal cyst and excluded any communication between the cyst and the collecting system

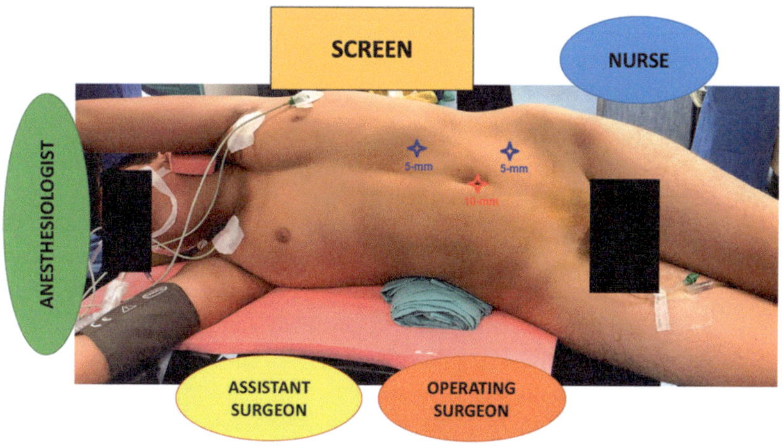

Fig. 29.3 Patient, ports, and surgical team positioning in laparoscopic approach to renal cysts

is positioned using sterile precautions and a nasogastric tube is placed, in order to keep the stomach empty during the procedure.

29.3 Positioning

Regarding patient's position, the patients are placed in the standard lateral kidney position rotating the operative side up by 30°–45° axially using silicone pads underneath the patient in both laparoscopic and robot-assisted approach.

Regarding trocars' positioning, three ports are placed in the laparoscopic technique: a 10-mm Hasson trocar is inserted transumbilically using the open technique for 30° 10-mm optic. After induction of pneumoperitoneum, two 5-mm operating trocars are introduced under vision along the midclavicular line in the upper and lower abdomen (in some cases, especially on the right side, a fourth trocar may be necessary to retract the liver) (Fig. 29.3).

Four ports are positioned in the robot-assisted technique: the first 8-mm robotic camera port is placed infra-umbilically using open Hasson technique for 30° 8-mm robotic optic. After induction of pneumoperitoneum, the two operative 8-mm robotic ports are placed under vision on the emiclavear line, one 2 cm under the subcostal arch, and the other 3 cm above the inguinal ligament.

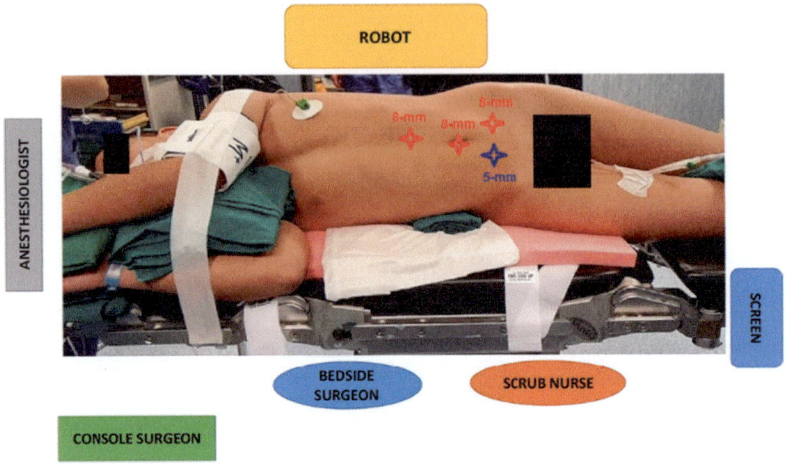

Fig. 29.4 Patient, ports, and surgical team positioning in robot-assisted approach to renal cysts

Finally, the fourth 5-mm assistant port is positioned on the pararectal line, mean 6 cm caudal to the robotic camera port (Fig. 29.4) and the da Vinci Xi robot is docked, using a three-arms configuration.

29.4 Instrumentation

Laparoscopic Technique:

- 5-mm laparoscopic atraumatic fenestrated grasping forceps
- 5-mm laparoscopic curved dissector
- 5-mm laparoscopic monopolar hook
- 5-mm laparoscopic peanut (optional)
- 5-mm Ligasure (optional)
- 5-mm laparoscopic needle
- 5-mm laparoscopic scissors
- 5-mm laparoscopic irrigation/suction device.

Robot-assisted Technique:

- 5-mm laparoscopic instruments (scissors, grasper, irrigation/suction device, glue applicator) to be used through the 5-mm assistant port
- 8-mm robotic monopolar curved scissors
- 8-mm robotic Cadiere grasper
- 8-mm robotic Maryland bipolar forceps.

29.5 Technique

29.5.1 Laparoscopic Technique

This approach can be accomplished via transperitoneal or retroperitoneal route.

29.5.1.1 Laparoscopic Transperitoneal Approach

After Toldt's line incision, the kidney is exposed and the cyst localized and freed from adhesions. The cyst dome is then opened and the wall excised using scissors and a monopolar hook. To better handle the edges of the cyst, a small amount of fluid (sent for cytological examination) can be aspirated using a transparietal or laparoscopic needle, in order to reduce the tension and to obtain a better grip. The wall of the cyst is excised circumferentially at its junction with the renal parenchyma using a monopolar hook and/or Ligasure, and the removed portion of the cyst wall is sent for histopathological exam. The portion of the cyst lying directly on the kidney surface is sealed using a monopolar hook to prevent fluid from being produced by the cyst lining. The cyst edges are sealed and the perirenal fat is placed on the bottom of the cyst (wadding technique). A drain is placed around the surgical site and trocars' orifices are closed using resorbable sutures.

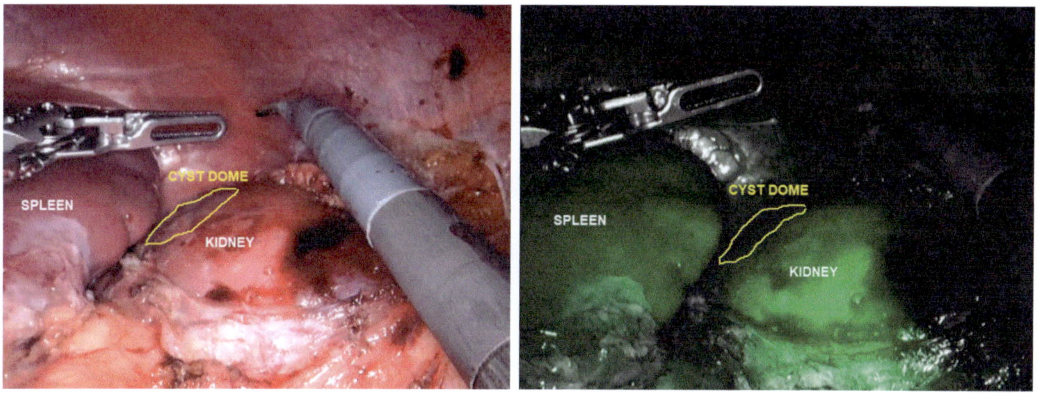

Fig. 29.5 ICG-enhanced fluorescence is very helpful to distinguish the "non-fluorescent" avascular cyst dome from the "fluorescent green" renal parenchyma

29.5.1.2 Laparoscopic Retroperitoneal Approach

A skin incision (2 cm) is made in the posterior axillary line midway between the iliac crest and the last rib. The incision is extended through the muscles and lumbar fascia. The index finger is then introduced to create sufficient space to accommodate the balloon trocar. Three ports are used routinely. A fourth port is added in some patients, usually those with anterior upper-pole cysts. Once identified, the cyst that can appear as a blue dome is dissected and its edge is delivered. The cyst contents are aspirated by a percutaneous or laparoscopic needle, and the aspirate is sent for cytological analysis. The roof of the cyst is then excised and the cyst edge is sealed by electrocautery, and the perirenal fat is finally placed over the base of the cyst. Finally, a tube drain is left and the wounds are closed using resorbable sutures.

29.5.2 Robot-Assisted Technique

After lowering of the colon, the Gerota fascia is opened to access the kidney. Pathological adhesions of epiploon to the parietal abdominal wall on the same side of the SRC are divided. Once the cyst is identified and exposed, it is punctured with a transparietal needle, the liquid content is evacuated and sent for cytological examination. For a better intra-operative identification of the cyst dome, the fluorescence imaging technology using indocyanine green (ICG) can be adopted intra-operatively. The ICG solution (2.5 mg/mL) is injected intravenously (dosage 0.3 mg/mL/kg), just after the division of the Gerota's fascia. In a matter of about 60 s following the injection, ICG-enhanced fluorescence allows to clearly distinguish the "non-fluorescent" area corresponding to the avascular cyst dome from the "fluorescent green" area corresponding to the normal perfused renal parenchyma (Fig. 29.5). The cyst roof is then resected using monopolar robotic scissors and sent for histological assessment (Fig. 29.6). The cyst edge is sprayed with a layer of chemical glue to dry the surgical site, and the cyst concavity is wadded using a pedicled flap of perirenal fat tissue (Fig. 29.7). A further layer of chemical

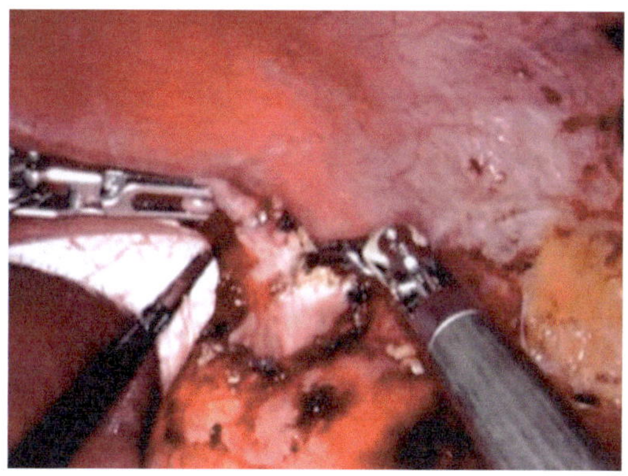

Fig. 29.6 The cyst roof is resected using robotic scissors

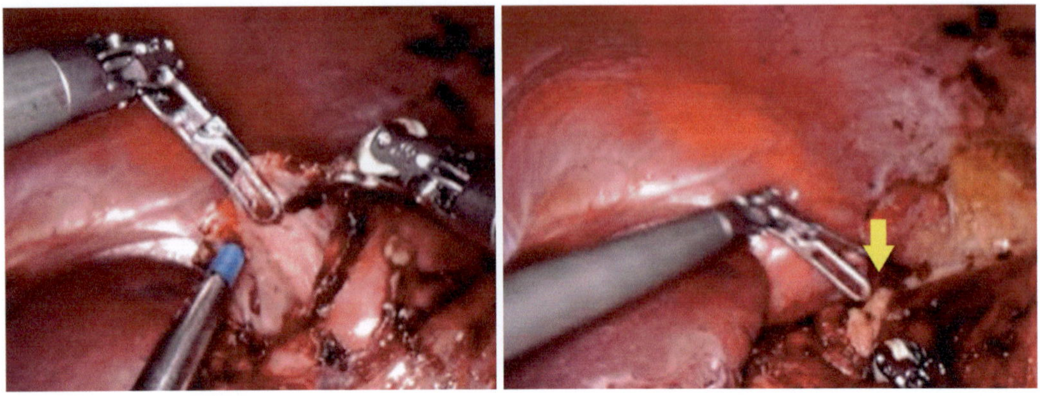

Fig. 29.7 The cyst concavity is sprayed with chemical glue and wadded with perirenal fat tissue flap (arrow)

glue is sprayed in order to secure the flap to the cyst cavity borders. A drain is left in the renal loggia and ports' orifices are closed using resorbable sutures.

29.6 Post-Operative Care

The bladder catheter is left in place for 24 h post-operatively and the drain is removed within 24–48 h postoperatively, provided that no urine leak is detected. Full oral feeding is resumed on the same day of surgery as tolerated. Pain control is obtained with oral analgesic medication (paracetamol 15 mg/kg/8 h).

Clinical and ultrasonographic follow-up is carried out at 1, 6, and 12 months postoperatively, and thereafter annually.

29.7 Results

As reported in our recently published experience [12], the median operative time was 50 min (range 35–90) for laparoscopic transperitoneal and retroperitoneal deroofing. The median operative time for robotic deroofing was 85 min (range 65–120) including surgical and docking time. There were no intra-operative complications. The median hospital stay was 2 days (range 1–4). All the patients remained asymptomatic during follow-up (2–42 months). At beginning of our experience, a small amount of liquid in the bottom of the cyst was detected on the postoperative US examination. Those cases were managed conservatively due to the absence of symptoms and size stability during follow-up. In the last patients treated with the fat tissue wadding technique, no liquid was detected postoperatively. The histological analysis consistently showed a cyst wall lining of a transitional epithelial type without evidence of malignity, compatible with the diagnosis of SRC.

Tips and Tricks

- An intra-operative challenge can be represented by the difficulty to correctly identify the cyst dome that has sometimes the same color as the renal parenchyma. ICG-enhanced fluorescence may be very helpful to distinguish the abnormal cyst dome that typically appears hypofluorescent relative to the remainder of the perfused renal parenchyma that appears fluorescent green. This tool is extremely easy to adopt; the fluorescence mode can be directly activated by the operating surgeon by pushing a foot-pedal in laparoscopy or a button on the console joystick in robotics and fluorescent vision appears almost instantaneously [14]. Using ICG-guided fluorescence, the cyst evacuation and deroofing can be safely performed.

- In case of middle-renal cysts, ipsilateral ureteral stenting with the bladder filled with methylene blue may be adopted intra-operatively in order to check the integrity of the collecting system after renal cyst's decortication.
- Use of sealing devices such as Ligasure or other in laparoscopy and retroperitoneoscopy and monopolar scissors or bipolar Maryland forceps in robotics may be very helpful to shorten the dissection time and reduce the risk of bleeding.
- The most frequent complication reported after renal cyst decortication is cyst recurrence [12]. It has been recommended to seal the portion of the cyst lying directly on the kidney surface using a monopolar hook to prevent fluid from being produced by the cyst lining [7, 15]. A useful trick that we adopt in our practice is to apply a little amount of chemical glue on the cyst edge in order to isolate this epithelial layer and prevent fluid leakage [12].
- A technical expedient to prevent cyst recurrence is to wad the cyst concavity with a flap of perirenal fat or omental tissue [7, 16, 17]. A useful trick that we adopt in our practice is to fix the flap to the cavity borders using a further layer of chemical glue in order to prevent its dislodgement [12]. We avoid use of sutures to fix the flap in order to prevent injuries to the underlying renal parenchyma.

29.8 Discussion

Treatment of symptomatic renal cysts is still controversial, and the pediatric literature is very poor in regard to this subject [6]. For asymptomatic cysts without complications, the "wait and see" strategy seems to be the better solution, especially in children [7]. A sudden increase in the size of the cyst, worsening of the pain, hematuria and recurrent colicky pain, or the onset of hypertension warrant a more invasive treatment [7]. A range of treatment options is now available: strict US surveillance, aspiration/alcoholization, or surgery. Percutaneous techniques with aspiration or injection of sclerosant agents have been associated with high recurrence rates ranging from 43% to 90% within 2 years [8, 9]. Furthermore, serious adverse effects secondary to the use of sclerosant agents, such as systemic absorption, calcification, or pain, have been described [12].

Laparoscopic management has become a valid alternative because it is minimally invasive and has a high success rate in terms of cyst recurrence [7, 15]. In a recent case series of laparoscopic management of renal cysts, the authors reported very good results in terms of efficacy, high success rate, minimal morbidity, operating time, and hospital stay [7, 15]. The cosmetic outcome in terms of patient satisfaction was also very encouraging. Pediatric cases of SRC deroofing have already been reported through either transperitoneal or retroperitoneal approach with good outcomes [7, 16–18]. More recently, robotic surgery has also been reported as a viable treatment option for SRC [11, 12]. However, there is very limited evidence in the current pediatric literature about MIS management of SRC, with only five cases of robotic treatment of SRC in pediatric patients published until now [11, 12]. Our group reported the largest experience with robot-assisted treatment and described two novel modifications to the traditional technique: the ICG-enhanced fluorescence to guide the procedure and the fat tissue wadding of the cyst to reduce the cyst recurrence after deroofing [12].

Concerning the surgical approach, the use of laparoscopy or robotics relied on SRC location, surgeon's experience, and availability of robot [12].

Laparoscopic transperitoneal SRC deroofing is probably the easiest surgical strategy [7, 15, 17]. However, posterior SRC may have a better access through retroperitoneoscopy [16, 18]. For those who have access to a surgical robot, robotics enables precise and careful tissue dissection and manipulation, comparable outcomes with laparoscopic approach, and superior ergonomics [11, 12]. Additionally, robot platform is already integrated with the ICG software Firefly® that can be instantaneously activated to improve intra-operative visualization of anatomic structures. A simple intravenous injection of ICG solution is required and real-time fluorescent images are obtained at any point during surgery [14]. In such indication, the ICG fluorescence was proved to be very helpful to distinguish the "non-fluorescent" avascular cyst dome from the "fluorescent" perfused renal parenchyma [12]. Consequently, SRC evacuation and deroofing are safely performed without major bleeding or injury to the renal parenchyma. This specific application of the ICG fluorescence is even more useful in giant SRC in which the renal architecture may be distorted [12].

Several authors have reported the fulguration of the cyst edge after deroofing as a means to prevent cyst recurrence [7, 15]. We believe that this maneuver must be performed using extreme caution considering the non-negligible risk of fistulization with the major renal vessels or collecting system [19]. In our experience, we prefer to apply a thin layer of chemical glue on the cyst base in order to isolate the secreting epithelial lining and also to fix the fat tissue flap that is adopted to wad the cyst cavity. Based upon our experience, we believe that both the chemical glue spraying and the fat wadding of the SRC may play a role in preventing cyst recurrence [12].

Analyzing the operating time, robotic is faster than laparoscopic approach, but patient installation, robot docking, and undocking times are still longer than standard laparoscopic preparation. Fast improvement of learning curve in robotics will shorten this gap [12].

Based upon the available evidence, we can outline the following considerations. Given the low risk of malignancy (<1%) and complications (<5%), conservative management should be the first choice for asymptomatic SRC [7]. The US modified Bosniak classification is a reliable tool to differentiate between stages III–IV and stages I–II SRC [20]. We suggest the follow-up of stages I–II SRC with serial US, in the absence of any change in the cyst morphology or patient symptoms [12]. All stages III–IV or symptomatic stages I–II SRC require surgical treatment [12]. Minimally invasive cyst deroofing and fat tissue wadding technique using both laparoscopic and robot-assisted approaches can be considered the gold standard treatment in case of symptomatic stages I–II SRC, reporting high success rate, low morbidity rate, and fast postoperative course [7, 12]. In case of stages III–IV SRC, complete excision of the lesion is mandatory to rule out histological malignancy [12].

Take-Home Points

- Accurate pre-operative imaging study is crucial to exclude cyst communication with the collecting system and to plan the surgical strategy.
- Laparoscopic or robot-assisted cyst deroofing is the first-line treatment for symptomatic Bosniak stages I–II renal cysts.
- Intra-operative ICG-enhanced fluorescence may be helpful to guide the evacuative puncture and the cyst deroofing, especially in giant cysts with distorted renal architecture.
- Perirenal fat tissue wadding technique is useful to reduce the cyst recurrence after deroofing.
- Chemical glue spraying may be useful to isolate the secreting epithelial lining in the cyst edge and to fix the fat tissue flap in order to prevent its dislodgement.

References

1. Bisceglia M, Galliani CA, Senger C, Stallone C, Sessa A. Renal cystic diseases: a review. Adv Anat Pathol. 2006;13(1):26–56.
2. Hanash KA, Al-Othman K, Mokhtar A, Al-Ghamdi A, Aslam M. Laparoscopic ablation of giant renal cyst. J Endourol. 2003;17:781–4.
3. Bosniak MA. The current radiological approach to renal cysts. Radiology. 1986;158:1–10.
4. Bosniak MA. The Bosniak renal cyst classification: 25 years later. Radiology. 2012;262:781–5.

5. Eroglu FK, Kargın Çakıcı E, Can G, Güngör T, Yazılıtaş F, Kurt-Sukur ED, Celikkaya E, Üner Ç, Çakmakçı E, Bülbül M. Retrospective analysis of simple and stage II renal cysts: pediatric nephrology point of view. Pediatr Int. 2018;60:1068–72.
6. Wang ZTP, Chan EP, Moreno NV, Filler G, McAleer I, Wehbi E, Chuang KW, Khoury A. What to do with renal cysts in children? Urology. 2020;140:138–42. https://doi.org/10.1016/j.urology.2020.03.001.
7. Marte A, Pintozzi L. Laparoscopic treatment of symptomatic simple renal cysts in children: single-center experience. Pediatr Med Chir. 2018;40(1) https://doi.org/10.4081/pmc.2018.168.
8. Cho YJ, Shin JH. Comparison of acetic acid and ethanol sclerotherapy for simple renal cysts: clinical experience with 86 patients. Springerplus. 2016;5:299.
9. Okeke AA, Mitchelmore AE, Keeley FX, Timoney AG. A comparison of aspiration and sclerotherapy with laparoscopic de-roofing in the management of symptomatic simple renal cysts. BJU Int. 2003;92:610–3.
10. Koutlidis N, Joyeux L, Méjean N, Sapin E. Management of simple renal cyst in children: French multicenter experience of 36 cases and review of the literature. J Pediatr Urol. 2015;11:113–7.
11. Wang YC, Xia JD, Zhang QJ, Chen C, Xue JX, Yang J, Qin C, Song NH, Wang ZJ. Robotic renal cyst decortication with calyceal diverticulectomy in a toddler—technical practicalities: a case report. J Med Case Rep. 2018;12:284.
12. Esposito C, Soria-Gondek A, Castagnetti M, Cerulo M, Del Conte F, Esposito G, Pecoraro C, Cicala D, Farina A, Escolino M. Laparoscopic or robotic deroofing guided by indocyanine green fluorescence and perirenal fat tissue wadding technique of pediatric simple renal cysts. J Laparoendosc Adv Surg Tech A. 2020;30:471–6. https://doi.org/10.1089/lap.2019.0650.
13. Israel GM, Hindman N, Bosniak MA. Evaluation of cystic renal masses: comparison of CT and MR imaging by using the Bosniak classification system. Radiology. 2004;231:365–71.
14. Esposito C, Del Conte F, Cerulo M, Gargiulo F, Izzo S, Esposito G, Spagnuolo MI, Escolino M. Clinical application and technical standardization of indocyanine green (ICG) fluorescence imaging in pediatric minimally invasive surgery. Pediatr Surg Int. 2019;35(10):1043–50.
15. Tuncel A, Aydin O, Balci M, Aslan Y, Atan A. Laparoscopic decortication of symptomatic simple renal cyst using conventional monopolar device. Kaohsiung J Med Sci. 2011;27(2):64–7.
16. Porpiglia F, Fiori C, Billia M, Renard J, Di Stasio A, Vaccino D, Bertolo R, Scarpa RM. Retroperitoneal decortication of simple renal cysts vs decortication with wadding using perirenal fat tissue: results of a prospective randomized trial. BJU Int. 2009;103:1532–6.
17. El-Shazly M, Allam A, Hathout B. Laparoscopic decortication of simple renal cyst with omental wadding technique: single-center experience. J Laparoendosc Adv Surg Tech A. 2012;22(9):886–8.
18. Tefekli A, Altunrende F, Baykal M, Sarilar O, Kabay S, Muslumanoglu AY. Retroperitoneal laparoscopic decortication of simple renal cysts using the bipolar PlasmaKinetic scissors. Int J Urol. 2006;13:331–6.
19. Hemal AK. Laparoscopic management of renal cystic disease. Urol Clin North Am. 2001;28(1):115–26.
20. Karmazyn B, Tawadros A, Delaney LR, Marine MB, Cain MP, Rink RC, Jennings SG, Kaefer M. Ultrasound classification of solitary renal cysts in children. J Pediatr Urol. 2015;11:149.e1–6.

30 Laparoscopic Radical Nephrectomy for Wilms' Tumors

Aurélien Scalabre, François Varlet, Aurore Bouty, Thomas Blanc, and Yves Heloury

Learning Objectives

- To describe step by step the technique of laparoscopic radical nephrectomy (LRN).
- To describe the robot-assisted LRN.
- To report the latest results of the review of literature.
- To show a video with the technique of LRN.

Supplementary Information The online version contains supplementary material available at [https://doi.org/10.1007/978-3-030-99280-4_30].

A. Scalabre · F. Varlet (✉)
Pediatric Surgery Department, Hôpital Nord, CHU de Saint-Etienne, Saint-Etienne Cedex 2, France
e-mail: aurelien.scalabre@chu-st-etienne.fr; francois.varlet@chu-st-etienne.fr

A. Bouty
Pediatric Surgery Department, University Femme-Mere-Enfant Hospital, Bron, France
e-mail: aurore.bouty@chu-lyon.fr

T. Blanc · Y. Heloury
University Necker-Enfant Malades Hospital, Paris, France
e-mail: thomas.blanc@aphp.fr; yves.heloury@aphp.fr

30.1 Introduction

According to International Society of Pediatric Oncology (SIOP) protocol, Wilms' tumors (WT) must be treated by neoadjuvant chemotherapy and open radical nephrectomy as a first step. The overall survival rate remains high since several decades, around 90%, and protocols tried to decrease the burden of chemotherapy and radiotherapy [1]. The same thinking was conducted by a few surgeons to decrease the burden of surgery with laparoscopic radical nephrectomy (LRN), especially about adhesion-related complication as postoperative small bowel obstruction and scars altering quality of life of long-term survivors [2–7]. Therefore, new SIOP-Umbrella protocols included indications to laparoscopic resection of WT: (1) surgery must adhere to oncological principles with transperitoneal radical nephrectomy including lymph nodes sampling, (2) only for small, central tumors with rim of "normal" renal tissue, (3) with extraction of the specimen in a bag without morcellation involving an adequate abdominal wall incision, (4) and open surgery is required if a nephron-sparing surgery is feasible. There are also laparoscopic contraindications in the protocol: (1) tumor infiltrating extrarenal structures are extended beyond the ipsilateral border of spinal column, (2) thrombus in renal vein or veina cava, (3) peripheral location of nephron-sparing surgery is not deemed feasible, (4) tumor without any response to chemotherapy due to the risk of tumor rupture, (5) and

C. Esposito et al. (eds.), *Minimally Invasive Techniques in Pediatric Urology*, https://doi.org/10.1007/978-3-030-99280-4_30

little or no experience in laparoscopic nephrectomy (consider transfer to another unit or obtain more experienced help) [8]. These SIOP-Umbrella criteria for LRN are conservative and safe but indications can be extended for teams experienced in surgical oncology and minimally invasive surgery [9]. However, it should be kept in mind to avoid any tumor rupture or uncontrolled spreading during laparoscopy, whatever radiotherapy will be required increasing burden of surgery [4, 10].

30.2 Preoperative Preparation

Thus, a good CT scan or MRI analysis with the radiologist before surgery and after chemotherapy is mandatory to assess if laparoscopy seems feasible. If a nephron-sparing surgery is feasible, it should be performed. Thrombus in renal vein or veina cava remains an undebatable contraindication. Obvious tumor-infiltrating extrarenal structures are also undebatable which needs open surgery, but the most often tumor infiltration is very difficult to assert definitely on CT scan or MRI before procedure. In this case, LRN can be started and quickly converted if there are criteria of contraindication. A WT with large lymph nodes is not indicated for laparoscopy (Fig. 30.1). When there is a tumor rupture at diagnosis, laparoscopy is debatable because the spillage is already done in abdominal cavity, and LRN was nevertheless done in one case with favorable outcome [11].

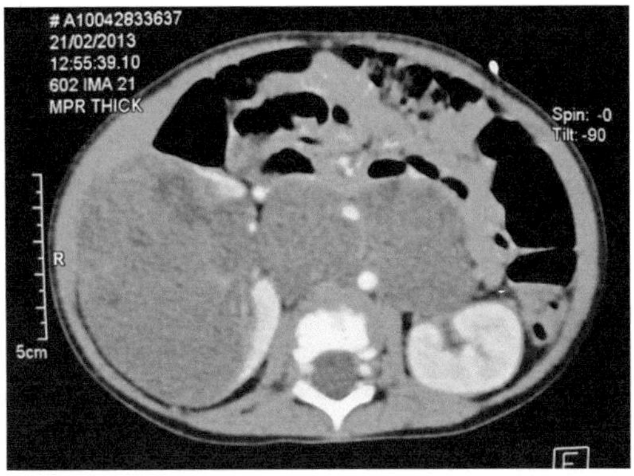

Fig. 30.1 Huge lymph nodes surrounding the great vessels after chemotherapy

The risk of laparoscopy, tumor rupture, great vessels injury, interest of lymph nodes sampling, and conversion are explained to the parents before to obtain consent.

30.3 Positioning

Before positioning, you have to draw the suprapubic incision for specimen extraction and the possible open approach in case of conversion. The patient was positioned at 45–60° lateral decubitus with the interest to have a good exposure of retroperitoneal area after colon releasing because of falling down (Fig. 30.2).

The video column is placed in the back of the patient and the surgeon stands at the front with his

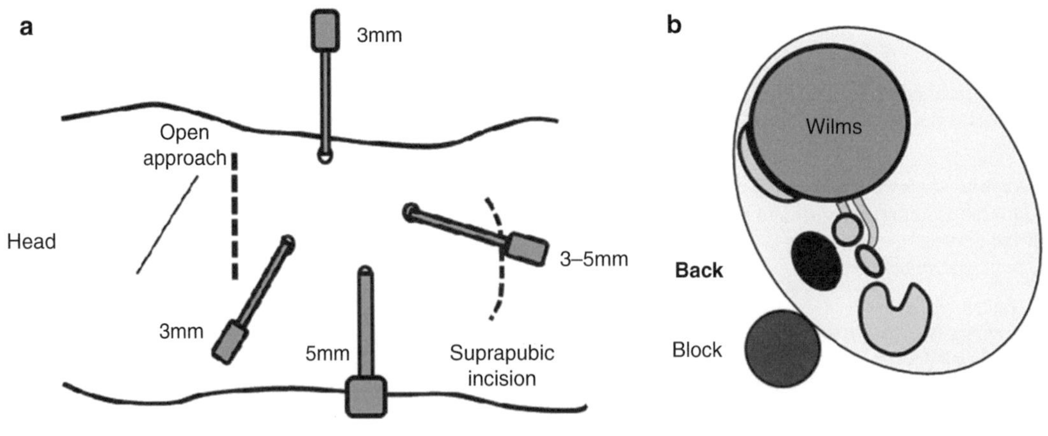

Fig. 30.2 (**a**) Trocars and incisions. (**b**) 45–60° lateral decubitus installation

assistant. Trocars placement is similar to every nephrectomy: one by trans-umbilical approach according to Hasson's technique, one in subcostal area, often replaced by a 5 mm one to introduce sealing devices, one in lower quadrant, and a fourth one just below xiphoid process to help maintaining liver or spleen or sometimes tumor retraction.

30.4 Instrumentation

A 30° lens is mandatory to ensure a good vision during the procedure. If using a 0° lens, the umbilical trocar must be changed by an upper location between umbilicus and flank. According to the child, a 5 mm or 10 mm telescope is required and 3 mm or 5 mm instruments can be used. The required instruments are scissors, atraumatic forceps, dissector, monopolar hook, bipolar forceps, sealing devices as Ultracision™ (Ethicon Endo-surgery, Cincinnati, Ohio, USA) or LigaSure™ (Valleylab, Boulder, Colorado, USA), atraumatic retractor, Hem-o-lock® (Teleflex, Morrisville, NC, USA), suction.

30.5 Technique

The aim is to do LRN with monobloc nephroureterectomy outside the Gerota's fascia with lymph nodes sampling, needing a wide dissection of vena cava on the right side and aorta on the left side for lymph nodes picking above the level of renal pedicle. In small tumors, guidelines imply to do first the ligation of renal pedicle and it is better performing artery ligation before renal vein to avoid swelling of the tumor, but sometimes the renal vein keeps the artery hidden and has to be dissected and ligated first. In bigger tumors, the best way is to begin dissection lower at the level of iliac vessels and when the ureter is identified, the dissection follow-up vena cava on the right and aorta on the left to reach the renal pedicle. If thin adhesions between tumor and diaphragm occur, the dissection may go through the diaphragm to remove a tumor extension. A conversion is required if adhesions are thick and infiltrate widely the muscle. A macroscopic complete resection (R0) is mandatory.

For a right WT, the steps are as following:

- Releasing of the colon from cecum to right flexure to obtain a good exposure of renal pedicle, good dissection of vena cava, and good access to pelvic ureter.
- Retracting the liver.
- Opening of retroperitoneum at the level of renal pedicle to free vein and artery before ligating artery first by Hem-o-lock® (Teleflex, Morrisville, NC, USA), two beside the aorta and one beside the kidney; the same ligation is done to the renal vein (Fig. 30.3).

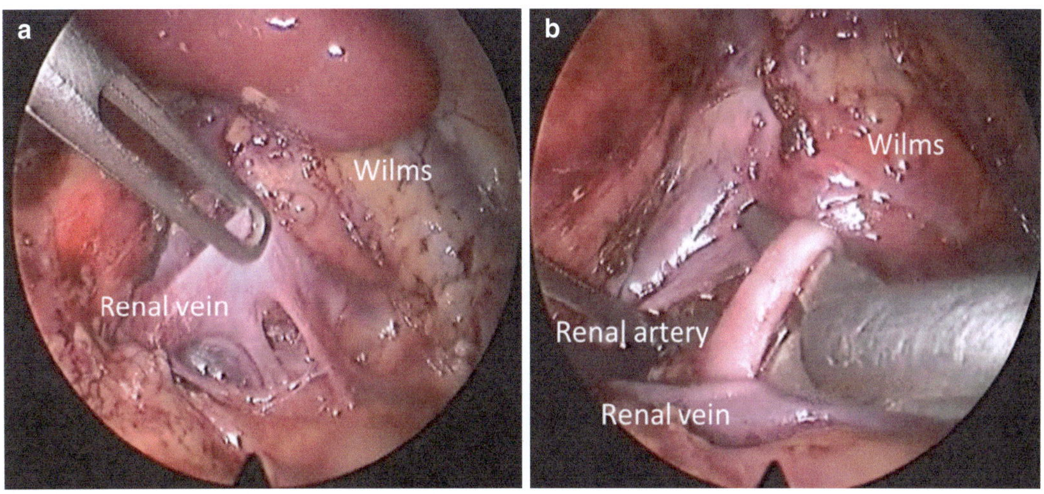

Fig. 30.3 Left Wilms' tumor. (**a**) Renal and genital veins. (**b**) Renal artery

- If the tumor is bigger and stops the retroperitoneal approach, the iliac vein is coming up before reaching vena cava and proceeding dissection cranially along it until above renal pedicle to have a good exposure of suprarenal vena cava. Right gonadal vessels may be spared, but they are ligated if necessary.
- Mobilization of duodenum and pancreas to see the left side of vena cava and the right side of aorta because guidelines impose to ligate renal artery close to the aorta and to sample lymph nodes between the great vessels above the level of renal pedicle.
- After renal pedicle ligation, releasing of kidney is performed along suprarenal vena cava, sparing or not the adrenal gland according to the decision of multidisciplinary meeting, most often removed when upper pole tumor, then around the Gerota's fascia close to psoas muscle. This latter step is much facilitated by new sealing devices, safely to avoiding bleeding.
- Dissecting down the ureter and ligating as low as possible.
- Performing the suprapubic incision and doing a small peritoneal hole to introduce the 15 mm-trocar for bag; thus, the pneumoperitoneum can be maintained and specimen placed in the bag with lymph nodes. Once this step is performed, the peritoneal hole is enlarged and the specimen is extracted by a mandatory adequate incision to avoid any tumor rupture.

For a left WT, the LRN is similar with few differences:

- The releasing of left colonic flexure and lateral edge of spleen must be done to have a good exposure on the kidney and adrenal gland because of falling down of the spleen and pancreatic tail during installation.
- In case of big tumor, the first approach of iliac vessels is done before dissecting aorta and following it above renal pedicle.
- Sampling of lymph nodes between aorta and vena cava with a good mobilization of spleen and pancreas, following splenic and renal veins.

Drainage is not mandatory but commonly left to show any postoperative bleeding or lymphatic suffusion.

Despite the lack of haptic feedback considered as a potential limitation, robot-assisted laparoscopy (RAL) has many advantages with 3D vision, seven degrees of freedom, and precise camera control. RAL can probably expand the possibilities of performing difficult operations, especially in case of deep and narrow field such as pediatric oncology surgery. For RAL total nephrectomy, patients were positioned in supine position and four robotic ports were inserted along the midline with one assistant port on the planned Pfannenstiel incision for subsequent specimen retrieval. Then, the same procedure described above is performed.

30.6 Post-Operative Care

At the end of procedure, bladder catheter and nasogastric tube can be removed. In case of peridural or morphinic analgesia, it is better to leave bladder catheter to avoid retention. Oral intake can be restarted 8–12 h after surgery. Level 1 analgesic is usually sufficient after 1 or 2 days. Drainage is removed after a few days, except in case of bleeding or effusion. The hospital stay is usually short, after assessing correct bowel movements and pain control. Most patients are discharged after 2 to 3 days.

30.7 Complications

Bleeding or lymphatic effusion can occur in the immediate postoperative course. Bleeding can require a redo in emergency. Drainage must be left during 1 or 2 weeks waiting for lymphatic effusion drying up. Pneumonia and bowel perforation have been reported justifying antibiotics or redo surgery.

Histological results are expected to confirm local disease stage I or II. Sometimes an unexpected small thrombus can be showed in the renal vein section or lymph nodes can be metastatic increasing WT in a stage III case and requiring radiotherapy. A tumor rupture leads to a similar treatment.

30.8 Results

A recent paper reported our results from 50 WT children between 2006 and 2018 [12]. With a median age of 38 months (6–181), children were treated according to SIOP 2001 or UMBRELLA SIOP-RTSG 2016 protocols receiving neoadjuvant chemotherapy and performing transperitoneal LRN. Sixteen tumors crossed the lateral border of spine of whom three crossed the midline (32%) and 6/16 required a conversion to open surgery. None of these WT was amenable to nephron-sparing surgery. No tumor rupture occurred and no tumor was upstaged even when conversion was required. After a median follow-up of 34 months (2–138), 47 patients were in complete remission. A local recurrence occurred in two patients at 7 and 9 months after LRN, both stage I and intermediate risk, requiring new chemotherapy and one presented with lung metastases 4 months after surgery, stage III and high risk; but there is no death among the 50 patients. About RAL, the results were reported in a few papers with good follow-up, but the number of patients is small and the follow-up is still short to analyze [4, 13–15].

Tip and Tricks

- Drawing future incisions before installation (Pfannenstiel, possible laparotomy).
- Positioning in semi-lateral decubitus and four trocars to have a good exposure.
- Dissecting cranially from iliac vessels along vena cava or aorta in case of big tumor.
- Wide suprapubic incision for extraction of specimen to avoid any rupture in the bag, as otherwise a proper staging is impossible to proof by histologist and surgeon if rupture occurred during laparoscopy or extraction.

30.9 Discussion

Open radical nephrectomy through a transverse transperitoneal incision and regional lymph node sampling is considered as the standard of treatment for most malignant renal tumors in children according to consecutive SIOP protocols. From 2003, nephron-sparing surgery in unilateral WT has been proposed for selected small tumors after chemotherapy and SIOP included this conservative surgery in its new protocols [16, 17]. The first reports of laparoscopic radical nephrectomies were published between 2004 and 2011 [2, 3, 11, 18] and laparoscopy was more and more done with good outcomes. Finally, laparoscopy was included in UMBRELLA SIOP-RTSG 2016 protocol with criteria for indications and contraindications. The series of 50 cases of LRN for unilateral WT, represented 19% of WT in the same time, demonstrated no death, a 3-year event-free survival of 94%, a rate of local relapse of 4% and a rate of conversion in open surgery of 12% without upstaging of the tumor [12]. Contraindications have to be discussed:

- About tumor infiltrating extrarenal structures, this contraindication is undebatable and needs open surgery, but the most often tumor infiltration is very difficult to assert definitely on CT scan or MRI before procedure. In this case, LRN can be started and quickly converted if laparoscopy is unable to remove safely the tumor with a macroscopic complete resection (R0).
- About extension of the tumor beyond the ipsilateral border of spinal column, we proposed in a first step to perform LRN only when WT did not cross lateral border of the spine for a safe procedure [4]. However, with training, we demonstrated in the series that the technique was feasible even in tumors crossing this line or sometimes the midline (16/50), with 6/16 conversions in open surgery without rupture [12]. But it is certainly better to begin LRN by small tumors.
- Thrombus in renal vein or vena cava remains a contraindication, but preoperative CT scan can miss a small remnant, and Doppler color

ultrasound seems to be more efficient [19]. An open conversion is required if a thrombus is discovered during LRN.

- Peripheral location of tumor, without rim of "normal" renal tissue, would be a contraindication, but the vast majority of WT has no rim of normal parenchyma around them, as in most series, without bad oncologic outcomes [2, 4, 11, 12, 18].
- Tumor without any response to chemotherapy due to the risk of tumor rupture is also debatable because we must never do any rupture by minimal invasive surgery as in open surgery. Several adenocarcinoma, renal cell carcinoma, and clear cell sarcoma were removed by laparoscopy without any rupture [4, 15].
- The last contraindication is undebatable, only trained oncologic and laparoscopic surgeons can perform LRN.

The place of nephron-sparing surgery in unilateral WT has no consensus but if partial nephrectomy seems feasible, it should be preferred. After neoadjuvant chemotherapy, WT can reduce dramatically and make nephron-sparing surgery feasible. Today, the best indication for nephron-sparing surgery seems to be a tumor lower than 4 cm, distant from the renal hilum and respecting at least 50% of the renal parenchyma. In a review of 294 nephron-sparing surgeries in literature, positive margins were higher with nephron-sparing surgery than radical nephrectomy (8.5% vs. 0.5% in radical nephrectomy). However, overall survival and event-free survival were similar, and the rate of mild to moderate renal function was higher after radical nephrectomy (42% vs. 10% after nephron-sparing surgery) [20]. A few laparoscopic nephron-sparing surgeries were reported and seemed to be feasible [15, 21]. New imaging such as 3D reconstruction with view of intrarenal vessels is expected and probably will allow selecting the best parameters for this surgery.

The local relapse occurred in 4% in the LRN series and similar results were reported in open surgery by SIOP 93/01 protocol (2.8%) [22] and National Wilms' Tumor Study 4 (4%) [23], and below than United Kingdom experience, with 7.9% but this series reported more stage III [24].

No small bowel obstruction was reported after LRN and rates of 2.5% and 5.4% were reported by SIOP and National Wilms' Tumor Study in open surgery [22, 25], but the follow-up is too short to conclude. The patients and their parents were very happy about cosmetic results with small visible scars on the abdominal wall and invisible suprapubic scar.

The RAL may overcome the difficulties of dissection of the renal pedicle in tumors crossing the midline rather than laparoscopy with maintaining of clear vision of the tumor limits, allowing easy and secure dissection of the involved organs and diaphragmatic repair, and sometimes performing caudal pancreatectomy, splenectomy, lymphadenectomy, and partial diaphragmatic resection to ensure R0 resection [15]. In adult renal cancer, tumor infiltration of extrarenal structures is not considered as contraindication to RAL nephrectomy [26].

Take-Home Points

- Preoperative CT scan or MRI has to be discussed with your radiologist to select children amenable to nephron-sparing nephrectomy, LRN, or RAL and open surgery.
- The aim of LRN is obtaining macroscopic complete resection (R0), the same as in open surgery.
- Direct access to renal pedicle is feasible in small WT. In bigger tumors, the dissection must start at level of iliac vessels and move up along vena cava on the right and aorta on the left.
- Lymph nodes sampling above renal pedicle and between vena cava and aorta is mandatory.
- Tight adhesions with liver, spleen or diaphragm, and venous thrombus lead to conversion in open surgery.

30.10 Conclusion

In selected patients, LRN is feasible and safe by trained laparoscopic surgeon with same overall survival and event-free survival than in open surgery. The rate of local recurrence is around 4% and today no small bowel obstruction was reported after LRN.

References

1. Nakamura L, Ritchey M. Current management of Wilms' tumor. Curr Urol Rep. 2010;11:58–65.
2. Duarte RJ, Denes FT, Cristofani LM, Giron AM, Filho VO, Arap S. Laparoscopic nephrectomy for Wilms' tumor after chemotherapy: initial experience. J Urol. 2004;172(4Pt1):1438–40.
3. Varlet F, Stephan JL, Guye E, Allary R, Berger C, Lopez M. Laparoscopic radical nephrectomy for unilateral renal cancer in children. Surg Laparosc Endosc Percutan Tech. 2009;19:148–52.
4. Varlet F, Petit T, Leclair MD, Lardy H, Geiss S, Becmeur F, Ravasse P, Rod J, de Lambert G, Braik K, Lardellier-Reynaud F, Lopez M. Laparoscopic treatment of renal cancer in children: a multicentric study and review of oncologic and surgical complications. J Pediatr Urol. 2014;10:505–10.
5. Bouty A, Burnand K, Nightingale M, Roberts A, Campbell M, O'Brien M, Heloury Y. What is the risk of local recurrence after laparoscopic transperitoneal radical nephrectomy in children with Wilms tumours? Analysis of a local series and review of the literature. J Pediatr Urol. 2018;14:327.e1–7.
6. Aguayo P, Ho B, Fraser JD, Gamis A, St Peter SD, Snyder CL. Bowel obstruction after treatment of intra-abdominal tumors. Eur J Pediatr Surg. 2010;20:234–6.
7. Kinahan KE, Sharp LK, Seidel K, Didwania A, Lacouture ME, Stovall M, Haryani A, Robison LL, Krull KR. Scarring, disfigurement and quality of life in long-term survivors of childhood cancer: a report from childhood cancer survivor study. J Clin Oncol. 2012;30:2466–74.
8. Van den Heuvel-Eibrink MM, Hol JA, Pritchard-Jones K, Van Tinteren H, Furtwängler R, Verschuur AC, Vujanic GM, Leuschner I, Brok J, Rübe C, Smets AM, Janssens GO, Godzinski J, Ramírez-Villar GL, de Camargo B, Segers H, Collini P, Gessler M, Bergeron C, Spreafico F, Graf N. Position paper: rationale for the treatment of Wilms tumor in the UMBRELLA SIOP-RTSG 2016 protocol. Nat Rev Urol. 2017;14:743–52.
9. Burnand K, Roberts A, Bouty A, Nightingale M, Campbell M, Heloury Y. Laparoscopic nephrectomy for Wilms' tumor: can we expand on the current SIOP criteria? J Pediatr Urol. 2018;14:253.e1–8.
10. Leclair MD. In: Esposito C, et al., (eds.), ESPES Manual of Pediatric Minimally Invasive Surgery. Springer Nature Switzerland AG; 2019. p. 429–33. https://doi.org/10.1007/978-3-030-00964-9_59.
11. Javid PJ, Lendvay TS, Acierno S, Gow KW. Laparoscopic nephroureterectomy for Wilms' tumor: oncologic considerations. J Pediatr Surg. 2011;46:978–82.
12. Bouty A, Blanc T, Leclair MD, Lavrand F, Faure A, Binet A, Rod J, O'Brien M, Sarnacki S, Nightingale M, Heloury Y, Varlet F, Scalabre A. Minimally invasive surgery for unilateral Wilms tumors: multicenter retrospective analysis of 50 transperitoneal laparoscopic total nephrectomies. Pediatr Blood Cancer. 2020;67:e28212.
13. Meignan P, Ballouhey Q, Lejeune J, Braik K, Longis B, Cook AR, Lardy H, Fourcade L, Binet A. Robotic-assisted laparoscopic surgery for pediatric tumors: a bicenter experience. J Robot Surg. 2018;12:501–8.
14. Cost NG, Liss ZJ, Bean CM, Geller JI, Minevich EA, Noh PH. Prechemotherapy robotic-assisted laparoscopic radical nephrectomy for an adolescent with Wilms tumor. J Pediatr Hematol Oncol. 2015;37:e125–7.
15. Blanc T, Pio L, Clermidi P, Muller C, Orbach D, Minard-Colin V, Harte C, Meignan P, Kohaut J, Heloury Y, Sarnacki S. Robotic-assisted laparoscopic management of renal tumors in children: preliminary results. Pediatr Blood Cancer. 2019;66(Suppl 3):e27867.
16. Haecker FM, von Schweinitz D, Harms D, Buerger D, Graf N. Partial nephrectomy for unilateral Wilms' tumor: results of study SIOP 93e01/GPOH. J Urol. 2003;170:939–44.
17. Cost NG, Lubahn JD, Granberg CF, Schlomer BJ, Wickiser JE, Rakheja D, Gargollo PC, Leonard D, Raj GV, Baker LA, Margulis V. Oncologic outcomes of partial versus radical nephrectomy for unilateral Wilms tumor. Pediatr Blood Cancer. 2012;58:898–904.
18. Barber TD, Wickiser JE, Wilcox DT, Baker LA. Prechemotherapy laparoscopic nephrectomy for Wilms' tumor. J Pediatr Urol. 2009;5:416–9.
19. Brisse HJ, Smets AM, Kaste SC, Owens CM. Imaging in unilateral Wilms tumour. Pediatr Radiol. 2008;38:18–29.
20. Tricarda T, Lacreuse I, Louis V, Schneider A, Chaussy Y, Soler L, Moog R, Lang H, Jacqmin D, Becmeur F. Is nephron-sparing surgery relevant for unilateral Wilms tumors? Arch Pediatr. 2017;24:650–8.
21. Piche N, Barrieras D. Minimally invasive nephron-sparing surgery for unilateral Wilms' tumor. J Pediatr Surg. 2012;47:e1–4.
22. Fuchs J, Kienecker K, Furtwängler R, Warmann SW, Bürger D, Thürhoff JW, Hager J, Graf N. Surgical aspects in the treatment of patients with unilateral Wilms tumor. A report from the SIOP 93-01/German society of pediatric oncology and hematology. Ann Surg. 2009;249:666–71.

23. Shamberger RC, Guthrie KA, Ritchey ML, Haase GM, Takashima J, Beckwith JB, D'Angio GJ, Green DM, Breslow NE. Surgery-related factors and local recurrence of Wilms tumor in National Wilms Tumor Study 4. Ann Surg. 1999;229:292–7.
24. Irtan S, Jitlal M, Bate J, Powis M, Vujanic G, Kelsey A, Walker J, Mitchell C, Machin D, Pritchard-Jones K. Renal Tumours Committee of the Children's Cancer and Leukaemia Group (CCLG). Eur J Cancer. 2015;51:225–32.
25. Ritchey ML, Kelalis PP, Etzioni R, Breslow N, Shochat S, Haase GM. Small bowel obstruction after nephrectomy for Wilms tumor. A report of the National Wilms' tumor Study-3. Ann Surg. 1993;218:654–9.
26. Peyronnet B, Seisen T, Oger E, Vaessen C, Grassano Y, Benoit T, et al. Comparison of 1800 robotic and open partial nephrectomies for renal tumors. Ann Surg Oncol. 2016;23:4277–83.

Robotic Approach for Kidney Tumors in Pediatric Patients

31

Thomas Blanc, Luca Pio, Enrico Brönnimann, Yves Heloury, and Sabine Sarnacki

Learning Objectives

- To describe step by step the technique of robotic approach for kidney tumors in pediatric patients.
- To describe tips and tricks of our technique.
- To report our latest results compared to the international papers.
- To show a video with the technique of robotic approach for kidney tumors.

31.1 Introduction

The application of minimally invasive surgery (MIS) in pediatric surgical oncology has encountered several concerns including limited tumor manipulation, challenges of vascular involvement, and risk of spillage.

The first series of Wilms' tumors (WT) treated by an MIS approach was reported in 2004 by Duarte et al. in children receiving neoadjuvant chemotherapy [1] and in 2009 by Barber et al. in children without preoperative treatment [2]. In 2014, the Renal Tumor Strategy Group of the International Society of Paediatric Oncology (SIOP) published the largest cohort of WT treated with MIS [3], and in the same year, SIOP released the Umbrella protocol with criteria for laparoscopic nephrectomy [4, 5]. In 2018, Bouty et al. analyzed 88 articles totaling more than 100 laparoscopic nephrectomies for WT in the world and showed that in highly selected cases, this approach did not worsen prognosis [6]. Recently, the same group has published an international multicenter review of MIS total nephrectomies for WT between 2006 and 2018 [7].

Robotic-assisted laparoscopy (RAL), with its 3D vision, seven degrees of freedom, tremor filtration, and precise camera control, has expanded the possibilities of performing and reproducing difficult operations, especially when there is a deep and narrow field and when fine dissection is required for delicate tissue manipulation, as is the case in pediatric oncology surgery. The lack of haptic feedback may be considered as a potential limitation, especially in tumors that cannot be fragmented, such as WT.

Supplementary Information The online version contains supplementary material available at [https://doi.org/10.1007/978-3-030-99280-4_31].

T. Blanc (✉) · L. Pio · E. Brönnimann · Y. Heloury
S. Sarnacki
Department of Paediatric Surgery and Urology, Necker-Enfants Malades University Children Hospital, AP-HP Centre—Université de Paris, Paris, France
e-mail: thomas.blanc@aphp.fr; lucakeats@hotmail.it; e_broennimann@hotmail.com; yves.heloury@gmail.com; sabine.sarnacki@aphp.fr

C. Esposito et al. (eds.), *Minimally Invasive Techniques in Pediatric Urology*,
https://doi.org/10.1007/978-3-030-99280-4_31

The first applications of RAL for pediatric renal tumors were reported by Cost et al., who described in 2012 transperitoneal partial nephrectomy [8] and in 2014 a nephrectomy in an adolescent with WT [9]. To date, fewer than 10 cases of robotic management of renal tumors in children have been reported in the literature [10, 11].

Recently, we published our preliminary experience of RAL management of renal tumors [12].

This chapter is focused on the operative technique of robotic approach for kidney tumors (nephroureterectomy and partial nephrectomy) in pediatric patients.

31.2 Pre-Operative Preparation

All the patients are operated under general anesthesia with orotracheal intubation, and they received a nasogastric tube and a bladder catheter before surgery.

31.3 Nephroureterectomy (Transperitoneal Approach)

31.3.1 Positioning

The procedure starts with a crucial element for success: proper positioning of the patient.

The patient is positioned supine on the TruSystem™ 7000dV—Trumpf Medical. The Integrated Table Motion enables the da Vinci® Xi™ Surgical System to connect to Trumpf Medical's TruSystem™ 7000dV OR Table so that the child can be dynamically positioned while the surgeon operates. The ability to reposition the operating table allows for the intra-abdominal contents to move away from the surgical site for optimal exposure and access to the target anatomy. No jelly roll, egg crates, pillows, or an infant-sized bean bag is used. For left kidney, a rectal tube is inserted to deflate the sigmoid.

The patient is secured to the table with wide tape across the nipple line of the chest and knees

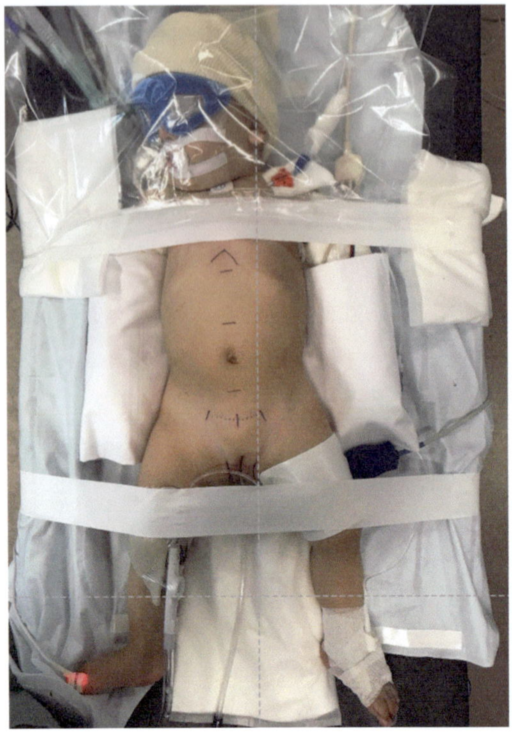

Fig. 31.1 Patient set-up for transperitoneal RAL nephrectomy

(Fig. 31.1). With the help of the anesthesiologist, proper positioning, and adequate access to the patient's airway and IV lines are confirmed before the start of the procedure.

31.3.2 Initial Access, Insufflation, and Trocar Placement

The access is performed with the open Hassan technique. A 8 mm optical trocar is placed under direct vision in the umbilical position allowing easy and safe access. The port position for robotic assisted laparoscopic will be in straight line (Fig. 31.2). The 8 mm robotic trocars are placed under direct vision. "Burping" of all ports gives additional intra-abdominal space needed in order to successfully perform the procedure on smaller children. The assistant port, 8-mm AirSeal® iFS System, is inserted in the iliac fossa, on the opposite side of the tumor. This system is advantageous in providing a stable

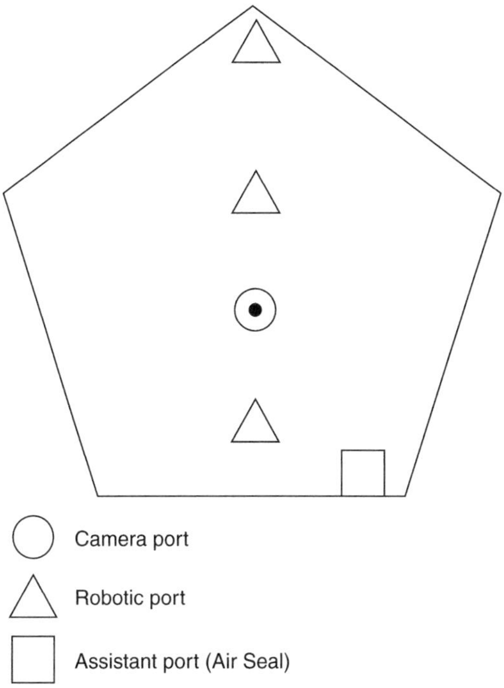

Fig. 31.2 Trocar positioning for right transperitoneal RAL nephrectomy

pneumoperitoneum, constant smoke evacuation, and valve-free access.

31.3.3 Docking with Xi System

Xi robotic system comes from the tumor side and is docked at the level of the umbilical port (camera site). The arms of the robot are rotated to adjust to the surgical site without moving the operating table.

Once the robot is docked, the table is tilted 20°.

31.3.4 Instrumentation

Robotic instruments used during the procedure include:

- Monopolar Curved Scissors/Hot Shears™.
- Fenestrated and Maryland Bipolar Forceps.
- Tip-Up Fenestrated Grasper.
- Vessel Sealer Extend.

31.3.5 Surgical Technique

For right kidney tumor, as shown in the video, the ascending colon and hepatic flexure are mobilized medially using monopolar curved scissors. A Kocher maneuver is performed to mobilize the duodenum until the vena cava is visualized. The ureter, located just lateral and deep to the gonadal vein, is ligated using a vessel sealer. The gonadal vein is ligated with a vessel sealer. The dissection of the right renal vein is then performed. The renal artery is identified and dissected free. A vessel loop is advanced to generate gentle traction on the renal artery to facilitate clip placement. The renal artery is clamped with Hemolocks and sectioned. Same technique is used for the vein. The renal hilar dissection is achieved with some minimal blood loss. Attachments between Gerota's fascia and the underlying musculature are divided with blunt dissection. The adrenal is left in situ if possible. The kidney and the peri-renal fat are dissected en bloc. Following completion of the nephrectomy and peri-hilar and peri-aortic lymph node sampling, the specimen is placed in a plastic bag. The tumor is extracted inside the plastic bag and without morcellation through a Pfannenstiel incision. No drain is placed.

31.4 Partial Nephrectomy (Retroperitoneal Lateral Approach)

31.4.1 Positioning

The procedure starts with a crucial element for success: proper positioning of the patient.

The child is placed in the lateral position close to the edge of the table, with minimum flexion, using lumbar padding to stretch the costo-iliac distance without flexing the operating table. Non-stretch adhesive banding secures this position and prevents displacement either forward or backward. The upper leg is stretched while the lower leg is flexed, with no contact between them to avoid compression.

31.4.2 Initial Access, Insufflation, and Trocar Placement

Three 8-mm robotic ports and one 12-mm AirSeal® iFS System assistant port are placed in an imaginary line drawn from the iliovertebral angle to the iliac fossa (Fig. 31.3).

- A first 15 mm incision is made in the mid axillary line, at a point between 1/3 and 2/3 extending from the iliac crest to the 12th rib and retroperitoneal access is achieved with a muscle splitting blunt dissection. The first trocar is fixed with a 0 PDS purse-string suture that is applied around the muscles to ensure an airtight seal and to allow traction with the Hasson cone in order to increase the working space. The retroperitoneal space is created with the camera (8-mm; 0°) by blunt dissection and gas insufflation dissection, with no need for finger or balloon dissection.

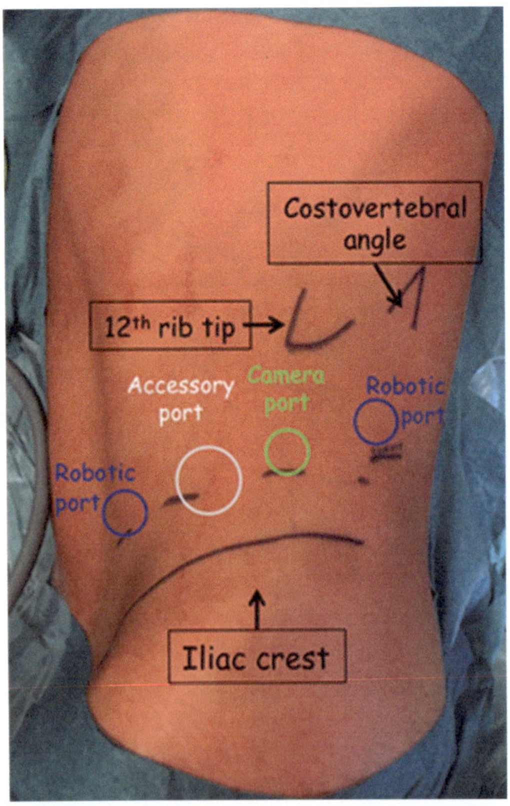

Fig. 31.3 Trocar positioning for left lateral retroperitoneal RAL partial nephrectomy

- The second port is inserted under direct vision at the angle of the iliac crest and the lateral border of the paraspinal muscles.
- To avoid transperitoneal insertion of the third 8-mm robotic port in the iliac fossa, on the edge of the rectus abdominis muscle, the retroperitoneal working space is fully developed by identifying the deep surface of the anterior wall muscles and pushing the peritoneum medially with a laparoscopic bipolar forceps.
- The 12-mm AirSeal AirSeal® iFS System (ConMed Corporation) assistant port is then inserted in between the camera port and the iliac fossa port. Insufflation pressure does not exceed 12 mmHg, and the CO_2 flow rate is 5 L/min.

The Hasson cone allows for stable and constant traction of the robotic camera port, which is a major advantage with a retroperitoneal limited working space and all the trocars are "burped" as much as possible upward and outward, to give an overall 1–2 cm space needed for safe maneuvering and to reduce the risk of breaching the peritoneum.

31.4.3 Docking with Xi System

Xi robotic system comes in the front of the children (Fig. 31.4). No table tilt is needed.

31.4.4 Instrumentation

Robotic instruments used during the procedure include:

- Monopolar Curved Scissors/Hot Shears™.
- Maryland Bipolar Forceps.
- Large Needle Driver.
- Scanlan clamp 3795-59.

31.4.5 Surgical Technique

After docking, when the instruments are inserted, the Gerota's fascia is widely opened in a caudo-cranial manner close to the quadratus lumborum muscle with the monopolar curved scissors. Insufflation and gravity push the kidney medially, which correspondingly appears on the upper section of the screen.

Dissection began on the posterior surface of the kidney with exposition of the renal hilum, with no kidney mobilization. The renal artery is dissected free to allow for later clamping. Vessel loop is advanced to generate gentle traction on the renal artery to facilitate clamp placement. The peripheral mass is easily identified on the posterior aspect of the kidney. Once delimitation of the tumor on the renal capsule is done, we place the bulldog clamp to maintain a bloodless field to optimize complete tumor excision and renorrhaphy. Direct tumor manipulation is carefully avoided. The tumor is resected en bloc using monopolar scissors. The proper plane between the nodule and normal renal parenchyma is determined in order to preserve an adjacent rim of normal parenchyma to ensure negative surgical margins (Fig. 31.5). The sliding-clip renorrhaphy technique is used with 4/0 PDS running suture and Hem-o-Lock clips,

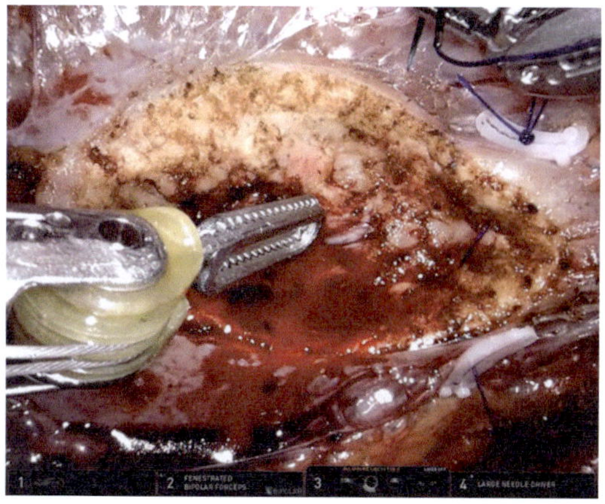

Fig. 31.5 Cone-shape defect after partial nephrectomy

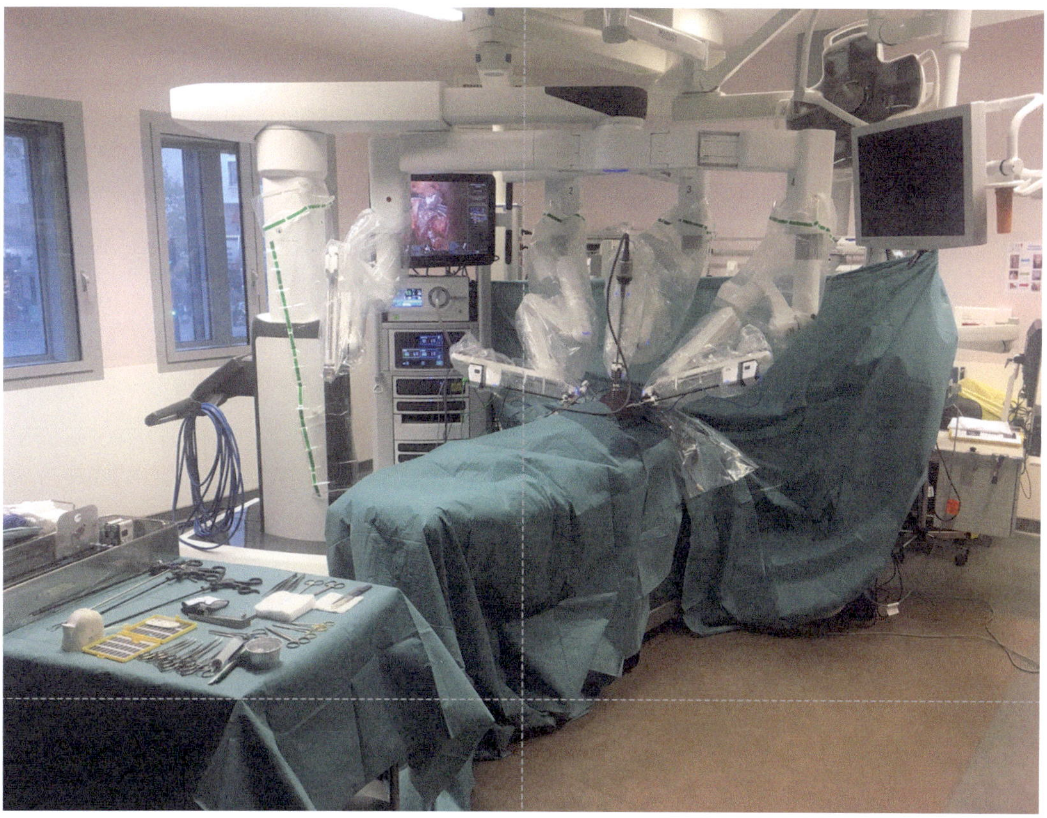

Fig. 31.4 Room set-up for left lateral retroperitoneal RAL partial nephrectomy

incorporating a small piece of Surgicel Fibrillar, to close the cone-shaped defect and ensure hemostasis (Fig. 31.6). The arterial clamp is then released after complete repair of the renal parenchyma defect and hemostasis is confirmed. The tumor is retrieved with an EndoCatch bag without morcellation through the robotic port incision.

No drain is placed.

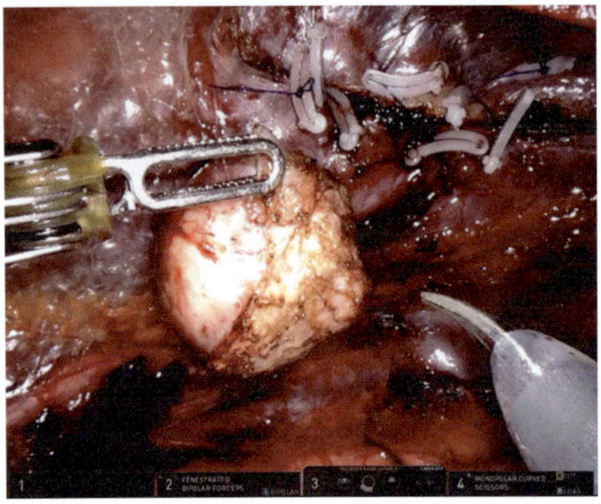

Fig. 31.6 Sliding-clip renorrhaphy technique with 4/0 PDS running suture and Hem-o-Lock clips

31.5 Results

From December 2016 to June 2020, 20 patients were treated by a RAL technique for renal tumors (Table 31.1). The median age was 5.5 years (7 months–14.1 years). During the same period, 325 RAL procedures for urology, general surgery, oncology, ENT surgery, thoracic surgery, and transoral robotic surgery were performed.

Fifteen total RAL nephrectomies were performed, 14 for WT and one for an LMNA/NTRK metastatic renal sarcoma. Eight WT out of 14, scheduled for RAL nephroureterectomy, had tumor extension beyond the ipsilateral border of the spinal column.

The median console time for nonconverted RAL total nephrectomy was 270 min (180–360 min). Median lymph nodes sampling was 8 (1–22). Three children needed a partial diaphragmatic resection. Four conversions occurred: in case #1: renal vein injury with no need for blood transfusion; in case #9 (renal sarcoma): difficult renal hilum dissection; in case #14: renal vein bleeding with emergency undocking, and in case #18: acute respiratory failure secondary to pneumothorax after partial diaphragmatic resection.

Table 31.1 Patient characteristics

#	Age	Past medical history	Approach	Surgery	Conversion	Pathology	LN
1	5.1	-	Trans	Nephrectomy	**Yes**	Wilms, stage 1	7
2	5.2	-	Trans	Nephrectomy	No	Wilms, stage 2	6
3	4.2	Nephroblastomatosis	Trans	Nephrectomy	No	Wilms, stage 3	2
4	3.6	-	Trans	Nephrectomy	No	Wilms, stage 2	2
5	4.7	Wilms (controlateral)	**Retro**	Partial nephrectomy	No	Wilms, stage 1	0
6	3.2	Nephroblastomatosis	**Retro**	Partial nephrectomy	No	Wilms, stage 1	0
7	14.1	Liver Tx for HBL	**Retro**	Partial nephrectomy	No	Tubulopapillary carcinoma	0
8	10.1	-	Trans	Nephrectomy	No	Wilms, stage 1	5
9	12.8	-	Trans	Nephrectomy	**Yes**	Sarcoma	10
10	3.5	-	Trans	Nephrectomy + splenectomy + distal pancreatectomy *	No	Wilms, stage 3 local (4)	15
11	9.8	Wilms (controlateral)	**Retro**	Partial nephrectomy	No	Wilms, stage 1	0
12	0.9	-	Trans	Nephrectomy	No	Wilms, stage 2	5
13	5	-	Trans	Nephrectomy	No	Wilms, stage 1	1
14	8.2	-	Trans	Nephrectomy	**Yes**	Wilms, stage 1	22
15	0.6	-	Trans	Nephrectomy	No	Wilms, stage 1	2
16	3.7	-	Trans	Nephrectomy	No	Wilms, stage 2	20
17	5.2	-	Trans	Nephrectomy	No	Wilms, stage 1	4
18	2.5	-	Trans	Nephrectomy *	**Yes**	Wilms, stage 3 local (4)	8
19	2.8	Nephroblastomatosis	Trans	Nephrectomy *	No	Wilms, stage 1	10
20	5.2	-	**Retro**	Partial nephrectomy	No	Nephrogenic rest	0

* partial diaphragmatic resection

Five RAL partial nephrectomies were performed for three WT, one tubulopapillary carcinoma and one nephrogenic rest. Tumor volume varied from 2 mL to 11.6 mL, console time from 110 to 140 min with the warm ischemia time from 19 to 40 min.

We did not experience any robot malfunction, system failures, or complications.

Macroscopic complete resection (R0) was achieved in all patients.

The median length of hospital stay was 4 days (2–7 days). Postoperative course was uneventful.

Tips and Tricks

- Gauze in the operating field in case of bleeding.
- Rectal tube to reduce the sigmoid distension.
- 20° tilt.

31.6 Discussion

We have recently reported our initial results of RAL total and partial nephrectomy and demonstrated its feasibility once oncological surgical ruled in carefully selected patients are adhered to [12]. Interestingly, transition from an open to a robotic assisted approach was carried out without the previous laparoscopic management of renal tumors in our institution. This cohort is, to our knowledge, the largest of RAL treatment of renal tumors in a pediatric population. This group represented 37% of the children that were operated for renal tumor during the same period in our department, a similar number to previous reports of laparoscopic nephrectomies for WT [3, 6]. All indications of the robotic approach were discussed at the tumor board. In eight cases, the tumor extended beyond the ipsilateral border of the spinal column, a criterion retained as a contraindication in the SIOP Umbrella protocol since the first publication of Varlet et al. on laparoscopic nephrectomy for renal tumors [13]. This was also reported in the recent series of laparoscopic nephrectomies of Burnand et al. who stressed the need of a high level of expertise in laparoscopic procedures to overcome this risk factor [4]. However, one of the authors (YH) underlined the superiority of RAL to overcome the difficulties of dissection of the renal pedicle in tumors crossing the midline. In case# 10, the benefit of the robotics when compared with laparoscopy were apparent; clear vision of the tumor limits was maintained, allowing easy and secure dissection of the involved organs and diaphragmatic repair. This patient had presented with hemoperitoneum at diagnosis before any treatment and therefore abdominal radiation therapy was planned regardless of intraoperative findings and histology. Enlarged nephrectomy including caudal pancreatectomy, splenectomy, lymphadenectomy, and partial diaphragmatic resection were performed to ensure R0 resection following neoadjuvant chemotherapy and it also indicated for open surgery. Finally, tumor infiltration of extrarenal structures is not considered a contraindication to RAL nephrectomy in adult renal cancer [14].

There was no upstaging due to the robotic procedure. The misdiagnosed renal vein thrombus in patient #3 was a complication related to the insufficiency of MRI and not to the type of surgery as it could have occurred during an open approach with the same consequence in terms of upstaging. This underlines the usefulness to systematically perform a Doppler US just before surgery, especially in the case of laparoscopic or RAL nephrectomy for WT. The conversion rate was 20% and was guided by safety in order to respect oncologic rules. The first case was due to a renal vein injury in the earlier days of our program in robotic surgery (14th case). With our current experience, this type of complication would now be managed while maintaining a robotic approach. Another conversion was due to a major bleeding on the renal vein and required an emergency undocking, the only one since the beginning of the multidisciplinary pediatric robotic program.

Lymph node sampling was facilitated by RAL, thereby minimizing the risk of understaging [3]. In this series, lymph node sampling was similar to the more recent series of MIS [1, 6] and compared favorably with open surgery [15]. Finally, we could reproduce the different steps of the open procedure and we were not hindered by the lack of haptic feedback, thanks to the 3D-HD vision.

NSS for unilateral WT has long been widely accepted in syndromic patients such as Denys–Drash, WAGR, and other WT1-related diseases and [16, 17] more recently applied to any unilateral WT that fulfilled the criteria of the Umbrella protocol [4]. In our experience, nephron-sparing surgery is usually performed by a transperitoneal open approach. With oncological input, a retroperitoneal approach was considered a better alternative in order to spare the peritoneal cavity (in case of new developing lesions) in these children already heavily treated. When margins are positive, this approach allows postoperative radiotherapy to be limited to retroperitoneal space avoiding in toto irradiation of the abdomen.

RAL nephrectomy and retroperitoneal robotic-assisted partial nephrectomy for pediatric renal tumors are feasible procedures in carefully selected patients after neoadjuvant chemotherapy. A high case selection was operated at our tumor board to identify patients eligible for RAL. This rigorous selection contributes to favorable outcome and shorter length of hospital stay. In our recent study, we have shown that, in comparison with the group of patients treated by an open approach, the hospital stay was shorter ($P = 0.01$). This procedure should be performed only once a robotic program is established and only by surgeons with significant experience in advanced oncological and MIS procedures. RAL surgery allows the surgeon to perform complex tasks in a minimally invasive manner and can reproduce all the steps of an open nephrectomy for renal tumor while maintaining the same rules of staging and oncologic dissection, with the advantages of a short hospital stay. Patient suitability is a major factor and requires an in-depth knowledge of pediatric cancer and ongoing multidisciplinary input particularly with medical oncologists and radiologists in order to avoid a widespread and uncontrolled application of the robotic approach.

Take-Home Points

- Required experience in advance laparoscopic and oncological procedure.
- High case selection at the tumor board to identify patients eligible for RAL.
- Bloodless field.

References

1. Duarte RJ, Dénes FT, Cristofani LM, Giron AM, Filho VO, Arap S. Laparoscopic nephrectomy for Wilms tumor after chemotherapy: initial experience. J Urol. 2004;172(4):1438–40. https://doi.org/10.1097/01.ju.0000138230.51134.65.
2. Barber TD, Wickiser JE, Wilcox DT, Baker LA. Prechemotherapy laparoscopic nephrectomy for Wilms' tumor. J Pediatr Urol. 2009;5(5):416–9. https://doi.org/10.1016/j.jpurol.2009.01.011.
3. Warmann SW, et al. Minimally invasive nephrectomy for Wilms tumors in children—data from SIOP 2001. J Pediatr Surg. 2014;49(11):1544–8. https://doi.org/10.1016/j.jpedsurg.2014.06.005.
4. Burnand K, Roberts A, Bouty A, Nightingale M, Campbell M, Heloury Y. Laparoscopic nephrectomy for Wilms' tumor: can we expand on the current SIOP criteria? J Pediatr Urol. 2018;14(3):253.e1–8. https://doi.org/10.1016/j.jpurol.2018.01.005.
5. Van Den Heuvel-Eibrink MM, et al. Position paper: rationale for the treatment of Wilms tumour in the UMBRELLA SIOP-RTSG 2016 protocol. Nat Rev Urol. 2017;14(12):743–52. https://doi.org/10.1038/nrurol.2017.163.
6. Bouty A, et al. What is the risk of local recurrence after laparoscopic transperitoneal radical nephrectomy in children with Wilms tumours? Analysis of a local series and review of the literature. J Pediatr Urol. 2018;14(4):327.e1–7. https://doi.org/10.1016/j.jpurol.2018.03.016.
7. Bouty A, et al. Minimally invasive surgery for unilateral Wilms tumors: multicenter retrospective analysis of 50 transperitoneal laparoscopic total nephrectomies. Pediatr Blood Cancer. 2020;67(5):e28212. https://doi.org/10.1002/pbc.28212.
8. Cost NG, Geller JI, Defoor WR, Wagner LM, Noh PH. A robotic-assisted laparoscopic approach for pediatric renal cell carcinoma allows for both nephron-sparing surgery and extended lymph node dissection. J Pediatr Surg. 2012;47(10):1946–50. https://doi.org/10.1016/j.jpedsurg.2012.08.017.
9. Cost NG, Liss ZJ, Bean CM, Geller JI, Minevich EA, Noh PH. Prechemotherapy robotic-assisted laparoscopic radical nephrectomy for an adolescent with wilms tumor. J Pediatr Hematol Oncol. 2015;37(2):e125–7. https://doi.org/10.1097/MPH.0000000000000193.

10. Meignan P, et al. Robotic-assisted laparoscopic surgery for pediatric tumors: a bicenter experience. J Robot Surg. 2018;12(3):501–8. https://doi.org/10.1007/s11701-017-0773-2.
11. Varda BK, Cho P, Wagner AA, Lee RS. Collaborating with our adult colleagues: a case series of robotic surgery for suspicious and cancerous lesions in children and young adults performed in a free-standing children's hospital. J Pediatr Urol. 2018;14(2):182.e1–8. https://doi.org/10.1016/j.jpurol.2018.01.003.
12. Blanc T, et al. Robotic-assisted laparoscopic management of renal tumors in children: preliminary results. Pediatr Blood Cancer. 2019;66(S3):e27867. https://doi.org/10.1002/pbc.27867.
13. Varlet F, et al. Laparoscopic treatment of renal cancer in children: a multicentric study and review of oncologic and surgical complications. J Pediatr Urol. 2014;10(3):500–5. https://doi.org/10.1016/j.jpurol.2013.11.005.
14. Peyronnet B, et al. Comparison of 1800 robotic and open partial nephrectomies for renal tumors. Ann Surg Oncol. 2016;23(13):4277–83. https://doi.org/10.1245/s10434-016-5411-0.
15. Ezekian B, et al. Comparing oncologic outcomes after minimally invasive and open surgery for pediatric neuroblastoma and Wilms tumor. Pediatr Blood Cancer. 2018;65(1):e26755. https://doi.org/10.1002/pbc.26755.
16. Rauth TP, Slone J, Crane G, Correa H, Friedman DL, Lovvorn HN. Laparoscopic nephron-sparing resection of synchronous Wilms tumors in a case of hyperplastic perilobar nephroblastomatosis. J Pediatr Surg. 2011;46(5):983–8. https://doi.org/10.1016/j.jpedsurg.2011.01.025.
17. Piché N, Barrieras D. Minimally invasive nephron-sparing surgery for unilateral Wilms tumor. J Pediatr Surg. 2012;47(7):e1. https://doi.org/10.1016/j.jpedsurg.2012.02.018.

MIS Management of Adrenal Tumors in Pediatric Patients

32

Luca Pio, Yves Heloury, Sabine Sarnacki, and Thomas Blanc

Learning Objectives

- To describe preoperative diagnostic setting and surgical preparation to the procedure.
- To describe step by step the various MIS approaches for pediatric adrenalectomy.
- To describe long-term outcomes of pediatric adrenalectomy.

32.1 Introduction

Adrenal tumors in children are neuroblastoma in the majority of pediatric case, with an incidence of 52% in the largest international series presented by Fascetti Leon in 2017 [1].

Other non-neuroblastic tumors originated from cortex or adrenal medulla have been described with a low incidence, and they are represented by pheochromocytomas, adrenocortical carcinoma, adenomas, and alveolar sarcoma.

Some rare macronodular and micronodular masses have been observed in case of syndromic diseases as Carney complex (an autosomical disease characterized by myomas, spotty skin pigmentation, and endocrine over-activity) and McCune Albright syndrome (characterized by peripheral precocious puberty, café-au lait skin spots, and endocrinopathies as acromegaly, hyperthyroidism, and ACTH-independent Cushing syndrome) [2, 3].

Clinical presentation of adrenal masses can range from asymptomatic patients to children with sweating, visual problems, behavioral alteration, headache, and glucocorticoid excess-related symptoms (malignant hypertension, coagulopathy, hyperlipidemia, obesity osteoporosis, impaired glucose tolerance, and diabetes).

Biochemical blood and urinary analysis play a crucial role in the differential diagnosis of adrenal masses, with the measurement of homovanillic acid (VMA) and homovanillic acid (HVA) and metanephrines.

As of now, several MIS approaches have been described, starting with the transperitoneal technique (which represents the surgical access of choice in more than 90% of cases) to the introduction of the retroperitoneal approach [4].

Supplementary Information The online version contains supplementary material available at [https://doi.org/10.1007/978-3-030-99280-4_32].

L. Pio (✉) · Y. Heloury · S. Sarnacki · T. Blanc
Pediatric Surgery Unit, Hôpital Necker-Enfants Malades, University of Paris, Paris, France
e-mail: luca.pio@aphp.fr; lucapio@gaslini.org; yves.heloury@aphp.fr; yves.heloury@gmail.com; sabine.sarnacki@aphp.fr; thomas.blanc@aphp.fr

C. Esposito et al. (eds.), *Minimally Invasive Techniques in Pediatric Urology*,
https://doi.org/10.1007/978-3-030-99280-4_32

32.2 Preoperative Preparation

Preoperative differential diagnosis of adrenal masses includes urine normetanephrine and norepinephrine tests and plasma renin activity, cortisol, aldosterone, adrenocorticotropic hormone (ACTH), dehydroepiandrosterone sulfate (DHEAS) in case of secreting mass.

Localizing imaging studies such as computed tomography (CT) scan (Fig. 32.1) and/or magnetic resonance imaging (MRI) (Fig. 32.2) are needed to evaluate the tumor size and the presence of radiological risk factors such as vascular or organ infiltration/contact in case of neuroblastic tumors [5].

In case of functional masses, a metaiodobenzylguanidine (MIBG) or a PET scan is needed to confirm a pheochromocytoma, adenoma, or neuroblastic secreting tumor.

In case of hypertension, a preoperative pharmacological preparation is mandatory, with a single treatment with alpha-blockers or in association with beta-blockers if the single pharmacological treatment is not sufficient [1, 6].

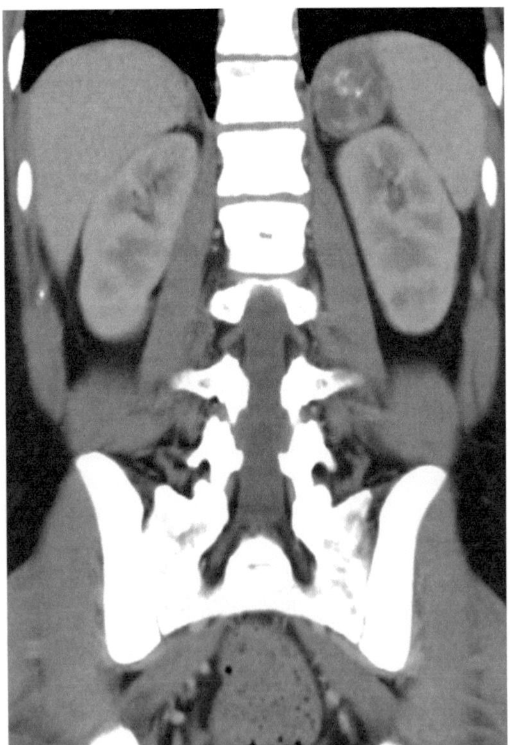

Fig. 32.1 Computed tomography scan with coronal plane: left adrenal mass

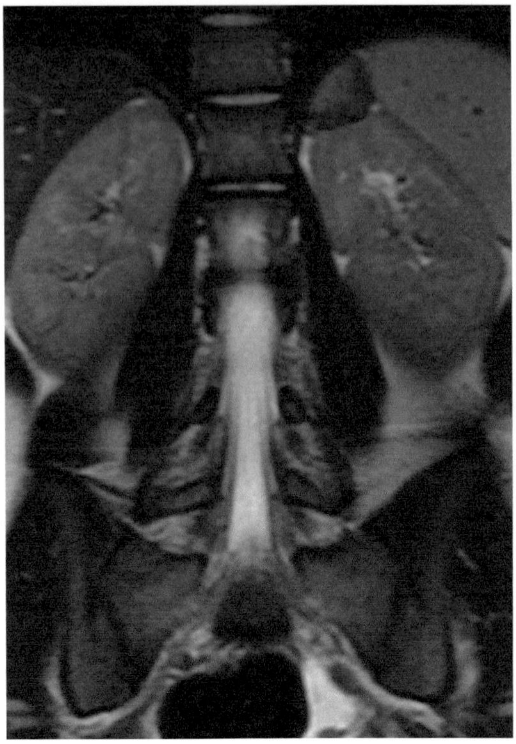

Fig. 32.2 Magnetic resonance imaging with coronal plane: left adrenal mass

An intestinal preparation is not necessary, and the pre-operative antibiotic prophylaxis with cephalosporine is sufficient to prevent postoperative infections [7].

General anesthesia is administered and a bladder catheter is not necessary. A nasogastric tube is placed in order to have a sufficient working space during the procedure.

32.3 Positioning

32.3.1 Positioning Depends on Surgical Approach

In case of transperitoneal approach, the patient is positioned in a lateral decubitus, elevated on a soft roll, a 10–12 mm or 5 mm (depending by child size) umbilical camera port was initially placed for a 30° camera, followed by 5-mm working ports placed in the epigastrium and in the right/left lower quadrant depending on tumor location to provide a good triangulation. 5-mm ports are preferred in order to provide the utilization of vessel sealer device. An additional 3 mm or 5 mm port was often required to provide liver or spleen retraction. Carbon dioxide insufflation is provided with 12 mmHg and 2 L/min pression.

For retroperitoneal approach, a first 10-mm port was placed in a half position between the 11th costal margin and the iliac crest via an open approach with a 2 cm incision until the Gerota's fascia without balloon system. The first operative 5 mm trocar is placed on the paravertebral side and the second one up to the iliac crest (Fig. 32.3).

Carbon dioxide insufflation was provided with 8 mmHg and 2 L/min pression.

Even if robotic surgery was previously described for pediatric abdominal tumors [8–10], this surgical approach was technically described only by Uwaydah [11]. The first optical 12 mm port was inserted in supraumbilical position, followed by a 8 mm trocar in the midline below the xiphoid and a second 8 mm operative port toward the anterior iliac crest, a fourth assistant port was placed suprapubically on the midline. Carbon dioxide insufflation is provided with 12 mmHg and 2 L/min pression.

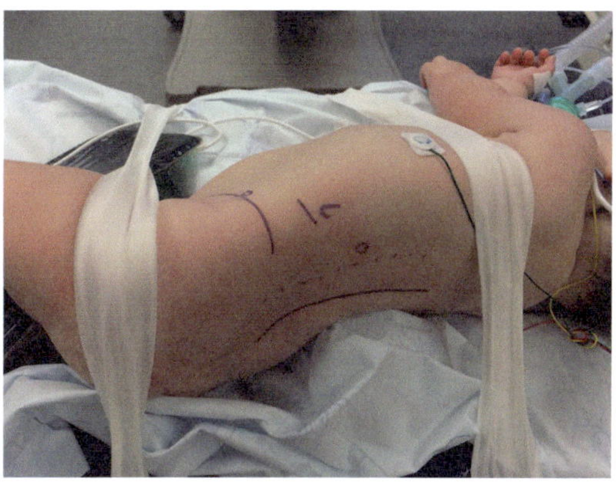

Fig. 32.3 Patient installation with retroperitoneal port position

32.4 Instrumentation

A 5-mm or 10-mm 30° optic and 5-mm instruments were used for conventional minimally invasive surgery (MIS). Instrumentation for conventional MIS (laparoscopy, retroperitoneoscopy) consisted in fenestrated grasping forceps, a curved dissector in case of vessel isolation, a monopolar hook 5 cautery to perform dissection, and a vessel sealer device (LigaSure™, Covidien, Boulder. CO, 80301–3299 USA) which is sufficient for the adrenal vessels dissection, laparoscopic clips are rarely necessary. A 10 mm endobag is normally sufficient to achieve tumor removal by umbilicus or suprapubic incision.

For robotic approach, monopolar curved scissor can provide the vast majority of tumor dissection, the other operative instrument can be fenestrated using bipolar forceps. A robotic vessel sealer device can provide an adequate vascular dissection.

32.5 Technique

In case of transperitonal approach, the phases of conventional MIS and robotic approach are the same.

The first step consisted of the access of the suprarenal space, which is possible opening the parietocolic peritoneum with a minimal displacement of the right/left colonic angle according to the tumor location.

The second step consisted of the adrenal dissection under the identification of the main vessels (vena cava for the right side and aorta for the left side). In case of right-sided adrenal masses, the duodenal identification is mandatory to avoid postoperative complications such as perforations during tumor dissection.

Adrenal vessels may originate from the renal vessels, aorta, vena cava, or from the diaphragm. Therefore, great care is taken in the dissection of the mass from these structures. Adrenal vessels are managed by a vessel sealer device.

When the tumor is freed, the mass can be placed in an endobag and extracted through the umbilical access or a suprapubic incision.

Retroperitoneal approach started opening the space between the Gerota's fascia and the lateral peritoneum (avoiding its opening), then the dissection was performed medially to laterally, starting with the vessel dissection using a sealing device. The tumor is removed through the camera port with an endobag or a first-finger surgical glove.

An indwelling abdominal drain is not usually necessary.

Morcellation of the tumor to achieve extraction is not advisable because of adequate margin assessment and to avoid bag rupture. Lymph node excision is performed only if enlarged local lymph nodes are identified.

32.6 Postoperative Care

Postoperative analgesia not required in opioid treatment and oral feeding is started the same day of the procedure. Length of hospital stay ranged from 2 to 4 postoperative days.

In case of bilateral adrenalectomy, a biological assessment with hormonal dosage is made daily at 1, 2, 3, 5, and at 7 days after surgery.

To avoid adrenal insufficiency, the intravenous cortisone supplementation was continued until feeding followed by progressive adaptation of oral treatment.

Postoperative control is planned together with oncologist, with a surgical control of 1 month postoperatively. Imaging control (CT scan or MRI) is planned according to the tumor histology.

32.7 Results

A recent European multicentric study [1] reported one of the largest series of pediatric adrenalectomy.

MIS is showed to be safe and effective to children with tumors up to 145 cc.

Presence of IDRFs such as renal pedicle contact is not related to postoperative recurrence and complications.

In this multicentric study, no conversion was observed. In bilateral tumor location, adrenal sparing resection has an elevated risk of tumor relapse, with 50% in the reported series and up to 38% in the previous reported studies [1, 12].

Transperitoneal surgery is the preferred approach, with a 92.8% incidence among the involved European pediatric surgeons.

Number of ports varied between 3 and 5 for unilateral location and 7–8 for bilateral tumors.

The multivariate analysis showed that number of ports is directly related to the increase in the length of hospital stay.

Clip-less approach was used in 58.4% of cases with a mean decrease of 35 min of operative time and a comparable bleeding control.

Univariate analyses showed a correlation between volume activity and length of hospital stay and operative time.

Robotic approach resulted to be feasible for reported series, but its indication is still debated and its superiority to conventional MIS has to be proved [8–11].

Tips and Tricks

- In case of secreting tumors, the preoperative pharmacological management is essential to ameliorate and to have a better control of perioperative anesthesia.
- Patient positioning is a crucial part of the perioperative procedure as it is necessary to achieve a good suprarenal area.
- The identification of vascular structures such as venal rein, vena cava, and aorta provide a safer tumor dissection (Fig. 32.4).
- Vessel sealer devices provide an adequate and safe vascular dissection as feeding tumor and adrenal vessels exceptionally have a diameter higher than 5–7 mm.
- Abdominal drain is not required; its absence ameliorates patient postoperative mobilization, reducing postoperative pain.

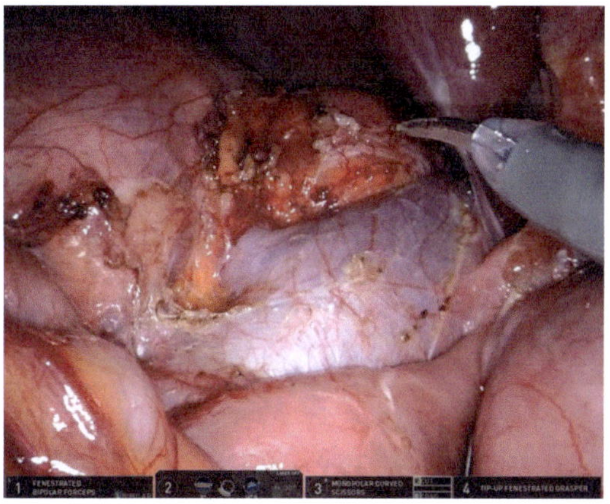

Fig. 32.4 Peri-operative robotic view: right adrenal tumor with IDRFs (contact with renal pedicle)

32.8 Discussion

MIS pediatric adrenalectomy became an accepted and established technique over the last decade [1, 4, 6]. Indications were established for a large spectrum of benign and malignant adrenal masses, including functional tumors.

MIS provides well-known advantages as less postoperative pain, image magnification, and best cosmetic results when compared to open surgery [13].

Several MIS approaches were described, based almost on the surgical center experience, with retroperitoneal approach preferred by pediatric urologist and the transperitoneal approach by the general pediatric surgeons.

Current literature supports the need of centralization of this type of procedure as centers with higher volume of patients have better surgical outcomes [1, 14], in addition to a MIS experience, surgeons must have surgical oncology skills, as the same surgical oncology principles must be respected.

An adequate preoperative management is mandatory to avoid pre-operative and post-operative complications related to the tumor ACTH or catecholamine secretion.

In the past, several surgical risk factors such as tumor size (>5 cm of diameter) and IDRFs were described [15, 16], but a recent multicentric study did not relate these surgical risk factors with an increased conversion rate of postoperative complications [1].

In case of bilateral location, the adrenal sparing procedure must be considered, as the need of life-long hormonal replacement therapy can be reduced in 78–90% of cases [17].

Technology advances provided several MIS devices which allow a good vascular control.

In the last years, robotic surgery gained more and more visibility also in pediatric surgical oncology [8, 9], but its advantages in terms of increase of indication and tumor operability of pre/postoperative outcomes compared to conventional MIS have to be defined.

In conclusion, MIS approaches are effective, providing good surgical and oncological outcomes. Future robotic innovations can improve MIS approach in terms of surgical indications and outcomes.

Take-Home Points

- Minimally invasive adrenalectomy requires surgical oncology skills and experience in laparoscopic procedures.
- Identification of vascular main structures of the working area allows to reduce perioperative complications.
- Sealing devices provide adequate vascular control, reducing operative time.

References

1. Fascetti-Leon F, Scotton G, Pio L, Beltrà R, Caione P, Esposito C, Mattioli G, Saxena AK, Sarnacki S, Gamba P. Minimally invasive resection of adrenal masses in infants and children: results of a European multicenter survey. Surg Endosc. 2017;31(11):4505–12.
2. Aarskog D, Tveteraas E. McCune-Albright's syndrome following adrenalectomy for Cushing's syndrome in infancy. J Pediatr. 1968;73(1):89–96.
3. Albiger M, Ceccato F, Zilio M, Sbarbot M, Occhi G, Rizzati S, Fassina A, Mantero F, Boscaro M, Iacobone M, Scaroni C. An analysis of different therapeutic options in patients with CS due to bilateral macronodular adrenal hyperplasia: a single-centre experience. Clin Endocrinol. 2015;82(6):808–15.
4. López PJ, Pierro A, Curry JI, Mushtaq I. Retroperitoneoscopic adrenalectomy: an early institutional experience. J Pediatr Urol. 2007;3(2):96–9.

5. Brisse HJ, McCarville MB, Granata C, Krug KB, Wootton-Gorges SL, Kanegawa K, Giammarile F, Schmidt M, Shulkin BL, Matthay KK, Lewington VJ, Sarnacki S, Hero B, Kaneko M, London WB, Pearson AD, Cohn SL, Monclair T, International Neuroblastoma Risk Group Project. Guidelines for imaging and staging of neuroblastic tumors: consensus report from the International Neuroblastoma Risk Group Project. Radiology. 2011;261(1):243–57.
6. International Pediatric Endosurgery Group. IPEG guidelines for the surgical treatment of adrenal masses in children. J Laparoendosc Adv Surg Tech A. 2010;20(2):7–9.
7. Pio L, Avanzini S, Paraboschi I, Wong M, Naselli A, Garaventa A, Conte M, Rosati U, Losurdo G, Fratino G, Martucciello G, Mattioli G, Castagnola E. Antibiotic prophylaxis in children undergoing abdominal surgery for neoplastic diseases. Infez Med. 2018;26(2):122–5.
8. Blanc T, Pio L, Clermidi P, Muller C, Orbach D, Minard-Colin V, Harte C, Meignan P, Kohaut J, Heloury Y, Sarnacki S. Robotic-assisted laparoscopic management of renal tumors in children: preliminary results. Pediatr Blood Cancer. 2019;66(Suppl 3):e27867.
9. Meignan P, Ballouhey Q, Lejeune J, Braik K, Longis B, Cook AR, Lardy H, Fourcade L, Binet A. Robotic-assisted laparoscopic surgery for pediatric tumors: a bicenter experience. J Robot Surg. 2018;12(3):501–8.
10. Mattioli G, Pini Prato A, Razore B, Leonelli L, Pio L, Avanzini S, Boscarelli A, Barabino P, Disma NM, Zanaboni C, Garzi A, Martigli SP, Buffi NM, Rosati U, Petralia P. Da Vinci robotic surgery in a pediatric hospital. J Laparoendosc Adv Surg Tech A. 2017;27(5):539–45.
11. Uwaydah NI, Jones A, Elkaissi M, Yu Z, Palmer BW. Pediatric robot-assisted laparoscopic radical adrenalectomy and lymph-node dissection for neuroblastoma in a 15-month-old. J Robot Surg. 2014;8(3):289–93.
12. Waguespack SG, Rich T, Grubbs E, Ying AK, Perrier ND, Ayala-Ramirez M, Jimenez C. A current review of the etiology, diagnosis, and treatment of pediatric pheochromocytoma and paraganglioma. J Clin Endocrinol Metab. 2010;95(5):2023–37.
13. Leclair MD, de Lagausie P, Becmeur F, Varlet F, Thomas C, Valla JS, Petit T, Philippe-Chomette P, Mure PY, Sarnacki S, Michon J, Heloury Y. Laparoscopic resection of abdominal neuroblastoma. Ann Surg Oncol. 2008;15(1):117–24.
14. Al-Shanafey S, Habib Z. Feasibility and safety of laparoscopic adrenalectomy in children: special emphasis on neoplastic lesions. J Laparoendosc Adv Surg Tech A. 2008;18(2):306–9.
15. Cecchetto G, Riccipetitoni G, Inserra A, Esposito C, Michelazzi A, Ruggeri G, Spinelli C, Lima M, Italian Group of Pediatric Surgical Oncology. Minimally-invasive surgery in paediatric oncology: proposal of recommendations. Pediatr Med Chir. 2010;32(5):197–201.
16. Irtan S, Brisse HJ, Minard-Colin V, Schleiermacher G, Canale S, Sarnacki S. Minimally invasive surgery of neuroblastic tumors in children: indications depend on anatomical location and image-defined risk factors. Pediatr Blood Cancer. 2015;62(2):257–61.
17. Lenders JW, Duh QY, Eisenhofer G, Gimenez-Roqueplo AP, Grebe SK, Murad MH, Naruse M, Pacak K, Young WF Jr, Endocrine Society. Pheochromocytoma and paraganglioma: an endocrine society clinical practice guideline. J Clin Endocrinol Metab. 2014;99(6):1915–42.

Part III

Ureter

Endoscopic Treatment of Primary Obstructive Megaureter

33

José María Angulo, Rubén Ortiz, Laura Burgos, Beatriz Fernández, Javier Ordoñez, and Alberto Parente

Learning Objectives

- To describe in detail the endoscopic balloon dilation technique in POM cases.
- To report our results, complications, and long-term outcomes of EBD.
- To report the updated results and outcomes of international papers concerning this technique.
- To show a video of EBD procedure step by step and modifications done along the last years.
- To describe tips and tricks for EBD in POM, suitable for other endourological techniques in children.

33.1 Introduction

Primary obstructive megaureter (POM) resolves spontaneously in most cases during early months of life, and only a minority of patients will need surgical treatment [1, 2].

However, the adequate treatment of POM remains controversial since it has been changing in the last two decades, especially regarding the outcomes of endoscopic approach compared to traditional techniques.

Ureteral reimplantation with or without ureteral tapering has been considered the gold standard procedure for these patients; but, reimplantation of a grossly dilated ureter in a small infant bladder entails difficulty and potential complications [3, 4].

In the last decade, endoscopic treatment with high-pressure balloon dilation of the vesicoureteral junction (VUJ) has been reported with good results and outcomes, closely to the standard surgical procedure. Several authors have reported that these outcomes are maintained in long-term

Supplementary Information The online version contains supplementary material available at [https://doi.org/10.1007/978-3-030-99280-4_33].

J. M. Angulo (✉) · R. Ortiz · L. Burgos
B. Fernández · J. Ordoñez
Pediatric Urology Unit, Department of Pediatric Surgery, Hospital Universitario Gregorio Marañón, Madrid, Spain
e-mail: jmangulo_@hotmail.com; josemaria.angulo@salud.madrid.org; Ruben.ortiz@salud.madrid.org; Laura.burgos@salud.madrid.org; bfbautista@salud.madrid.org; javier.orodnez@salud.madrid.org

A. Parente
Pediatric Urology Unit, Department of Pediatric Surgery, Hospital Universitario Gregorio Marañón, Madrid, Spain

Pediatric Urology Department, Reina Sofia University Hospital, Córdoba, Spain
e-mail: alberto.parente@salud.madrid.org

C. Esposito et al. (eds.), *Minimally Invasive Techniques in Pediatric Urology*,
https://doi.org/10.1007/978-3-030-99280-4_33

with low and acceptable complication rate, which makes endoscopic balloon dilation a preferred treatment option for the surgical management of POM even in small infants [5–7].

This chapter is focused on the endoscopic high-pressure balloon dilation technique in POM cases with surgical criteria, reporting updated results, complications, outcomes, and controversies of this procedure.

33.2 Pre-Operative Preparation

Preoperative examinations are focused on the diagnosis of POM ruling out other urological conditions. Primary obstructive megaureter is defined and managed according to the international guidelines and consensus statement of this entity [8]. Ultrasound is used to measure the anteroposterior diameter of the renal pelvis, calyces, renal parenchyma, and ureter. Ureterohydronephrosis (UHN) grade is defined according to the guidelines of the Society of Fetal Urology Classification and Urinary Tract Dilatation Grading System [9].US scan is done at birth (in cases of prenatal diagnosis), at 1 month of life, and then every 3 months under conservative surveillance with low-dose antibiotic prophylaxis. Vesicoureteral reflux is ruled out in all patients with voiding cystourethrography. MAG-3 diuretic renal scan is done to reveal renal function and ureteral drainage, considering washout half time T1/2 > 20 min after furosemide injection as obstruction, with progressive cumulative radiotracer in ureteral area.

Surgery is indicated in those symptomatic POM cases with febrile UTI despite antibiotic prophylaxis, in those with loss of renal function or in cases of ureterohydronephrosis worsening with renal parenchyma thinning during expectative surveillance.

Parents have to sign a specifically formulated informed consent before the procedure. Patients receive midazolam (0.3–0.5 mg/k) 30 min before the intervention, and then general anaesthesia with laryngeal mask. Preoperative antibiotic prophylaxis (amoxicillin-clavulanic acid 30 mg/k) is administered during anaesthesia induction.

33.3 Positioning

The patient is placed in lithotomy position, with a foam roller (appropriate for infant's size) under each leg in infants and children under 15 k or adequate leg loops for bigger children. A heating wrap or blanket is used to cover the patient's body. The surgeon and the assistant stand at the edge of the surgical bench with access to the patient's urethra. The fluoroscopy c-arm is disposed on one side of the bench, the cystoscopy monitor on the other side, and the x-ray monitor in front of the surgeon (Fig. 33.1).

33.4 Instrumentation

Regarding the cystoscopy, we use a 9.5 f cystoscope with 5f working channel. In case we want to perform a retrograde pyelography prior to the

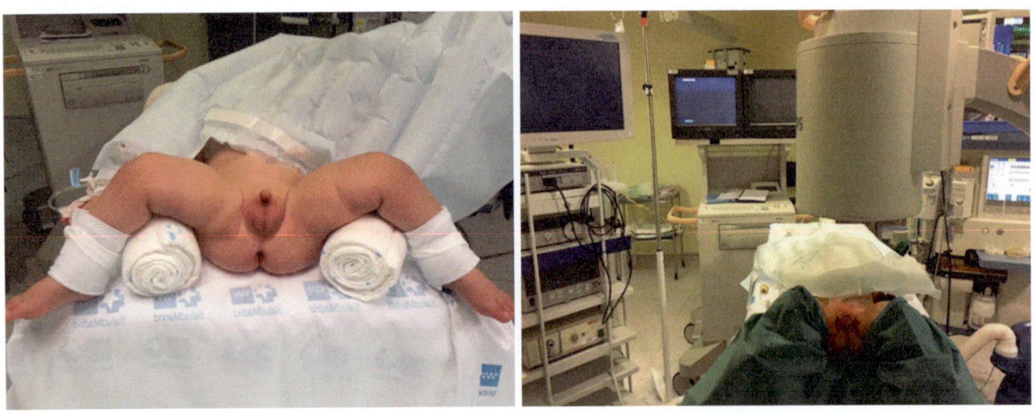

Fig. 33.1 Patient position

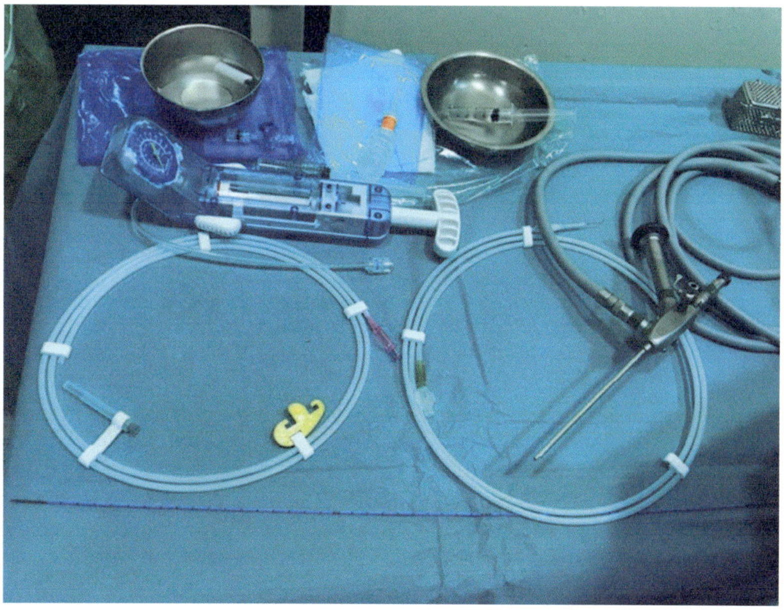

Fig. 33.2 Material needed: Cystoscope (9.5Fr), ureteral catheter (3Fr), guide-wire (0.014″–0.018″), endoscopic balloon catheter, pressure inflation pump, radiologic contrast agent, double J stent

EBD, a perforated 3f ureteral catheter and radiological contrastagent are needed (we dilute it 50% with saline).

Passing a guide through the affected vesicoureteral junction is mandatory prior to performing the dilation. Guide-wires should be hydrophilic and soft on the tip. We usually adopt 0.018″ (*Radiofocus, Terumo*®) or 0.014″ (*Choice PT* ™ *J-tip, Boston Scientific*). It is important to take care to use guide-wires by which the catheter balloon can easily progress. The balloons we choose for the dilation procedure are semi-compliant 3.1Fr high-pressure balloon catheters with nominal balloon diameter from 5 to 7 mm and 2 cm length (*RX Muso*™*, Terumo*). These low-profile balloons easily run through the cystoscope working channel and allow to do the dilation procedure under cystoscopic vision. Other catheter balloons with profile >5Fr are useful for the technique too, but they don't run through the cystoscope and may complicate the procedure. A pressure inflation pump is required to fill the balloons.

After EBD is done, a double-J stent catheter is placed. In infants under 1 year old, we are used to placing 3Fr, 8–12 cm long (*Sof-Flex Multi-Length Ureteral Stents Cook Medical Europe*™) and in children between 1 and 3 years old, 3Fr–14 cm long stents and over 3 years 4.8Fr 16–20 cm (Fig. 33.2).

33.5 Technique

We start doing the cystoscopy, checking the urethra in males and the normal position of ureteral meatus. For some early cases of our series, a retrograde pyelography was performed before dilation, using contrast through a 3Fr ureteral catheter (Fig. 33.3).

A hydrophilic guide-wire (0.014″–0.018″) is introduced through the VUJ, followed by the dilating balloon. When the balloon is located at the VUJ, it is filled with radiologic contrast to its nominal pressure (14–16 atm) with a pressure inflation device, under direct and fluoroscopic control until the complete disappearance of the stenosis. Successful dilation is considered when the stenotic notch completely disappears, and the balloon is removed immediately after (see Figs. 33.3 and 33.4).

After dilation, the cystoscope is introduced through the distal ureter to assess the VUJ and a double J stent is placed. A bladder catheter is left after the procedure during 24 h to prevent complications.

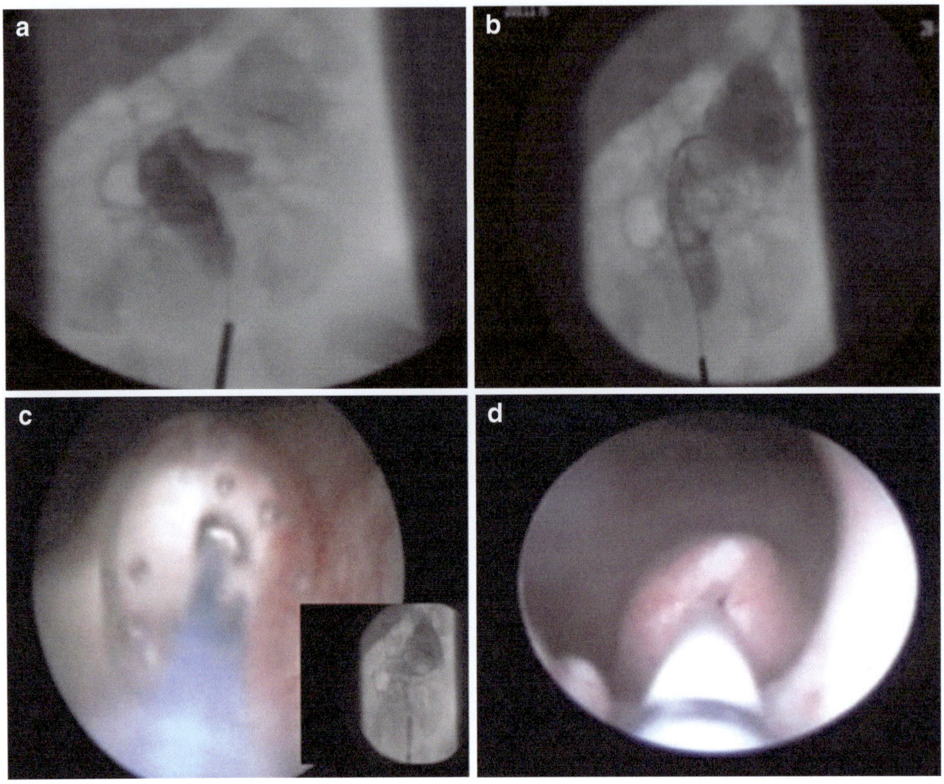

Fig. 33.3 Retrograde pyelography and EBD under fluoroscopic guidance. (**a**) Radiological contrast is introduced through a ureteral catheter showing the megaureter. (**b**) Passing the wire to the renal pelvis. (**c**) The balloon is located at the VUJ and inflated under radioscopic guidance. (**d**) Double J stent placement (renal pelvis bladder)

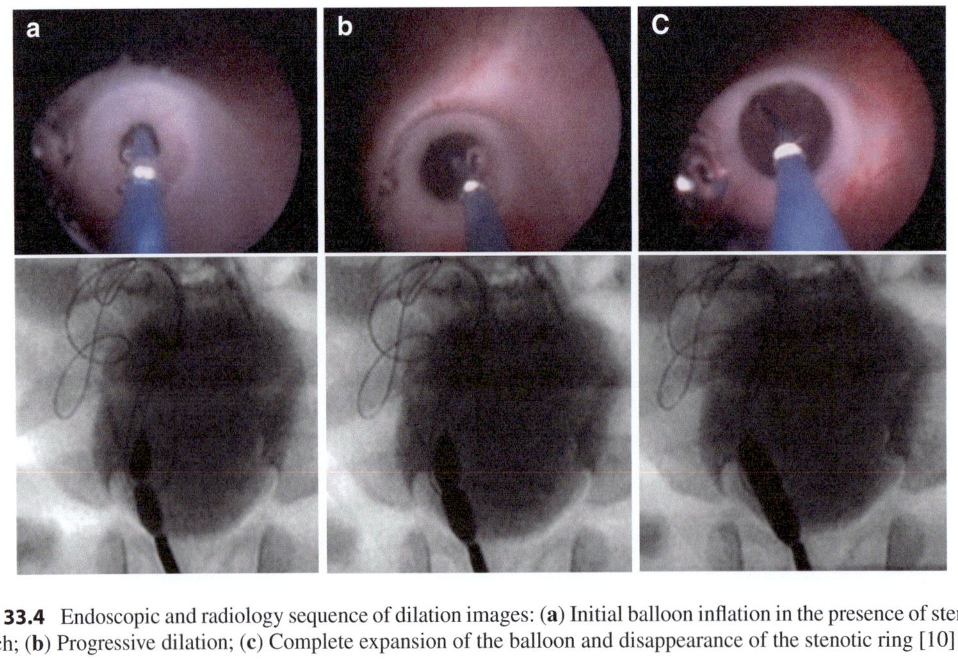

Fig. 33.4 Endoscopic and radiology sequence of dilation images: (**a**) Initial balloon inflation in the presence of stenotic notch; (**b**) Progressive dilation; (**c**) Complete expansion of the balloon and disappearance of the stenotic ring [10]

33.6 Postoperative Care

Patients start oral feeding 1–2 h after the procedure. Analgesic drugs required are metamizole (10–40 mg/k) or Paracetamol (10–15 mg/k) at 8 h interval. Bladder catheter is usually withdrawn at 24 h and patients are discharged from hospital after spontaneous micturition with oral analgesia and antibiotic prophylaxis.

Double-J stents are removed at 4–6 weeks in a second cystoscopy. At this time, the VUJ is calibrated by distal ureteroscopy.

Follow-up protocol consists of clinical reviews with US at 3, 6, 12, and 18 months after double-J stent removal, and then annually. MAG-3–furosemide renogram scan is performed at 6 and 18 months. Antibiotic prophylaxis is stopped when US showed improvement in UHN or adequate renal drainage at the postoperative diuretic renogram. In the last years, renogram at 18-postoperative month was not done if UHN had significantly reduced. Cystography is only indicated in symptomatic patients who present UTI during follow-up or persistent urinary tract dilatation without obstruction at the MAG-3 renogram.

33.7 Results

We have recently reported the experience of our institution since year 2004 in 79 consecutive POM cases with a median follow-up of 5.6 years (1.5–13.5) [10].

Median age at surgery was 4 months (0.5–44), with median operating time of 20 min (10–60) and median hospital stay of 1 day (1–7). Intraoperative complications occurred in four cases (5.1%). EBD could not be performed because of failure of the guide-wire to pass through the VUJ in two children who underwent ureteral reimplantation thereafter, and troublesome dilation with false path occurred in other two, requiring temporary nephrostomy and then open ureteral reimplantation. Early complications were reported in six cases (7.8%), being UTI after the endoscopic procedure or after Doube J stent removal in five (Clavien–Dindo 1). The other patient presented postoperative ureteral double J stent migration and developed early severe re-stenosis with pyonephrosis, requiring nephrostomy (Clavien–Dindo 3) and subsequent open ureteral reimplantation weeks later.

Ureterohydronephrosis grade significantly improved after endoscopic balloon dilatation, showing progressive decrease in urinary tract dilation and renal parenchyma improvement in those with thinned renal parenchyma detected prior to the intervention. Significant preoperative–postoperative differences were reported in hydronephrosis grade, ureteral diameter and renal parenchyma thinning that were maintained in the long-term (Table 33.1).

Statistical analysis revealed significant differences in renal drainage on the MAG-3 diuretic renogram before and after endoscopic treatment ($T1/2 > 50$ min vs. 9.8 ± 4.5 min, $p < 0.001$ *T*-test) and in the renal function (mean DRF 44.4% ± 6.3 vs. 46.2 ± 5.9 $p < 0.05$) with no subsequent function deterioration in any case.

Postoperative secondary vesicoureteral reflux (VUR) was detected during long-term surveillance in 17 cases (21.5%). Endoscopic treatment with sub-ureteral injection of *Deflux*™ was successful in 13 patients (76.4%) and failed in 4 (23.6%) on whom open surgery was indicated.

Long-term re-stenosis occurred in nine cases (12.2%). A new EBD procedure was successfully done in eight cases (88.9%) at a median postoperative period of 9.5 months (5–63). Only one patient developed re-stenosis recurrence and finally required ureteral reimplantation.

Endoscopic approach of POM had a long-term success rate in our series of 69/79 (87.3%). We considered failure of the technique in those

Table 33.1 Renal US findings after successful EBD [10]

	Pre-operatory	Early p.o. US	Long-term p.o. US	*p* Value
Mean pelvis diameter (mm) ($n = 74$)	19.2 ± 4.9	10.3 ± 5.5	5.2 ± 3.5	<0.001 (*T*-test)
Mean ureteral diameter (mm) ($n = 74$)	14.9 ± 2.9	9.2 ± 4.2	6.6 ± 6.5	<0.001 (*T*-test)
Mean parenchyma thickness (mm) ($n = 49$)	4.1 ± 1.6	5.5 ± 2.2	8.3 ± 2.4	<0.001 (*T*-test)

Table 33.2 Comparison between fluoroscopic guidance or not during the EBD procedure [10]

	Initial failure	Early p.o. complication	2° VUR	Long-term re-stenosis	Long-term ureteral reimplantation	Final outcome (failure/success)
Fluoroscopic ($n = 43$)	2	3[a]	10	5	3	6/37
No fluoroscopic	2	3	7	4	2	4/32
($n = 36$)	4	6	17	9	5	10/69

[a]Early postoperative complications were 5 UTI and 1 severe re-stenosis with JJ migration and pyonephrosis that required open ureteral reimplantation (fluoroscopic group)
Spearman's correlation test $p > 0.05$.

cases that required ureteral reimplantation ($n = 10$). Five were early failures of the technique, and the other five were long-term reimplantation due to refractory secondary reflux ($n = 4$) and re-stenosis recurrence ($n = 1$). Nevertheless, if we focus on ureteral obstruction resolution, the long-term outcomes for normalization of urinary drainage and preserving initial renal function were 92.4% (73 of 79).

We treated a total of 43/79 POM under the original EBD technique described with fluoroscopic guidance until year 2011. Since then, 36/79 underwent dilation procedure of the VUJ without radioscopic control being double J catheters left on the dilated ureter instead. Statistical analysis did not reveal significant differences comparing the use of fluoroscopic guidance at the procedure in technical failure, postoperative complications, secondary VUR, re-stenosis, long-term ureteral reimplantation, and final outcome (Table 33.2).

Tips and Tricks

- Once the technique was consolidated after overcoming an important learning curve, we realized that the procedure could be performed only under cystoscopic vision, avoiding unnecessary radiation in the majority of patients. For this reason, since year 2011, we have been doing the balloon dilation without fluoroscopic control. Performing a retrograde ureteropyelography through a narrow meatus may be challenging and produce mucosal inflammation, oedema, or bleeding that may complicate the subsequent endoscopic procedure. In the same way, overtaking the ureteral loops with the guide-wire may be technically demanding, time-consuming, and it implies unnecessary radiation exposure for the baby. Therefore, the guide-wire and the double J stent are not meant to reach the renal pelvis, but they are left in the dilated ureter instead. We actually obviate the retrograde pyelography, the wire is directly introduced into the ureter and the EBD is done only under cystoscopic vision, with no radiological exposure during the procedure. After the complete release of the stenosis, the cystoscope is progressed to the distal ureter, the balloon is removed and a double j stent is left "in situ" between the dilated ureter and bladder (Fig. 33.5).
- However, the success of the EBD technique lies in the use of adequate endoscopic material according to paediatric age. The selection of appropriate hydrophilic guide-wires (0.014″–0.018″), balloon catheters with low profile (3F), and double-J stents suitable for patient's age and size are crucial both for the success of the technique and to avoid complications. It is a common error to think that any endourologic material can be useful for this approach, and often leads to technical difficulty, complications, and failure.

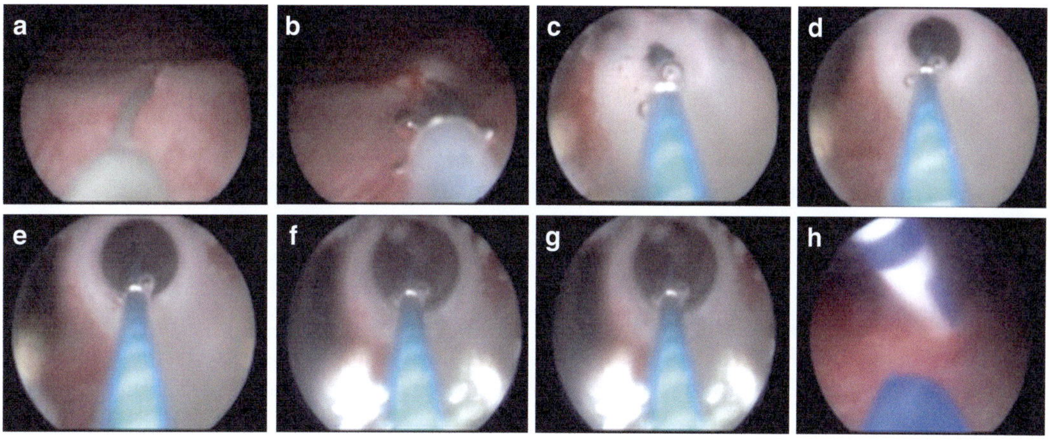

Fig. 33.5 Endoscopic balloon dilatation with no fluoroscopic guidance. (**a**) Inserting the guide-wire into the ureter. (**b**) Progressing the balloon through the wire and locating it at VUJ. (**c–f**) Balloon dilatation procedure under cystoscopic vision. (**g**) Distal ureteroscopy and balloon removal. (**h**) Double-J stent placement (ureter bladder)

33.8 Discussion

Less-invasive procedures such as endoscopic approaches have emerged aiming to avoid the challenge of reimplantation of a grossly dilated ureter in a small infantile bladder and its potential complications [3, 4], becoming so popular in the last decades.

Endoscopic balloon dilation was first described by Angulo et al. [11] in 1998 as initial treatment for children with complicated POM. Since then several publications with few patients and short follow-up periods proved that EBD was a feasible, safe, and less-invasive procedure for the initial management of POM with surgical criteria even for very young patients. In 2007, Angerri et al. [12] reported their initial experience with six patients in whom urinary obstruction disappeared without associated complications in a median follow-up of 31 months. Torino et al. [13] presented five cases treated below 1 year of age, with resolution of the obstruction after a mean follow-up of 23.8 months. Christman et al. [14] reported in 2012 their experience after the treatment of 17 children with a follow-up of 3.2 years. These authors added a laser incision in cases of ureteral stenosis greater than 2 cm and placed two double J stent in the ureter simultaneously, reporting good long-term outcome with disappearance of hydroureteronephrosis in 71% of the series. García-Aparicio et al. [15] presented a series of 13 patients with a medium-term success rate of 84.6% (11/13), requiring ureteral reimplantation in three patients (2 persistence of UHN and 1 refractory secondary VUR).

Recent publications have focused on establishing long-term effectiveness of EBD as definitive treatment of POM, confirming good outcomes with minimal associated morbidity. Romero et al. [5] reported in 2014 the experience of our institution in 29 patients treated until 2010, with a median follow-up of 47 months. It was concluded that the patients who had a favourable evolution with disappearance of the UHN and adequate renal drainage confirmed by renogram remained asymptomatic and with stable situation during the subsequent follow-up. Bujons et al. [6] reported in 2015 excellent results in 19 patients, with a long-term success of 90% after the initial dilatation procedure and a follow-up of 6.9 years. One patient required a second dilatation due to re-stenosis, and another one endoscopic treatment of 2° VUR, both with good outcome. Casal et al. [7] reported in 2018 good outcomes in a short series of 13 patients, but with an important median follow-up of 10.3 years (4.7–12.2), asserting the value of balloon dilation as a definitive treatment for POM. A multicentric study carried out by four referral French centres has been recently published by Kassite et al. [16], presenting their initial experience with 42 ureters treated by endoscopic HPBD between 2012 and 2017. They reported only four cases that required surgical treatment, so ureteral reimplantation was avoided in 90% cases with a median follow-up of 24 months. They reported 50% complications rate mainly related to double J stents.

Technical variations to the initial EBD procedure have been proposed with encouraging results. Capozza et al. [17] published the dilation of the VUJ with cutting-balloon™ in three patients with persistence of the stenotic ring during the previous endoscopic high-pressure balloon dilation, obtaining a complete resolution of the stenosis and good mid-term postoperative course.

Despite the advantages described of EBD, the endourological management of POM remains controversial. The aspects to be discussed focus on secondary VUR, the possibility of re-stenosis, and the use of radiation. Additionally, it is difficult to assess its value as a definitive treatment in POM attending to the short experience reported in the literature and the absence of prospective comparative studies.

Regarding secondary VUR, García-Aparicio [18] analysed it in his group of patients, reporting 27% (6 cases of 22 POM treated). The author concluded that the coexistence of ipsilateral paraureteral diverticulum is a risk factor for developing secondary VUR; however, the number of cases was very low (2 of 4). In the series published by Bujons et al. [6], only 1 case of 19 presented secondary VUR, and it was resolved endoscopically. We reported a 23% of secondary VUR, being successfully treated by endoscopic injection in 13 patients (76.4%). Three of these patients who developed secondary reflux had an ipsilateral para-meatal diverticulum, but only one required reimplantation. In our experience, the presence of para-meatal diverticulum was not a bad prognosis factor for the endoscopic management of POM, since 10 of 12 cases of the series had good outcome [10]. Kassite et al. [16] have not reported any case of secondary reflux in their multicentric study, but a longer follow-up period is needed.

Romero RM has recently exposed the IDEAL framework model as tool for the systematic review of POM treated by endoscopic high-pressure balloon dilatation [19]. The IDEAL framework and recommendations allowed a systematic analysis of the evidence quality of the reported experience in endoscopic balloon dilation of the VUJ in POM. The available evidence demonstrates that HPBD is an effective treatment in POM, with low morbidity and long-term success rate of 87.7%.

Take-Home Points

- Endoscopic high-pressure balloon dilation is a safe, feasible, and really less-invasive technique for POM.
- The use of adequate endourologic material according to the paediatric age and size is essential both for the success of the technique and to avoid complications.
- It is required a moderate experience in endourologic approaches. However, it is a relatively simple technique, reproducible with a short learning curve compared to other procedures.
- This technique avoids bladder surgery in the majority of cases. Nevertheless, it doesn't invalidate ureteral reimplantation in case of failure.

References

1. Di Renzo D, Aguiar L, Cascini V, Di Nicola M, McCarten KM, Ellsworth PI, et al. Long-term followup of primary nonrefluxing megaureter. J Urol. 2013;190:1021–6. https://doi.org/10.1016/j.juro.2013.03.008.
2. Braga LH, D'Cruz J, Rickard M, Jegatheeswaran K, Lorenzo AJ. The fate of primary nonrefluxing megaureter: a prospective outcome analysis of the rate of urinary tract infections, surgical indications and time to resolution. J Urol. 2016;195(4 Pt 2):1300–5. https://doi.org/10.1016/j.juro.2015.11.049.
3. Hendren WH. Complications of megaureter repair in children. J Urol. 1975;113:238–54. https://doi.org/10.1016/S0022-5347(17)59454-9.

4. Perdzynski W, Kalicinsky ZH. Long-term results after megaureter folding in children. J Pediatr Surg. 1996;31:1211–7.
5. Romero RM, Angulo JM, Parente A, Rivas S, Tardaguila AR. Primary obstructive megaureter: the role of high pressure balloon dilation. J Endourol. 2014;28:517–23. https://doi.org/10.1089/end.2013.0210.
6. Bujons A, Saldana L, Caffaratti J, Garat JM, Angerri O, Villavicencio H. Can endoscopic balloon dilation for primary obstructive megaureter be effective in a long-term follow-up? J Pediatr Urol. 2015;11:37.e1–6. https://doi.org/10.1016/j.jpurol.2014.09.005.
7. CasalBeloy I, Somoza Argibay I, García González M, García Novoa MA, Míguez Fortes LM, Dargallo CT. Endoscopic balloon dilatation in primary obstructive megaureter: long-term results. J Pediatr Urol. 2018;14:167.e1–5. https://doi.org/10.1016/j.jpurol.2017.10.016.
8. Farrugia MK, Hitchcock R, Radford A, Burki T, Murphy F, et al. British Association of Paediatric Urologists consensus statement on the management of the primary obstructive megaureter. J Pediatr Urol. 2014;10:26–33. https://doi.org/10.1016/j.jpurol.2013.09.018.
9. Braga LH, McGrath M, Farrokhyar F, Jegatheeswaran K, Lorenzo AJ. Society for Fetal Urology Classification vs urinary tract dilation grading system for prognostication in prenatal Hydronephrosis: a time to resolution analysis. J Urol. 2018;199(6):1615–21.
10. Ortiz R, Parente A, Perez-Egido L, Burgos L, Angulo JM. Long-term outcomes in primary obstructive megaureter treated by endoscopic balloon dilation. Experience after 100 cases. Front Pediatr. 2018;6:275. https://doi.org/10.3389/fped.2018.00275.
11. Angulo JM, Arteaga R, Rodriguez Alarcon J, Calvo MJ. Role of retrograde endoscopic dilatation with balloon and derivation using double pig-tail catheter as an initial treatment for vesico-ureteral junction stenosis in children. Cir Pediatr. 1998;11:15–8.
12. Angerri O, Caffaratti J, Garat JM, Villavicencio H. Primary obstructive megaureter: initial experience with endoscopic dilatation. J Endourol. 2007;21:999–1004. https://doi.org/10.1089/end.2006.0122.
13. Torino G, Collura G, Mele E, Garganese MC, Capozza N. Severe primary obstructive megaureter in the first year of life: preliminary experience with endoscopic balloon dilation. J Endourol. 2012;26:325–9. https://doi.org/10.1089/end.2011.0399.
14. Christman MS, Kasturi S, Lambert SM, Kovell RC, Casale P. Endoscopic management and the role of double stenting for primary obstructive megaureters. J Urol. 2012;187:1018–22. https://doi.org/10.1016/j.juro.2011.10.168.
15. Garcia-Aparicio L, Rodo J, Krauel L, Palazon P, Martin O, Ribo JM. High pressure balloon dilation of the ureterovesical junction–first line approach to treat primary obstructive megaureter? J Urol. 2012;187:1834–8. https://doi.org/10.1016/j.juro.2011.12.098.
16. Kassite I, Renaux Petel M, Chaussy Y, Eyssartier E, Alzahrani K, Sczwarc C, Villemagne T, Lardy H, Braik K, Binet A. High pressure balloon dilatation of primary obstructive megaureter in children: a multicenter study. Front Pediatr. 2018;6:329. https://doi.org/10.3389/fped.2018.00329.
17. Capozza N, Torino G, Nappo S, Collura G, Mele E. Primary obstructive megaureter in infants: our experience with endoscopic balloon dilation and cutting balloon ureterotomy. J Endourol. 2015;29:1–5. https://doi.org/10.1089/end.2013.0665.
18. García-Aparicio L, Blázquez-Gómez E, de Haro I, et al. Postoperative vesicoureteral reflux after high-pressure balloon dilation of the ureterovesical junction in primary obstructive megaureter. Incidence, management and predisposing factors. World J Urol. 2015;33(12):2103–6. https://doi.org/10.1007/s00345-015-1565-9.
19. Romero RM. Management of Primary Obstructive Megaureter by Endoscopic High-Pressure Balloon Dilatation. IDEAL framework model as a new tool for systematic review. Front Surg. 2019;6:20. https://doi.org/10.3389/fsurg.2019.00020.

Laparoscopic Management of the Primary Obstructive Megaureter

34

Manuel Lopez, Romy Gander, Gloria Royo, and Marino Asensio

Learning Objectives

- To describe step by step the technique of LUER.
- To report long-term results of and compare with existing literature.
- To present our evolution in technique.
- To describe tips and tricks.
- To show a video of LUER technique.

34.1 Introduction

Primary obstructed megaureter (POM) constitutes 10% of uropathies, with clinical significance detected prenatally. The overall incidence is in the range of 1:1500–1:2000. Currently, the ureters with retrovesical diameter < 7 mm from 30 weeks' gestation onward are considered abnormal [1].

The guidelines propose that an initial differential renal function (DRF) below 40%, or a drop in DRF of 5% on serial scans, and an increasing dilatation on serial ultrasound scans are considered suggestive of obstruction [2]. The majority of cases of POM are managed with conservative treatment, making this approach the current option for initial medical care [2–4]. Historically, ureteral reimplantation and tapering by extravesical or transvesical approach have been the surgical treatment of choice [5]. Distal ureteral tailoring is often necessary to achieve an adequate length-to-diameter ratio that is required for successful non-refluxing reimplantation.

Today, there are multiple possibilities for minimal invasive treatment, including endoscopic, laparoscopic, and robotic approaches. Laparoscopic repair for POM can be performed transvesically or extravesically. Kutikov et al. described the first report of laparoscopic repair for POM in 2006. Subsequently, different reports have described, and the corresponding success rate proved to be similar to the open procedure, making these approaches promising for the treatment of POM [6–10].

This chapter is focused on the operative technique of Laparoscopic-Assisted Extracorporeal Ureteral Tapering Repair (EUTR) and

Supplementary Information The online version contains supplementary material available at [https://doi.org/10.1007/978-3-030-99280-4_34].

M. Lopez (✉)
Department of Pediatric Surgery and Urology, University Hospital of Vall d'Hebron, Barcelona, Spain

Universidad Autonoma de Barcelona, Barcelona, Spain
e-mail: manuel.lopez@vhebron.net

R. Gander · G. Royo · M. Asensio
Department of Pediatric Surgery and Urology, University Hospital of Vall d'Hebron, Barcelona, Spain
e-mail: rgander@vhebron.net; Gloria.royo@vhebron.net; Marino.asensio@vhebron.net

C. Esposito et al. (eds.), *Minimally Invasive Techniques in Pediatric Urology*,
https://doi.org/10.1007/978-3-030-99280-4_34

Laparoscopic Ureteral Extravesical Reimplantation (LUER), and also the evolution of our technique.

34.2 Preoperative Preparation

Preoperatively, all patients undergo a renal ultrasound, voiding cystourethrogram (VCUG), and diuretic renogram mercaptoacetyltriglycine (MAG3). In the current practice, indicators for surgical intervention are initial differential renal function <40% associated, worsening dilatation, degradation of renal function, and/or clinical symptoms, such as febrile urinary tract infection, pain, or stones.

Patients are admitted to the hospital on the same day of surgery. A preoperative enema is advisable but not essential and can be administered at home. It is strongly recommended in patients with history of constipation, allowing better visualization and exposition of the distal ureter. Preoperative antibiotic prophylaxis should always be administered within 60 min before surgery.

34.3 Positioning

Under general anaesthesia, the patient is placed in supine position with legs apart; a urine catheter is inserted at the beginning of the surgery. It is connected to a 60 mL syringe in order to allow inflation and emptying of the bladder during the procedure.

The surgeon is positioned at the head of the patient, the assistant to the left or right depending on the side, and the nurse to the right or left. The monitor is place at the lower end of the table. The operating table is place in Trendelenburg position.

Three ports were used in all cases: 5 mm 30° for the telescope, inserted through a transumbilical incision and two 3 mm trocars placed at the left and right lower abdomen. (Fig. 34.1).

34.4 Instrumentation

To perform the LUER, we used 3 mm instruments including two atraumatic grasping forceps, a curve dissector, scissors with monopolar coagulation, needle holder, and 3 mm vessel sealer (Bolder surgical).

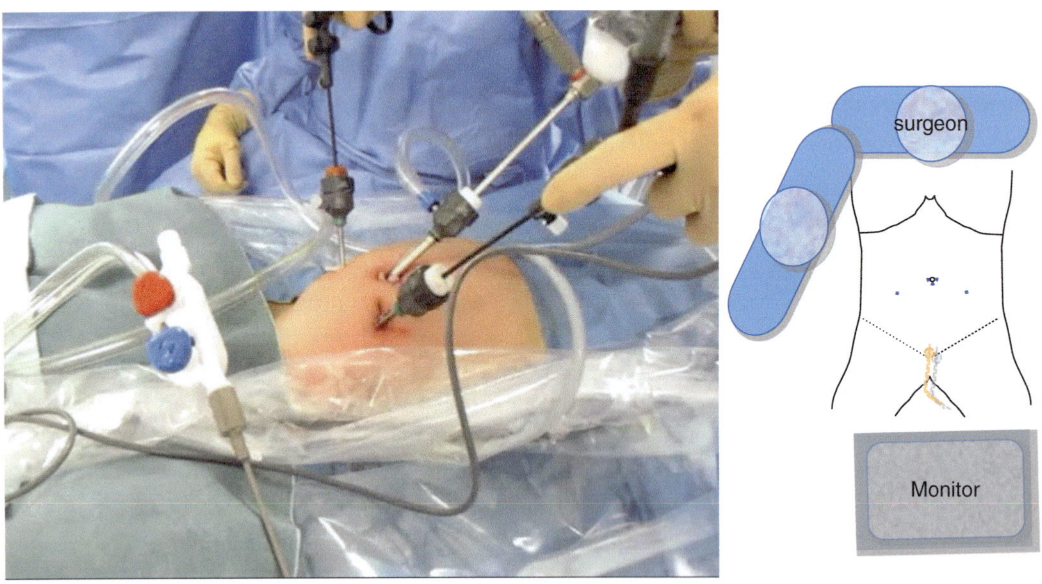

Fig. 34.1 Trocars and surgeons position

34.5 Sutures, Tape and Stent

Exposition of Vesical-Ureteral Junction (VUJ): two stay sutures are inserted through the abdominal wall and placed on each side of the posterior bladder to pull the anterior wall of the bladder up and to expose the VUJ. Long needles are recommended to go through the abdominal wall depending on the age and thickness of the wall as 19, 24, or 27 mm poliglactin suture.

Ureterovesical anastomosis: 5-0 or 6-0 Polydioxanone suture.

Re-approximation of the Detrusor: 3-0 polyester.

Umbilical tape: Placed around the ureter to avoid excessive handling during ureteral dissection.

Blue-Stent/pipi-salle stent (Urosoft-Bard) is inserted percutaneously through the bladder in intraoperative and under laparoscopy. The ureteric stent catheter directly drains the kidney through the ureter. The distal part of the stent is left outside. It usually exits to the abdomen through the bladder wall in the suprapubic region. The stent is removed at first week after surgery without anaesthesia.

34.6 Surgical Technique

Step 1. The retroperitoneum is incised starting below the iliac vessels toward the VUJ. The distal ureter is identified and isolated; an umbilical tape is passed around it precociously for traction. It avoids excessive handling of the ureter during the dissection.

The ureter is mobilized to achieve sufficient freedom for a tension-free reimplantation. During ureteral dissection, preservation of generous periureteral adventitia and limited use of thermal energy are crucial to avoid complications. When coagulation is necessary, the use of 3 mm vessel sealer system, monopolar or bipolar forceps is advisable.

Step 2. In males, VAS deferent is identified and mobilized for avoiding injury. In females, opening of peritoneum in front of the round ligament is necessary to dissect distal ureter.

Step 3. Two stay sutures are inserted through the abdominal wall and placed on each side of the posterior bladder to pull the anterior wall of the bladder up and to expose the UVJ.

Once the stenotic part of the ureter is completely dissected, the bladder is filled with air. Using the monopolar scissors, the peritoneum is incised to expose the detrusor and to create an optimal tunnel with a length that is about four times the size of the ureter (Paquin law). At that moment, the bladder is filled with air, and then the detrusor muscle fibbers are cautiously divided vertically, with scissors, to create a submucosal tunnel until the mucosa is exposed. (Fig. 34.2).

Step 4. The distal ureter is transected at the level of the stenosis. The ureteral stump is then closed with a simple stitch only in case of preexisting vesico ureteral reflux (VUR); otherwise it can be left open.

Step 5. In cases of ureteral tapering, the technique used is the Hendren procedure, with exteriorization of the ureter through the ipsilateral port, which had been enlarged to avoid tearing. Using continuous absorbable 6/0 polydioxanone suture, ureteral tailoring is performed.

Step 6. Vesicoureteral anastomosis is carried out after opening the bladder mucosa, at the top of the new tunnel (Fig. 34.3). The anastomosis is done using two continuous 6/0 polydioxanone sutures. A double polyurethane pigtail soft stent (Urosoft-Bard) is inserted percutaneously through the bladder in intraoperative and under laparoscopy. The ureteric stent catheter directly drains the kidney through the ureter. The distal part of the stent is left outside; it usually exits to the abdomen through the bladder wall in the suprapubic region (Fig. 34.4). The ureter is placed in the new tunnel, and then the detrusor muscle is reapproximated with non-absorbable sutures 3-0 polyester (Fig. 34.5). A non-peritoneal drain was used.

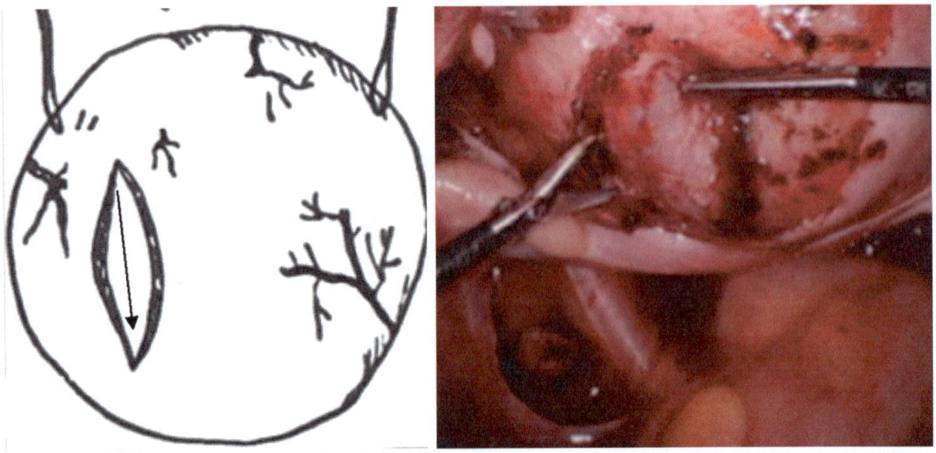

Fig. 34.2 Detrusor-myotomy is performed from the top to VUJ

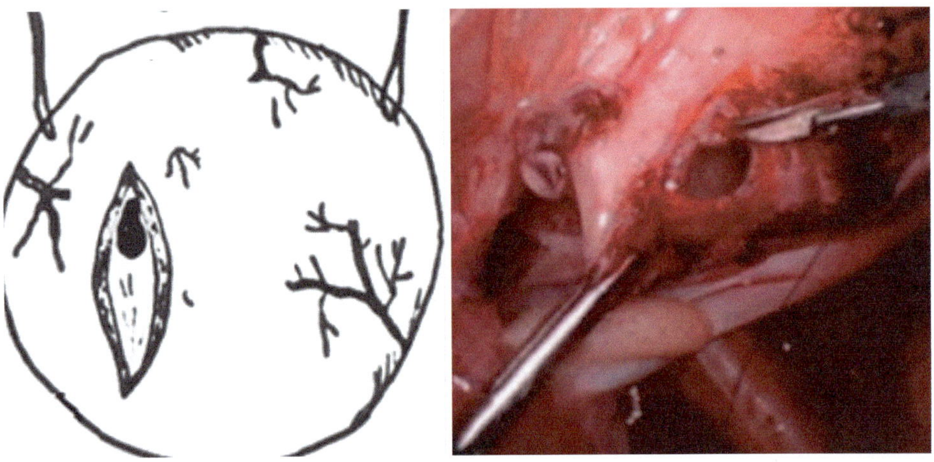

Fig. 34.3 Bladder mucosa is opened at the top of the tunnel

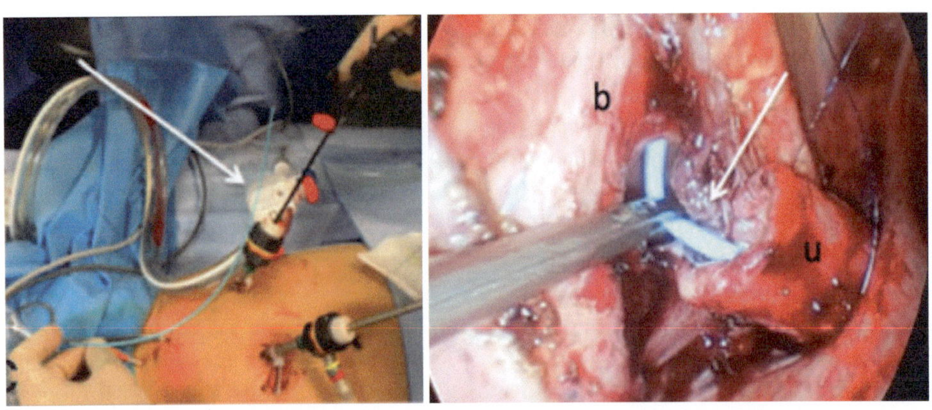

Fig. 34.4 A double polyurethane pigtail soft stent is inserted percutaneously through the bladder (b) in intraoperative and under laparoscopy. The ureteric stent catheter directly drains the kidney through the ureter (u). The distal part of the stent is left outside (arrow); it usually exits to the abdomen through the bladder wall in the suprapubic region

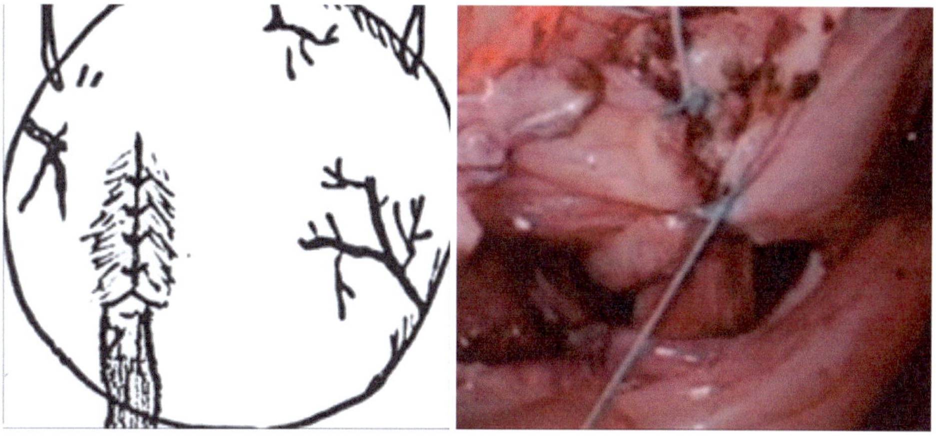

Fig. 34.5 The detrusor is reapproximated over the reimplanted ureter

34.7 Evolution of the Technique

Different modifications were observed that are necessary to improve the technique.

The first is the need to change the insertion point of the ureter into the bladder. During the first description, one of the most challenging aspects of the technique was to perform the anastomosis in the lower part of the new tunnel because it is very laborious and time-consuming. In order to reduce these technical difficulties, the insertion point of the ureter into the bladder was moved to the top of the new tunnel.

The second important point is to avoid a second intervention to remove the stent. Currently, we are using a double polyurethane pigtail soft stent; it is inserted percutaneously through the bladder in intraoperative and under laparoscopy. It is removed at 1 week after surgery, without anaesthesia, and during the first consultation.

More recently, a simplified technique has been introduced using the principle of Shanfield procedure. It allows to reduce the length of the detrusor myotomy; only 2 or 3 cm is enough to create the tunnel because the antireflux depends only on the valvular mechanism of the ureteral segment introduced into the bladder. Once the bladder mucosa is opened at the top of the tunnel, 1–1.5 cm of the distal ureter is introduced into the bladder. Afterwards, the ureter is fixed to the bladder mucosa by four cardinal stitches of absorbable sutures, reducing and facilitating the time of suturing (Fig. 34.6). In case of ureteral tension, it can be fixed using a U-Stitch to the detrusor muscle facilitating the anastomosis. Finally, the detrusor is reapproximated with non-absorbable sutures using 3-0 polyester. Neither a peritoneal drain nor ureteral stent is used. Ureteral tailoring is not necessary in this technique.

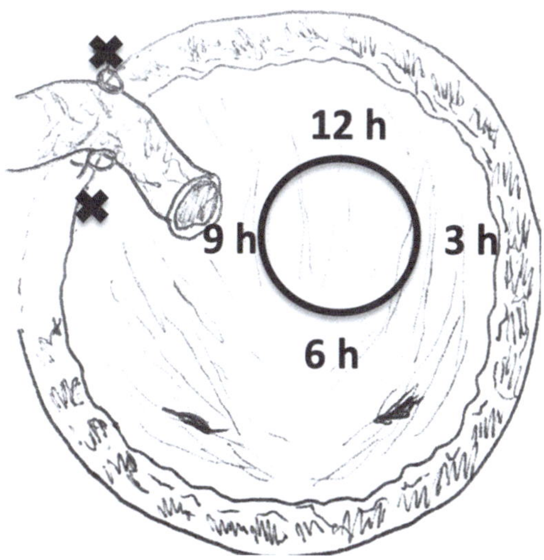

Fig. 34.6 Modified Shanfield Procedure. 1–1.5 cm of the distal ureter is introduced into the bladder to create a valve-like mechanism which prevents reflux. The ureter is fixed to the bladder mucosa by four cardinals stitches

34.7.1 Postoperative Care

Children are started on oral liquids feeds within 3 h after surgery. Postoperative analgesia is performed with metamizole and paracetamol. Usually bladder catheter is removed 48 h after surgery. In the first 14 cases, the double J stent was removed under general anaesthesia 1 month postoperatively, and in 12 cases "pipi salle" stent was removed at 7 days postoperatively without anaesthesia. In all patients, antibiotic prophylaxis by trimethoprim/sulfamethoxazole was administered until the stent was removed.

Follow-up appointments are scheduled at 1, 3, and 6 months post-discharge. A renal ultrasound is done at 1 and 3 months, thereafter VCUG and diuretic renogram MAG-3 are performed to rule out VUR and obstruction. Success is defined as improved hydronephrosis and absence of VUR and obstruction postoperatively.

34.8 Results

Laparoscopic approach was done in 32 patients without conversion. The first 26 patients underwent LUER with or without extracorporeal ureteral tapering, following Lich Gregoir technique. On seven of them vesicoureteral anastomosis was performed in a lower part of the new tunnel. In the remaining 19 cases, the anastomosis was done at the top of the new tunnel.

In 20 patients, laparoscopic-assisted EUTR was carried out. The mean operative time was 141 (130–170) min. In six patients, ureteral tapering was not necessary because the diameter of the ureter was inferior to 2 cm. The mean operative time was 100 (75–120) min. A vertical detrusor myotomy was done in all cases. There were no intraoperative complications. The mean hospital stay was 2–4 days (1–4 days). The mean follow-up period was 40 (7–84) months. No urinary leakage occurred in the postoperative period. None of the patients experienced postoperative voiding dysfunction. At 3 months postoperatively, one patient presented a febrile UTI, and VUR grade III was diagnosed by VCUG. A redo laparoscopic surgery was performed, showing partial disassembling of reimplantation; consequently, the tunnel was extended to increase the length of antireflux and LUER, following Lich Gregoir technique was performed with uneventful outcomes. At medium-term follow-up, all patients were asymptomatic without recurrence of POM or VUR.

The last six cases underwent LUER following modified Shanfield technique. The anastomosis was done at the top of the new tunnel. The mean operative time was 144 min (120–160). Ureteral tapering was not necessary in this technique. There were no intraoperative or postoperative complications. The mean follow-up was 15.83 months; all patients were asymptomatic without recurrence of POM or VUR.

Tips and Tricks

- Traction by grasping directly the ureter should be strongly avoided. Unnoticed ureteral injuries that may cause serious postoperative complications can thereby be prevented.
- Use air to fill the bladder, it allows major mucosal resistance during VU anastomosis.
- While performing the detrusor myotomy, it is easier to start from the top to Vesico-Ureteral Junction.
- Open the bladder mucosal at the top of the tunnel, it allows performed an easier VU anastomosis.
- In cases of LUER following Lich Gregoir technique, ureteric stent catheter directly drains the kidney through the ureter. "Pipi salle" stent avoid a second anaesthesia to remove it.
- In cases of LEUR following modified Shanfield technique, four cardinal stiches are enough. U-stich to the detrusor allows to perform the anastomosis without tension. Ureteral tapering is not necessary when you use this technique.

34.9 Discussion

Conservative treatment in POM avoids surgical correction in more than 80% of patients reported in different series [2–4]. The decision which favoured surgical correction was based on absolute renal function.

The gold standard for the treatment of POM includes open surgery, excision of the aperistaltic and/or narrow ureteral segment, reduction of calibre of the distal dilated ureter, and ureteral reimplantation into the bladder in an antireflux manner, with success rates around 90–96% in different reports.

Laparoscopic and robotic-assisted techniques have been developed as an alternative to open surgery. Different techniques of ureteral reimplantation demonstrating feasibility have been reported to be beneficial in terms of results, decreased postoperative pain, allowing shorter hospital stay, and a quicker return to normalcy. Nevertheless, purely laparoscopic reconstructive surgery can be technically challenging, even for the most experienced laparoscopic surgeons [6–10]. In 2006, Kutikov et al. described the first five cases for POM by pneumovesicoscopy. Ureteral strictures at the neo-ureterovesical anastomosis were observed in one patient after excisional tapering [6]. Same group suggests that intravesical laparoscopic reimplantation is challenging in small bladders, where the capacity is less than 130 cc, particularly when ureteral tapering is required. Jayanthi et al. used pneumovesicoscopy approach when tapering would not be necessary. In children under 2 years old, it decreased working space and made the procedure technically less demanding [11].

In 2015, Kim et al. reported laparoscopic intravesical detrusorrhaphy with ureteral plication in 11 patients with primary unilateral megaureter. The mean follow-up was 12.6 months. In all patients, improvement was noticed in the dilatation of the pelvicalyceal system and the ureters [12].

The transperitoneal approach provides a large operative space for reimplantation and does not limit the manipulation of the urinary bladder and ureter.

In 2006, Ansari et al. reported the first three cases of LUER following Lich Gregoir technique, with extracorporeal tailoring of the ureter, using the Hendren technique. After a 1-year follow-up, no patients presented VUR, and the renal function was preserved in all cases [9]. In 2012, Abraham et al. reported 13 cases of POM that had undergone LUER. In all cases, there was a decrease in ureteral and upper tract dilatation, as well as improved drainage [13].

The largest series of LUER for POM has been reported in 2020 by Bondarenko, based on a multi-institutional study on 78 ureters in 76 patients. Thirty-four of them were tailored, neither the type of reimplantation (tailored or non-tailored) nor age of patients influenced the success rate of LUER. 10.5% of patients presented postoperative complications, two ureteral obstruction, and 7 VUR [14].

Our previous experience in LUER for VUR was the basis for the development of LUER for the management of POM [15–17]. At the beginning of our initial experience for POM, we performed the ureteral anastomosis in the lower part of the new tunnel. Seven cases underwent LUER and EUTR following Lich Gregoir procedure, nevertheless it was very laborious and technically demanding [18]. To become technically less demanding, the insertion point of the ureter into the bladder was moved to the top of the new tunnel, reducing the operative time and probably improving the quality of the anastomosis.

Another important point during surgical correction is the use of the stent. From the beginning, we used a standard double J stent placed intraoperatively by laparoscopy and removed at 6 weeks postoperatively under general anaesthesia. Currently, to avoid a second anaesthesia, we are using a double polyurethane pigtail soft stent (pipi salle stent); it is inserted percutaneously through the bladder and under laparoscopy draining the kidney. The distal part of the stent is left outside. It can be removed without anaesthesia at 1 week during the first consultation after surgery. In our series, all 26 patients benefited from LUER with or without EUTR, with a success rate of 96%. One of the 26 patients (3.84%) presented a febrile UTI at 3 months postoperatively and a unilateral VUR grade III was diagnosed by VCUG. In this case, a redo laparoscopic extravesical ureteral reimplantation following Lich Gregoir technique was done with uneventful consequences in a long-term follow-up [19].

The last evolution in our technique has been based on the principle of Shanfield technique. 1 or 1.5 cm of the distal ureter is introduced into the bladder to create a valve-like mechanism which prevents reflux. This avoids not only the need for a complex vesicoureteral anastomosis but also the need for ureteral tailoring because the antireflux mechanism depends mainly on the valve mechanism of the ureteral tip introduced into the bladder and not entirely on the length of the submucosal tunnel, only 2 or 3 cm of detrusor myotomy is sufficient. Six patients underwent this procedure, and resolution of hydronephrosis, obstruction, and VUR were achieved in all cases [20].

In our experience, all cases were unilateral POM; the procedure was completed laparoscopically without conversion. No patient presented urinary leakage or experienced voiding difficulty. We found that the patient's age was not a limiting factor for performance. We operated on patients younger than 1-year old with similar results to those of older patients. After long-term follow-up, all patients were asymptomatic without recurrence of POM or VUR. In conclusion, we believe that LUER for POM treatment is an alternative to open procedure with a similar success rate. It seems to be a promising technique since it offers high success rate within a single intervention, and it can be practiced in all age groups with excellent outcomes. However, the limitation of this approach is that the surgeon needs training in laparoscopic reconstructive surgery. Nevertheless, further randomized clinical trials are needed to confirm these favourable outcomes.

Take-Home Points

- You to start to perform laparoscopic for POM only after prolonged experience in LEUR for VUR.
- Use umbilical tape around the ureter for avoiding excessive handling.
- Stay sutures allow good exposition of VU junction.
- 30° telescope is absolutely necessary to perform this procedure.
- A long-term outcome is crucial to evaluate the efficacy.

References

1. Thomas D, Duffy P, Rickwood A. Essentials of Paediatric Urology. 2nd ed. London: Informa Healthcare; 2008. p. 73–91.
2. Farrugia M, Hitchcock R, Radford A, Burki T, Robb A, Murphy F. BAPU consensus statement on the management of the primary obstructive megaureter. J Pediatr Urol. 2014;10:26–33.
3. Mc Lellan DL, Retik AB, Bauer SB, et al. Rate and predictors of spontaneous resolution of prenatally diagnosed primary nonrefluxing megaureter. J Urol. 2002;168:2177–80.
4. Ranawaka R, Hennayake S. Resolution of primary nonrefluxing megaureter: an observational study. J Pediatr Surg. 2013;48:380–3.
5. Hendren WH. Complications of megaureter repair in children. J Urol. 1975;113:238–54.
6. Kutikov A, Guzzo TJ, Canter DJ, Casale P. Initial experience with laparoscopic transvesical ureteral reimplantation at the Children's Hospital of Philadelphia. J Urol. 2006;176:2222–5.
7. Yeung CK, Sihoe JD, Borzi PA. Endoscopic crosstrigonal ureteral reimplantation under carbon dioxide bladder insufflation: a novel technique. J Endourol. 2005;19:295–9.
8. Bi Y, Sun Y. Laparoscopic pneumovesical ureteral tapering and reimplantation for megaureter. J Pediatr Surg. 2012;47:2285–8.
9. Ansari MS, Mandhani A, Khurana N, Kumar A. Laparoscopic ureteral reimplantation with extracorporeal tailoring for megaureter: a simple technical nuance. J Urol. 2006;176:2640–2.

10. Peters CA, Woo R. Intravesical robotically assisted bilateral ureteral reimplantation. J Endourol. 2005;19:618–21.
11. Jayanthi V, Patel A. Vesicoscopic ureteral reimplantation: a minimally invasive technique for the definitive repair of vesicoureteral reflux. Ther Adv Urol. 2008;2008:973616.
12. Kim SW, Lim NL, Lee YS, Han SW, Im YJ. Laparoscopic intravesical detrusorrhaphy with ureteral plication for megaureter: a novel technique. Urology. 2015;86:187–91.
13. Abraham GP, Das K, Ramaswami K, Siddaiah AT, George D, Abraham JJ, Thampan OS. Laparoscopic reconstruction for obstructive megaureter: single institution experience with short- and intermediate-term outcomes. J Endourol. 2012;26:1187–91.
14. Dubrov V, Smnyrov O, Kagantsov I, Kulaev A, Bondarenko S. Laparoscopic extravesical transverse ureteral reimplantation for megaureter in children: results from a multi-institutional study. J Pediatr Endosc Surg. 2020;2:21–7.
15. Lopez M, Varlet F. Laparoscopic extravesical transperitoneal approach following the lich-gregoir technique in the treatment of vesicoureteral reflux in children. J Pediatr Surg. 2010;45:806–10.
16. Lopez M, Melo C, Francois M, Varlet F. Laparoscopic extravesical transperitoneal approach following the lich gregoir procedure in refluxing duplicated collecting systems: initial experience. J Laparoendosc Adv Surg Tech A. 2011;21:165–9.
17. Soulier V, Scalabre AL, Lopez M, et al. Laparoscopic vesico-ureteral reimplantation with lich-gregoir approach in children: medium term results of 159 renal units in 117 children. World J Urol. 2017;35:1791–8.
18. Lopez M, Gander R, Royo G, Varlet F, Asensio M. Laparoscopic-assisted extravesical ureteral reimplantation and extracorporeal tapering repair for primary obstructive megaureter in children. J Laparoendosc Adv Surg Tech A. 2017;27:851–7.
19. Lopez M, Perez-Etchepare E, Bustangi N, Godik O, Juricic M, Varlet F, Gutierrez R, Gomez Culebras M, Gander R, Royo G, Asensio M. Laparoscopic extravesical reimplantation in children with primary obstructive megaureter. J Laparoendosc Adv Surg Tech A. 2020; https://doi.org/10.1089/lap.2019.0396.
20. Gander R, Asensio M, Royo GF, López M. Laparoscopic extravesical ureteral reimplantation for correction of primary and secondary megaureters: preliminary report of a new simplified technique. J Pediatr Surg. 2020;55:564–9.

Robot-Assisted Laparoscopic Tapered Ureteral Reimplantation (RAL-TUR)

35

Waleed Eassa and Ramnath Subramaniam

Learning Objectives
- To describe step by step our technique of (RAL-TUR) in children.
- To show the results of the technique.
- To review previous reports and compare them to ours.
- To show a video for (RAL-TUR) in children.
- To describe tips and tricks of our technique of (RAL-TUR) in children.

35.1 Introduction

Megaureter was first described by Caulk in 1923 [1]. In children, It is defined as a retrovesical ureteric diameter more than 7 mm from 30 weeks' gestation onward [2]. Initially classified by Smith into three categories, (1) obstructed, (2) refluxing, and (3) non-refluxing/ non-obstructing, each category was sub-grouped into either primary or secondary [3]. A more practical revision for this classification was done by King adding a fourth refluxing/obstructing category [4]. A primary obstructed megaureter (POM) constitutes 23% of cases of antenatal hydronephrosis. Several explanations have been suggested for the pathogenesis, which is described as a functional obstruction. Suggestions include excessive collagen deposition, segmental changes of muscle cells, a band of circumferential tissue, and dense nonadrenergic innervation in the ureteral smooth muscle collar [5]. Others proposed that it is a delayed fetal ureteral maturation process that involves the differentiation of smooth muscle cells and interstitial cells of Cajal which starts mid ureter and extends cranially and caudally; this theory explains the spontaneous resolution in many cases [6].

Nowadays, hydroureteronephrosis is mostly diagnosed antenatally. An early postnatal US is usually requested followed by MCUG to excluded reflux and BOO. After that, MAG3 is done to diagnose the obstruction and evaluate the renal function [7].

Most of POM cases are managed conservatively. Indications for surgical intervention are initial DRF <40% (especially when associated

Supplementary Information The online version contains supplementary material available at [https://doi.org/10.1007/978-3-030-99280-4_35].

W. Eassa
Sabah Al-Ahmad Urology Center (SAUC), Shuwaikh, Kuwait City, Kuwait
e-mail: weassa@moh.gov.kw

R. Subramaniam (✉)
Leeds Teaching Hospitals NHS Trust, University of Leeds, Leeds, UK
e-mail: ramnath.subramaniam@nhs.net

C. Esposito et al. (eds.), *Minimally Invasive Techniques in Pediatric Urology*,
https://doi.org/10.1007/978-3-030-99280-4_35

with massive hydroureteronephrosis) or failure of conservative management (breakthrough febrile UTIs, pain, worsening dilatation or deteriorating DRF on serial scans) [7].

Although open ureteral reimplantation with or without tapering is the gold standard for surgical correction, in a survey of 123 pediatric urologists from 30 countries, one-third of them will offer minimally invasive surgical (MIS) techniques for their patients [8].

Conventional laparoscopic ureteral reimplantation has a steeper learning curve, causes considerable musculoskeletal strain on the surgeon (exacerbated in smaller children), and its outcomes were not compatible with the open surgery results. With the introduction of daVinci Surgical System® (Intuitive Surgical, Sunnyvale, CA), minimally invasive surgery has now allowed surgeons to perform increasingly complex procedures with a faster learning curve and better outcomes, thanks to the three-dimensional visualization, the articulating instruments with 270° range of movement, the elimination of tremors, and ergonomically surgeon friendly. Thus, the outcomes of robotic-assisted laparoscopic ureteral reimplantation (RAL-UR) for correction of vesicoureteral reflux (VUR) became comparable to open surgery [9].

Tapering of dilated ureters for reimplantation was described as early as 1957 by Bischoff followed by Hendren in 1969 [10]. Weiss and Biancani explained the mechanical rational behind tapering as the narrower lumen helps to generate higher intraluminal pressure to transport urine [11].

Robot-assisted Laparoscopic Tapered Ureteral Reimplantation (RAL-TUR) is technically demanding and is classified as a complex robot-assisted procedure [12].

Limited numbers of publications describe the technique of Robotic-Assisted Laparoscopic Tapered Ureteral Reimplantation (RAL-TUR) in children for correction of POM. This chapter explains our operative technique of (RAL-TUR) step by step.

35.2 Preoperative Preparation

Usually US, MCUG, and MAG3 studies are sufficient for complete diagnosis of POM. MRU helps to accurately delineate the anatomy.

We are not particular about any special bowel preparation, enemas, or special diet preoperatively. We instruct for NPO starting 6 h—only clear fluids are allowed until 2 h—before surgery. Sensitivity test for the selected preoperative antibiotic prophylaxis is done early in the morning of surgery. We usually use third-generation cephalosporin if there are no prior positive cultures for guidance. Oral midazolam (0.5 to 1 mg/kg) is given 1 h before taking the child to OT as it helps to decrease separation anxiety and facilitate induction of anesthesia.

Vascular access is established at OT, and the preoperative antibiotic prophylaxis is administrated.

Cystoscopy ± retrograde ureteropyelography may be needed if we still have doubts regarding the anatomy or if MRU was not done. A Foley catheter is fixed and kept sterile.

35.3 Positioning, Docking, and Port Placement

We place the child in complete supine position. We bring the distal end of the sterile Foley catheter in our sterile field to be handy to control bladder filling during the procedure. We start port placement by the insertion of 12 mm camera port just below the xiphisternum, using Hasson open technique. Then the 30° camera is advanced through the port to inspect the peritoneal cavity and identify our anatomical landmarks. This is followed by under vision placement of two 8 mm arms' bilaterally at the mid-clavicular lines just below the costal margins (Fig. 35.1). We do not use assistant ports. We use the Da Vinci Si Robot, the cart is brought to the left side of the patient and docked parallel to the table with the arms directed cranially and medially to be in alignment with the ports "side docked" (Fig. 35.1).

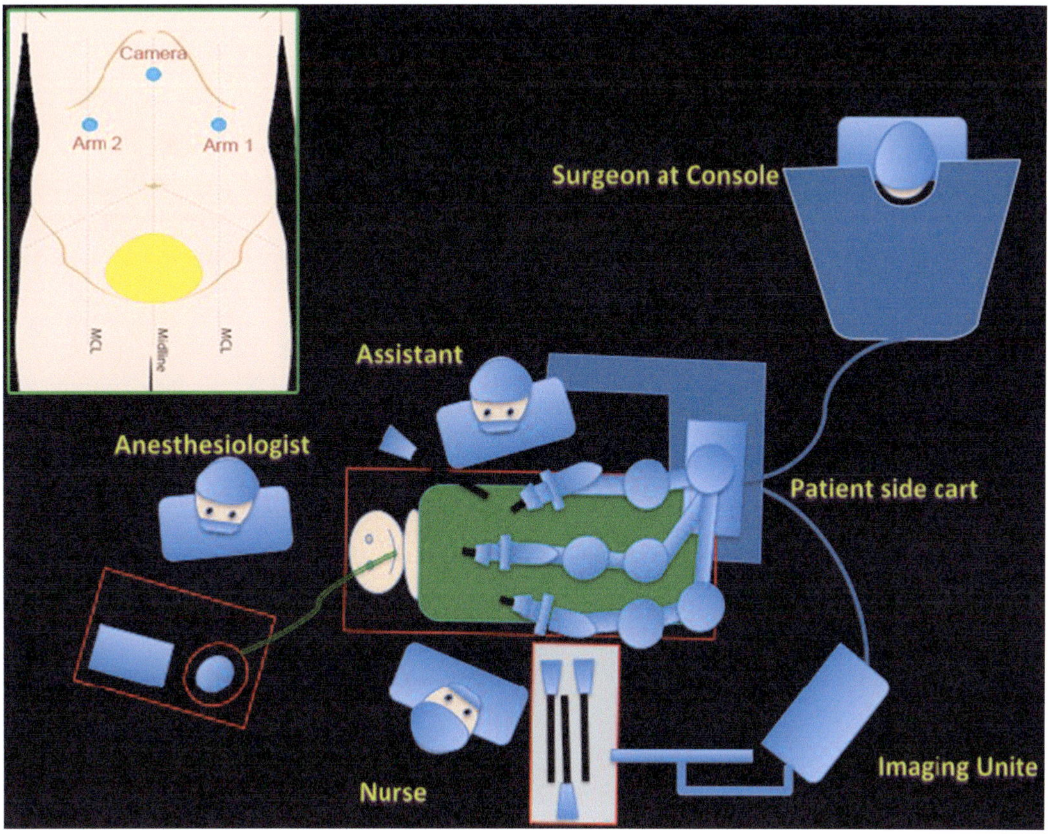

Fig. 35.1 Patient position, port placement, and side docking of the robot

35.4 Instrumentation

Dissection: we usually use a grasping instrument (a Prograsp® forceps) in the left arm and a dissecting instrument (a Maryland bipolar forceps or EndoWrist® PK Dissecting Forceps) in the right arm.

Trimming of the ureter and incising the bladder mucosa: a monopolar scissor is used. Suturing: a Black diamond® micro forceps and large needle driver were used.

35.5 Step-by-Step Technique

35.5.1 Dissection

The bladder is hitched up to the abdominal wall and the posterior peritoneum is opened just distal to the left round ligament in girls and distal to the vas in boys. After identification of the ureter, it is dissected meticulously until the ureterovesical junction and the narrow distal segment were clearly identified together with the dilated segment proximal to the narrowing.

35.5.2 Detrusorotomy

Detrusorotomy of an adequate size to accommodate the ureter is performed from the vesico- ureteric junction vertically upwards allowing the bladder mucosa to bulge. We partially fill the bladder at this step. Detrusor muscle is dissected free on both sides of the detrusorotomy to ensure adequate width to wrap around the ureter for the extravesical reimplant.

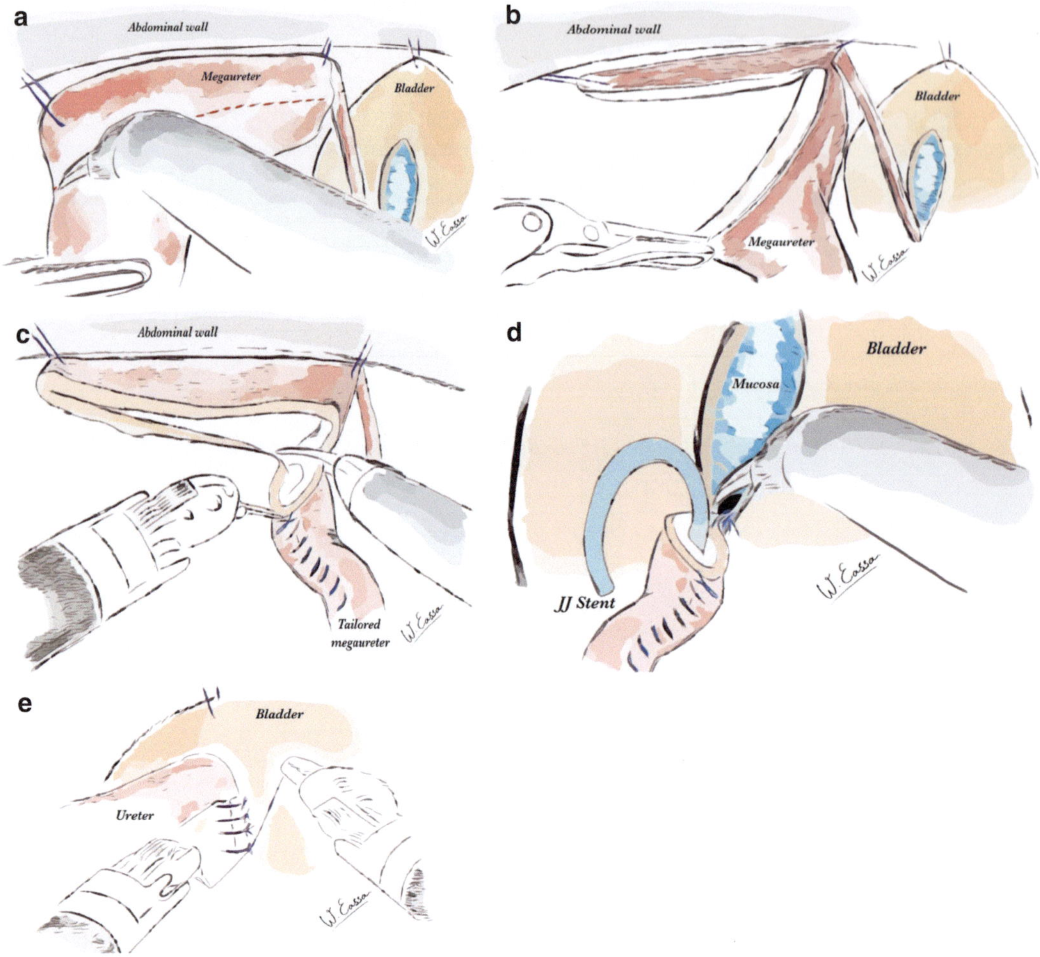

Fig. 35.2 Steps of robot-assisted laparoscopic tapered ureteral reimplantation (RAL-TUR) in children. (**a**) After dissection of the stenotic ureteral segment and detrusorotomy, the segment for trimming is identified, hitched, and the incision line is marked. (**b**) Trimmed megaureter. (**c**) Tailored megaureter, which will be stented percutaneously. (**d**) Fashioning of the neo-ureterovesicostomy. (**e**) Creation of detrusor wrap. Illustration by Syed Salahuddin

35.5.3 Trimming

The mega ureter is dissected proximally to identify the segment for tailoring which is then fixed to the anterior abdominal wall using two hitch stitches. Our line of incision is demarcated followed by excisional tapering of the ureter (Fig. 35.2a, b). The trimmed portion is tailored using running 5/0 PDS II® suture (Fig. 35.2c). The stenotic distal ureter is divided at the level of the native ureterovesical junction.

35.5.4 Stenting

Using a wide bore cannula passed through the abdominal wall, a guide-wire is advanced into the trimmed ureter, then a DJ stent was threaded on the wire through the abdominal wall after cannula removal.

35.5.5 Neo-Ureterovesicostomy

The distal end of the tailored ureter is hitched at 6 o'clock to the distal (lower) end of the detrusorotomy at the site of the neo-ureterovesicostomy by a 5-0 Vicryl® or PDS II® stitch then the mucosa at this site is opened to create the neo-ureterovesicostomy (Fig. 35.2d). The lower coil of the DJ stent is passed into the bladder. After that, the anastomosis is carried out using 5-0 Vicryl® or PDS II® sutures.

35.5.6 Detrusor Wrap

The detrusor muscle at the edges of detrusorotomy is wrapped around the tailored ureter using interrupted 5-0 Vicryl® or PDS II® sutures. The proximal stitch at the apex of the detrusorotomy is hitched to the ureter so as to ensure adequate tunnel for the reimplanted ureter. Then, closure of the detrusor is continued distally (from above downwards) using interrupted Vicryl® or PDS II® sutures until completely burying the tailored ureter in a tunnel with a length: width ratio of at least of 3:1 (Fig. 35.2e).

35.6 Postoperative Care

The child resumes oral intake after the return to the ward as tolerated, starting with fluids. Analgesia is rarely needed; postoperative oral paracetamol of 15 mg/kg is usually prescribed every 8 h PRN. Antibiotic is given orally for 7 days, then a prophylactic dose is maintained as long as the DJ stent is in place. The child can return to activity as soon as he/she can; usually at the same evening or next morning. The Foley catheter is removed in the next morning and the child can be sent home. After 4 weeks, the child is readmitted for removal of the DJ stent, a KUB is usually done to make sure that the DJ stent did not migrate proximally. After removal of the stent, the child is discharged the same day. We continue the prophylactic antibiotic until the third month postoperatively, when we request a follow- up US. If the hydroureteronephrosis is stable or improved, we stop the prophylactic antibiotic and plan to repeat the US every 3 months in the first year then biannually and then annually until complete improvement (frequency of follow-up can be planned according to each case and rate of resolution of hydroureteronephrosis).

35.7 Results

The video we present for our technique is that of an 8 years old female. She was presented to us with frequent left loin pain and was diagnosed with left POM. Left Split Renal Function (SRF) was 22%.

Console time was 126 min. There was no blood loss. She was fully mobile in the following morning. Foley catheter was removed after 1 day. LOH was 30 h. The Double J stent was removed after 8 weeks, Ultrasonography 3 months later showed receding hydroureteronephrosis and the MAG3 study showed resolution of obstruction and improvement of SRF 28%. Total follow-up period was 18 month (Fig. 35.3).

In total, we have experience of this technique of RAL-TUR in seven children, three for refluxing megaureter and four for POM; four girls and three boys. The mean age was 4.2 years (1.5 to 8 years), all were unilateral. Their presentation was recurrent UTIs and all with deteriorating renal functions. Mean console time was 113 min (93 to 148), blood loss was negligible in all cases. All the patients were discharged home next day following the procedure once feeds were established and patient was mobilizing well.

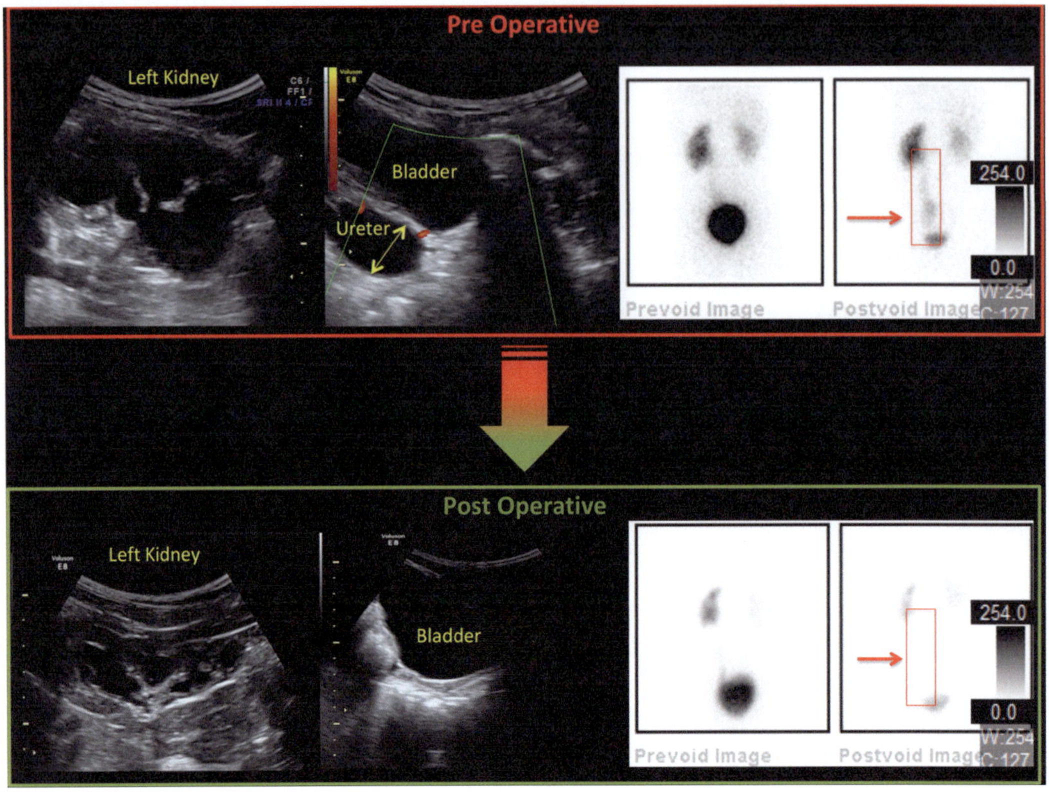

Fig. 35.3 Pre- and post-operative images of an 8 years old female child who underwent (LAP-TUR) for left POM

We measured our surgical success by resolution of hydroureteronephrosis by US, improved renal function or drainage by MAG3. In our series, all cases showed one or more of our success criteria and none needed any further surgery.

Tips and Tricks

- We prefer supine position; do not tilt the table or use lithotomy position. This obviates the need for any strappings. It is also the most preferable position by anesthesiologist.
- Side docking is better than conventional docking especially in children, as it allows the access for genital region for any retrograde manipulations—if needed— without undocking.
- We prefer using the 8 mm instruments as they offer better range of movement than the 5 mm ones; the cosmetic difference in port scars is negligible.
- Because of the small abdominal cavity of the children, any mild gas leakage will rapidly lead to loss of pressure and dislodgement of arms. This is why we apply a 2-0 subcutaneous cerclage stitch around the camera port, tied firmly to it, and the tie is extra secured by applying Steri-Strips™.
- To gain extra space after complete docking, the camera port is lifted gently to elevate the abdominal wall.
- It is important to keep bladder partially filled during detrusorotomy to avoid injuring the tenuous bulging bladder mucosa.
- Creation of good detrusor muscle troughs on both sides of the detrusorot-

omy is important also to avoid narrowing of the tunnel.

- For stenting, usage of a wide-bore cannula to pass the wire is a simple and fast trick. A snip with a scalpel tip in the skin at the site of cannula may be needed to allow threading large stents.
- The Paquin's ration of at least 1:3 (ureteral width to tunnel length) should be respected to avoid reflux by creating a flap valve antireflux mechanism.
- Detrusor wrap is created from proximal to distal (above to downwards when the bladder is hitched as seen in the video). The first stitch is the most important as it holds the ureter in place.

35.8 Discussion

Most of publications regarding robotic-assisted ureteral reimplantation (RAL-UR) in children are about using the technique for correction of VUR. It shares similar approach with (RAL-TUR) but much easier in terms that it lacks dismemberment and tapering, both of which are technically demanding steps. Few case reports described the technique of (RAL-TUR) for correction of POM.

The first reports of (RAL-TUR) for repair of POM were of adult cases. In 2009, Hemel et al., reported their experience including eight reimplants in seven patients (mean age was 28 years). They positioned their patients in low dorsal lithotomy position with steep Trendelenburg.

Trimming was done intracorporeally in six patients and extracorporeally after undocking in two patients. They used 12 mm camera port (umbilical) and other 4 ports (three robotic arms and one 5 mm assistant port). Mean console time was 127 min and mean LOH was 3.2 days. Their success rate was 100% with respect to drainage and preservation of renal function with a follow-up duration of 16 months. They concluded that the technique is feasible, safe, and effective for treatment in POM highlighting the advantages of RAL over traditional laparoscopy as well as the advantages of intracorporeal trimming over the extracorporeal one because of the nuisance of the undocking and re-docking of the robot [13].

Two years later, Goh et al. described their (RAL-TUR) technique in a 51-year-old adult patient. They also used the same dorsal lithotomy position and same number of total 5 ports. Tapering was done intracorporeally. Total operative time was 262 min with blood loss of 150 mL and LOH was 4 days [14].

The first example of (RAL-TUR) in children was a case report published by Faasse et al. in 2014. But it was done for a correction of refluxing megaureter (not obstructed) in a 9 year old child, so dismemberment was not done. In contrast to adults, the child was placed in supine position with slight Trendelenburg and the authors used only 3 ports (12 mm umbilical one for camera and other two 8 mm ports at mid-calvicular lines) just below the level of umbilicus. To facilitate trimming, they inserted a ureteric stent preoperatively in the ureter and placed several stay sutures anteriorly in the ureteral segment designated for trimming.

They sequentially lifted the stay stitches from proximal to distal to stabilize the megaureter during trimming which was done using CO_2 laser [15].

In our series, we put the patient in complete supine position which is convenient for both the surgeons and nurses and also the anesthesia team. We also use only 3 ports, but we prefer to place the ports higher in the abdomen. We believe this is advantageous in giving us more room for the robotic arms especially in small children where the bladder is relatively closer to the umbilicus in also preventing clashing. We do not stent the ureter preoperatively, which could be difficult in cases of POM if there is severe narrowing. Sometimes even the ureteral orifice cannot be detected. In our described technique, we stabilize the ureter to the abdominal wall by two hitch stitches, which is more easier and faster than applying several stay stitches, besides this frees one arm for use during trimming. We use robotic monopolar scissor for cutting which is more practical than using CO_2 laser.

In 2015, Villanueva published another case report for a (RAL-TUR) in an 11 year old child, but this time it was done for obstructed megaureter. He placed the child in lithotomy position and did the tapering extracorporeally. He applied hidden incision endoscopic surgery (HIDES) to achieve good cosmesis by making the incisions at the bikini line [16]. But still he has to undock and re-dock the machine, a time-consuming step that is spared in our technique.

Lastly a video published in 2017, demonstrating surgical technique of (RAL-TUR) in a series of 14 refluxing and obstructed ureters, it was very short reporting as there were no data regarding positioning, docking, or how many ureters were obstructed. They used the same technique reported by Faasse et al. which includes stenting the ureter preoperatively and placing a series of interrupted stay sutures along the anterior ureteral wall for manipulation [17].

Many surgeons create their detrusor wrap in RAL-UR surgeries starting distally at the site of the neo-ureterovesicostomy (down to top). We perform our detrusorrhaphy (top-down) with a suturing technique which is quick to perform and eliminates the need to manipulate the ureter at this step [18].

35.9 Conclusion

As far as we know, our series is the first to fully and systemically report a (RAL-TUR) for obstructed megaureter in children. Our described technique obviates a lot of complexities of previous reported cases as it doesn't need special positioning of the patient or preoperative stenting. Side docking is fast and away from the perineum so retrograde manipulation is easy to perform at any time during surgery. Tapering is intracorporeal, fast with minimal ureteral manipulation. A complex procedure like (RAL-TUR) for obstructed megaureter in children is feasible and safe with outcomes comparable to the gold standard open procedure if step-wise standardized technique is followed.

Take-Home Points

- RAL-TUR in children is feasible and has an outcome comparable to open surgery.
- Secure trocars as rapid loss of pressure and dislodgment of trocars and can easily happen in children.
- Partially fill the bladder during detrusorotomy and create good detrusor flaps.
- Hitch the megaureter to facilitate trimming and decrease manipulation.
- Stent can be threaded on a wire passed through the skin in children.
- Respect the Paquin's ration of at least 1:3 (ureteral width to tunnel length).
- Proximal to distal detrusor wrap obviates excess ureteral manipulation.

References

1. Caulk JR. Megaloureter: the importance of the uretero-vesical valve. J Urol. 1923;9:315–30. https://doi.org/10.1016/S0022-5347(17)73776-7.
2. Cussen LJ. Dimensions of the normal ureter in infancy and childhood. Investig Urol. 1967;5:164–78.
3. Smith ED. Report of working party to establish an international nomenclature for the large ureter. Birth Defects Orig Artic Ser. 1977;13:3–8.
4. King LR. Megaloureter: definition, diagnosis and management. J Urol. 1980;123:222–3. https://doi.org/10.1016/S0022-5347(17)55867-X.
5. Shokeir AA, Nijman RJM. Primary megaureter: current trends in diagnosis and treatment: primary megaureter. BJU Int. 2001;86:861–8. https://doi.org/10.1046/j.1464-410x.2000.00922.x.
6. Babu R, Vittalraj P, Sundaram S, Shalini S. Pathological changes in ureterovesical and ureteropelvic junction obstruction explained by fetal ureter histology. J Pediatr Urol. 2019;15:240.e1–7. https://doi.org/10.1016/j.jpurol.2019.02.001.
7. Farrugia M-K, Hitchcock R, Radford A, Burki T, Robb A, Murphy F. British Association of Paediatric Urologists consensus statement on the management of the primary obstructive megaureter. J Pediatr Urol. 2014;10:26–33. https://doi.org/10.1016/j.jpurol.2013.09.018.
8. Sanchez O, Lumpkins K, Silay S, Peycelon M, Gopal M, Smith C, et al. The megasurvey: international survey on the current practices in surgical management of primary obstructed megaureter. Eur

Urol Suppl. 2017;16:e1283. https://doi.org/10.1016/S1569-9056(17)30795-9.

9. Weiss DA, Shukla AR. The robotic-assisted ureteral reimplantation. Urol Clin N Am. 2015;42:99–109. https://doi.org/10.1016/j.ucl.2014.09.010.
10. Henderson BM. Operative repair of megaureter in children. J Pediatr Surg. 1969;4:584. https://doi.org/10.1016/0022-3468(69)90139-0.
11. Weiss RM, Biancani P. Rationale for ureteral tapering. Urology. 1982;20:482–7. https://doi.org/10.1016/0090-4295(82)90118-2.
12. Arlen AM, Broderick KM, Travers C, Smith EA, Elmore JM, Kirsch AJ. Outcomes of complex robot-assisted extravesical ureteral reimplantation in the pediatric population. J Pediatr Urol. 2016;12:169.e1–6. https://doi.org/10.1016/j.jpurol.2015.11.007.
13. Hemal AK, Nayyar R, Rao R. Robotic repair of primary symptomatic obstructive megaureter with intracorporeal or extracorporeal ureteric tapering and ureteroneocystostomy. J Endourol. 2009;23:2041–6. https://doi.org/10.1089/end.2009.0103.
14. Goh AC, Link RE. Robot-assisted tapered ureteral reimplantation for congenital megaureter. Urology. 2011;77:742–5. https://doi.org/10.1016/j.urology.2010.05.051.
15. Faasse MA, Lindgren BW, Gong EM. Robot-assisted laparoscopic ureteral reimplantation with excisional tailoring for refluxing megaureter. J Pediatr Urol. 2014;10:773.e1–2. https://doi.org/10.1016/j.jpurol.2014.01.023.
16. Villanueva CA. Extracorporeal ureteral tailoring during HIDES laparoscopic robotic- assisted ureteral reimplantation for megaureter. J Pediatr Urol. 2015;11:362–3. https://doi.org/10.1016/j.jpurol.2015.08.006.
17. Li B, Lindgren BW, Liu DB, Gong EM. Robot-assisted laparoscopic megaureter tapering with ureteral reimplantation: tips and tricks. J Pediatr Urol. 2017;13:637–8. https://doi.org/10.1016/j.jpurol.2017.09.013.
18. Silay MS, Baek M, Koh CJ. Robot-assisted laparoscopic extravesical ureteral reimplantation in children: top-down suturing technique without stent placement. J Endourol. 2015;29:864–6. https://doi.org/10.1089/end.2014.0815.

36 Retrocaval Ureter in Pediatric Patients

María Santos, Carolina Acuña, and Pedro-José Lopez

Learning Objectives

- To describe step by step the transperitoneal laparoscopic approach for retrocaval ureter.
- To describe tips and tricks for the transperitoneal laparoscopic approach.
- To describe generalities of retrocaval ureter in order to recognize this pathology.

36.1 Introduction

Retrocaval ureter (RU) is a rare congenital anomaly, where the ureter deviates medially, passes behind the inferior vena cava (IVC), and surrounds it coming back to the corresponding ipsilateral side by passing in afore (Fig. 36.1). It is found in approximately 1 of every 1000 patients, and the male to female ratio is 3:1 [1, 2]. Being infrequent in pediatric population, normally present in the third or fourth decades [1], it occurs more commonly on the right side and can be associated with

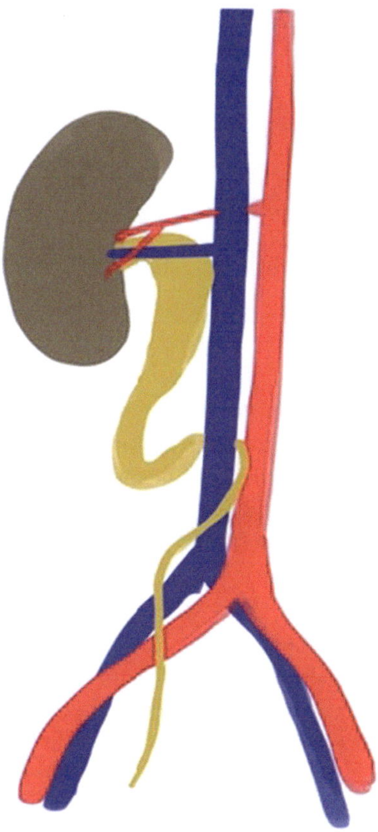

Fig. 36.1 Retrocaval ureter

Supplementary Information The online version contains supplementary material available at [https://doi.org/10.1007/978-3-030-99280-4_36].

M. Santos · C. Acuña
Pediatric Surgery Unit, Clinica Alemana, Universidad del Desarrollo, Santiago, Chile
e-mail: mariasantosc@gmail.com; caroacuna@gmail.com

P.-J. Lopez (✉)
Pediatric Urology Service, Hospital Exequiel Gonzalez Cortes and Clinica Alemana, Santiago, Chile
e-mail: pejotalopez@gmail.com

C. Esposito et al. (eds.), *Minimally Invasive Techniques in Pediatric Urology*,
https://doi.org/10.1007/978-3-030-99280-4_36

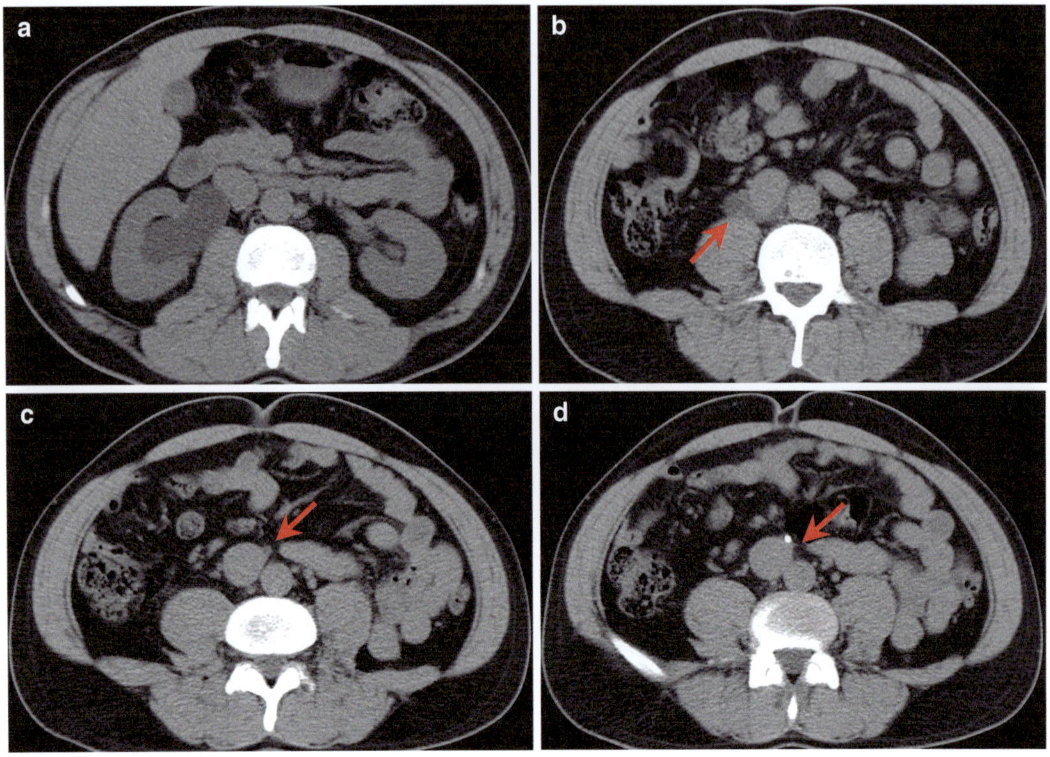

Fig. 36.2 Abdominal computed tomography showing right retrocaval ureter. (**a**) right hydronephrosis (**b**) right ureter next and behind inferior vena cava (**c**) right ureter on the left side of IVC (**d**) lithiasis in right ureter

other IVC or renal anomalies [1, 2]. Most cases are detected during routine radiologic imaging, being asymptomatic. When symptomatic, it can be present with abdominal colic pain, urinary tract infection, or hematuria. On ultrasound, it can be detected by a dilated tortuous proximal ureter or hydronephrosis (HN) secondary to pseudo-ureteral obstruction [2]. The aetiology is assumed to be abnormal embryologic development of the IVC due to the abnormal persistence of the right posterior subcardinal vein ventral to the ureter [3].

There are two types of retrocaval ureter: type I or "low loop" form, where the ureter curves back in the shape of a reverse "J" in front of the third of the fourth lumbar vertebra passing behind the IVC. This is the most common form and causes moderate to severe HN. Type II or "high loop" is rare and normally doesn't cause HN. Here the ureter has as a sickle-shaped ureteral curve, as the renal pelvis and upper ureter pass behind the IVC at the level of, or just above, the ureteropelvic junction [4].

The management in symptomatic patients consists in transection and relocation of the ureter anterior to the IVC. The first cases were treated with the Anderson–Hynes dismembered pyeloplasty but now minimally invasive surgery is the method of choice [4, 5]. The laparoscopic approach is the gold standard, having transperitoneal access easier than retroperitoneal. Robotic assisted surgery has shown good results and, if available, it is a very good option too.

This chapter is focused on the operative technique of laparoscopic transperitoneal resolution for retrocaval ureter in children.

36.2 Pre-Operative Preparation

Imaging studies are required to diagnose and classify RU. Intravenous pyelogram and retrograde pyelography are the most common studies. A combination with cavography has also been used when the diagnosis cannot be established by intravenous pyelogram.

During the last few years, Uro-CT scan (Figs. 36.2 and 36.3) or Uro-MRI have replaced

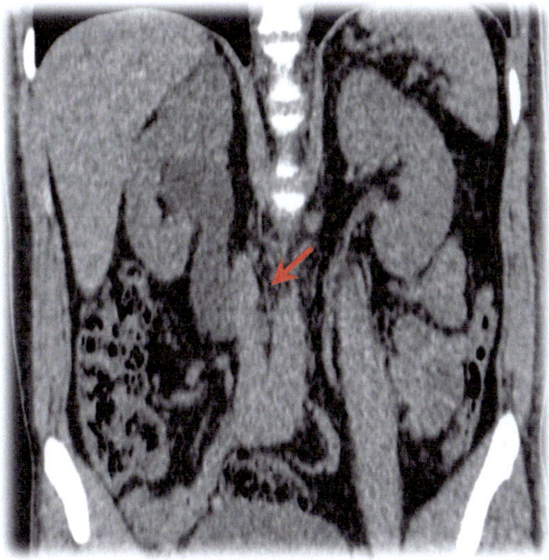

Fig. 36.3 Abdominal computed tomography showing right retrocaval ureter

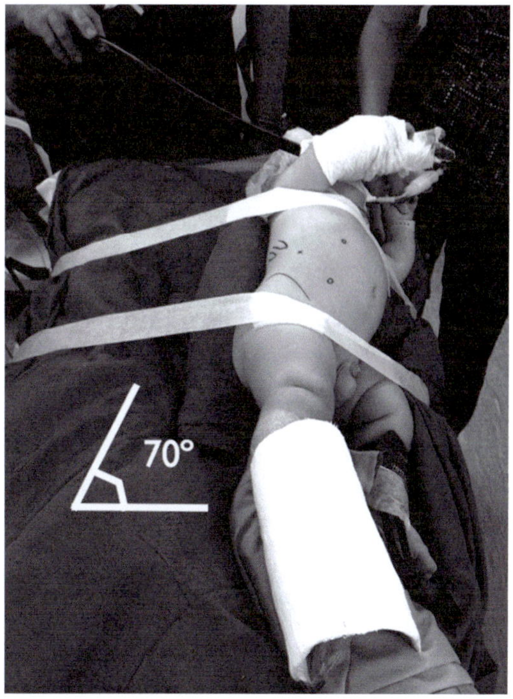

Fig. 36.4 Patient position

the use of invasive techniques, being less invasive these studies give more detailed anatomic information. Diuretic renogram could be useful to evaluate the degree of functional obstruction [2].

36.3 Positioning

The transperitoneal laparoscopic approach with three trocars is preferred. In comparison to the retroperitoneal approach, it offers a larger working space in the peritoneal cavity improving visualization and maneuverability. The ureter may be accessed in its entirety, dissected properly and it facilitates intracorporeal suturing and knotting [6]. The patient is placed in a lateral 75° decubitus position with the affected kidney on top, facing the surgeon, at the edge of the operating table and is secured with adhesive tapes (Fig. 36.4). This facilitates free movements of the instruments without hindrance from the table. The laparoscopic stack system with the screen should be placed opposite to the surgeon, at the back of the patient, making one line (surgeon–patient–stack). The camera is inserted through the umbilical port (5 mm) and two small ports (3 or 5 mm) will be introduced; one at the right iliac fossae (if approaching a right ureter) and the other on the costal margin on the mammary line with ergonomic criteria.

36.4 Instrumentation

The instrumentation needed will depend on the age of the patient. For younger patients 5 mm 30° optic and two 3-mm ports will be used. In older children, 10 mm 30° optic and two 5-mm ports could be used.

The complete laparoscopic instrument set needed contains:

- One 5- or 10-mm Hasson port.
- 2 ports for 3- or 5-mm instruments
- 1 bowel grasper
- 1 right angle dissector
- 1 Metzenbaum scissor
- 1 pyeloplasty scissor
- 1 diathermy hook
- 1 needle holder (3 mm).

1 suction/irrigation device.

5/0 resorbable suture for the ureteroouretero anastomosis.

14G Branula.

3.7 to 5.2 Fr 8 cm to 20 cm multi length silicone double J stent and guide-wire.

Foley catheter.

36.5 Technique

General anesthesia is administered and a Foley catheter is inserted before starting surgery leaving the bladder in free drainage. The first port is placed by an open technique (Hasson) in the region of the umbilicus and secured with a skin suture. This incision could be done longitudinal using all the umbilicus scars. The gas flow starts at 1 L/min until the peritoneal cavity is insufflated and then it can be raised until 8 L/min. The abdominal pressure is set at 10–12 mmHg. Two working ports are inserted under direct vision: one under the costal margin and the other in the ipsilateral iliac fossa. The position of this latter port (# 3), which is used for the needle holder, is crucial, as it has to be in line with the anastomosis to facilitate suturing.

The kidney is identified by reflecting the colon medially or through a transmesenteric window in the left side in suitable cases. Meticulous dissection with cutting rather than coagulation of the ureter is done, taking care of not damaging its vascularization and mobilizing the lower ureter sufficiently to achieve a tension-free ureteroureteral anastomosis. The anterior surface of the kidney should be left intact to keep its adherence; dissecting the posterior surface of the mid and lower pole is sufficient to expose the upper ureter. The hardest part is the dissection between the ureter and the IVC, where a blind dissection could be finding the correct plane between these two structures. Then, a horseshoe technique is done letting the ureter move freely behind the IVC. When the ureter is released completely, sectioning of the retrocaval segment is done. If the ureter is too close to the IVC and is not completely liberated, the ureter should be sectioned as close to the IVC as possible and then released. The retrocaval segment is mobilized and transposed anterior to the IVC (Fig. 36.5). Proximal and distal ends should be spatulated in an opposite way prior to the anastomosis. A “hitch stich” can be used to give stability and to facilitate the suturing, by passing a straight needle (3/0 or 4/0 Prolene) or a regular 5/0 Prolene in small infants, passing directly through the abdominal wall, and/or through a branula. Sometimes a fourth 3 mm trocar could be inserted for this maneuverer. If the ends of the ureters are wide, the anastomosis should be done in two running sutures, on the anterior side (the one facing the surgeon) and other on the posterior side of the ureter (the one distal from the surgeon). If there is some doubt regarding further stenosis, interrupted stiches are a good option too.

When the posterior side of the anastomosis is complete, a double J stent is inserted directly through the abdominal wall through a 14G branula. The guide-wire is passed down the ureter with Vaseline oil and into the bladder. Then the double J stent is advanced over the guide-wire and placed between the renal pelvis and the bladder. The double J stent is inserted anterogradely, first to the bladder and then into the kidney. In our experience, it’s been easier this way with good results.

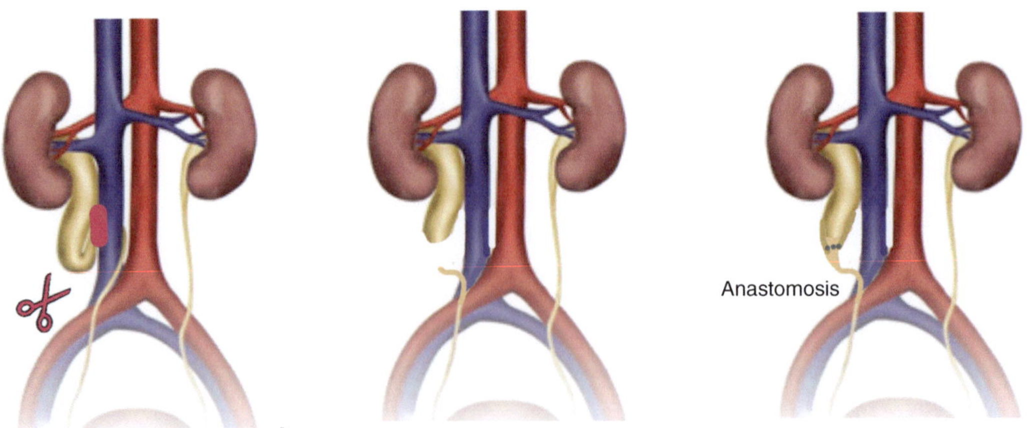

Fig. 36.5 Section and anastomosis of ureter

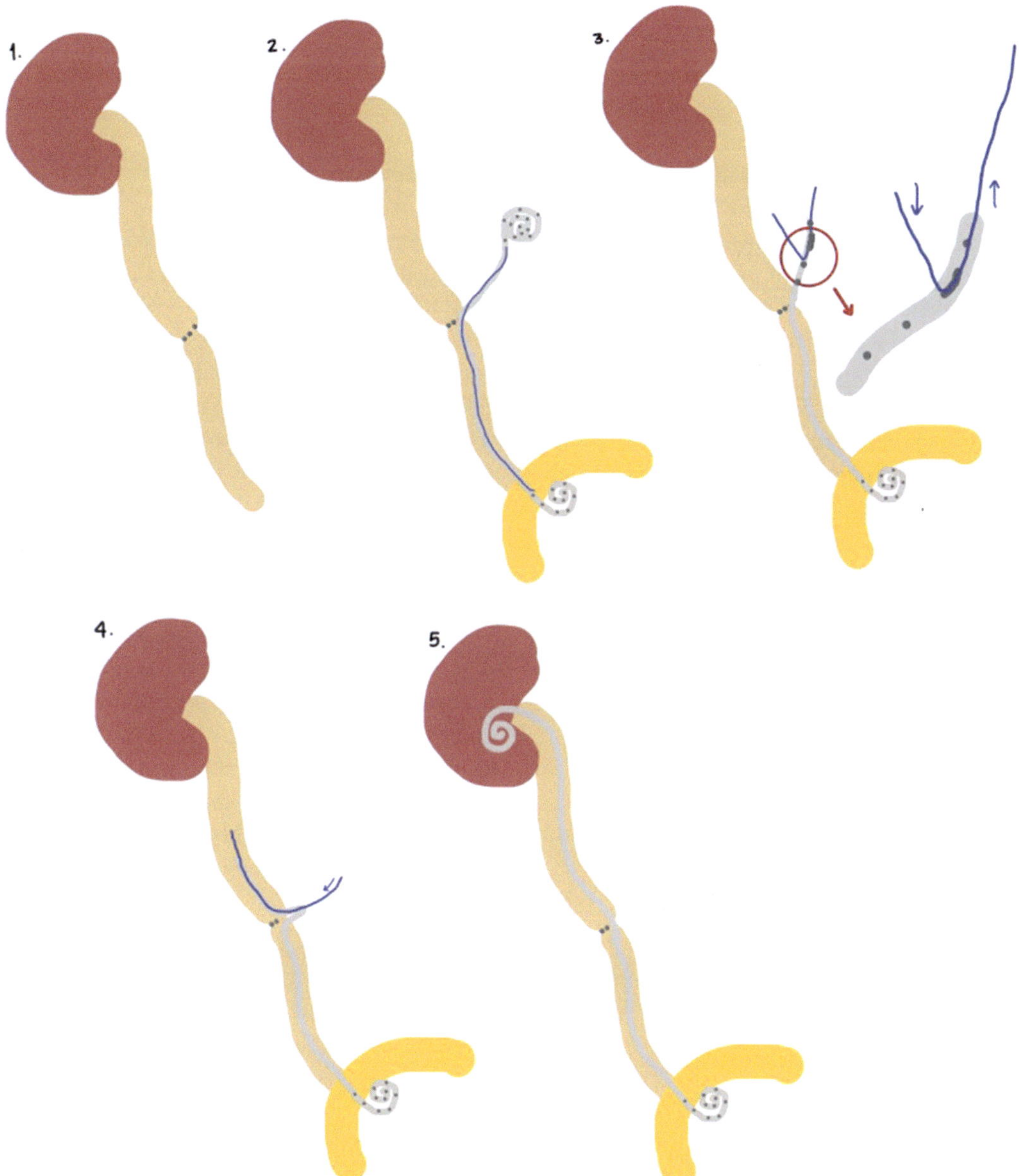

Fig. 36.6 Tips and tricks of insertion of JJ stent trough anastomosis (1). Anastomosis of posterior wall (2). Insertion of JJ stent and guidewire to the bladder (3). Insertion of guidewire through the dilated fenestration of JJ stent (4). Introduction of guidewire and JJ stent to the kidney (5). JJ stent in its correct position

An important trick to help with this technique is prior inserting of the double J stent through the branula; one of the fenestrations of the end that will be inserted in the kidney should be dilated (ideally the second or third distal fenestration). So, the double J stent is inserted with the guide-wire through the anastomosis into the bladder and then the guide-wire is removed. Then the guide-wire is inserted through the dilated fenestration and grabbed at the free end of the double J stent. Finally, the guide-wire is inserted with the double J stent through the proximal ureter to the kidney. When the double J stent is introduced completely, the guide-wire is carefully pulled out (Fig. 36.6).

To check that the double J stent is in the bladder, you can either have a full bladder and check that there is urine coming out from the stent or fill the bladder with methylene blue and corroborate that methylene blue comes out and up from the stent.

After the double J stent is in place, the anterior suture line of the anastomosis is completed. If the ends of the ureter are narrow, interrupted sutures can be done, and a knot pusher can be used to facilitate knotting. The anastomosis can be done with 5-0 or 6-0 poliglecaprone 25 (Monocryl) or 6-0 PDS.

The "hitch stitch" is removed, and the anastomosis is placed in the "new" normal anatomical position. The colon is replaced without a suture, and the mesenteric window could be closed if a trans-mesenteric approach was used.

Hemostasis is checked carefully. No additional perirenal drain is necessary. Ports are removed under direct vision, and the incisions are closed with 3/0 Vicryl to the fascia and 5/0 Monocryl or Dermabond to the skin.

The Foley catheter is left in free drainage for 2–3 days postoperatively.

36.6 Postoperative Care

Patients start oral feeding a few hours after surgery. Analgesics are administered orally and intravenously only if needed. Oral paracetamol (15 mg/kg) is given for the first 3 days.

Patients are discharged on the next day, but if the surgery is done at first time in the morning, it could be a day case surgery.

Foley catheter is left for 2–3 days after surgery and double J stent is taken out by cystoscopy 6 to 8 weeks after surgery. There are institutions that leave the double J stent for 10–14 days, with the pulling threads coming out of the urethra.

Prophylactic antibiotics are given until 24 h after the double J stent is been removed.

US controls should be done 1, 3, 6, and 12 months postoperatively to evaluate relief of obstruction. MAG 3 should only be done if ultrasound shows signs of persistent dilatation.

36.7 Results

As retrocaval ureter is a rare anomaly and not much is described in the literature; we do not have enough patients to make a series of cases descriptive cohort. The results shown in the literature and the few cases that we have experienced are very good. The most possible complication could be urine leak and ureteral obstruction. Peycelon et al. describe five patients in which a retroperitoneal approach was done and conclude that it is a safe and effective technique [7]. Escolino et al. compare open vs laparoscopic technique, and they observed better postoperative results with laparoscopic approach in terms of analgesic requirements, hospitalization, and cosmetic results. All of the patients reported had complete resolution of obstruction and only one, in the laparoscopic group, presented a complication (stenosis at the ureteral anastomosis) which was resolved in a redo surgery [4]. Other case reports have been published and report no complications added to resolution of the obstruction with transperitoneal approach [8, 9].

Our experience with the laparoscopic transperitoneal approach has been successful, with no complications and resolution of obstruction.

Tip and Tricks

- Ureteroureteral laparoscopic anastomosis is challenging but some tricks can help making it easier. Meticulous dissection with the hook in the cutting mode and not coagulation is our first tip to avoid ureteral damage and further stenosis. The hitch stich to fix the ureter and avoid extra mobilization would help to do the anastomosis. Another trick that will help in small ureters in which the ends are too narrow is to make the anastomosis with interrupted sutures instead of a continuous suture.
- Dilating one of the fenestrations of the proximal end (kidney end) of the double J stent will help to insert the guide-wire and introduce the stent into the kidney.

- Finally using only three ports and introducing the double J stent through a branula helps as there is no need of using a fourth port, which could be very useful especially during learning curve.

36.8 Discussion

Retrocaval ureter is a rare finding or cause of ureteral obstruction. Correction of this anomaly should be done only when symptomatic and/or with moderate to severe HN resulting from ureteral obstruction. Correction can be done by an open, laparoscopic or robotic approach. Minimally invasive surgery (MIS) could be retroperitoneal or transperitoneal. Independently of which way to approach the ureter, there are two main techniques that can be done, ureteroureterostomy or ureteropelvic anastomosis. As we all know, advances in laparoscopic approach during the last years have grown, hence allowing surgical correction of retrocaval ureter by MIS. The retroperitoneal technique is described in the literature and was used in nearly half of the published cases. They describe no differences regarding results between the retroperitoneal and transperitoneal approach [7]. However, in our opinion, the transperitoneal laparoscopic technique provides a better exposure, allowing an adequate space for dissection of the ureter, taking care of its vascularization, which is one of the most critical steps of this surgery. If the dissection is not done carefully and the vascularization is damaged, ureteral stenosis may be observed in the follow-up. On the other hand, the transperitoneal approach allows a smooth learning curve.

Take-Home Points

- Surgery is indicated only when symptomatic or when moderate to severe HN occurs.
- Nowadays, MIS is the way to perform this surgery, where transperitoneal laparoscopic approach is an excellent technique that offers good exposure of the ureter and the IVC for both beginners and advanced surgeons.
- One of the critical steps of the procedure is to be watchful of ureteral vascularization avoiding its damage and future stenosis of the ureteral anastomosis.

Acknowledgements Nathalie Web and Juan Bortagaray, Monash Hospital from Melbourne, for sharing the video.

Anibal Espinoza and Jorge Ortiz, Clínica Alemana Santiago, for sharing the CT scans.

References

1. Soundappan SVS, Barker AP. Retrocaval ureter in children: a report of two cases. Pediatr Surg Int. 2004;20:158–60.
2. Acharya SK, Jindal B, Yadav DK, Singha S, Bagga D. Retrocaval ureter: a rare cause of hydronephrosis in children. J Pediatr Surg. 2009;44:846–8.
3. Sun J-S, Zhang G, Lin T. Retrocaval ureter in children: a report of eight cases. West Indian Med J. 2015;64(4):397.
4. Escolino M, Masieri L, Valla JS, Lopez PJ, Tokar B, Mushtaq I, Esposito C. Laparoscopic and robotic-assisted repair of retrocaval ureter in children: a multi-institutional comparative study with open repair. World J Urol. 2019;37(9):1941–7. https://doi.org/10.1007/s00345-018-2577-z.
5. Anderson JC, Hynes W. Retrocaval ureter: a case diagnosed preoperatively and treated successfully by a plastic operation. Br J Urol. 1949;21:209.
6. Celis S, López P-J. Transperitoneal laparoscopic pyeloplasty: more room, more feasibility. Dial Pediatr Urol. 2012;33(6):20–2.
7. Peycelon M, Rembeyo G, et al. Laparoscopic retroperitoneal approach for retrocaval ureter in children. World J Urol. 2020;38(8):2055–62. https://doi.org/10.1007/s00345-019-02849-w.
8. Kadar A, Vatra L, Avram A, Stoica D, Oancea M. Laparoscopic repair of a left retrocaval ureter in a 16-year-old girl. Eur J Pediatr Surg Rep. 2018;6:e104–7.
9. Fernández-Fernández JA, Pachano-Arenas FE. Laparoscopic-assisted correction of a retrocaval ureter. J Pediatr Surg. 2008;43:1560–2.

Minimally Invasive Treatment of Ureteric Stones in Children

37

Lorenzo Masieri, Giulia Bortot, Simone Sforza, Chiara Cini, and Alberto Mantovani

Learning Objectives

- To give an overview of the approach to the patient with ureteric stone.
- To explain rationale of Medical Expulsive Therapy and surgical treatment.
- To describe ureteroscopy and its steps, complications, and stone-free rate.
- To underline controversy in the current literature.

37.1 Introduction

Nephrolithiasis among children has rapidly increased its prevalence in the last decades. Moreover, around 20% of children with nephrolithiasis will experience stone recurrence over a mean follow-up of 3 years [1]. Those data underline the importance to develop centres of expertise where resources can be continuously allocated to form surgeons with a special interest in this field who can treat patients adequately and promptly and follow-up on them carefully. Ureteric stones can typically present as an emergency, with pain, haematuria, and a new-onset upper-tract dilatation. Usually they can be first approached with Medical Expulsive Therapy (MET), especially when ureteric stones are <10 mm in size. Alpha-adrenergic blockers are mostly used (Doxasozin-Tamsulosin) associated or not with NSAIDs. In children, MET has shown to significantly increase the odds of spontaneous passage of ureteric stones [2]. Doxasozin is given at a dose of 0.03 mg/kg/die, Tamsulosin at a dose of 0.4 mg/die for patients >4 years-old and 0.1–0.2 mg/die for younger children. Stone passage usually happens within few days from the beginning of the treatment [3]. If spontaneous passage is not achieved in a reasonable time, or patient comorbidities are contraindications to MET, ureteroscopy (URS) is indicated (Table 37.1). Moreover, stones >10–12 mm usually do not respond to MET. Ureteroscopy can be performed in different ways depending on patients' age and surgeon experience. In particular, the approach to ureteric stones can be with or without pre-stenting the ureter. The safest approach is to place a double-J stent and plan URS on an elective basis within few weeks. The double-J stent will allow upper-tract drainage and temporary resolution of symptoms. Moreover, the ureter will improve its compliance which will help the definitive proce-

Supplementary Information The online version contains supplementary material available at [https://doi.org/10.1007/978-3-030-99280-4_37].

L. Masieri (✉) · G. Bortot · S. Sforza
C. Cini · A. Mantovani
Pediatric Urology Department, Meyer's Children Hospital, Florence, Italy
e-mail: lorenzo.masieri@meyer.it; giulia.bortot@meyer.it; simone.sforza@unifi.it; chiara.cini@meyer.it; alberto.mantovani@meyer.it

C. Esposito et al. (eds.), *Minimally Invasive Techniques in Pediatric Urology*,
https://doi.org/10.1007/978-3-030-99280-4_37

Table 37.1 General criteria for MET and double-J stent/URS

MET	Stones <10 mm	Double-J stent/URS	Stones ≥10 mm unlikely to pass spontaneously
	Distal-ureteric stones[a]		Failed MET (beyond at least 8 days)
	Good pain control		Uncontrolled pain
	No IVU		IVU or suspect of infected stones
	Unilateral condition		Single kidney patient
	No upper tract dilatation		Upper tract dilatation[b]

[a] Mid-ureteric and proximal-ureteric stone can also be treated with MET, but with less chances of spontaneous resolution

[b] At the beginning of the pain episodes, the dilatation can be modest. However, one has to consider it as a new-onset dilatation representing obstruction

dure. The ureteric orifice will also undergo passive dilatation. Ureteric stones less frequently affect small children as they are more common in late childhood or adolescence and beyond. At those ages, the ureter can be often approached with URS without pre-stenting, especially in case of distal ureteric stones. Of note, paediatric ureteric stones (especially if located in the proximal ureter) can also be treated with extracorporeal shock-wave lithotripsy (ESWL) under general anaesthesia, even if this approach is not routinely adopted by the authors.

37.2 Preoperative Preparation

For the elective procedure, the child is admitted on the day of the operation. A negative urine culture must be recorded at pre-assessment. No particular bowel preparation is usually required. At induction, the patient will receive adequate antibiotic prophylaxis. We suggest a broad-spectrum cephalosporin, such as Cefixime. Sometimes patients have a history of UTIs. In this scenario, previous antibiogram will guide the choice of the best antibiotic prophylaxis.

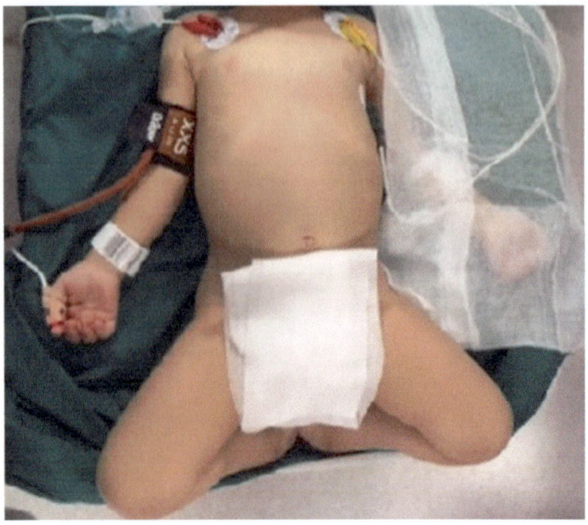

Fig. 37.1 Frog-leg position in an 18-months-old girl who underwent URS for a stuck distal ureteric stone

37.3 Positioning

The patient is placed in frog-leg or dorsal lithotomy position (Fig. 37.1). Some surgeons like to slightly lower and extend the leg of the side affected, in order to optimize the alignment of the ureter during the endoscopic procedure. Anti-Trendelenburg position helps the stone fragments not to migrate up to the renal pelvis during fragmentation. Before starting the operation, take care the C-arm reaches the kidney without interfering with the table.

37.4 Instrumentation

Instrumentation is indicative and varies according to surgeon experience and department availability.

– *Semi-rigid ureteroscope*.

  - Diameter: 7 Fr.
  - Working length: 34–43 cm.
  - Allowed instruments: 3–4 Fr.

– *Hydrophilic guide-wire*: 0.035 in. (0.89 mm)–150 cm length, with straight tip (ask for the angled tip only if required). Rarely small

guide-wire might be necessary: 0.025–0.018 in.
- *Fixed core guide-wire*: 0.035 in. (0.89 mm)–145 cm, with straight or angled tip.
- *Open-end ureteral catheter*: 4 Fr–70 cm.
- *Ureteric double-J* (various size/types).
- *Urethral catheter* (various size/types).
- *Laser fibres*: 230 μm (1.5 Fr) – most commonly used in children. There are also bigger fibres like 365 μm (2 Fr)/600 μm (3 Fr).
- *Tipless Nitinol Basket*: diameter 1.9 Fr (wire), 12 mm (basket) – length 120 cm.
- *Flexible ureteroscope*: diameter 7.5 Fr, 67 cm length.

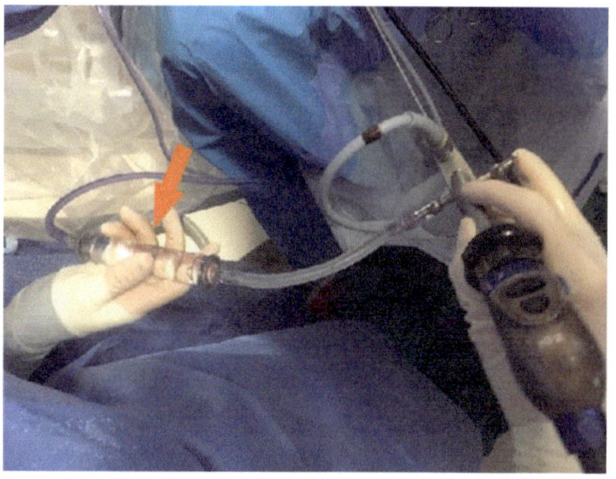

Fig. 37.2 Hand-held pump device (orange arrow)

37.5 Technique

The ureteric orifice is identified at cystoscopy. First of all, a retrograde study is performed through a ureteric stent to confirm the position of the stone and to view the upper tract anatomy. A hydrophilic 0.035 guide-wire is passed through the ureteric orifice up to the pelvis. The position of the guide-wire is checked with fluoroscopy and, when correctly in place, the redundant guide-wire is fixed outside within the sterile field. At this point, one can proceed with the ureteroscope. If the alignment of the ureter is insufficient, we suggest to place another 0.035 guide-wire to better view the ureteric lumen. With two guide-wires in place and fixed, the ureteroscope can eventually safely advance along the ureter, between the two guide-wires, up to the level of the stone. During the procedure, it is better to keep a urethral stent open in order to avoid bladder overdistension. Usually a small urethral catheter is enough and, unless very small babies, this can be placed aside the guide-wires and ureteroscope. If it is not possible to place a 5–10 Fr suprapubic catheter, leaving it open during the procedure is a choice.

Once the stone is viewed optimally, check that the flow for irrigation through the ureteroscope is enough to properly wash out the debris during fragmentation as usually the pressure at the exit of small instruments is poor. To improve the pressure, one can use a pressure bag or, alternatively, a three-way connection along the washing channel, which can be handled by the assistant for high-pressure, controlled, intermittent washing only when requested. Another technique for irrigation is to use hand-held pump device without three-way connection, managed by the assistant (Fig. 37.2). The authors found the last to be the best way to maintain an optimal view during the procedure.

Stone fragmentation and retrieval is a combination of laser and basket techniques, respectively. Holmium-YAG laser is currently the laser of choice. Dusting, fragmentation, and 'pop-corn' techniques can be combined to obtain the best effect. A 230-μm (1.5 Fr) fibre is usually enough to fragment ureteric stones in a timely manner in children. The more effect is achieved, the more the stone fragments will move off the laser field, at a point where shots will have to be given in the lumen of the ureter to achieve random final fragmentation ('pop-corn'). To retrieve stone fragments, the basket is usually the best option, and the stones collected can be left within the bladder until the end of the URS (Fig. 37.3a, b).

The aim of the procedure is to remove all significant fragments, and subsequently resolve the obstruction. At the end of the operation, small stone dust usually remains within the ureter, but this will be eventually washed out spontaneously. Once URS is completed, it is useful cleaning the stone fragments left within the bladder and leave a new double-J stent. A useful method to estimate double-J length is 10+ patient's age in centime-

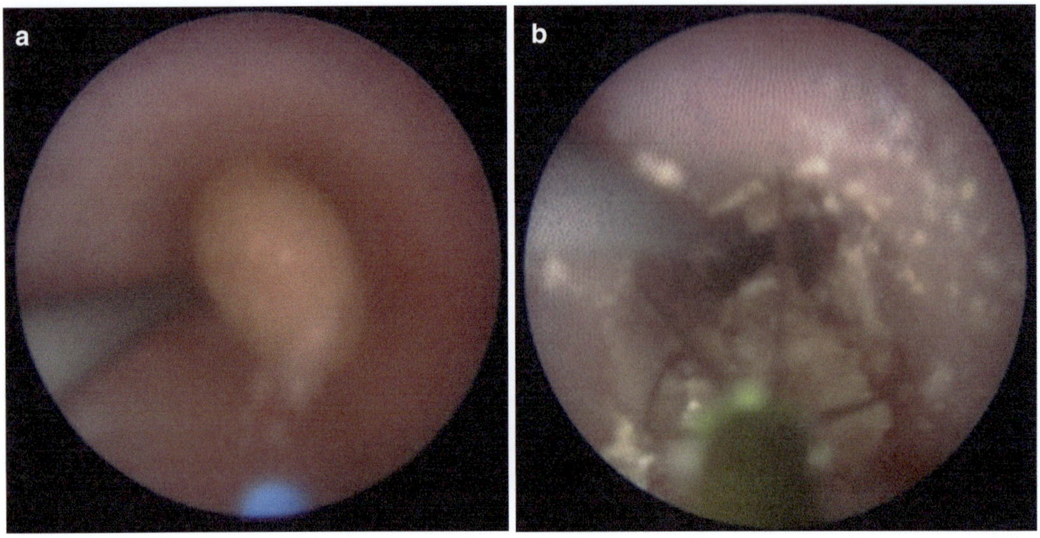

Fig. 37.3 (**a** and **b**) Ureteric stone before and after fragmentation in the same 18-months-old female patient. Basket was used to retrieve final fragments

tres. A urethral catheter is left as well at the end of the operation: if the child is old enough, an open-end catheter should provide better final washout during the post-op.

It is important to keep a flexible ureteroscope ready in case of stone migration or proximal stones not properly reached with semi-rigid ureteroscope. The detailed technique is described in the RIRS chapter (Refer to Video 37.1)

37.6 Post-Operative Care

The patient is allowed to eat and drink once well awake, generally a couple of hours after the end of the general anaesthesia. Antibiotic treatment should be continued for at least 3 days. During the recovery at 100% maintenance, I.V. fluid is given in order to improve kidney washout. Urethral catheter is removed once haematuria has resolved, usually after 2–3 days. The patient is then discharged on prophylaxis until double-J stent removal, which is planned in 3–4 weeks.

Renal-US is the imaging modality of choice during follow-up. Metabolic screening for paediatric nephrolithiasis is undertaken, and the involvement of paediatric nephrologist in a multidisciplinary setting is guaranteed.

37.7 Results

Reported stone free-rate (SFR) after URS for ureteral stones in children varies widely, but generally it is as high as 80–98% [4–7]. In a recent multicentric retrospective review including authors' center, 149 pediatric patients with ureteric stones who underwent URS with dusting technique (Holmium-YAG laser) reached an overall SFR of 97.3%. The median stone burden was 10.3 mm (range 5–17). Intra-operative complications included five bleedings (3.3%) and seven stone migration (4.7%). Post-operative complications included two cases of stent migration (1.3%) and four residual stone fragments (2.7%). Proximal location was associated with the need of re-treatment [8]. Another recent retrospective, large volume, single center review suggested a higher complication rate for proximal ureteric stones, while higher SFR was expected for distal ureteric stones, single stones, and children older than 36 months [9]. In a systematic review on URS in children published by Ishii et al. in 2015, including 83% of ureteric stones, age $\leq$ 6-years-old was associated with an overall complication rate of 24%, compared with the 7.1% reported for older children [10].

Tip and Tricks

- Remember to check the double-J stent position with X-ray or Ultrasound before stent removal, as sometimes it can be displaced. Moreover, the X-ray can identify small residual stones along the ureter, especially if the double-J stent has remained in place longer than expected. If this is suspected, keep more theatre space for stent removal, alert fluoroscopy and ask theatre staff to keep URS instruments ready, as the double-J stent might be stuck and another ureteroscopy will be then necessary. Do not force pulling the stent if this does not come out easily as ureteric damage or avulsion are likely to occur.
- The authors find the 0.035 guide-wires very versatile. However, they tend to slide down if not well fixed and regularly checked. If the ureter has a good compliance, a stiff (fixed core) guidewire can be used instead which is potentially more traumatic but maintains the position much better.
- The guide-wires usually bypass the stone easily, but long-lasting stones might be enclosed within the ureteric urothelium, not allowing the guidewire to pass beyond. This is an unusual scenario which requires very expert endourologist to look for the correct passage by attempting multiple times and often with different guide-wires, and eventually with direct fragmentation of the stone. It is important to frequently check with fluoroscopy where the instruments are as they make a false passage underneath the mucosa is not a rare event. If an enclosed stone is found, the URS should be limited to the position of the double-J stent, and stone fragmentation postponed on an elective basis.

37.8 Discussion

MET should be the first approach whenever possible, especially for ureteric stones <10 mm. Mokhless et al. reported an expulsion rate of 87.8% in the group of patients treated with Tamsulosin compared with 64.2% in patient managed with analgesic only, with a mean stone burden of around 8 mm. Moreover, days to expulsion were significantly lower in the alpha-blocker group (8.2 vs. 14.5) [11]. MET is contraindicated in case of big ureteric stones unlikely to pass spontaneously, infected stones, single kidney, or immunocompromised patients. If ESWL is available, this can also represent a valid option for ureteric stones. Lu et al. reported SFR of 95% on 115 children treated for ureteric stones (mean stone burden 7.4 mm, range 4–21) with ESWL, with 16% requiring re-treatment. No significant complications were reported and ESWL was adopted for stones located anywhere along the ureter [12]. The authors do not adopt ESWL for ureteric stones, and if MET fails, URS is the next step. When URS is indicated, there is still debate about what is the best strategy, with many centres in favour of pre-stenting the affected ureter before definitive surgery: this seems to lower the complication rate and increase SFR [13, 14]. The choice largely depends on surgeon experience, stone size, and location. Generally, large-size and proximal stones are more safely treated after pre-stenting.

Operative time is an important factor in stones treatment. Even if evidence about a strong direct correlation between operative time and complications is lacking for URS in children, this has been better shown for kidney stones, especially for the ones treated with the percutaneous approach, where the longer the operative time, the higher the complication rate, especially febrile UTIs, as a consequence of prolonged exposure of the pelvis and calyx to high pressures during the procedure [15]. In the authors' multicentric cohort, median operative URS time was 29.8 min (20–95).

In the paediatric population, the general indication is to place a double-J stent at the end of ureteroscopy. However, in adult experience, this has been questioned and it appears that uncomplicated ureteroscopy might not need a double-J stent at the end. In their systematic review, Tang et al. showed that patients discharged without stent had less urinary symptoms and haematuria compared with the stented group, in the face of similar analgesia requirement, UTIs, ureteral strictures, and SFR [16]. In children, the suggestion remains to stent the ureter at the end of URS, especially for toddlers. Conversely, pre-pubertal and pubertal patient may not need a double-J after an uncomplicated URS. The decision might also depend on degree of oedema and trauma at the ureteric orifice. If double-J is not placed, a short corticosteroid treatment can help to limit the oedema.

Take-Home Points

- MET is an option for ureteric stone <10 mm, if not contraindicated for comorbidities. Alpha-blockers are used with or without associated NSAIDs.
- URS represents a widely accepted treatment for ureteric stones. Pre-stenting the ureter is almost always a safe temporary solution but stone fragmentation can be also performed as first and definitive treatment in expert hands.
- Distal, small ureteric stones in older children seem to carry less risk of complications and higher stone-free rate compared with proximal, big ureteric stones and stones in very young patients.

References

1. Pietrow PK, Pope JC 4th, Adams MC, Shyr Y, Brock JW 3rd. Clinical outcome of pediatric stone disease. J Urol. 2002;167(2 Pt 1):670–3.
2. Velázquez N, Zapata D, Wang HH, Wiener JS, Lipkin ME, Routh JC. Medical expulsive therapy for pediatric urolithiasis: systematic review and meta-analysis. J Pediatr Urol. 2015;11(6):321–7.
3. Aydogdu O, Burgu B, Gucuk A, Suer E, Soygur T. Effectiveness of doxazosin in treatment of distal ureteral stones in children. J Urol. 2009;182(6):2880–4.
4. Minevich E, Defoor W, Reddy P. Ureteroscopy is safe and effective in prepubertal children. J Urol. 2005;174:276–9.
5. Dogan HS, Onal B, Satar N. Factors affecting the complication rates of ureteroscopic lithotripsy in children: results of multi-institutional retrospective analysis by Pediatric Stone Disease Study Group of Turkish Pediatric Urology Society. J Urol. 2011;186:1035–40.
6. Atar M, Sancaktutar AA, Penbegul N. Comparison of a 4.5 F semi-rigid ureteroscope with a 7.5 F rigid ureteroscope in the treatment of ureteral stones in preschool-age children. Urol Res. 2012;40:733–8.
7. Nerli RB, Patil SM, Guntaka AK. Flexible ureteroscopy for upper ureteral calculi in children. J Endourol. 2011;25:579–82.
8. Esposito C, Masieri L, Bagnara V, Tokar B, Golebiewski A, Escolino M. Ureteroscopic lithotripsy for ureteral stones in children using holmium: yag laser energy: results of a multicentric survey. J Pediatr Urol. 2019;15(4):391.e1–7.
9. Çitamak B, Mammadov E, Kahraman O, Ceylan T, Doğan HS, Tekgül S. Semi-rigid ureteroscopy should not be the first option for proximal ureteral stones in children. J Endourol. 2018;32(11):1028–32.
10. Ishii H, Griffin S, Somani BK. Ureteroscopy for stone disease in the paediatric population: a systematic review. BJU Int. 2015;115(6):867–73.
11. Mokhless I, Zahran AR, Youssif M, Fahmy A. Tamsulosin for the management of distal ureteral stones in children: a prospective randomized study. J Pediatr Urol. 2012;8:544–8.
12. Lu J, Sun X, He L, Wang Y. Efficacy of extracorporeal shock wave lithotropsy for ureteral stones in children. Pediatr Surg Int. 2009;25(12):1109–12.
13. Gokce MI, Telli O, Akinci A, Esen B, Suer E, Ozkidik M, Hajiyev P, Soygur T, Burgu B. Effect of prestenting on success and complication rates of ureterorenoscopy in pediatric population. J Endourol. 2016;30(8):850–5.
14. Jessen JP, Breda A, Brehmer M, Liatsikos EN, Millan Rodriguez F, Osther PJ, Scoffone CM, Knoll T. International collaboration in endourology: multicenter evaluation of prestenting for ureterorenoscopy. J Endourol. 2016;30(3):268–73.
15. Kaygısız O, Satar N, Güneş A, Doğan HS, Erözenci A, Özden E, Pişkin MM, Demirci D, Toksöz S, Çiçek T, Gürocak S, Kılıçarslan H, Nazlı O, Kefi A, İzol V, Beytur A, Sarıkaya Ş, Tekgül S, Önal B. Factors predicting postoperative febrile urinary tract infection following percutaneous nephrolithotomy in prepubertal children. J Pediatr Urol. 2018;14(5):448.
16. Tang L, Gao X, Xu B, Hou J, Zhang Z, Xu C, Wang L, Sun Y. Placement of ureteral stent after uncomplicated ureteroscopy: do we really need it? Urology. 2011;78(6):1248–56.

38 Minimally Invasive Treatment of Rare Ureteral Pathologies in Pediatric Patients

S. Gerocarni Nappo and S. F. Chiarenza

Learning Objectives

- To describe the mini-invasive approach to the upper, mid, and lower ureter.
- To describe the mini-invasive treatment of rare congenital ureteral pathologies such as fibroepitelial polyps, ureteral stenosis, and valves.
- To describe the mini-invasive treatment of rare acquired ureteral pathologies such as ureteric trauma, acquired ureteric stenosis.
- To describe laparoscopic ureteroureterostomy in duplex system as alternative option to hemnephroureterectomy and show the technique.
- To describe how to retrieve a migrated double J stent and show the technique.

Supplementary Information The online version contains supplementary material available at [https://doi.org/10.1007/978-3-030-99280-4_38].

S. G. Nappo (✉)
Simona Gerocarni Nappo, Paediatric Urology, "Regina Margherita" Children's Hospital, Turin, Italy
e-mail: sgerocarninappo@cittadellasalute.to.it

S. F. Chiarenza
Simona Gerocarni Nappo, Paediatric Urology, "Regina Margherita" Children's Hospital, Turin, Italy

Department of Pediatric Surgery and Pediatric Minimally Invasive Surgery and New Technologies, San Bortolo Hospital, Vicenza, Italy
e-mail: fabio.chiarenza@aulss8.veneto.it

38.1 Position of the Patient

For endoscopic procedures on the ureter, the patient is placed in full lithotomic position, supine with bent and spread legs laying on stirrups. The surgeon is placed between the patient legs, the assistant to the side of the surgeon, endoscopic monitor in front of the surgeon, X-Ray monitor lateral to the endoscopic monitor. Pediatric cystoscopes 5, 8, and 9.5 Fr with straight operative channel and if necessary pediatric semirigid ureteroscopes size 4,5/6,5, 6,5/7, 5, or 8/9,8 are required. Several laparoscopic procedures require first preoperative ureteric stenting.

For laparoscopic transperitoneal procedures directed to the upper and mid ureter, the patient is placed in a modified flank position, at 30°–45° degree with a pillow under the flank. Contralateral arm is extended on an arm board. The ipsilateral arm is parallel to the other arm on an elevated arm rest or on a pillow. The surgeon and assistant both face the patient, the monitor is behind the back of the patient (see position for transperitoneal pyeloplasty). Port placement is as follows: camera at umbilicus, second trocar cephalad to the camera port in the epigastric area on the midline, third trocar in the ipsilateral flank or midline below the umbilicus, fourth trocar if necessary in the ipsilateral hypocodrium. The camera port can be placed in either an open Hasson technique, which is favored by most pediatric laparoscopic surgeons, or with a Verres needle.

C. Esposito et al. (eds.), *Minimally Invasive Techniques in Pediatric Urology*,
https://doi.org/10.1007/978-3-030-99280-4_38

For transperitoneal procedures to the lower ureter, the patient is supine in Trendelemburg position, surgeon and assistant are on both sides toward the head of the patient, monitor at the feet. Port placement is as follows: camera at umbilicus, second and third port in the right and left flanks (see position for laparoscopic ureteric reimplantation).

Quick access to the proximal left ureter can be obtained, if the anatomy of the patient is favorable, through a transmesocolic approach. Access to the mid and lower left ureter, or to the right ureter, is gained after incision of the white line of Toldt and medial reflection of the colic flexure and the descending or ascending colon, respectively. Careful and delicate handling of the ureter is always mandatory.

For retroperitoneoscopic procedure, the patient is placed in full flank position, surgeon and assistant both at the back at the patient, monitor in front of the patient. Port placement is as follows: camera at the apex of XII rib, second trocar at the costovertebral angle, third trocar at the iliac crest mid-axillary line (see position for retroperitoneoscopic pyeloplasty). As an alternative, trocar can be placed in line below the XII rib on the anterior, posterior, and mid axillary line.

For robotic-assisted procedures to the upper and mid ureter, the position is the same as for laparoscopic procedure. Alternatively, the patient can be placed supine and the table rotated to elevate the pathologic side. Careful padding of all the pressure points is mandatory. The patient is always flattened for port placement. The camera port is placed first, usually at the umbilicus. Then other ports are placed under visual control. For Da Vinci Si, ports must be placed in triangulation, with one working port cephalad to the camera port and the other in the flank. Ideally, ports should be spaced about one hand from each other in order to avoid clushing. For Si, camera needs a 12 mm trocar, second and third trocar be either 5 or 8 mm according to instrument size. For da Vinci Xi, camera and working ports are all 8 mm and optimal port placement is in line. In small children, ports can be placed in the midline, thus maximizing the working space. An additional port is placed for the assistant [1].

38.2 Ureteric Stenting

Ureteric stenting can be required as the only procedure, or be performed at the beginning or at the end of an endoscopic or laparoscopic procedure. The ureter can be cannulated in a retrograde manner, from the bladder during cystoscopy or in an antegrade fashion during a laparoscopic procedure (both trans or retroperitoneal).

Double J stents used in children are of reduced size and length compared to adults. They are available in size 3, 3.7, 4, and 4.8 Fr, fixed length from 10 to 26 cm, or variable length from 8 to 20 cm. Ten and 12 cm, 3 ch are used in newborns and infants. In older children, the correct length for the patient can be calculated according to Palmer and Palmer as catheter length in cm = age in years + 10 [2] or according to Forzini et al. as age in years + 12 [3].

In retrograde placement, a cystoscope 8 or 9.5 ch with straight operative channel 5 ch is used. With the bladder half filled with saline, the ureteric orifice is negotiated with an open tip ureteric catheter 3–5 ch, and contrast medium is injected for retrograde pyelogram, in order to visualize the ureteric anatomy and presence of lesions. During retrograde, pyelogram care must be taken to avoid creating false routes while negotiating the UVJ and inducing high pressure in the upper tract. After the pyelogram, a guide-wire is inserted in the ureteric orifice. Guide-wires are available in different materials, hydrophilic, with hydrophilic tip or non-hydrophilic, and different size (0.025′ or 0.035′ generally used in children). If possible, the guide-wire can be inserted within the open-tip ureteric catheter already in place, in order to minimize the risk of traumatic lesions at the VUJ (0.025′ guide-wire fits in a 4 ch ureteric catheter, 0.035′ guide-wire in a 5 ch). Once the guide-wire is in place, the double J, properly lubricated, can be gently pushed over the guide-wire. Correct position of the proximal end of the double J is seen on X-ray of the distal end in the bladder by direct endoscopic view.

In the antegrade placement of a double J stent, the urinary tract (ureter or renal pelvis) is opened during the laparoscopic surgery. Under direct vision, a 14 gauge cannula is placed percutaneously, the guide-wire is inserted through the cannula in the proximal ureter and pushed into the bladder with laparoscopic instruments. Then the double J is gently pushed over the guide-wire. The correct position of the distal end in the bladder can be assessed with the use of diluted methylene blue filling the bladder: once the stent is in proper place, blue drops will come from the proximal end.

38.3 Ureteric Trauma

The ureter is located deep in the abdomen, running along the psoas muscle, is thin and elastic. Lesions of the ureter following a trauma are therefore very unusual in children. Penetrating trauma are uncommon, but even rarer are blunt trauma, in which the mechanism of action is often deceleration (car accidents, fall from a height, etc.). Lesions occurring after blunt trauma can be favored by a pre-existing urinary tract malformation and are often accompanied by lesions of other intra-abdominal organs.

The vast majority of ureteric traumas are indeed iatrogenic in nature, occurring during open, endoscopic, or laparoscopic surgery. In case of iatrogenic lesion, especially if the ureteric lesion is incomplete, immediate cystoscopy and double J stent placement is recommended [4–6].

Lesions occurring after blunt or penetrating trauma are more subtle to uncover. Diagnosis is often reached because the patient complains of abdominal/lumbar pain, swelling, or fever a few days after the trauma. Abdominal US shows anechoic or mixed anechoic collection in the retroperitoneum. CT scan with contrast medium is required in order to differentiate urinoma from hematoma and identify the ureteric lesion. In case of a longstanding but still incomplete ureteric lesion, attempt at double J stent placement and prolonged bladder drainage are recommended. Retroperitoneal drainage can be associated [4, 6].

If the ureteric lesion is complete, temporary nephrostomy is required. Subsequent surgery will be: ureteric reimplantation with or without Boari flap or psoas hitch for lower ureteric lesions, ureteroureteтero direct anastomosis for mid-ureteric lesions or even ureteral substitution if required. This kind of reconstructive surgery is generally performed open. Recently laparoscopic/robotic ureteral substitution with appendix has been described in few cases in children as rescue therapy, alternative to nephrectomy or kidney autotransplantation (see Sect. 38.9).

38.4 Ureteric Polyp

Fibroepithelial polyps of the ureter are a rare cause of upper urinary tract obstruction. They are benign mesenchymal tumors made histologically by a core of fibrous stoma leaned by normal appearing urohelium. Etiology is unknown, but recurrent infections, trauma, lithiasis, and immunologic disturbances have been proposed [7]. Fibroepithelial polyps occur mostly in school-age children, in males from 58% to 98% of cases and on the left side in 75% of cases [8]. Clinical presentation include intermittent flank pain, hematuria, and hydronephrosis, therefore UPJ obstruction can be misdiagnosed, with correct diagnosis often occurring at surgery. Adey et al. report the finding of fibroepithelial polyp in 0.5% of children operated for UPJ obstruction [8]. Urinary ultrasound is rarely diagnostic. In case of suspicion, the polyp can be easily visualized at CT or RMI or at preoperative retrograde pyelogram. The majority of polyps are located at the UPJ or in the proximal ureter, but they can also be found in the mid ureter, or distal ureter, or have multiple locations as well. Correct preoperative diagnosis is warranted for adequate treatment.

While earlier literature advocated open surgery excision, antegrade and retrograde endoscopic management of ureteral polyps with the use of Holmium laser and baskets has been described with high success rate [9]. However, the risk of subsequent ureteral stenosis or recurrence is not negligible and the endoscopic treatment is not suitable for large or multifocal polyps.

More recently, cases of laparoscopic treatment of ureteric polyps in children, both transperitoneally [10] and retroperitoneally [11], or robotic assisted have been published with good results [12]. Laparoscopic dismembered or flap pyeloplasty seems to be a good option for polyps of the upper ureter, while partial ureterectomy and direct ureteroureteroanstomosis have been advocated for mid-ureteric lesions. Complete preoperative imaging is warranted in order to avoid unnecessary extensive ureteric resection. Double J stenting is also recommended in order to reduce the risk of postoperative ureteric stenosis [12].

38.5 Congenital Ureteric Valves and Stenosis

Congenital ureteric valves and stenosis are other rare causes of ureteric obstruction. They have similar diagnostic issues and mini-invasive treatment and are therefore discussed together.

Valves were defined in 1952 by Wall and Watcher [13] as anatomically demonstrable transverse folds of ureteral mucosa containing bundles of smooth muscle fibers and causing obstructive changes in the urinary upper tract in the absence of other possible causes. Rabinowitz modified these standards stating that a true valve exist even when muscle fibers are found only at the base of the valves, as long as the urothelium is normal and the these criteria are met [14].

The embryogenesis of ureteral valves remains unclear [15]. Three theories exist: the persistence of Chwalla's membrane which explains the valves of the distal ureter, the persistence of the physiologic fetal folds, and abnormal ureteral embryogenesis. This last theory is enforced by the high incidence, up to 57% [14] of associated urinary anomalies, including vesicoureteric reflux, duplex system or ectopic ureter.

The distribution of valves within the ureter in children is reported as 50% in the proximal ureter, 17% in mid ureter, and 33% in the distal ureter [14].

Congenital ureteric strictures are characterized at histology by the finding of increased, decreased, or disorganized arrangement of the ureteric musculature, with or without fibrosis, with true narrowing of the ureteric lumen in the absence of valves [16]. The hypothesis is that stenosis results from relative ischemia during development, possibly by malformation of medial branched artery when the stenosis is at the level of mid ureter or due to compression by the vas deferens at the level of pelvic ureter. Prenatal diagnosis of hydronephrosis and progressive worsening of dilatation in the postnatal period is a frequent clinical presentation [17]. As for fibroepithelial polyps, both ureteric valves and congenital ureteric stenosis can be misdiagnosed preoperatively for UPJ obstruction, when located in the proximal ureter, or UVJ obstruction, when located in the distal ureter, and correct diagnosis is often made at surgery. In case accurate US and MAG3 scan suspect ureteric valves or stenosis, correct diagnosis is better confirmed preoperatively at RMI, CT scan, or retrograde pyelogram (Fig. 38.1). Intraoperative retrograde pyelogram is always recommended by some authors in order to better assess the patency of the distal ureter [16].

Traditionally treated with open surgery, congenital ureteric valves and stenosis can be successfully treated with mini-invasive surgery (Fig. 38.2). For stenosis of short segments, repair with Heinecke–Mikulicz procedure can be adequate. For longer stenosis, cases of laparoscopic repair of ureteric stricture have been described both in adults and in children [17]. A few technical consideration are worth mentioning: correct triangulation of the port according to the site of the stenosis is essential for easy suturing. Stabilization of the proximal ureter with a transabdominal stay suture, as in pyeloplasty, may help the suture. Manipulation of the distal, nondilated ureter should be reduced to the minimum, caring for accurate preservation of ureteric vascularization. After complete resection of the stenotic segment, the distal ureter must be spatulated avoiding any rotation or spiraling, and the spatulation made wide enough to match the diameter of the proximal ureter, avoiding at the same time any tension on the anastomosis. The anastomosis can be performed with 5/0 sutures over a double J of adequate size. Drain is not deemed necessary if the procedure is uneventful. As for pyeloplasty, a Foley transurethral catheter

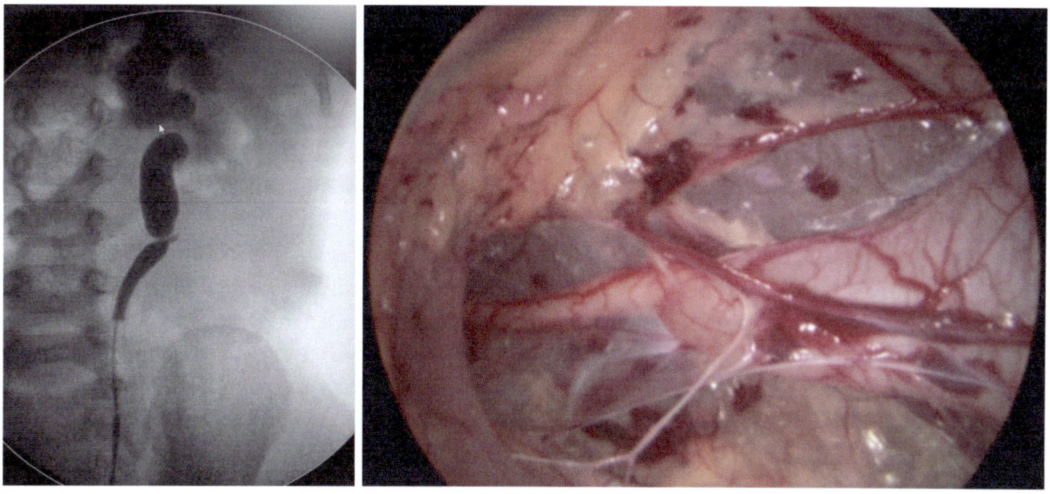

Fig. 38.1 Proximal ureteric valve: view at retroperitoneoscopy

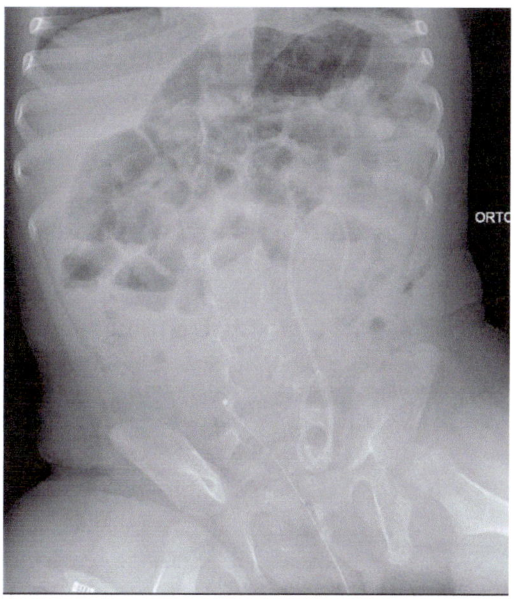

Fig. 38.2 Double J stent migrated in the distal ureter in an infant after pyeloplasty

is left in place for 48 h. Chandrasekhram reported seven patients <1 year of age with congenital mid ureteric stenosis treated with laparoscopic excision of the stenotic segment and direct uretero-ureteroanastomosis: average operative time was 87 min; at a median follow-up of 18 months; all patients showed improvement of hydronephrosis with an excellent cosmetic result.

38.6 Ureterocalicostomy for Recurrent UPJ Obstruction

Ureterocalicostomy is a potential option in patients with UPJ obstruction and significant dilatation of the lower calyx. First described in 1932 by Neuwirt, it is generally reserved to patient after failed pyeloplasty, with significant scarring at the UPJ, an intrarenal pelvis, and a dilatation of the lower calyx.

Laparoscopic and robotic ureterocalicostomy techniques were described with small case series in adults with favorable results in the majority of cases [18, 19]. In children, Casale et al. first reported robotic assisted ureterocalicostomy in 9 children aged 3–15 years with recurrent UPJ obstruction. Mean operative time was 168 min, mean hospital stay was 21 h, and all patients showed resolution of obstruction at MAG3 scan performed at 6–12 months follow-up [20]. The laparoscopic technique resembles the open ones. Cystoscopy and ureteric stenting are recommended as first step, in order to identify the ureter in the scarred tissue. Trocars are placed as for pyeloplasty. After incision of the white line of Toldt, wide mobilization of the colon and opening of the Gerota, the ureter is isolated at the level of the iliac vessels and traced up to the stenotic segment. Care is taken to preserve ureteric vasculature. The stenotic UPJ is transected and sutured. The hilar vessels can be prepared (though clamping is almost never necessary). After clearing the lower pole of the kidney from the perinephric fat, the parenchyma at the lower pole is widely excised with cautery and the mucosa of the lower calyx is exposed. Bleeding may occur at this stage. The proximal ureter is widely spatulated on the lateral side (since vascularizaton is situated medially) and directly sutured to the everted mucosa of the lower calyx in interrupted sutures. Casale et al. described using running 5/0 polyglycolic acid sutures for the posterior anastomosis and interrupted sutures for the anterior anastomosis, after placing the double J in an antegrade fashion. Careful evertion of the calyceal mucosa in the suture is of utmost importance. Recurrent stenosis may however occur.

Recently in adults, the use of near-infrared fluorescent (NIRF) imaging and intravenous IGC has been suggested during robotic-assisted calycoureterostomy, in order to assess adequate vascularity of the proximal ureter and prevent recurrent stenosis [21].

38.7 Ureteroureterostomy in Duplex System

Duplex renal system is found in 1% of the general population. It can be associated with anomalies of either the upper pole (ureterocele, ectopic ureter) or the lower pole (vesicoureteric reflux). Recurrent UTI, incontinence due to ureteric ectopia or persistent significant urinary dilatation, may require surgical correction. In such instances, surgery may follow reconstructive or ablative principles and different technical procedures have been described, including ureteric reimplantation, heminephrectomy, pyeloureterostomy, or ureteroureterostomy. The selection of the procedure is generally based on the function of the involved moiety, the presence of vesicoureteric reflux on the other moiety, the width of the ureter, surgeon, and parental preference.

Ureteroureterostomy (low) or pyeloureterostomy (high) are both valid alternatives to heminephrectomy [22], with no significant complication reported after low anastomosis due to the feared "Yo-Yo effect" [22]. Both techniques have been described either as laparoscopic-assisted, laparoscopic, or robot-assisted procedures [23–27].

Liem et al. described a single trocar retroperitoneoscopic-assisted ureteroureteroanastomosis with a technique mutated from the single trocar laparoscopic-assisted pyeloplasty. After creation of retroperitoneum, with a single 10 mm trocar and an operative camera, both ureters are isolated distally for a short segment, placed on a loop and exteriorized through the port access. The anastomosis is then performed in an open fashion. The authors used the technique in nine children with a mean operative time of 78 min, mean postoperative hospital stay of 2.6 days and functional and cosmetic good results in all patients [23].

As far as laparoscopic and robotic-assisted procedures, Lee et al. compared 25 children undergoing robotic-assisted ureteroureterostomy with 19 open procedures and found no difference in terms of operative time and complication rate [24]. Tip and tricks of the procedure are as follows. The first step is cystoscopy and placement of a double J stent in the good moiety. Then the patient is turned for the laparoscopic procedure. For high pyeloureteroanastomosis, trocar placement is like in pyeloplasty. For mid or low ureteroureterostomy, trocars are placed on the midline. Ureters are isolated as minimally as possible. The "recipient" ureter is longitudinally cut on the lateral aspect and a termino-ureteral anastomosis is performed between the "donor" ureter and the "recipient" one in 5/0 or 6/0 polydioxanone running suture. The donor ureter can be tapered in case of width discrepancy with the recipient [27]. The double J stent previously placed during cystoscopy is mobilized across the anastomosis. The foley catheter is left indwelling for about 48 h. No drain is generally deemed necessary [24–27].

The case series published in children show the technique to be easy and with a low complication rate. McLeod et al. reported a retrospective review of 41 ureteroureterostomie, 12 laparoscopic, with two complications, one requiring heminephroureterectomy [27]. Furthermore, long-term follow-up of ureteroureterostomy performed open in state in the past shows that no complication occurs at long-term follow-up related to the preservation of the dysplastic low-functioning upper pole, provided that arterial blood pressure is monitored [27]. Laparoscopic or robotic-assisted ureteroureteroanastomosis in duplex kidney can therefore be considered a valid alternative to laparoscopic heminephrectomy, irrespective of the function of the pole, the site high or low of the anastomosis and the size of the donor ureter. The rare complications described are mostly stenosis at the ureteroureteroanastomosis requiring subsequent laparoscopic heminephroureterectomy [27].

38.8 Retrieval of Migrated Double J Stent in Infants

Double J stents are frequently left in place as temporary internal drainage after several urological open or mini-invasive procedures. Migration of the tip of the double J stent from the bladder into the distal ureter is an infrequent but boresome complication. It is reported to occur in adults in 1–4% of cases [28], while its incidence in children is unknown. Risk factors are higher in short double J, misplacement at the time of initial positioning, a long-standing double J, location of the proximal curl in the upper calyx, and inadequate distal curl. The typical case is an infant who has undergone pyeloplasty, with a coexistent undetected UVJ obstruction: in such case, the double J is not found in the bladder at the time of the planned endoscopic retrieval, generally 3–6 weeks after placement.

The migrated double J in adults is universally retrieved by ureteroscopy or by endoscopic technique under fluoroscopic control: the use of different grasping forceps, helical basket, or ureteral balloon dilator tip has been described. However, if these grasping instruments are used blindly, there is a definite potential of ureteral damage.

While in older children ureteroscopy is feasible, in infants and young children, which represents the vast majority of children undergoing reconstructive procedures in pediatric urology, the ureteric orifice can be impossible to negotiate. In such instance, Koral et al. suggested an antegrade technique through a nephroscopic approach in three infants [29], and Jakumar et al., described in three patients the use of a goose neck snare under radiologic control [30]. Personal experience of one of the authors (SGN) is to dilate the UVJ with a high pressure balloon catheter, as for the endourologic treatment of primary obstructed megaureter, allowing the temporary insertion of a ureteroscope or small cystoscope in the distal ureter and retrieval of the migrated double J under direct vision. A single J is generally left indwelling for 24 h after the UVJ dilatation. The technique was used in eight cases <3 years of age, with success in all cases (personal unpublished data). A great advantage of the technique is that it leaves unchanged the cystoscopic approach planned with the parents of the child. The only concern is the potential development of vesico-ureteric after dilatation at the VUJ, but this occurrence has been reported only rarely after EHPBD in primary obstructed megaureter.

38.9 Ureteric Substitution

Ureteric defects are a rare and dramatic event occurring after failed surgery at the UPJ and/or UVJ or after ureteric trauma. Short and distal ureteric defects can be corrected with technique such as Boari flap psoas hitch, but the reconstruction of large ureteric defects is always a challenge for the pediatric urologist. In recent years, ureteric substitution has become a viable alternative treatment for adults and children with long ureteric defects, using appendix or ileum according to Yang-Monti technique.

The use of mini-invasive surgery for such procedures in children has been described anecdotically. Cao et al. [31] recently reported successful laparoscopic ureteric replacement with appendix in four patients with a mean age of 2 years. Mean ureteric stricture length was 4.5 cm, 2 right-sided, 2 left-sided. Trocars were placed on the midline. After colic mobilization, the stenotic ureter and the pelvis were dissected. The appendix was carefully mobilized, with special attention given to avoid twisting the mesoappendix. The distal end of the appendix was resected and the appendiceal lumen was irrigated with saline. The appendix was then sutured to the pelvis on one side and the lower ureter on the other side in 6/0 sutures. A double J was inserted in an antegrade fashion. Mean operative time was 238 min, mean hospital stay was 7.3 days, two patients had UTI and patency of the anastomosis was assessed in all cases at 2 month follow-up.

In case of unavailable appendix (previous appendectomy, inadequate appendix mobilization for left side ureteric defect), ileal ureteric replacement or Young-Monti ileal channel for ureteric replacement have both been described with robotic-assisted technique, with rapid recovery and little trauma. Liu et al. [32] reported robotic-assisted Young-Monti channel in six children with a mean age of 8 years and a mean ureteric defects of 5.8 cm. The procedure was successfully accomplished robotically, with an average operative time of 314 min. However, data are only initial, follow-up is short, advantages of the robotic procedure are yet to be demonstrated. Furthermore, complications of ileal ureteric substitution are nor negligible (UTI, mucous production) and the procedure should be reserved to carefully selected patients when no other option is available.

Take-Home Points

- Congenital ureteric pathologies, such as polyps, valves, or stenosis, and acquired disease, such as traumatic lesions or stenosis, are rarely encountered in daily practice of pediatric urology. Diagnosis is not always easy and may require retrograde pyelogram, CT, RMI, etc.
- Data from the literature show that it is feasible to treat these pathologies successfully by mini-invasive surgery, but the small numbers of the case series make impossible to draw conclusion on the real advantages.
- Mini-invasive technique on the ureter could be considered in the daily armamentarium of pediatric laparoscopist in selected complex cases. Laparoscopic/robotic pyeloureteric anastomosis and ureteroureteroanastomosis can been considered alternatives to heminephrectomy or ureteroneocystostomy, and similarly laparoscopic ureterocalicostomy is an option in case of recurrent UPJ obstruction.
- When embarking on mini-invasive surgery on the ureter, one should keep in mind that this is however a particularly delicate surgery. The surgeon should be an expert reconstructive laparoscopist, at ease with dissection of upper abdomen, lower abdomen, and precise suturing of pyeloplasty. Handling of the ureter should be particularly careful in order to minimize trauma and ischemic injuries, and stay sutures be used for suspension and to avoid ureteric torsion. These conditions should be always fulfilled for a successful laparoscopic reconstructive surgery on the ureter.

References

1. Bilgutay AN, Kirsch AJ. Robotic ureteral reconstruction in the pediatric population. Front Pedaitr. 2019;7:85. https://doi.org/10.3389/fped.2019.00085.
2. Palmer JS, Palmer LS. Determining the proper stent length to use in children: age +10. J Urol. 2007;178:1566.9. https://doi.org/10.1016/j.juro.2007.03.191.
3. Forzini T, Demouron M, Uhl M, Mesureur S, Renard C, Klein C, Heraux E. Computer tomography evaluation of ureteral length in children. J Pediatr Urol. 2019;15:555.e1–5. https://doi.org/10.1016/j.jpurol.2019.06.011.
4. Mariotto A, Zampieri N, Cecchetto M, Camoglio FS. Ureteral rupture after blunt trauma in a child with unknown horseshoe kidney. Pediatr Med Chir. 2015;37:110.
5. Lee Van E, Zmora O, Cazzulino F, et al. Management of pediatric blunt renal trauma: a systematic review. J Trauma Acute Care Surg. 2016;80(3):519–28.

6. Bryk DJ, Zhao LC. Guideline of guidelines: a review of urological trauma guidelines. BJU Int. 2016;117:226–34.
7. Cassar Delia E, Joseph VT, Sherwood W. Fibroepitehlial polyps causing ureteropelvic junction obstruction in children-case report and review article. Eur J Pediatr Surg. 2007;17:142–7.
8. Adey GS, Vargas SO, REtik AB, et al. Fibroepithelial polyps causing ureteroplevic junction obstruction in children. J Urol. 2003;169:1834–6.
9. Childs MA, Umbreit EC, Krambeck AE, et al. Fibropeithelial polyps of the ureter—a single institutional experience. J Endourol. 2009;23:1415–9.
10. Bian Z, Liu X, Hua Y, et al. Laparoscopic management of multiple ureteral polyps in children. J Urol. 2011;186:1444–9.
11. Dai LN, Chen CD, Lin XK, et al. Retroperitoneal laparoscopy management for ureteral fibroepitelial polyps causing hydronephrosis in children: a report of five cases. J Pediatr Urol. 2015;11:257.e1–5.
12. Osbun N, Ellison JS, Lendvay TS. Robot-assisted laparoscopic excision of ureteral and ureteropelvic junction fibroepithelial polyps in children. J Endourol. 2016;30(8):896–900.
13. Wall B, Wachter E. Congenital ureteral valve: its role as a primary obstructive lesion: classification of the literature and report of an authentic case. J Urol. 1952;68:684–90.
14. Rabinowitz R, Kingston TE, Wesselhoeft C, Caldamone AA. Ureteral valves in children. Urology. 1998;51(Suppl 5A):7–11.
15. Maizels M, Stephens FD. Valves of the ureter as a cause of primary obstruction of the ureter: anatomic, embryologic and clinical aspects. J Urol. 1980;123:742–7.
16. Hwang AH, McAleer AM, Shapiro E, et al. Congenital mid ureteral stricture. J Urol. 2005;174:1999–2002.
17. Chandrasekhram VVS. Laparoscopic repair of congenital midureteric stricture in infants and children. J Pediatr Surg. 2015;50:1909–13.
18. Gill IS, Cherullo EE, Steinberg AP, et al. Laparoscopic ureterocalicostomy: initial experience. J Urol. 2004;171:1227–30.
19. Schimpf MO, Wagner JR. Robotic-assisted laparoscopic ureterocalicostomy with long term followup. J Endourol. 2009;23(2):293–5.
20. Casale P, Muchsavage P, Resnik M, Kim SS. Robotic ureterocalicostomy in the pediatric population. J Urol. 2008;180:2643–8.
21. Ramanitharan M, Narayanan DL, Sreenivasan SR, et al. Outcome of robot-assisted ureterocalicostomy in secondary ureteropelvic junction in adults: initial experience using Da Vinci xi system with near-infrared fluorescence imaging. J Laparoendosc Adv Surg Tech A. 2020;30(1):48–52.
22. Chacko JK, Koyle MA, Mingin GC, et al. Ipsilateral uretero-ureterostomy in the surgical management of the severely dilated ureter in ureteral duplication. J Urol. 2007;178:1689–92.
23. Liem NT, Dung LA, Viet ND. Single trocar retroperitoneoscopic assisted ipsilateral ureteroureterostomy for ureteral duplication. Pediatr Sureg Int. 2012;28:1031–4.
24. Lee NG, Corbett ST, Cobb KC, et al. Bi-institutional comparison of robot-assisted laparoscopic versus open uretero-ureterostomy in the pediatric population. J Endourol. 2015;29(11):1237–41. https://doi.org/10.1089/end.2015.0223.
25. Storm D, Modi A, Jayanthi VR. Laparoscopic ipsilateral ureteroureterostomy in the management of ureteral ectopia in infants and children. J Pediatr Urol. 2011;7:529–33.
26. Passerotti CC, Diamond DA Borer JG, et al. Robotic-assisted laparoscopic ureteroureterostomy: description of technique. J Endourol. 2008;22:581–5.
27. McLeod DJ, Alpert SA, Ural Z, Jayanthi VR. Ureteroureterostomy irrespective of ureteral size or upper pole function: a single center experience. J Pediatr Urol. 2014;10:616–9.
28. Livadas KE, Varkarakis IM, Skolarikos A, Karagiotis E, Alivizatos G, Sofras F, Deliveliotis C, Bissas A. Ureteroscopic removal of mildly migrated stents using local anesthesia only. J Urol. 2007;178(5):1998–2001. https://doi.org/10.1016/j.juro.2007.07.027. Epub 2007 Sep 17. PMID: 17869304.
29. Koral K, Desai D, Gargollo P, Snodgrass W. Antegrade retrieval of double J with capture of the bladder end in three young children. Clin Imaging. 2012;36:626–8.
30. Sivasankar J, Marjan M, Wong K, Bolia A, Ninan GK. Retrieval of proximally migrated double J ureteric stents in children using goose neck snare. J Indian Assoc Pediatr Surg. 2012;17(1):6–8.
31. Cao H, Zhou H, Yang F, Ma L, Zhou X, Tao T, et al. Laparoscopic appendiceal interposition pyeloplasty for long ureteric strictures in children. J Pediatr Urol. 2018;14(6):551.e1–5.e5. https://doi.org/10.1016/j.jpurol.2018.06.017.
32. Liu D, Zhou H, Hao X, Cao H, Ma L, Zhou X, et al. Laparoscopic Yang-Monti ureteral reconstruction in children. Urology. 2018;118:177–82. https://doi.org/10.1016/j.urology.2018.04.034.

Part IV

Bladder

Minimally Invasive Techniques in Pediatric Urology: Vesicoureteral Reflux Endoscopy

39

Hiroyuki Koga, Hiroshi Murakami, and Atsuyuki Yamataka

Learning Objectives

- To master the technique for endoscopic Deflux® treatment (DT) using step-by-step instructions.
- To understand the effectiveness of DT by reviewing mid-term results.
- To have up-to-date knowledge of the latest reports about DT in the literature.
- To reinforce understanding of DT by watching a video.

39.1 Introduction

Vesicoureteral reflux (VUR) is one of the most frequently detected urinary tract abnormalities, affecting approximately 1–2% of the pediatric population and 25–40% children presenting with a history of febrile urinary tract infection (UTI) [1, 2]. There is a range of severity of VUR and management regimes that incorporate a spectrum of philosophies and modalities ranging from observation with or without continuous antibiotic prophylaxis to active surgical intervention [3]. Essentially, the optimal treatment for VUR is yet to be established because not all cases require intervention. The indications for those who will benefit from intervention include the grade of VUR, history of recurrent UTI, and parental preference. However, whether intervention should be an open surgical procedure is currently controversial because of the major change in treating VUR that followed Puri's first clinical report about an endoscopic procedure they called STING, published in 1984 [4]. Since then, STING has been modified to improve VUR cure rates, for example, by introducing the hydrodistention implantation technique (HIT) [5] and double HIT [6]. Several tissue augmenting substances have been used for subureteral injection, such as polytetrafluoroethylene, collagen, silicone, autologous chondrocytes, and Deflux® [7], followed by a succession of new substances; for example, in 2010, the preliminary results of a prospective multicenter study of a new substance "polyacrylate polyalcohol copolymer (PPC/Vantris®)" was published [8]. While Deflux® is still the most widely used implant agent, recently, DT has been implicated as a potential cause of ureteral obstruction.

The goals of treating a child with VUR are: (1) to prevent febrile UTI; (2) to prevent renal damage; and (3) to: "to maximize improvement

Supplementary Information The online version contains supplementary material available at [https://doi.org/10.1007/978-3-030-99280-4_39].

H. Koga (✉) · H. Murakami · A. Yamataka
Department of Pediatric General and Urogenital Surgery, Juntendo University School of Medicine, Tokyo, Japan
e-mail: h-koga@juntendo.ac.jp; hmuraka@juntendo.ac.jp; yama@juntendo.ac.jp

C. Esposito et al. (eds.), *Minimally Invasive Techniques in Pediatric Urology*,
https://doi.org/10.1007/978-3-030-99280-4_39

with minimal physical/emotional stress" [3]. Here, we describe our technique for the endoscopic treatment of VUR and a simple noninvasive maneuver that we pioneered to identify post-DT ureteral obstruction and at-rsik patients for ureteral obstruction, especially late-onset ureteral obstruction.

39.2 Preprocedural Preparation

Preoperative ultrasonography is performed as the initial imaging study to determine the shape of the kidney and confirm the presence of scarring. If scarring is considerable, or renal parenchymal volume is reduced, or the kidney is hyperechoic, or cortico-medullary junctions are obscure, 99mTc-dimercaptosuccinic acid (DMSA) renal scintigraphy is performed to further assess preoperative function and drainage. If function is poor (<10%), consideration should be given to removing the kidney and ureter rather than correcting VUR. Prior to any surgical intervention for VUR, cystography is mandatory using either classical cystography, which allows the morphology of the bladder and the ureters to be confirmed with detailed delineation of VUR for accurate classification but associated with high radiation exposure or cystoscintigraphy that has the advantage of less radiation exposure but less accurate representation of morphology and potential for less accurate classification of VUR.

39.3 Materials

39.3.1 Implant Substances

Deflux®: A suspension of dextranomer microspheres in sodium hyaluronate solution developed by Stenberg and Lackgren. Currently, it is the most widely used injectable implant substance. In most cases, a volume of 0.5 to 1.5 mL is effective for correcting VUR.

Cystoscopes and Needles.

We prefer to use an 8.0 or 9.5 Fr pediatric cystoscope (Karl Storz, Inc., Tuttlingen, Germany) with an offset lens for injecting Deflux® because the offset lens permits direct passage of a 3.7 Fr needle in line with the ureter, so there is no need to bend the Deflux® needle.

39.4 Patient Positioning

General anesthesia is induced conventionally and maintained by endotracheal intubation or a laryngeal mask airway with no special additional requirements. The patient is placed supine with the legs lowered slightly and spread wide enough apart for the treating surgeon to access a very lateral ureteral orifice or stand between the patient's legs if required. Special imaging equipment is not required (Fig. 39.1).

39.5 Technique

After cystoscopy, the bladder is drained to provide just enough distention to allow inspection of the trigone. When the bladder is less full, ureteral orifices and intramural tunnels are easier to identify. We insert a soft-tip epidural anesthesia catheter (20 gauge, Perifix®) (B. Braun, Melsungen AG, Germany) through a side channel of the cystoscope. Once the epidural catheter has been inserted into the ureter, the cystoscope is withdrawn, leaving the epidural catheter in the ureter and the urethra (Fig. 39.2). The cystoscope is then carefully reinserted into the urethra with the epidural catheter in situ, and a needle is inserted through the side channel of the cystoscope. The needle is then advanced enough to support the trigone but not so far as to result in injection outside Waldeyer's sheath into the detrusor or extravesical space. The needle must be just submucosal. After confirmation that the Deflux® needle is in the desired position, Deflux® is injected submucosally according to the original technique reported by O'Donnell [4]. Initially, injection should be inserted very gently to assess where the injected material is going. Immediately following this, 1~3 mL of 20% indigo carmine solution is injected through the epidural catheter, and passage of dye from the treated ureteral orifice into the bladder within a reasonable time is confirmed

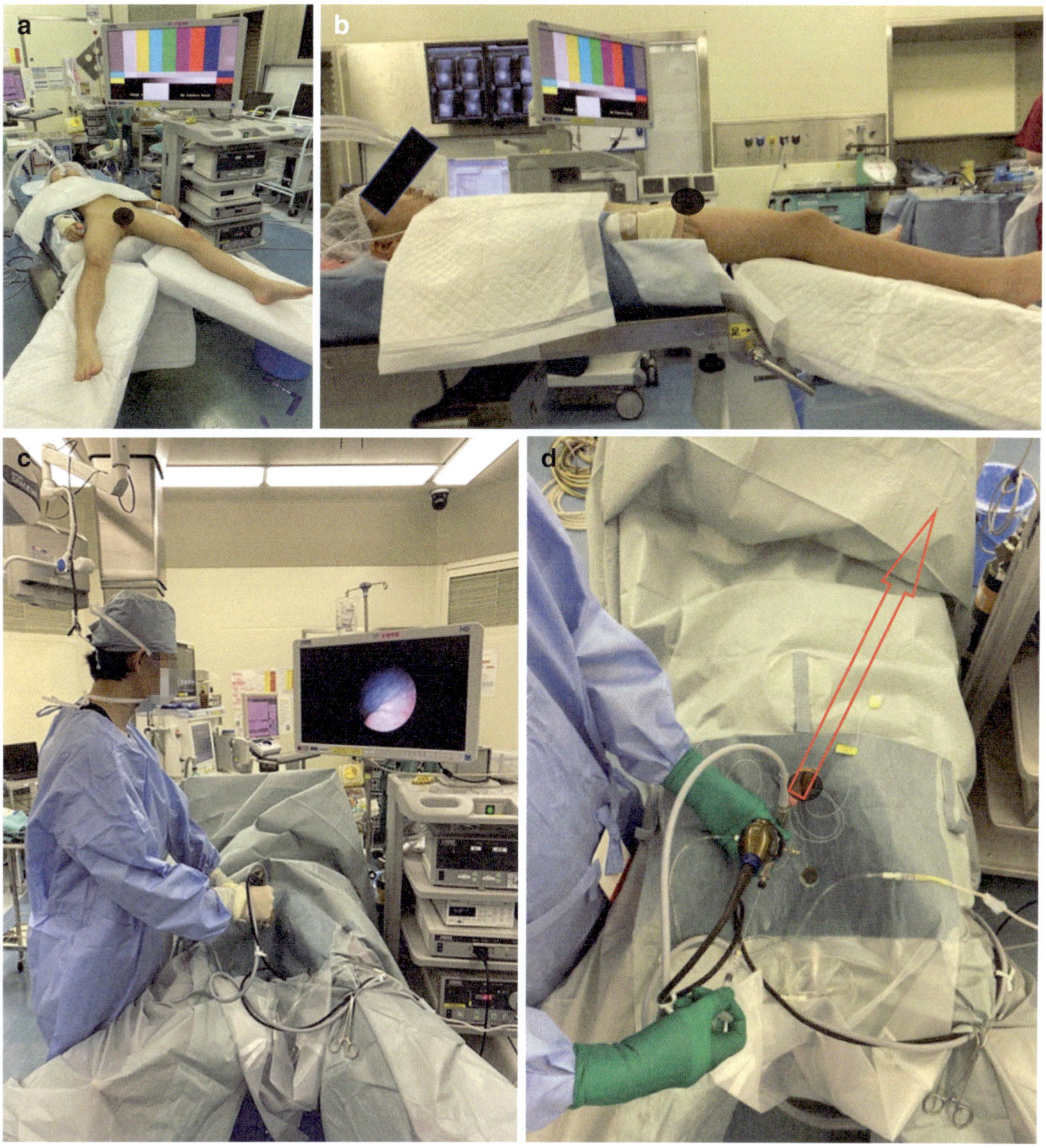

Fig. 39.1 Standard operating room layout. (**a**) This figure shows a standard operating room layout for a left DT procedure. (**b**) The patient's feet are positioned slightly lower than the torso to help use the cystoscope better. (**c**) The operating surgeon will stand on the right side of the patient for a left DT, and on the left side of the patient for a right DT, and between the patient's legs for bilateral DT procedures. (**d**) The surgeon's direction of view and the orientation of the cystoscope are the same (large red arrow)

before the epidural catheter is removed (Fig. 39.3). If there is no passage of dye after at least 15 min of observation, the epidural catheter is not removed and clamped because the patient is at risk for ureteral obstruction, and the patient is transferred back to the ward with the epidural catheter in situ overnight. If dye is observed in the urine the next day, the patient may be discharged, but if no dye is observed, ultrasonography is performed to check for hydronephrosis which is a pathognomonic sign of ureteral obstruction. If there are no signs of ureteral obstruction on ultrasonography, the epidural catheter is removed in the ward the next day. If there are signs of ureteral obstruction on ultrasonography, a double J stent is inserted into the ureter. Renal and bladder ultraso-

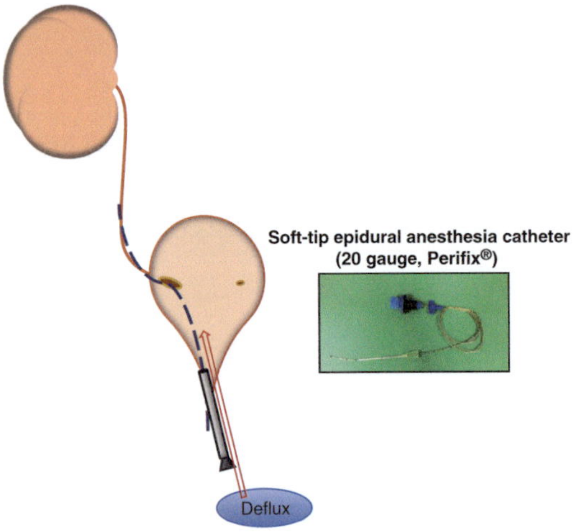

Fig. 39.2 Diagram of our epidural catheter maneuver. This maneuver involves inserting an epidural catheter into the ureter treated by Deflux® and injecting a solution of indigo carmine to observe for passage of dye

nography are organized for the first routine outpatient clinic follow-up visit, 3 weeks after discharge from hospital.

39.6 Postprocedural Care

Patients are prescribed antibiotic prophylaxis for 3 months, at which time voiding cystography is performed. If VUR has been cured, antibiotic prophylaxis is ceased, and the patient is advised to be wary of early signs of UTI. Voiding cystography is not performed routinely unless required. Ultrasonography of the kidneys and bladder is performed annually to assess the position, size, and location of implants. It is essential that the patient and caregivers are aware that VUR may relapse if there is migration or breakdown of an

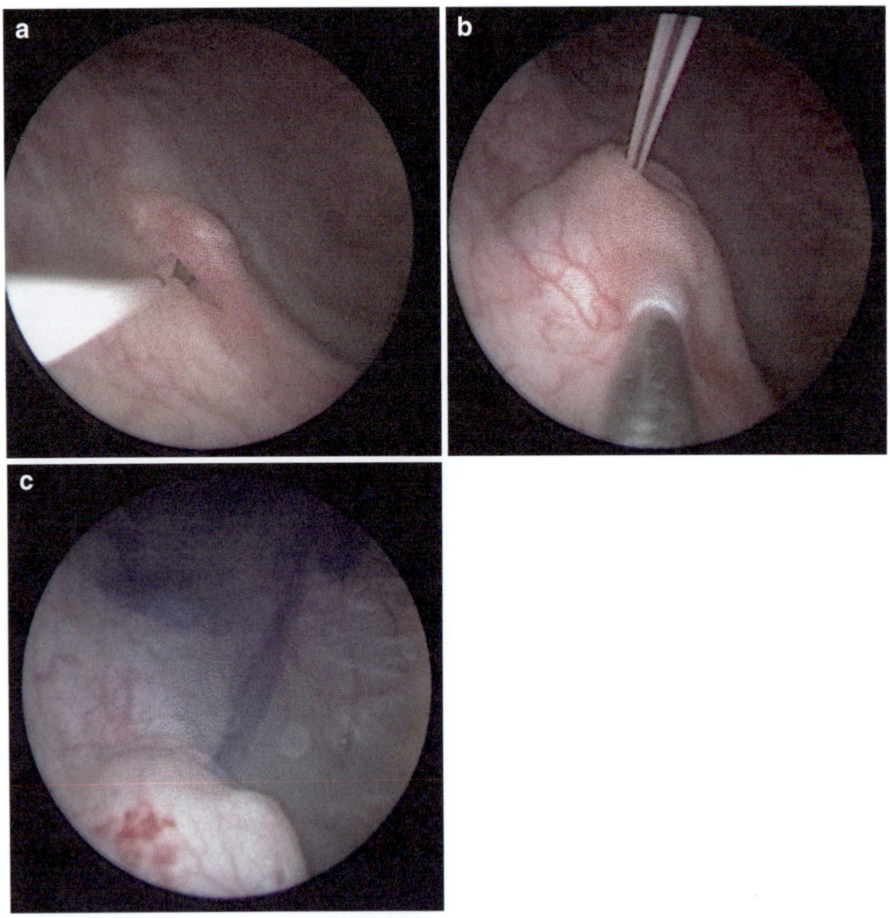

Fig. 39.3 Our epidural catheter maneuver being performed. Our epidural catheter maneuver. An epidural catheter is inserted into the ureter (**a**), then a Deflux® needle is inserted at the 6 o'clock position and Deflux® is injected (**b**). There is flow of dye from the treated ureteral orifice into the bladder (**c**)

implant. Caregivers are instructed to return for immediate assessment if there is any cause for concern or any evidence of UTI.

39.7 Results

We have treated 259 ureters with grades II to V VUR in 175 patients using the technique we described between 2011 and 2019. Of these, 109 were male and 66 were female. VUR severity in our series of 259 ureters was grade II in 50 (19.3%), grade III in 84 (32.4%), grade IV in 103 (39.7%), and grade V in 22 (8.4%). Mean age at the first DT was 4.7 years (range: 0.7–29.8 years). Mean operative time was 29.4 min (range: 9–45 min). Mean duration of postoperative follow-up was 5.9 years (range: 0.2–9.3 years).

"Cure" was defined as complete disappearance of VUR or downgrading to grade I. Overall "cure" after one DT was 58.3%, 78.8% after two DT, and 84.2% after three DT (Table 39.1). As per original grade of VUR, "cure" after one DT was 72.0% for grade II; 63.1% for grade III; 51.5% for grade IV; and 40.9% for grade V; two DT was 90.0% for grade II; 75.0% for grade III; 84.4% for grade IV; and 59.1% for grade V; and 92.0%; three DT was 92.0% for grade II; 82.1% for grade III; 87.4% for grade IV; and 59.1% for grade V (Table 39.2). The mean number of DT required to "cure" grade II was 1.35 times; 1.39 times for grade III; 1.52 times for grade IV; and 1.80 times for grade V.

Of the 259 ureters treated in this series, there was no passage of dye observed after 15 min in six cases (2.3%). Of these, two required surgical intervention. One case was a 10-year-old boy whose catheter was left in situ because there was no dye flow after 15 min of observation, however, when the catheter was clamped, he developed flank pain and significant hydronephrosis was identified on ultrasonography the next day, requiring insertion of a double J stent with complete resolution of pain and hydronephrosis. The stent was removed after 1 month. He has been pain-free with stable follow-up since then. The other case was a 1-year-old boy whose epidural catheter was removed before confirming dye flow and required insertion of a double J stent because of gross hydronephrosis caused by Deflux® (Fig. 39.4). The stent currently remains in situ.

Table 39.1 Overall "cure" rates with respect to number of Deflux treatments (DT)

	After one DT	After two DT	After three DT
Overall "cure"	151/259 (58.3%)	204/259 (78.8%)	218/259 (84.2%)

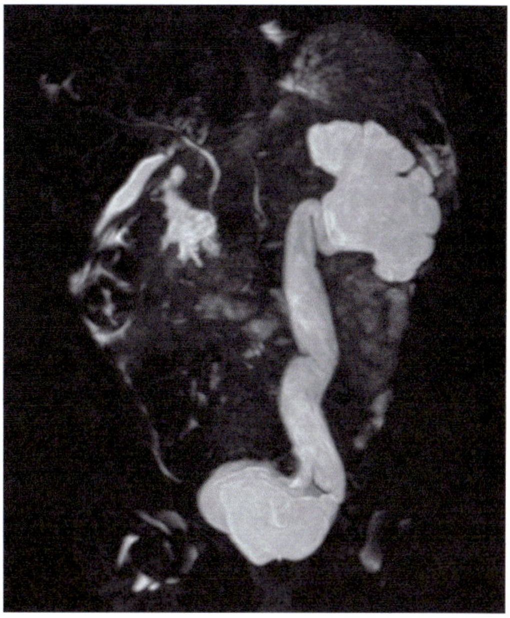

Fig. 39.4 Magnetic resonance urography appearance of ureteral obstruction after Deflux®. MR urography appearance of ureteral obstruction in a patient who had DT without confirmation of dye passage

Table 39.2 "Cure" rates with respect to grade of VUR and number of DT

VUR Grade	After one DT	After two DT	After three DT	Overall "cure" after three DT
II	36/50 (72.0%)	36 + 9/50 (90.0%)	45 + 1/50 (92.0%)	46/50 (92.0%)
III	53/84 (63.1%)	53 + 10/84 (75.0%)	63 + 6/84 (82.1%)	69/84 (82.1%)
IV	53/103 (51.5%)	53 + 34/103 (84.4%)	87 + 3/103 (87.4%)	90/103 (87.4%)
V	9/22 (40.9%)	9 + 4/22 (59.1%)	13 + 0/22 (59.1%)	13/22 (59.1%)

DT = Deflux treatments

Tips and Tricks

- The patient should be positioned with their legs spread as wide apart as is comfortable. The operating surgeon will stand on the patient's right side for a left DT and on the patient's left side for a right DT and between the patient's legs for bilateral cases. The operating surgeon's direction of view and the orientation of the cystoscope are the same.
- If the needle is removed too quickly after injection during DT, Deflux® will leak from the injection site. The needle should be maintained steadily at the injection site for at least 60 s after injection to prevent leakage of Deflux®. Nevertheless, a minute amount of leakage is unavoidable and will cease spontaneously.
- If there is no bulging during injection, the needle may be too deep and periureteral rather than submucosal. The injection should be abandoned, the needle removed, and the injection repeated in the correct place with a fresh dose of Deflux®.
- If bulging during injection is not in the correct place, do not remove the needle. Change the angle of the needle or rotate the needle and try injecting again very carefully, checking if the bulge is located more favorably.
- Practice makes perfect. Successful DT depends on the expertise and experience of the operating surgeon as Kirsch et al. reported; outcome of DT is a correlation between location of injected material and experience [9].

39.8 Discussion

Although various options are available for the treatment of children with VUR, endoscopic DT is now a well-accepted technique for treating VUR. Although ureteral reimplantation has been the gold standard for the treatment of high grade VUR for many years, it is invasive, requiring extended hospitalization, and is associated with complications such as vesicoureteral obstruction. Endoscopic treatment of VUR is a minimally invasive procedure with low reported rates of complications requiring surgical intervention, of the order of less than 1% [10] and reported rates of postoperative ureteral obstruction of less than 1% of treated cases, which appears be independent of the injected bulking agent, volume, and technique. Of interest is that ureteral obstruction has also been reported to be caused by perioperative edema alone. A recently published report about late-onset ureteral obstruction, defined as newly developed or progressive hydronephrosis 8 weeks or more after Deflux® or Vantris® injection, found the rate of late ureteral obstruction after Deflux® or Vantris® injection was 1.9% and that the mean time taken for late ureteral obstruction to occur was 13.4 months [11]. To date, we have not had any development of late-onset ureteral obstructions even though our mean follow-up (5.9 years) is longer than the mean time for late-onset ureteral obstruction to develop, as reported recently (1.1 years) [11].

A randomized controlled trial conducted on 203 children with grade III to IV VUR revealed that endoscopic Deflux® injection resulted in resolution or downgrading in most instances [12]. A meta-analysis conducted by Elder et al. showed success rates of 57% to 77% for a single injection of the four most widely used substances with an overall resolution rate of 72% [13, 14]. In other words, about 50% of children with high grades of VUR will not be cured without multiple injections. Friedmacher et al. emphasized that endoscopic injection with Deflux provides a high-resolution rate in grades IV and V VUR. Additional injection treatments can easily be repeated in cases of failure, with a high subsequent resolution rate. Elder's meta-analysis reported a success rate of 85% with multiple treatments [13, 14]. Therefore, this minimally invasive procedure was included as an option in the 2010 AUA (American Urological Association) guidelines for the management of primary VUR in children [3].

As a result, the majority of parents clearly prefer DT over invasive open surgery, even if the cure rate dose not equal that of open surgical intervention and additional anesthesia is required, while a growing number prefer it over prophylactic antibiotic use [5]. Indeed, a survey of 100 counseled caregivers of children with VUR found that 80% opted for endoscopic injection rather than surveillance with prophylactic antibiotics or open reimplantation surgery, when given the choice [15]. Thus, the demand for DT is likely to increase and the prevention of complications becomes a major issue.

We believe our epidural catheter maneuver effectively identifies patients at risk for ureteral obstruction, both acute and late-onset. If dye flow is delayed or absent, our protocol defines what should be done specifically so that early diagnosis, early treatment, and appropriate follow-up are all organized appropriately.

With continued acceptance, success, and minimal to no side effects from the use of injectable implant material, minimal invasive endoscopy will continue to maintain its prominent place as a first-line treatment for VUR.

Take-Home Points

- Creation of an elevated, coapted mound correlates with VUR resolution, regardless of injection volume and technique.
- Failure of DT is usually associated with poor wound formation due to loss of injected material or migration of material from under the ureteral orifice.
- DT can be repeated safely in cases of failure, with a high subsequent resolution rate.
- Our epidural catheter maneuver effectively identifies patients at risk for ureteral obstruction, both acute and late-onset.
- Due to the sudden boom in DT for VUR, most institutions are yet to accumulate sufficient data to assess long-term outcome, objectively. In particular, the stability of injectable implant material as well as their degeneration/degradation, migration, and possible chemical reactions are all issues that could prove to be problematic over time but are only just starting to find their way into the literature.

References

1. Kirsch AJ, Arlen AM, Lackgren G. Current trends in dextranomer hyaluronic acid copolymer (Deflux) injection technique for endoscopic treatment of vesicoureteral reflux. Urology. 2014;84(2):462–8.
2. Skoog SJ, Peters CA, Arant BS Jr, Copp HL, Elder JS, Hudson RG, et al. Pediatric vesicoureteral reflux guidelines panel summary report: clinical practice guidelines for screening siblings of children with vesicoureteral reflux and neonates/infants with prenatal hydronephrosis. J Urol. 2010;184(3):1145–51.
3. Peters CA, Skoog SJ, Arant BS Jr, Copp HL, Elder JS, Hudson RG, et al. Summary of the AUA guideline on management of primary vesicoureteral reflux in children. J Urol. 2010;184(3):1134–44.
4. O'Donnell B, Puri P. Treatment of vesicoureteric reflux by endoscopic injection of Teflon. 1984. J Urol. 2002;167(4):1808–9. discussion 10
5. Kirsch AJ, Perez-Brayfield M, Smith EA, Scherz HC. The modified sting procedure to correct vesicoureteral reflux: improved results with submucosal implantation within the intramural ureter. J Urol. 2004;171(6 Pt 1):2413–6.
6. Cerwinka WH, Scherz HC, Kirsch AJ. Dynamic hydrodistention classification of the ureter and the double hit method to correct vesicoureteral reflux. Arch Esp Urol. 2008;61(8):882–7.
7. Puri P, Pirker M, Mohanan N, Dawrant M, Dass L, Colhoun E. Subureteral dextranomer/hyaluronic acid injection as first line treatment in the management of high grade vesicoureteral reflux. J Urol. 2006;176(4 Pt 2):1856–9. discussion 9–60
8. Ormaechea M, Ruiz E, Denes E, Gimenez F, Denes FT, Moldes J, et al. New tissue bulking agent (polyacrylate polyalcohol) for treating vesicoureteral reflux: preliminary results in children. J Urol. 2010;183(2):714–7.
9. Friedmacher F, Colhoun E, Puri P. Endoscopic injection of dextranomer/hyaluronic acid as first line treatment in 851 consecutive children with high grade vesicoureteral reflux: efficacy and long-term results. J Urol. 2018;200(3):650–5.
10. Romain J, Fourcade L, Centi J, Blanc P, Masselin MC, Lescure V, et al. Delayed-onset ureteral obstruc-

tion and calcification masquerading as renal colic following deflux injection. Urology. 2016;94:218–20.
11. Ben-Meir D, Bahouth Z, Halachmi S. Late-onset uretero-vesical junction obstruction following endoscopic injection of bulking material for the treatment of vesico-ureteral reflux. Urology. 2017;101:60–2.
12. Holmdahl G, Brandstrom P, Lackgren G, Sillen U, Stokland E, Jodal U, et al. The Swedish reflux trial in children: II. Vesicoureteral reflux outcome. J Urol. 2010;184(1):280–5.
13. Elder JS, Diaz M, Caldamone AA, Cendron M, Greenfield S, Hurwitz R, et al. Endoscopic therapy for vesicoureteral reflux: a meta-analysis. I. Reflux resolution and urinary tract infection. J Urol. 2006;175(2):716–22.
14. Elder JS, Peters CA, Arant BS Jr, Ewalt DH, Hawtrey CE, Hurwitz RS, et al. Pediatric Vesicoureteral Reflux Guidelines Panel summary report on the management of primary vesicoureteral reflux in children. J Urol. 1997;157(5):1846–51.
15. Capozza N, Lais A, Matarazzo E, Nappo S, Patricolo M, Caione P. Treatment of vesico-ureteric reflux: a new algorithm based on parental preference. BJU Int. 2003;92(3):285–8.

40 Vesico-Ureteric Reflux (VUR): Laparoscopic Lich–Gregoir Repair

François Varlet, Aurélien Scalabre, and Sophie Vermersch

40.1 Introduction

Vesico-ureteral reflux (VUR) is defined as a permanent or intermittent intrusion of bladder urine into the upper urinary tract due to a defective uretero-vesical junction. The pathophysiology of VUR remains unclear, but there is a general consensus that intrarenal reflux of infected urine can cause renal damage (reflux nephropathy). VUR can be the result of a morphological abnormality at the level of the vesico-ureteral junction (primary malformative VUR) or secondary to lower urinary tract dysfunction. Primary malformative VUR can be diagnosed prenatally when associated with urinary tract dilatation. It is more frequent in boys and the regression rate is low. VUR secondary to lower urinary tract dysfunction is more common. It usually occurs in girls with poor bladder and bowel function. Its resolution rate is high with education regarding good micturition and medical treatment against constipation. There is currently no consensus regarding indications for surgery in children with VUR [1, 2]. However, repeated pyelonephritis despite bladder educational treatment or antibioprophylaxis and decreasing renal function on isotope studies are strong arguments for surgical treatment.

Different techniques are available for the surgical treatment of VUR. The Cohen technique described in 1969 is often considered the gold standard [3]. Minimally invasive surgery techniques were recently developed in order to reduce postoperative pain, avoid postoperative haematuria, and shorten hospitalization. They include endoscopic treatment, vesicoscopy, and laparoscopic vesico-ureteral reimplantation.

The Lich–Gregoir technique is an extravesical ureteral reimplantation described by Lich et al in 1962 and Gregoir in 1964 [4, 5], more recently adapted for laparoscopic approach [6]. This technique is often used for unilateral reflux, but concerns regarding the risk of postoperative urinary retention have limited its indications for bilateral cases [7]. Nevertheless, bilateral reimplantation is possible as laparoscopy allows an easy approach to the posterior bladder wall with a limited dissection sparing bladder innervation [8, 9].

Supplementary Information The online version contains supplementary material available at [https://doi.org/10.1007/978-3-030-99280-4_40].

F. Varlet (✉) · A. Scalabre · S. Vermersch
Pediatric Surgery Department, University Hospital, Saint-Etienne Cedex 2, France
e-mail: francois.varlet@chu-st-etienne.fr; aurelien.scalabre@chu-st-etienne.fr; sophie.vermersch@chu-st-etienne.fr

40.2 Pre-Operative Preparation

Renal isotope study, ultrasonography, and voiding cystography are realized before treatment. Voiding cystourethrogram (VCUG) is the

C. Esposito et al. (eds.), *Minimally Invasive Techniques in Pediatric Urology*, https://doi.org/10.1007/978-3-030-99280-4_40

standard method to identify and grade VUR in children with recurrent febrile urinary tract infections. Indications for surgery are discussed upon the clinical history and results of renal ultrasonography and isotope studies, but there is currently no consensus when medical or surgical therapy should be used among paediatric urologists and nephrologists. The different techniques available for the treatment of VUR and their potential complications are explained to the patients and their parents before surgery. A bacteriologic urine exam is performed a few days before surgery to ensure that urine is sterile.

40.3 Anaesthesia

General endotracheal anaesthesia is complemented by caudal anaesthesia. A broadspectrum antibiotic is routinely administered intravenously on induction of general anaesthesia.

40.4 Initial Cystoscopy

A cystoscopy may be performed initially if bladder control is required, especially in children with a duplex system, to assess the location of the ureteral orifices and to check the anatomy. In children with asymmetric bilateral VUR, endoscopic treatment of a contralateral low-grade reflux can be performed before the unilateral Lich–Gregoir procedure.

40.5 Positioning

The patient is placed in a supine position with the arms lying along the body. The surgeon stands at the head of the patient and the assistant and the nurse on one side, usually opposite to the refluxing ureter. The video column is placed at the feet of the patient (Fig. 40.1). When the child is too tall, the surgeon must stand laterally, on the right side for the left ureter and on the left side for the right ureter.

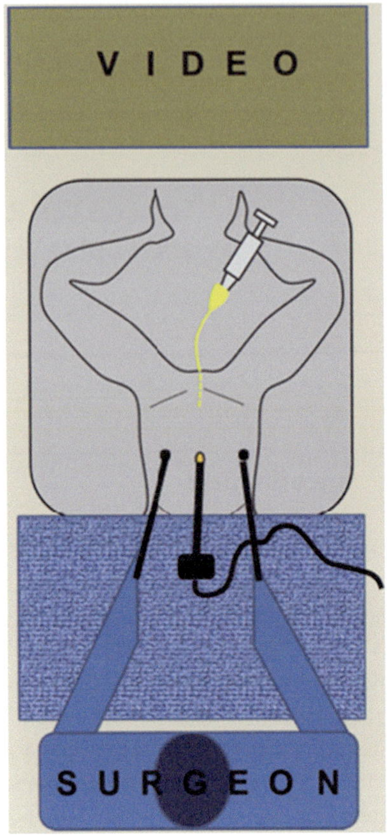

Fig. 40.1 Positioning of the patient, the surgeon, and video column

40.6 Instrumentation

After preparation of the abdominal wall, a bladder catheter is placed. It must be accessible during the procedure to fill or to empty the bladder according to the step of procedure. A 5-mm-30° lens and 3-mm instruments are used: blunt grasper, bipolar forceps, hook, needle holder, and scissors.

40.7 Technique

A transperitoneal approach is used. A 5-mm port is inserted through a lateral or transumbilical incision under vision to avoid vis-

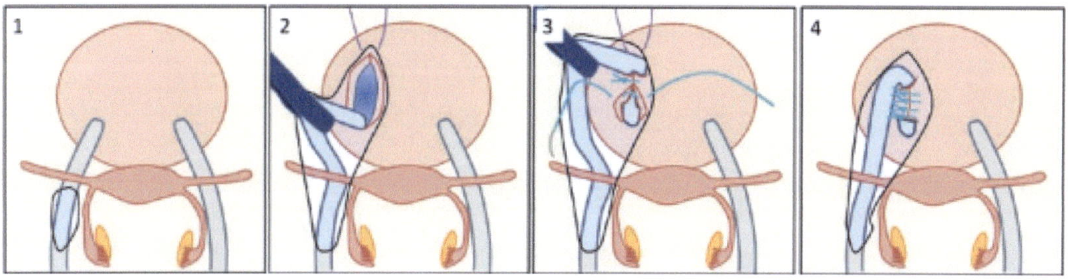

Fig. 40.2 Opening of the peritoneum (1); detrusorotomy (2); detrusororrhaphy (3); finished reimplantation (4). With permission from: Esposito C. et al (2019) ESPES Manual of Pediatric Minimally Invasive Surgery, Springer

ceral damage. Two 3-mm trocars are inserted in the left and right flanks under direct vision. They are inserted at the umbilicus level in children before 2 years old and lower in older children. At the beginning of procedure, the bladder is emptying and a Trendelenburg position is done to obtain a good exposure of the pelvic cavity.

40.7.1 Ureteral Dissection

The ureter is easily identified where it crosses the external iliac vessels. The peritoneum is opened down to the uretero-vesical junction (Fig. 40.2).

To avoid excessive handling of the ureter, a large surgical loop is wrapped around the ureter and used for manipulation (Fig. 40.3). In boys, the vas deferens is teased away from the ureter. In girls, the broad ligament is opened and the ureter is pulled up through this opening. The ureter is mobilized to achieve sufficient freedom for a tension-free reimplantation. We recommend a gentle and soft dissection of tissues around the lower ureteral part and no extensive coagulation for sparing bladder nerves, especially in bilateral procedure to avoid urinary retention reported by open surgery.

The bladder dome is suspended to the anterior abdominal wall with a transparietal stay suture in order to expose the uretero-vesical junction.

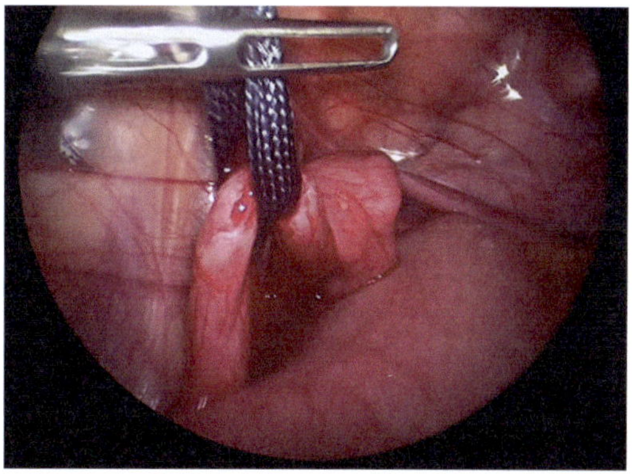

Fig. 40.3 The ureter is manipulated using a soft band wrapped around it

40.7.2 Detrusorotomy and Exposure of the Bladder Mucosa

The bladder is filled with saline to get a good exposure of its posterior wall and the telescope is turned by 180°. The direction and length of the muscular trench is outlined with the unipolar coagulation following the Paquin's rule: the length of the submucosal tunnel should be at least four or five times the ureteric diameter. The muscular fibres are coagulated and divided with scissors or monopolar hook to reach the bladder mucosa (Fig. 40.4).

The trench is ended at the level of the terminal part of the ureter. Lateral dissection of the bladder should be limited to avoid damage to pelvic nerves. In case of mucosal tear, we favour closure

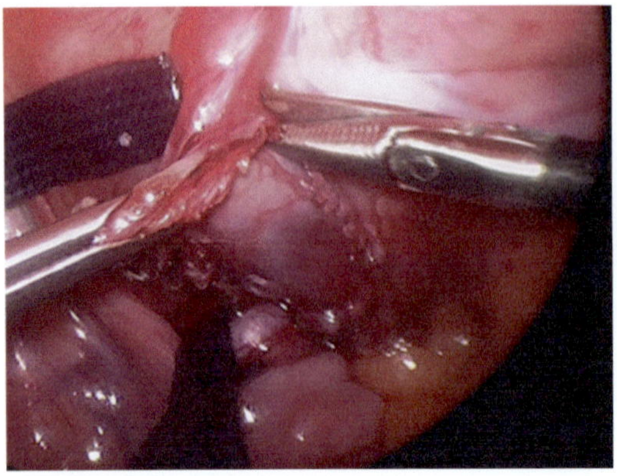

Fig. 40.4 Detrusorotomy

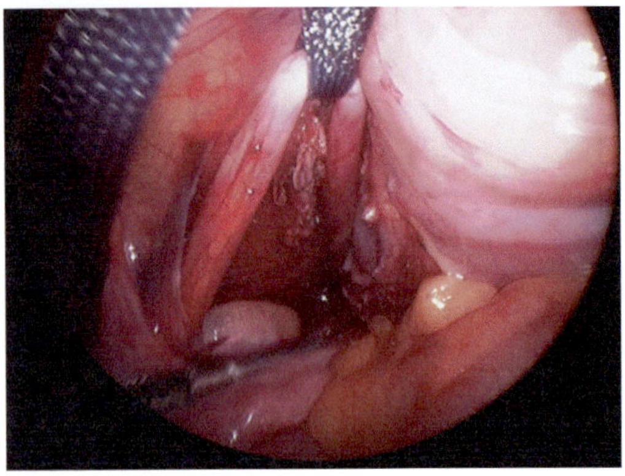

Fig. 40.5 The ureter is placed in position along the muscular trench

by an endoloop rather than direct suture (requiring an empty bladder).

40.7.3 Detrusororrhaphy

The ureter is laid between the two edges of the muscular trench and kept in this position with a third transparietal stay suture through the soft band used for mobilization of the ureter (Fig. 40.5).

In case of ureteral duplication, both ureters are dissected and laid into the trench together. The detrusor is then reapproximated over the ureter with three to four stitches of 3/0 or 4/0 sutures, either absorbable or not (Fig. 40.6). We usually start by the lower stitch. When all stitches are done, the transperitoneal suspensions are

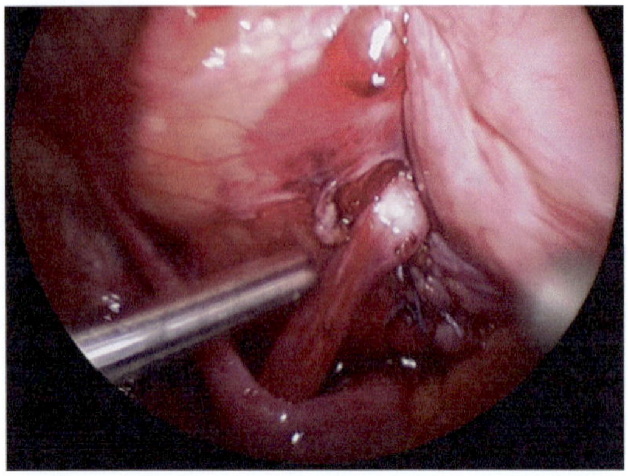

Fig. 40.6 Finished reimplantation

removed. The new ureteral entry in the bladder must be large enough to avoid ureteral obstruction. In case of excessive tension, the ureter is released proximally.

40.8 Closure

Drainage is not mandatory. The trocars are removed, their orifices stitched, and the bladder catheter removed. It is possible to leave 100–150 mL of saline serum in the bladder to allow a quick postoperative micturition before discharge in an outpatient setting.

40.9 Bilateral Reimplantation

The same procedure can be done on both sides by laparoscopy with special attention to avoid any coagulation during dissection of the distal parts of the ureters (Fig. 40.7).

40.9.1 Postoperative Care

Unilateral reimplantation following this technique can be performed as day-case, the patient being discharged after complete micturition. Only standard painkillers are needed. For bilateral reimplantation, we prefer to keep the patient hospitalized until the next day, to be sure there is no urinary retention. The child is kept off school for

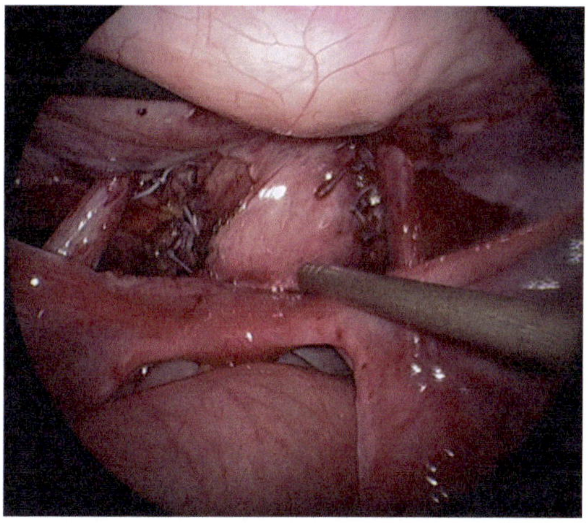

Fig. 40.7 Finished bilateral reimplantation in a girl

8 days with no sport for 1 month. An ultrasound scan is performed 1 month later. As for open surgery, VCUG is not routinely performed [10].

40.10 Results

We operated on 145 children (203 renal units) over the past 13 years. We managed 58 bilateral and 87 unilateral VUR. Bilateral VUR were treated by bilateral Lich–Gregoir procedure in 37 patients, and by unilateral Lich–Gregoir procedure and contralateral endoscopic sub-ureteral injection during the same procedure in 21 patients. Then 182 ureters were treated by Lich–Gregoir procedure in this period with only one tapering for a megaureter and one uretero-ureterostomy for a duplex system. Thirty-one patients had a duplex system with VUR in the lower pole including five bilateral VUR. Eight patients had Hutch diverticulum treated by doing a precautionary suture in the lower part of the bladder channel. The mean operative time was around 90 minutes for unilateral and 2 hours for bilateral reimplantation. In six cases, a mucosal perforation occurred during the detrusorotomy, treated immediately by an endoloop repair.

The mean hospital stay was between 24 and 30 hours, and 15 children could be recently treated in day-case surgery for unilateral procedure with an uneventful postoperative course.

Three temporary urinary retentions occurred after bilateral reimplantation. A supra-pubic catheter was placed under general anaesthesia and removed 10 days later with uneventful recovery. None had a long-term bladder paresis. At the beginning of our experience, two patients needed reintervention for a ureteral perforation, 7 and 15 days after surgery. One was treated by Cohen procedure and one by double J stent and ureteral suturing.

A recent long-term review of our patients found eight failures of Lich–Gregoir procedure (5.5% of children), revealed by a new pyelonephritis and confirmed by VCUG. Two failures with bilateral VUR occurred from one bilateral procedure and one unilateral procedure with contralateral endoscopic injection. Six failures with unilateral VUR occurred from two bilateral and four unilateral Lich–Gregoir procedures. They were managed by endoscopic injection (3), Lich–Gregoir redo (2), Cohen procedure (1), and watching (2).

The resolution rate, in terms of no further febrile urinary tract infection (UTI), accounted to 91.4% (131/145 patients). The UTI occurred in the eight surgical failures, but also in four children with bowel and urinary dysfunction despite a good medical management; two other patients had a transitory UTI a few months after surgery but none after 5 to 10 years of follow-up.

Tips and Tricks

- The two ureteral perforations at the beginning of our experience made us slightly modify the surgical technique. We reviewed the surgery videos but did not find the traumatic cause for these perforations. We assume that possible causes were ischemia caused by excessive handling of the ureter, a burn with the monopolar hook dissection or an excessive closing of the detrusor trench. To avoid this complication, we opted to wrap a soft band around the ureter for its manipulation and to limit the amount

and duration of cautery. No more ureteral perforation occurred since we made these modifications (>120 cases).
- Suspension of the bladder by transparietal stay suture is a good way to obtain correct exposure of the posterior wall and bladder trench without adding unnecessary trocars, and we regularly use this technique for other surgeries. Sometimes a second transparietal suspension allows a better exposure of the posterior wall of the bladder.
- To prevent postoperative urinary retention, the surgeon must be really careful avoiding any extensive monopolar cautery, especially on the lower part of the ureter, surrounded by bladder nerves.
- In case of mucosal perforation, the mucosa can be closed immediately by using an endoloop.
- It is also important to check that the final trench is not too obstructive after reimplantation. If the tunnel seems too tight, the proximal stitch must be removed.
- All our laparoscopic interventions are video-recorded, which help sharing our experience and techniques with students, residents, and colleagues. We also review and criticize our procedures afterward to improve our technique when we confront complications.

40.11 Discussion

VUR management is controversial. There is no strong consensus about prophylactic antibiotic treatment, operative indications, and age of surgery or follow-up management [1]. According to AUA recommendations, we decided to operate on children by Lich–Gregoir procedure with VUR grade III or more, with renal dysfunction (DMSA<40%) or renal scarring demonstrated on isotope renography, and children developing recurrent pyelonephritis despite optimal medical treatment.

The goal of any anti-reflux procedure is to restore anti-reflux mechanism of the uretero-vesical junction. Open uretero-vesical reimplantation by the Cohen procedure is often considered to be the gold standard for ureteral reimplantation, with a success rate over 98% [11]. However, the Lich–Gregoir technique is also associated with a high success rate with some advantages including lower pain, shorter recovery and hospital stay, and excellent cosmetic results [2, 8, 9, 12]. This technique avoids postoperative bladder spasms and adverse effects of bladder opening like haematuria. Furthermore, the ureteral meatus is still in its initial position, allowing easier endourology in the future if necessary.

The main issue with this approach is the 8 to 15% reported incidence of urinary retention after bilateral extravesical reimplantation by open approach [7]. This might be a result of neurovascular injury during wound handling and ureteral and bladder dissection. A nerve-sparing technique proposed by David in 2004 allows reducing this complication (2% of transitory bladder retention) [6]. In 2012, Bayne et al. reported a cohort of patients undergoing extravesical ureteral reimplantation by laparoscopy with the Lich–Gregoir technique with a 6.5% incidence of urinary retention after bilateral reimplantation [13]. In our experience, only three patients presented with a transitory bladder emptying difficulty after a bilateral reimplantation. Lateral dissection of the ureter and bladder should be limited to avoid damage to pelvic nerves [6], and we recommend a gentle and soft tissue dissection around the lower ureter with no extensive coagulation. In our opinion, no bladder catheter is needed during the post-operative period. In addition, faster recovery compared to open surgery allows discharge a few hours after surgery [8, 9, 14]. Today, the robot-assisted extravesical reimplantation is an interesting alternative with the same good results [15, 16].

One of the most common operative complications in laparoscopic extravesical reimplantation is ureteral injury or obstruction (ischemia) owing to excessive handling of the ureter or excessive closure of the trench. Lakshmanan and Kasturi in 2000 and 2012, respectively, reported 6.3% (3/47) and 0.6% (1/150) intra-abdominal urinary leak requiring drainage and bilateral pigtail stents for 2 months [17, 18]. Bayne et al observed a 2.04% rate of ureteral leakage [13] and Esposito et al showed a 1.33% of the same complication in open Cohen procedures [11]. We recommend a limited use of the monopolar coagulation and handling of the ureter by a soft band to avoid this complication. After more than 120 cases treated using this soft band, no more ureteral perforation occurred.

The open Lich–Gregoir technique for unilateral VUR is also done with good results as an outpatient procedure [12, 14]. Advantages of laparoscopy over open surgery in this context are a better bladder wall exposition and less scaring.

The results of laparoscopic Lich–Gregoir reimplantation are comparable with pneumovesicoscopic reimplantation [19, 20]. However, it is technically challenging to obtain a correct pneumovesicum with bladder sealing at the start of the procedure. Moreover, pneumovesicoscopic reimplantation requires postoperative drainage. On the other hand, the pneumovesicoscopic approach allows treatment of ureteroceles and Hutch diverticula, whereas only small diverticula can be treated by laparoscopy.

40.12 Conclusion

Laparoscopic extravesical ureteral reimplantation with the Lich–Gregoir technique is a safe and effective procedure for the treatment of VUR in children. Its results are comparable to open procedures. The technique results in reduced hospital stay and recovery period. It can be applied to unilateral VUR, bilateral VUR, and duplex system. With cautious dissection, the risk of urinary retention following bilateral reimplantation is low.

References

1. Peters CA, Skoog SJ, Arant BS, Copp HL, Elder JS, Hudson RG, et al. Summary of the AUA guideline on management of primary vesicoureteral reflux in children. J Urol. 2010;184(3):1134–44.
2. Hajiyev P, Burgu B. Contemporary management of vesicoureteral reflux. Eur Urol Focus. 2017;3(2–3):181–8.
3. Cohen MH, Rotner MB. A new method to create a submucosal ureteral tunnel. J Urol. 1969;102(5):567–8.
4. Lich R, Howerton LW, Davis LA. Ureteral reflux, its significance and correction. South Med J. 1962;55:633–5.
5. Gregoir W. The surgical treatment of congenital vesico-ureteral reflux. Acta Chir Belg. 1964;63:431–9.
6. Casale P, Patel RP, Kolon TF. Nerve sparing robotic extravesical ureteral reimplantation. J Urol. 2008;179:1987–90.
7. Fung LC, McLorie GA, Jain U, Khoury AE, Churchill BM. Voiding efficiency after ureteral reimplantation: a comparison of extravesical and intravesical techniques. J Urol. 1995;153:1972–5.
8. Lopez M, Varlet F. Laparoscopic extravesical transperitoneal approach following the Lich-Gregoir technique in the treatment of vesicoureteral reflux in children. J Pediatr Surg. 2010;45:806–10.
9. Soulier V, Scalabre AL, Lopez M, Li C-Y, Thach S, Vermersch S, et al. Laparoscopic vesico-ureteral reimplantation with Lich-Gregoir approach in children: medium term results of 159 renal units in 117 children. World J Urol. 2017;35:1791–8.
10. Grossklaus DJ, Pope JC, Adams MC, Brock JW. Is postoperative cystography necessary after ureteral reimplantation? Urology. 2001;58:1041–5.
11. Esposito C, Escolino M, Lopez M, Farina A, Cerulo M, Savanelli A, et al. Surgical management of pediatric vesicoureteral reflux: a comparative study between endoscopic, laparoscopic, and open surgery. J Laparoendosc Adv Surg Tech A. 2016;26:574–80.
12. Palmer JS. Extravesical ureteral reimplantation: an outpatient procedure. J Urol. 2008;180(4 Suppl):1828–31.
13. Bayne AP, Shoss JM, Starke NR, Cisek LJ. Single-Centre experience with pediatric laparoscopic extravesical reimplantation: safe and effective in simple and complex anatomy. J Laparoendosc Adv Surg Tech A. 2012;22:102–6.
14. Wicher C, Hadley D, Ludlow D, Oottamasathien S, Wallis MC, Devries C, et al. 250 consecutive unilateral extravesical ureteral reimplantations in an outpatient setting. J Urol. 2010;184:311–4.
15. Esposito C, Masieri L, Steyaert H, Escolino M, Cerchione R, La Manna A, Cini C, Lendvay TS. Robot-assisted extravesical ureteral reimplantation (revur) for unilateral vesico-ureteral reflux in children: results of a multicentric international survey. World J Urol. 2018;36:481–8.
16. Sahadev R, Spencer K, Srinivasan AK, Long CJ, Shukla AR. The robot-assisted extravesical anti-reflux surgery: how we overcame the learning curve. Front Pediatr. 2019;7:93.
17. Lakshmanan Y, Fung LC. Laparoscopic extravesicular ureteral reimplantation for vesicoureteral reflux: recent technical advances. J Endourol. 2000;14:589–94.
18. Kasturi S, Sehgal SS, Christman MS, Lambert SM, Casale P. Prospective long-term analysis of nerve-

sparing extravesical robotic-assisted laparoscopic ureteral reimplantation. Urology. 2012;79:680–3.
19. Yeung CK, Sihoe JDY, Borzi PA. Endoscopic cross-trigonal ureteral reimplantation under carbon dioxide bladder insufflation: a novel technique. J Endourol. 2005;19:295–9.
20. Valla JS, Steyaert H, Griffin SJ, Lauron J, Fragoso AC, Arnaud P, et al. Transvesicoscopic Cohen ureteric reimplantation for vesicoureteral reflux in children: a single-Centre 5-year experience. J Pediatr Urol. 2009;5:466–71.

Technique of Pneumovesicoscopy

41

Jean Stephane Valla

Learning Objectives
- To describe step-by-step how trocars should be introduced into the bladder.
- To describe how the orifices should be closed at the end of the procedure.
- To show a video illustrating all tips and tricks.

41.1 Introduction

Bladder insufflation with carbon dioxide (CO2) for cystoscopic diagnostic purpose in adults was first described in 1966 [1]. In children, suprapubic access of a liquid-filled bladder via a trocar and a scope was described in 1986 [2] for antegrade ablation of posterior valves and later for the injection of bulking agents. Such a suprapubic access was also used to perform ureteroscopy or ureteral catheterization in patients with altered ureteral position, for example, after cross-trigonal reimplantation or renal transplantation. In reality, pediatric urologists were the first to use pneumovesicum as a true operative technique: at the beginning of the 2000s, CK Yeung, PA Borzi, and JS Valla collaborated to develop this new approach [3, 4]. If the transperitoneal approach have been used at the beginning of a minimally invasive surgery for upper and lower urinary tract diseases, it was not the preferred route for classical open urologic surgery. Besides retroperitoneoscopy, the pneumovesicoscopic approach is specifically urological: it allows introduction of a telescope and operating instruments into the bladder and the performance of all procedures that need a large bladder opening in classical surgery. So mastery of retroperitoneoscopy and pneumovesicoscopy enables the management of all diseases of the urinary system from the adrenal gland to the bladder neck and without violating the peritoneal cavity and without disturbing the digestive tract. This idea seems logical, but putting it into practice turned out to be difficult; that explains why the adoption of this technique was only progressive.

The principle of pneumovesicoscopy (Fig. 41.1) is based on two facts:

- Filling the bladder with a gas provides a clear intravesical vision, much better than the vision in a liquid-filled bladder.
- Introduction of the telescope through the bladder dome provides "a familiar forward intravesical view towards the trigone and the

Supplementary Information The online version contains supplementary material available at [https://doi.org/10.1007/978-3-030-99280-4_41].

J. S. Valla (✉)
Professeur de Chirurgie Pediatrique, Nice, France
e-mail: jeff.valla@gmail.com

C. Esposito et al. (eds.), *Minimally Invasive Techniques in Pediatric Urology*,
https://doi.org/10.1007/978-3-030-99280-4_41

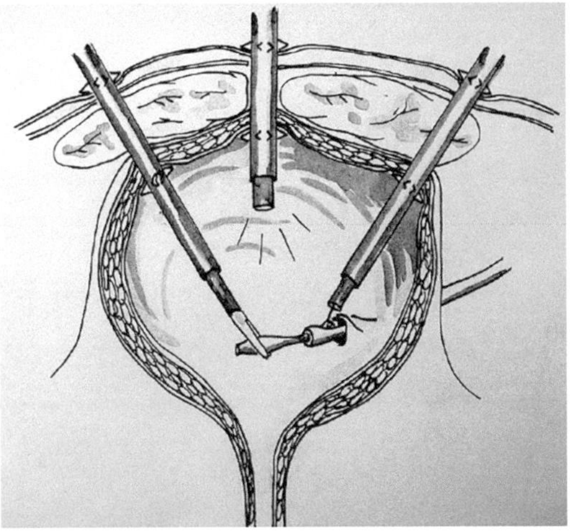

Fig. 41.1 Principle of pneumovesicoscopy: bladder insufflated with CO_2, one telescope, two operating instruments introduced through the abdominal and bladder wall. Illustration by Valla

ureteric orifices that is similar to that obtained with an open bladder incision" [3].

- So vision and ergonomic position are well related.

41.2 Limitations and Contraindications

- Related to the Patient. The major limiting factor is the bladder capacity. The smaller the bladder, the more restricted the working space. Even though our youngest patients were 4 months old, the decreased working space does make the procedure more technically demanding and may obviate the advantages of vesicoscopic repair. Hence, this method may be difficult to apply in patients under 1 year of age or in patients with bladder of less than 100-mL volume. That explains why the use of the robot, even if it seems a theoretically good solution, is not in fact the way to solve the problem [5]

  Another limiting factor is the bladder wall condition: in case of markedly thickened or inflamed bladder wall, the procedure could be quite difficult.

  However, previous failed injection therapy or previous intra- or extravesical surgery should not be considered a contraindication. This technique is also workable in patients with an augmented bladder.
- Related to the Surgeon. All vesicoscopic procedures are challenging. Expertise in intracorporeal suturing in a confined space with a fine 5/0 or 6/0 thread is essential; there is a tremendous learning curve: in short, these reconstructive procedures are reserved for good laparoscopic pediatric surgeons.

41.3 Preoperative Preparation

Preoperative investigations include all the necessary exams concerning the disease: ultrasound, cystogram, MRI, renal scintiscan, cystoscopy, urodynamics, etc.

Detailed information is given to the parents and, if possible, the patient regarding the technique used, the possible technical difficulties and complications, and the possibility of intraoperative conversion to the open technique. An informed consent is obtained.

There is no specific preoperative preparation. As with open surgery, preoperative urine samples confirm that no urinary infection is present. In case of associated constipation, the rectum can be emptied with a fleet enema, usually given the evening before.

The patient is prepared for general anesthesia with endotracheal intubation; a caudal anesthesia could be performed according to the anesthesiologist's preference; muscle relaxation is essential to ensure a good bladder insufflation. A broad-spectrum antibiotic is routinely given intravenously on induction of anesthesia. A nasogastric tube is usually not necessary.

41.4 Positioning

- The patient is placed in the modified lithotomy position with the thighs abducted. Small patients are placed transversally on the operating table (Fig. 41.2); taller patients are placed at the end of the operating table (Fig. 41.3). The abdomen and genitalia are

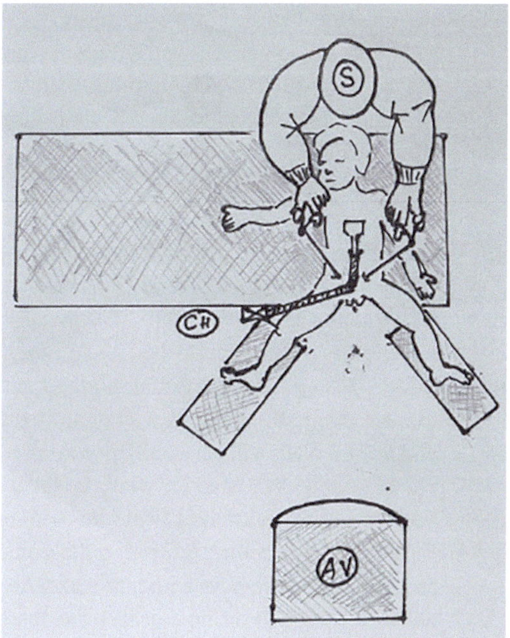

Fig. 41.2 Positioning a small child transversally on the operating table; the surgeon stands at the head in a perfect ergonomic position. Adapted by permission from Springer, Videochirurgia pediatrica, by C. Esposito et al (eds), 2010

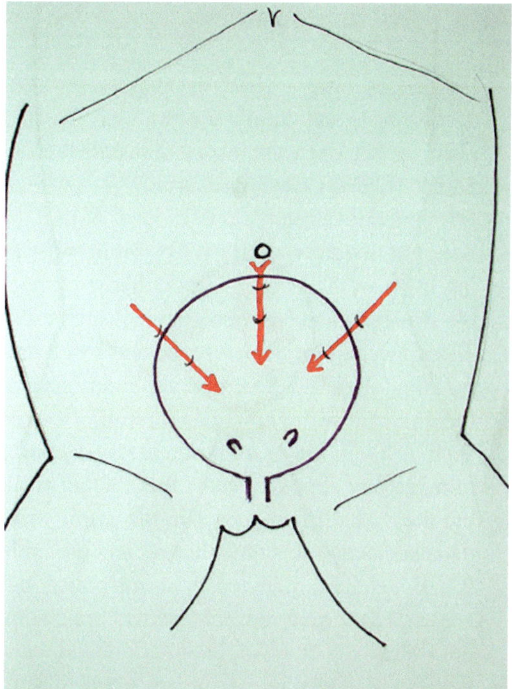

Fig. 41.4 Entrance point and direction of trocars in a child under 3 or 4 years of age. Adapted by permission from Springer, ESPES Manual of Pediatric Minimally Invasive Surgery, by C. Esposito et al. (eds.), 2019

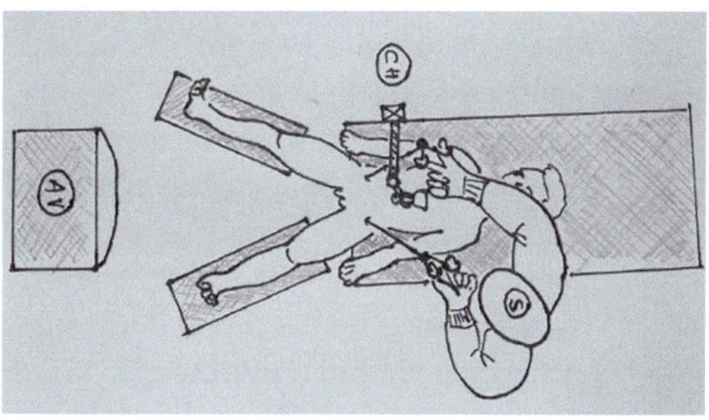

Fig. 41.3 Positioning a tall child on the operating table; the surgeon stands on the lateral edge of the table. His position is not so ergonomic for his back and his shoulder. Adapted by permission from Springer, Videochirurgia pediatrica, by C. Esposito et al (eds), 2010

prepared and wrapped. The pelvis is tilted with a padding just below the buttock. The patient is strapped on the table to prevent slipping during movements of the table (Trendelenburg position).

– The position of the surgeon changes twice during the procedure: during the first step (cystoscopy), the surgeon stands between the patient's legs with the video column on the left side of the patient (Fig. 41.4); during the second pneumovesicoscopic step, the position of the surgeon varies according the child's size—a more ergonomic position for the surgeon is to stand at the head of the child in the axis of the bladder trigone and the video column which is positioned between the patient's legs, with the cables coming from the patient' left side and fixed to the superior part of the operative field (Fig. 41.2). The camera holder is fixed on the right side of the table, but this position is possible only in the case of small children (under 5 years of age). In older children, the surgeon is positioned similar to when performing open bladder surgery: the surgeon (if right handed) positions on the left side of the patient, with the monitor next to the patient's right leg (Fig. 41.3).

41.5 Instrumentation

- For cystoscopy, a rigid cystoscope is used according to the child's urethra size. To suspend the bladder wall, a special needle (suture passer 1GSPO1 Gore) is useful.
- For pneumovesicum, a telescope 5 mm or 3 mm in diameter, at 0° or 30°, 3-mm operating instruments, hook, grasper, dissector, needle holder, and suction device are used. Trocars, 5 mm for the telescope and 5 or 3 mm for the operative instruments, and special locking trocars with self-retaining devices such as a balloon or umbrella are very useful to avoid any slippage out of the bladder wall, but they are difficult to get in the 3-mm size; disposable self-expandable trocars are safe (blunt needle), quite easy to introduce but expensive; normal reusable trocars are cheap, but sharp, so it must be manipulated cautiously. At any time during the procedure, a third 3-mm operating instrument or a catheter for suction or flushing can be passed through the urethra if needed. A camera holder, mechanical or pneumatic or robotic, is useful to ensure a stable vision, especially when suturing: as for all reconstructive surgery in a confined space, this point seems crucial.

41.6 Technique

- How to Begin.
  1. Cystoscopy and introduction of the first median trocar.

     After having emptied the bladder (transurethral catheter + Credé maneuver), pneumovesicum is created by insufflating CO2 through the irrigation channel of the rigid cystoscope at a maximal pressure of 8 to 10 mm Hg. Once the bladder is distended, the dome is fixed to the abdominal wall under vision control. There are several possibilities: if the abdominal wall is thin, a percutaneous transfixing 2/0 or 0/0 suture with a curved needle is sufficient, quick, and effective; in case of a thick abdominal wall, more time and special instruments are needed. Yeung [2] has described the technique using two 18-gauge long needle, one to introduce a strong monofilament and the other to introduce a loop that allows to extract the hitch stitch; personally I use a suture passer to introduce and extract the thread and an endoscopic grasper introduced through the operating channel of the cystoscope in order to manipulate the thread into the bladder. Another possibility, described by Abraham [6], is to use a curved urethral dilatator and to push inside the bladder wall against the abdominal wall; a T-bar could also be used [7, 8]. Once the bladder wall is firmly secured to the abdominal wall, the median 5-mm port is introduced through the dome and secured to the skin with a thread. Then the cystoscope is removed and the team and the video column prepare for the second pneumovesicoscopic step.
  2. Pneumovesicoscopy and introduction of the two lateral trocars.

     The bladder is insufflated via the dome port (pressure 8–12 mmHg, volume 2 to 3 L/min); there is no or few gas leak through the urethra even in girls, so there is no need to occlude it during the procedure; on the contrary, a 3-mm operating instrument could be introduced through the urethra, in girls as well as in boys, to replace cystoscopic grasping forceps. The vision provided by the 5-mm telescope is much better than the cystoscopic vision; the surgeon stands in line with the trigone and the screen. The position selected for insertion of the lateral ports could vary according to the size of the patients and the size of the bladder: in small children less than 4 years old, the bladder is located in a more superior position, and the trocars are more close to the umbilicus, carrying the risk of peritoneal perforation (Fig. 41.5), so it can induce a pneumoperitoneum which must be exufflated by introducing a transumbilical Veress needle. In older children, the bladder is deeper and lower in the pelvis; the penetrating points

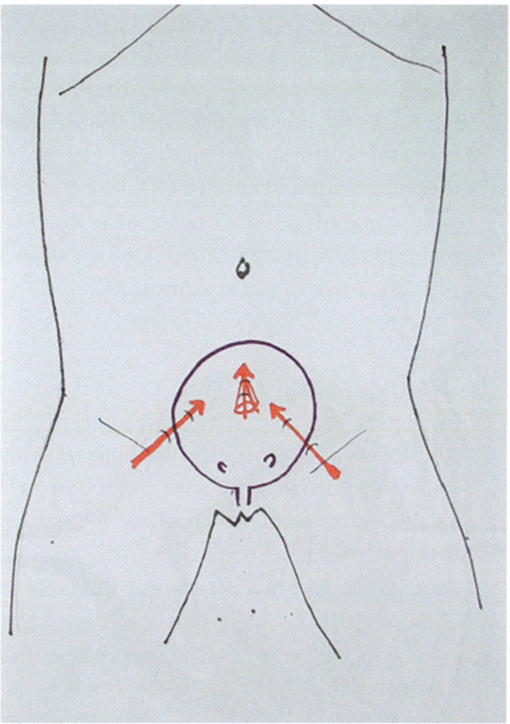

Fig. 41.5 Entrance point and direction of trocars in a child up to 5 years of age. Adapted by permission from Springer, ESPES Manual of Pediatric Minimally Invasive Surgery, by C. Esposito et al. (eds.), 2019

of lateral ports are close to the bikini line, carrying the risk of epigastric vessel injury. Concerning the lateral ports, the penetration point in the bladder must be chosen carefully, because if they are introduced at a too low level, the tip of the cannulas will be too close to the ureteral orifice making dissection difficult. Introducing a fine needle before the lateral trocar enables visualization of the right direction and the right depth and puts the trocar in the right position at the first attempt, avoiding multiple mucosal perforation. The suspension of the lateral bladder wall to the lateral abdominal wall is done according the same technique as for the median port: direct percutaneous transfixing thread, manipulation of two needles, suture passer, or T-bar.

Again the lateral cannulas must be firmly fixed to the abdominal skin.

- How to Finish.
  Closing the trocar wounds is done in the reverse order to that of the introduction.
- The lateral trocars are extracted first; it may seem possible to leave this port's hole open, reckoning on spontaneous healing with time and bladder drainage. My position is not so optimistic and more qualified: concerning the 3-mm lateral holes, especially if the trocar course through the bladder wall is oblique, that is to say that the mucosal hole is out of line with the detrusoral hole, I agree to leave it open; but all 5-mm mucosal wounds, whatever the patient's age or the bladder wall thickness, must be closed to avoid any urine leakage during the postoperative period. Some surgeons [3] recommend placing the suspension suture around the trocar at the beginning of the procedure and just tying it at the end; personally I recommend using the suture passer under vision control by the telescope.

The third median trocar is then extracted. There is no need to reintroduce a cystoscope because this 5-mm hole could be closed under direct vision; continuous bladder insufflation through the urethral catheter facilitates spotting the mucosal edges. After tying the knot, if no gas leak is audible, the maneuver is considered successful. In case of difficulty in closing this median hole, the safety maneuver is to leave a 10- or 12-Fr catheter as suprapubic drainage for few days. No perivesical drain is needed. The skin wounds are closed with 5/0 subcuticular absorbable monofilament suture.

41.7 Postoperative Care

The duration of the bladder drainage varies from case to case, for 1–4 days, normally 2 days. Persistent mild hematuria is usual. As a result of caudal anesthesia, postoperative pain is usually mild and oral analgesics suffice. Postoperative antibiotic therapy is given according the preoperative urinalysis. Patients start feeding a few hours postoperatively and are discharged on the second or third day after the procedure. In the case of ureteric stenting with pigtail catheter, for example, after a difficult bilateral ureteral reimplantation, the use of a ureteric-cutaneus stent avoids a second general anesthesia to remove it.

The distal follow-up is scheduled according to the severity of the initial disease and the possible postoperative complications; in any case, an ultrasound is performed at 1 and 6 months.

41.8 Discussion

In this chapter, the discussion is limited to the technique and its complications; the discussion about the possible indications will be discussed in a next chapter.

- Why choose to fill the bladder with gas at the beginning of the procedure? Of course, filling the bladder with liquid is more classical and offers a stronger counterpressure when introducing a trocar; it could be an advantage because the bladder wall is particularly flexible in infants and can be distorted and pushed away by the trocar tip before being entered. However, we changed to CO_2 insufflation for two reasons: first, blood oozing from the bladder hole can cloud the cystoscopic fluid, and second, liquid extravasation out of the bladder can occur and lead to collapse of the bladder resulting in poor visibility; gas leakage, on the other hand, will be absorbed in few minutes.
- Introduction of the trocars is critical because some complications are directly related to this approach. The specific problem, when introducing the ports, is to go through two walls, first, the abdominal wall, only thin and aponeurotic in the midline but thick and muscular laterally (Fig. 41.1), and then the bladder wall and not to be stuck in the extravesical space. That is why suspending the bladder firmly to the abdominal wall is of utmost importance.
- During the procedure, the main reason for conversion is port displacement; any inadvertent dislodgment out of the bladder is a source of difficulty: so again, the trocars must be firmly secured to the skin.
- What is the risk of CO_2 insufflation in the bladder? Contrary to the peritoneum, the urothelial lining is relatively impermeable to carbon dioxide; there are minimal physiological disturbances due to CO_2 absorption. The gas escape in the perivesical space is usually minimal; it could explain some cases of moderate suprapubic or scrotal emphysema. The pneumovesicum, even in case of CO_2 reflux in the upper urinary tract, does not appear to affect renal arteries or venous blood flow, nor does it introduce a risk of gas embolism [9].
- What are the advantages of pneumovesicum?

1. Excellent visibility.
2. Reduction of abdominal wall trauma.
3. Reduction of bladder wall trauma: no wide cystotomy, no mucosal irritation with gauze swabs, no intravesical retractors; that means less postoperative hematuria, less mucosal edema, and less bladder spasms than that in open surgery.
4. No complications or physiological changes that may occur in transperitoneal laparoscopy.
5. No neuromuscular injury of the detrusor, so no risk of voiding dysfunction or postoperative urinary retention.

Take-Home Points

- It is imperative to start pneumovesicoscopy only after an extensive experience in laparoscopy, especially if you intend to perform reconstructive surgery.
- Do not forget the limitations due to the bladder capacity in infants.
- Pneumovesicoscopy is only a new endovesical therapeutic approach between pure endoscopic and classical open approaches. Do not change your indications.
- It is now proven that this approach is as safe and as efficient in expert hands than that of open surgery.
- Some progress remains to be made to simplify the technique and to achieve the “ideal” minimally invasive bladder surgery, that is to say, real day surgery without drainage.

References

1. Wear JP. Cystoscopy with carbon dioxide irrigation. J Urol. 1966;96:828.
2. Zaontz MR, Firlit CF. Percutaneous antegrade ablation of posterior ureteral valves in infants with small caliber urethras: an alternative to urinary diversion. J Urol. 1986;136:247–8.
3. Yeung CK, Sihoe JB, Borzi PA. Endoscopic cross-trigonal reimplantation, under carbon dioxide bladder insufflation. A novel technique. J Endourol. 2005;19:295–9.
4. Valla JS, Steyaert H, Griffin SJ, Lauron J, Fragoso AC, Arnaud P, et al. Transvesicoscopic Cohen ureteric reimplantation for vesicoureteral reflux in children: a single-center 5-years experience. J Pediatr Urol. 2009;5:466–71.
5. Thakre AA, Bailly Y, Sun LW, Van Meer F, Yeung CK. Is a smaller working space a limit for robot performance in laparoscopy? J Urol. 2008;179:1042–3.
6. Abraham MK, Viswanath N, Bindu S, Kerari P, et al. A simple and safe technique for trocar positioning vesicoscopic ureteric preimplantation. Pediatr Surg Int. 2011;27:1223–6.
7. Yagis B, Balci O. A novel technique for bladder wall fixation in pneumovesicoscopic surgery: T-bar. J Laparoendosc Adv Surg Tech A. 2020;2(10):1089.
8. Lau CT, Lan LCL, Wong KKY, Tam P. Pneumovesical ureteric preimplantation using T-fastener: a modification for bladder wall anchorage. J Pediatr Urol. 2017;13:326–8.
9. Xiang B, Liu JX, Sung HB, Yan B, Cheng W. The effect of CO2 pneumovesicum on upper urinary tract. J Pediatr Surg. 2010;45:1863–7.

42 Robot-Assisted Extravesical Ureteral Reimplantation (REVUR) for Vesico-Ureteral Reflux in Children

Ciro Esposito, Lorenzo Masieri, Fulvia Del Conte, Giuseppe Autorino, Vincenzo Coppola, Mariapina Cerulo, and Maria Escolino

Learning Objectives

- To describe step-by-step the technique of REVUR.
- To present long-term outcomes of this technique.
- To report the latest results of major international papers about REVUR.
- To show a video of the REVUR technique.
- To describe tips and tricks of REVUR.

42.1 Introduction

In the past 30 years, the therapeutic approach to children with vesicoureteral reflux (VUR) has undergone a dramatic evolution from a mainly surgical approach, as soon as VUR was detected, toward a conservative approach with antibiotics, to a minimally invasive approach using an endoscopic or laparoscopic approach or, in the last 10 years, using laparoscopy and robotic-assisted surgery [1].

Robot-assisted extravesical ureteral reimplantation (REVUR) was first described more than 10 years ago, and since then, it has become the preferred approach for complex VUR cases instead of pure laparoscopic extravesical ureteral reimplantation (LEVUR), in particular for the technical challenges of laparoscopic intracorporeal suturing and knotting [2, 3].

Analyzing the results of the international literature, it seems that REVUR presents a success rate absolutely comparable to the results of open ureteral reimplantation [4, 5].

This chapter is focused on the technique of robot-assisted extravesical ureteral reimplantation according to the Lich-Gregoir procedure (REVUR).

42.2 Preoperative Preparation

The preoperative workup included ultrasonography (US), voiding cystourethrogram (VCUG) or cysto-scintigraphy, and renal scan to analyze renal function in each patient [6].

Supplementary Information The online version contains supplementary material available at [https://doi.org/10.1007/978-3-030-99280-4_42].

C. Esposito (✉) · F. Del Conte · G. Autorino
V. Coppola · M. Cerulo · M. Escolino
Pediatric Surgery Unit, Federico II University of Naples, Naples, Italy
e-mail: ciroespo@unina.it; fulvia.delconte@unina.it; autorino.giuseppe@gmail.com; vincenzocoppola1992@gmail.com; mariapina.cerulo@unina.it; maria.escolino@unina.it

L. Masieri
Pediatric Urology Unit, Meyer Children Hospital, Florence, Italy
e-mail: lorenzo.masieri@meyer.it

C. Esposito et al. (eds.), *Minimally Invasive Techniques in Pediatric Urology*,
https://doi.org/10.1007/978-3-030-99280-4_42

All patients and their parents have to sign a specifically formulated informed consent before the procedure. Patients receive general anesthesia with orotracheal intubation and myorelaxation. A Foley catheter is left in place during surgery to fill and empty the bladder using sterile precautions during the procedure [6].

42.3 Positioning

The patient should be placed in a supine position with the table at 15° Trendelenburg position. The surgeon is positioned on the robotic console, the bedside surgeon and the nurse stand on both sides of the table, and the monitor for the bedside surgeon and nurse is positioned at the feet of the patients (Fig. 42.1). We always adopt three 8-mm robotic trocars and a 5-mm trocar for the bedside surgeon. The trocars are positioned in triangulation with the optic in order to achieve better ergonomics (Fig. 42.2) [7, 8].

42.4 Instrumentation

Regarding the robotic procedure, we adopt an 8-mm 30-degree optic, two other 8-mm robotic instruments (needle holder, scissors, curved Maryland, and fenestrated forceps). We also adopt a 5-mm trocar for the bedside surgeon to

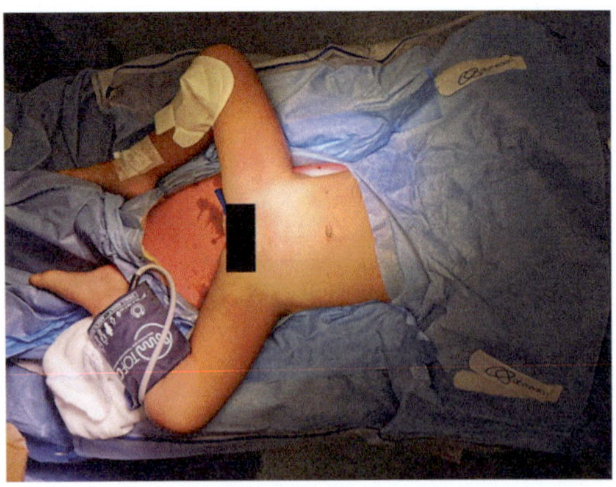

Fig. 42.1 The patient position

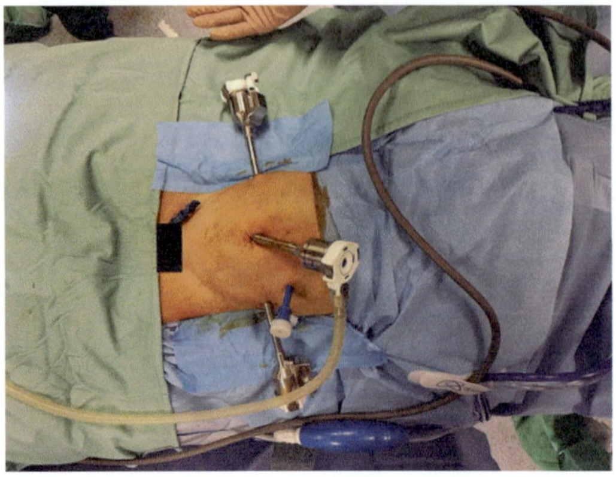

Fig. 42.2 Trocar position

introduce and remove the needles, cut the suture, and expose or retract tissues [8]. We adopt a vessel loop or an umbilical tape to manage the ureter to avoid grasping it. In general, for a standard REVUR it is not necessary to position a JJ stent. In case of paraureteral diverticulum or if you have to taper the ureter, we position a JJ stent in the ureter and in the bladder [7, 9].

42.5 Technique

All procedures were performed under general anesthesia with orotracheal intubation. The patient was placed in the Trendelenburg position and the da Vinci robot was docked over the patient's feet [6, 10]. In all cases, two surgeons and a scrub assistant started the procedure, and then the main surgeon, after the trocars were positioned, moved to the robotic console and the bedside surgeon remained at the operative table to change instruments, insert needles, and cut sutures [10]. As for the surgical technique, an incision is made in the peritoneum just above the posterior bladder wall on the affected side and then the ureter is dissected. The ureter is mobilized by careful dissection to avoid injuring the vas deferens or the uterine artery (Fig. 42.3). A polyglactin acid suture hitch stitch may be placed to draw the bladder to the opposite side and enhance visualization (Fig. 42.4). The bladder is filled with saline and a 2.5- to 3-cm detrusor inci-

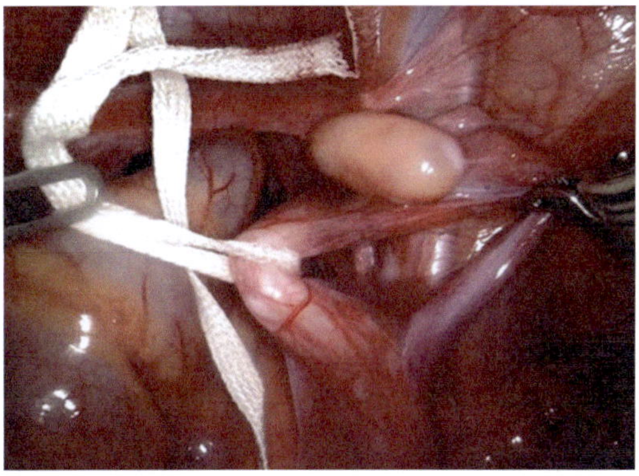

Fig. 42.3 Bladder suspension

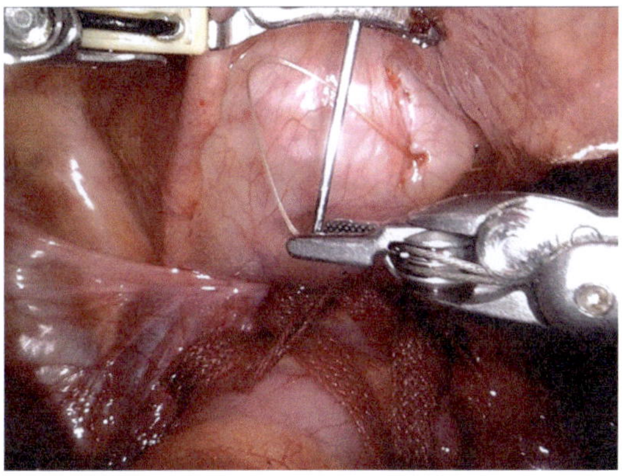

Fig. 42.4 Standard REVUR ureteral isolation

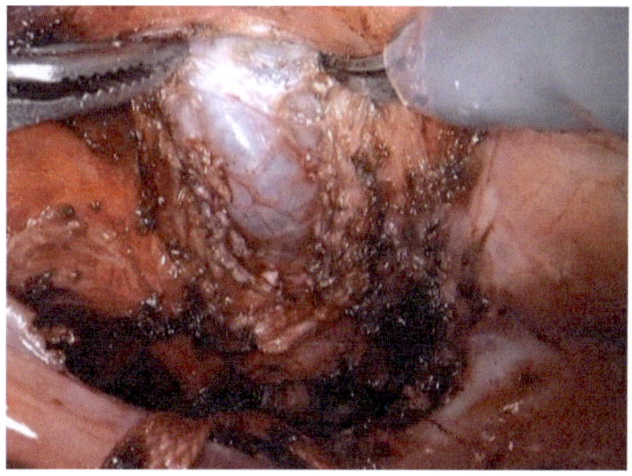

Fig. 42.5 Standard REVUR ureteral reimplantation

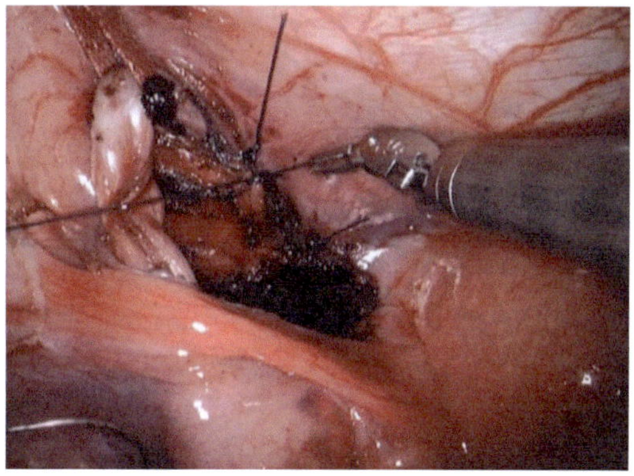

Fig. 42.6 Ureteral remodeling

sion is made to the level of the mucosa. The detrusor muscle is then separated from the mucosa laterally, establishing the muscular flaps used to create the detrusor tunnel (Fig. 42.5). The detrusor flaps are then wrapped around the ureter and reapproximated using a 4–0 polyglactin running suture (Fig. 42.6). In duplex systems, both the ureters are reimplanted in the same way in a common detrusor sheath. In case of bilateral VUR, the same procedure is performed on the contralateral side. In case of standard REVUR, only a Foley catheter is left in place [5, 7].

In case of a megaureter or in case of paraureteral diverticulum, the ureter must be detached from the bladder, to resect and to remove the diverticulum or to remodel the ureter with a running suture in case of a megaureter [9, 11]. Then the ureter is sutured to the bladder mucosa orifice and then it is reimplanted as previously described. If the ureter is detached from the bladder before reimplantation a JJ stent must be positioned in the ureter and bladder [9].

The working ports are removed and the trocar orifices are finally closed using interrupted stitches. A bladder catheter is left in place postoperatively in all cases. No other drains are left after surgery [5, 8, 12].

42.6 Postoperative Care

Patients start oral feeding a few hours postoperatively. Analgesic therapy is rarely necessary; paracetamol (dosage 15 mg/kg at an 8-h interval) is usually administered in the first 12–24 h postoperatively [13]. A Foley catheter is removed on the first postoperative day. Patients are discharged 24–72 h after surgery whether they received ureteral tapering or not [6, 9]. Postoperative clinical controls are scheduled on the 7th and 30th POD and thereafter annually. Patients continue an antibiotic prophylaxis for about 1 month after surgery. An US exam is performed 3 months after surgery and voiding cystourethrogram (VCUG) 9–12 months after surgery [8].

- The role of the bedside surgeon is crucial to introduce and remove needles, cut the suture, and help the surgeon during the procedure.
- We always prepared a laparoscopic kit in case of conversion from robotics to laparoscopy.

42.7 Results

The average robot docking time was 16.2 ± 3.4 min (range 5–30 min). The average total operative time, calculated once port incisions were made, was 92.2 ± 8.6 min (range 50–170 min) [12, 14, 15].

No conversion to laparoscopic or open surgery, major bleeding, or other intraoperative complications were reported [12, 14, 16].

The average pain score, measured using the Visual Analogue Scale (VAS) during the first 24 h after surgery, was 2.9 ± 1.2 (range 1–6) [13].

The postoperative VCUG showed that the reflux had been resolved in more than 96% of patients.

We finally analyzed the costs of surgery and recorded an average cost of 14,100 euro (€) for each robotic procedure [6, 12].

Tips and Tricks

- Regarding the patient's position, a 15° Trendelenburg position is a crucial point for the success of the procedure; indeed, using this patient's positioning, the loops slide down and you have an excellent exposure of the bladder and ureters. It is important to fix the bladder to the abdominal wall to obtain a good exposure of the bladder during the reimplantation phase [5].
- It is also important to train the robotic team (surgeons and nurses) to reduce docking time [8].

42.8 Discussion

Laparoscopic extravesical Lich-Gregoir reimplantation (LEVUR) has gained a widespread acceptance in the last 15 years, and several papers have reported resolution rates of 87–100% using this technique. However, this procedure requires very advanced laparoscopic skills, in particular for intracorporeal suturing and knot-tying; in addition, it is associated with very bad ergonomics for the surgeon, especially for bilateral repairs. For this reason, LEVUR had a scanty diffusion among pediatric urologists [2, 14].

In the past 10 years, robot-assisted extravesical ureteral reimplantation according to the Lich Gregoir procedure (REVUR) has gained acceptance as a means of minimizing the morbidity associated with formal open intravesical reimplantation, including lower frequencies of postoperative hematuria, bladder spasms, shorter hospital stay, and bladder catheterization time compared to intravesical procedures [4]. In addition, REVUR is technically easier to perform compared to LEVUR.

In general, extravesical ureteral reimplantation allows to retain a normal ureteral anatomy, which might prove useful later in life if the child needs to undergo ureteroscopic procedures for stone disease or other indications [7, 15].

REVUR has been utilized by an increasing number of pediatric surgeons since the first series published by Peters et al. in 2004.

The published series have reported a success rate ranging from 77 to 100% [10, 14].

On the basis of our personal experience, it seems that REVUR is a very easy, safe, and fast procedure to perform with a reported shorter operative time compared to that of the laparoscopic Lich-Gregoir procedure [8, 10].

The second consideration is that you can also adopt this technique for duplex renal systems and you can perform reimplantation of both the ureters with the same good results as for a standard single ureter.

As for the learning curve, after a mandatory period of training on a simulator, the learning period is short, thanks to the possibility of having two consoles in the operative theater; moreover, for beginners, REVUR is very easy to perform with the help of an expert proctor [8].

The postoperative period was absolutely painless and quick as reported for the standard LEVUR. Patients after surgery had no hematuria and no bladder spasms and the length of hospital stay was very short (average of 2–3 days).

In our series, the success rate was excellent (96.3%) [3, 10, 14].

The main disadvantages of REVUR are the docking time, still takes too long for pediatric patients, and above all the diameter of robotic trocars; in fact, 8-mm trocars were adopted to perform REVUR, whereas 3-mm trocars were usually adopted to perform LEVUR [6, 17].

However, the worst criticism for robotics is the high cost of the procedure and the limited life of robotic instruments. In fact, in our experience, we noted that robotic instruments lost quality in their performances after the 6th–7th life, for example, robotic scissors began to cut very badly.

In addition, the robot is very big for a small baby; for this reason, the pediatric patient has to be well positioned and fixed on the operative table and the trocars have to be fixed to the skin using Steri-Strips or sutures in order to avoid dislodgement [8, 14].

Above all, REVUR is indicated in complex cases such as a megaureter or paraureteral diverticulum [9, 11]. This way, thanks to the 6 degrees of freedom of robotic instruments, it is easier when compared to that of laparoscopy to detach the ureter from the bladder to taper it and then to reimplant it into the bladder.

In the surgeons' opinion, robotic surgery is an amazing experience to perform for all the surgical team and robotic surgery changes difficult and long-lasting procedures such as Lich-Gregoir reimplantation into very easy and fast operations.

In conclusion, REVUR is a safe, effective, and successful procedure to adopt in patients with primary unilateral VUR with a reported 96% success rate in our series [8, 10, 18].

Using 3D robotic technology, the technique is easy and fast to perform thanks to the 6 degrees of freedom of robotic arms. The postoperative period is uneventful and painless as previously reported for endoscopic and laparoscopic procedures [13].

The learning curve is short, and it is useful to start the robotic experience with a surgeon expert in robotic surgery as a proctor on the second robotic console.

The high cost and the diameter of instruments remain the main challenges of robotic applications in pediatric urology.

Take-Home Points

- Before starting REVUR, it is important to have a preliminary experience in LEVUR.
- A team (surgeons and nurses) well trained in robotic surgery is essential before starting robotic procedures.
- During the learning curve period it's preferable to work with an expert surgeon on the second robotic console.
- The role of the bedside surgeon is crucial for the success of the procedure.
- In case of standard REVUR, we left only a Foley catheter, while in the case of a megaureter or ureteral diverticulum, we prefer to position a JJ stent in the bladder and ureter.

References

1. Elder JS, Diaz M, Caldamone AA, Cendron M, Greenfield S, Hurwitz R, Kirsch A, Koyle MA, Pope J, Shapiro E. Endoscopic therapy for vesicoureteral reflux: a meta-analysis. I Reflux resolution and urinary tract infection. J Urol. 2006;175:716–22.

2. Sung J, Skoog J. Surgical management of vesicoureteral reflux in children. Pediatr Nephrol. 2012;27:551–61.
3. Esposito C, Escolino M, Lopez M, Farina A, Cerulo M, Savanelli A, La Manna A, Caprio MG, Settimi A, Varlet F. Surgical management of pediatric vesicoureteral reflux: a comparative study between endoscopic, laparoscopic, and open surgery. J Laparoendosc Adv Surg Tech A. 2016;26(7):574–80.
4. Lendvay T. Robotic-assisted laparoscopic management of vesicoureteral reflux. Adv Urol. 2008;2008:732942. https://doi.org/10.1155/2008/732942.
5. Grimsby GM, Dwyer ME, Jacobs MA, Ost MC, Schneck FX, Cannon GM, Gargollo PC. Multi-institutional review of outcomes of robot-assisted laparoscopic extravesical ureteral reimplantation. J Urol. 2015;193(5 Suppl):1791–5.
6. Stanasel I, Atala A, Hemal A. Robotic assisted ureteral reimplantation: current status. Curr Urol Rep. 2013;14:32–6.
7. Gundeti MS, Kojima Y, Haga N, Kiriluk K. Robotic assisted laparoscopic reconstructive surgery in the lower urinary tract. Curr Urol Rep. 2013;14:333–41.
8. Gundeti MS, Boysen WR, Shah A. Robot-assisted laparoscopic extravesical ureteral reimplantation: technique modification contribute to optimized outcomes. Eur Urol. 2016;70:818–23.
9. Goh AC, Link RE. Robot-assisted tapered ureteral reimplantation for congenital megaureter. Urology. 2011;77:742–5.
10. Marchini GS, Hong YK, Minnillo BJ, Diamond DA, Houck CS, Meier PM, Passerotti CC, Kaplan JR, Retik AB, Nguyen HT. Robotic assisted laparoscopic ureteral reimplantation in children: case matched comparative study with open surgical approach. J Urol. 2011;185(5):1870–5.
11. Noh PH, Bansal D. Pediatric robotic assisted laparoscopy for paraureteral bladder diverticulum excision with ureteral reimplantation. J Pediatr Urol. 2013;9:28–30.
12. Chalmers D, Herbst K, Kim C. Robotic-assisted laparoscopic extravesical ureteral reimplantation: an initial experience. J Pediatr Urol. 2012;8:268–71.
13. Harel M, Herbst KW, Silvis R, Makari JH, Ferrer FA, Kim C. Objective pain assessment after ureteral reimplantation: comparison of open versus robotic approach. J Pediatr Urol. 2015;11:82–e1.
14. Castillo OA, Zubieta R, Yañez R. Laparoscopic surgery of vesicoureteral reflux: an experience in 42 patients with the lich- Gregoir extravesical technique. Actas Urol Esp. 2013;37(10):630–3.
15. Akhavan A, Avery D, Lendvay TS. Robot-assisted extravesical ureteral reimplantation: outcomes and conclusions from 78 ureters. J Pediatr Urol. 2014;10:864–8.
16. Dindo D, Demartines N, Clavien PA. Classification of surgical complications. A new proposal with evaluation in a cohort of 6336 patients and results of a survey. Ann Surg. 2004;240:205–13.
17. Casale P, Patel RP, Kolon TF. Nerve sparing robotic extravesical ureteral reimplantation. J Urol. 2008;179:1987–90.
18. Arlen AM, Broderick KM, Travers C, Smith EA, Elmore JM, Kirsch AJ. Outcomes of complex robot-assisted extravesical ureteral reimplantation in the pediatric population. J Pediatr Urol. 2016;12:169–e1.

Minimally Invasive Treatment of Ureterocele

43

Marco Castagnetti and Nicola Capozza

Learning Objectives

- To describe the possible technical alternatives for endoscopic decompression of ureterocele.
- To show a video with the technique of endoscopic decompression of ureteroceles.
- To describe tips and tricks and the new technologies available in pediatric urology that can be adopted to perform endoscopic decompression of a ureterocele.
- To discuss the indications for secondary surgery after endoscopic decompression of a ureterocele.
- To present long-term outcomes reported in the literature after endoscopic decompression for the management of ureterocele.

43.1 Introduction

The ureterocele is a cystic dilatation of the terminal portion of the ureter. The condition is rare and most pediatric urology centers are expected to treat less than ten cases per year [1].

The etiology is unknown. The most accredited embryologic mechanism is a failure of the spontaneous reabsorption of the Chawalla membrane present at the ureteral orifice during fetal development.

The ureterocele can be associate with a single or a duplex system. In the latter, the ureterocele invariably involves the upper pole moiety. Based on its extension, a ureterocele can be classified as intravesical, if entirely confined within the bladder, or ectopic, if it encroaches on the bladder neck or posterior urethra. Duplex system ureteroceles (DSUs) are the most common variant and are almost invariably ectopic. This variant is also called fetal ureterocele, as 80% are detected prenatally. Under these circumstances, the patient is asymptomatic by definition at birth. The initial management of this group of patients is the most challenging and controversial [2].

From a pathophysiologic point of view, the ureterocele determines an obstruction in the uretero-

Supplementary Information The online version contains supplementary material available at [https://doi.org/10.1007/978-3-030-99280-4_43].

M. Castagnetti (✉)
Department of Surgical, Oncological and Gastrointestinal Sciences, University Hospital of Padova, Padua, Italy

Pediatric Urology Unit, Bambin Gesù Children Hospital and Research Center, Rome, Italy
e-mail: marco.castagnetti@unipd.it; marco.castagnetti@opbg.net

N. Capozza
Pediatric Urology Unit, Bambin Gesù Children Hospital and Research Center, Rome, Italy
e-mail: nicola.capozza@opbg.net

C. Esposito et al. (eds.), *Minimally Invasive Techniques in Pediatric Urology*,
https://doi.org/10.1007/978-3-030-99280-4_43

cele moiety which can cause variable degrees of renal function impairment of the affected renal unit ranging from a multicystic dysplasia to an almost normal function [2]. In DSU, the ureterocele moiety is generally dysplastic and function of the upper pole ureterocele moieties negligible [3]. At bladder level, the ureterocele determines a compression atrophy of the surrounding muscular wall and, therefore, behaves as a defect in the detrusor and trigon in the intravesical variants and also in the bladder neck and posterior urethra in the ectopic variants [2]. As such, the ureterocele can have variable consequences on trigonal function, potentially being associated with variable degrees of obstruction or vesicoureteral reflux (VUR) in associated (ipsilateral and contralateral) moieties, and on bladder function, potentially being associated with variable degrees of detrusor underactivity, bladder outlet obstruction (BOO), and/or bladder neck insufficiency. These functional abnormalities are risk factors for urinary tract infections (UTI) and incontinence, the two major clinical issues reported in ureterocele patients [2].

Different surgical strategies do exist for the treatment of ureterocele ranging from watchful waiting to total reconstruction [2]. The latter includes ureterocele excision, reconstruction of the bladder base/neck, and ipsilateral ureteral reimplantation with or without upper pole partial nephrectomy in case of a DSU [4, 5]. Minimally invasive treatment options, instead, include a range of upper urinary tract surgeries (such as upper pole partial nephrectomy, upper to lower pole ureteropyelostomy, clipping of the obstructed moiety, or upper-to-lower pole ureteroureterostomy) which can be performed using a laparoscopic, retroperitoneoscopic, or robotic-assisted technique, and endoscopic decompression of the ureterocele [6]. Criteria proposed to select management include patient characteristics, e.g., patient age at diagnosis, presentation and degree of upper tract dilatation (both in ureterocele and associated moieties), surgeon preference, and expected goals of treatment. Nevertheless, there is no definitive evidence one approach to be superior to the others [5].

Present chapter will mainly focus on the endoscopic management of the ureterocele, whereas the reader is referred to other chapters for upper tract surgeries.

43.2 Preoperative Preparation

In patients presenting with a febrile UTI, the medical treatment of the infection is the mainstay. Urinary diversion is generally unnecessary. Ureterocele puncture to allow drainage of the infected urines entrapped in the upper tract (Fig. 43.1) can be considered if medical treatment fails. Otherwise, elective surgical treatment is recommended whenever possible [7].

Initial conservative management is also recommended in the asymptomatic neonate with a ureterocele. We generally recommend to start these patients on antibiotic prophylaxis soon after birth [8].

This period allows for the accomplishment of a comprehensive evaluation. The latter typically includes an ultrasound (US) of the upper urinary tract and bladder to assess the degree of upper urinary tract dilatation and confirm the presence of a ureterocele within the bladder (Fig. 43.1), a voiding cystourethrography (VCUG) including a low

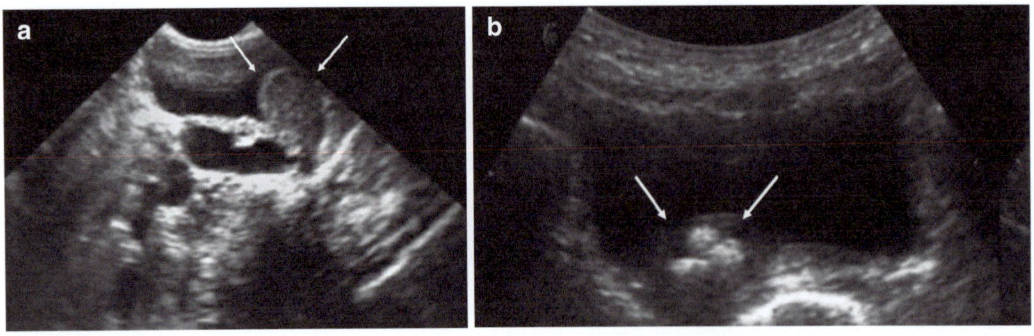

Fig. 43.1 US of the bladder. (**a**) Ureterocele full of debris; (**b**) Ureterocele with stones inside

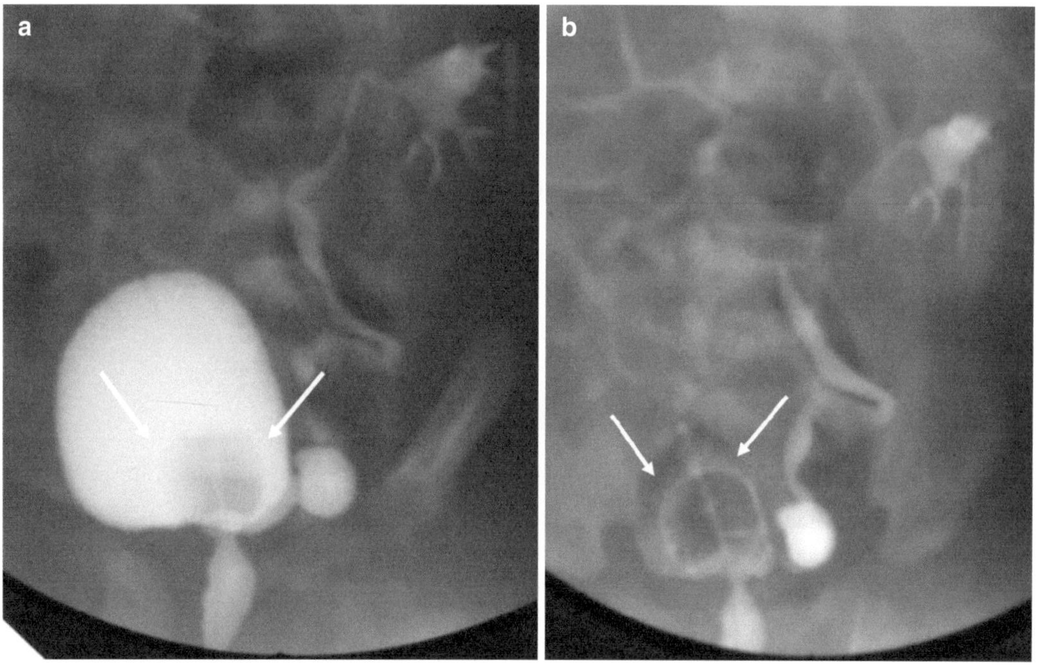

Fig. 43.2 VCUG (**a**) With full bladder; (**b**) At low bladder filling

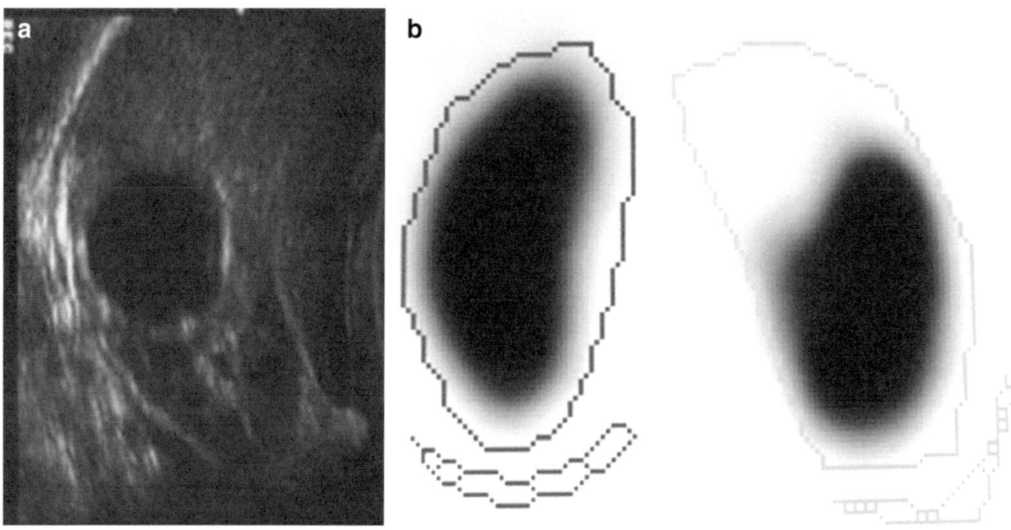

Fig. 43.3 Appearance of a right nonfunctioning, dilated upper pole on US (**a**) and renal nuclear scan (**b**)

filling phase to assess ureterocele extension and rule out the presence of VUR or BOO (Fig. 43.2), and a renal scintigraphy to assess ureterocele moiety function (Fig. 43.3) [2]. In our practice we prefer a (99 m)Tc-mercaptoacetyltriglycine, MAG3, diuretic renography for this purpose.

The actual need for a preoperative VCUG could be questioned in neonates, if the presence of VUR is not considered a factor driving the decision-making. Indeed, the VUR status can greatly change after ureterocele decompression, and therefore, postponing this investigation after surgery may be reasonable from a clinical point of view. Going further, the VCUG might also be limited only to patients developing UTI after endoscopic decompression. In the same way, also the renal scintigraphy could be avoided if the surgeon policy is to decompress any dilated ureterocele moiety irrespective of moiety function as the latter is often negligible and, as discussed below, preserving/improving ureterocele moiety function might not be a goal of ureterocele decompression.

43.3 Positioning

The procedure is performed with the patient in a lithotomy position or a frog-leg position in infants. As for any cystoscopy, the main goal of positioning is to have the legs spread enough to allow for unimpaired lateral movements of the cystoscope to assess the whole bladder.

The procedure can be performed using a caudal anesthesia plus sedation. A single dose of intravenous antibiotics at induction is generally recommended.

Before starting the endoscopy, the perineum should be assessed in females to check whether the ureterocele protrudes via the urethral orifice.

43.4 Instrumentation

An 8 Fr to 9.5 Fr cystoscope is adequate for most of the patients, but in the exceptional case of an older male, due to the urethral length.

A variety of instruments have been used for endoscopic ureterocele decompression including the Bugbee electrode, ureteral catheter stylet wire, Collin knife, and laser [9]. In all cases, the ureterocele can either be punctured or incised. In our opinion, the main goal is to create the smallest possible opening allowing for a satisfactory decompression [10–12]. Therefore, the ideal instrument should allow for the creation of a very precise and pin point hole in the ureterocele [12]. Tiny laser fibers are probably the most precise instrument for this purpose (Video 43.1). Fibers

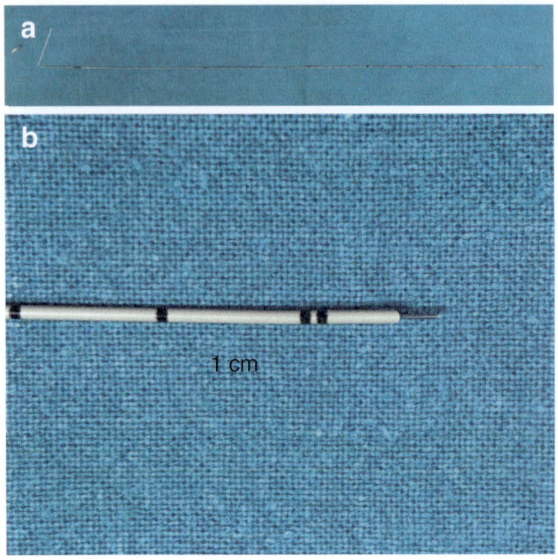

Fig. 43.4 Preparation of the stylet wire of a 3 Fr ureteral catheter for endoscopic decompression. (**a**) Full catheter with cut tip. (**b**) Close up of the wire coming out from the catheter tip

as small as 272 microns are available. To make such a small fiber stronger and easier to manipulate, passing it into a 4F open tip ureteral catheter can be helpful [12]. Using the holmium-YAG laser, power setting should include high frequency, 10–20 Hz, and low energy, around 1 Joule [13]. This allows for a net puncture with minimal energy dispersion around the incision spot. The real drawbacks of laser includes its limited availability and the high cost. For this reason, an alternative option, still widely used at one of the authors' institution, is the use of the stylet wire of a 3 Fr ureteral catheter [11]. In order to reduce the risk of damage to surrounding tissues and improve precision, the wire is pushed 4–5 mm out from the cut tip of the 3 Fr ureteral catheter (Fig. 43.4). Monopolar energy is applied connecting the proximal part of the stylet wire to the power cable. The recommended setting is high-voltage (such as 80 W) pure cutting energy. This instrument is widely available and almost inexpensive. Under this circumstance, however, the use of monopolar current makes the puncture less precise and causes more thermic damage around the puncture site (Fig. 43.5), possibly increasing the risk of hole closure.

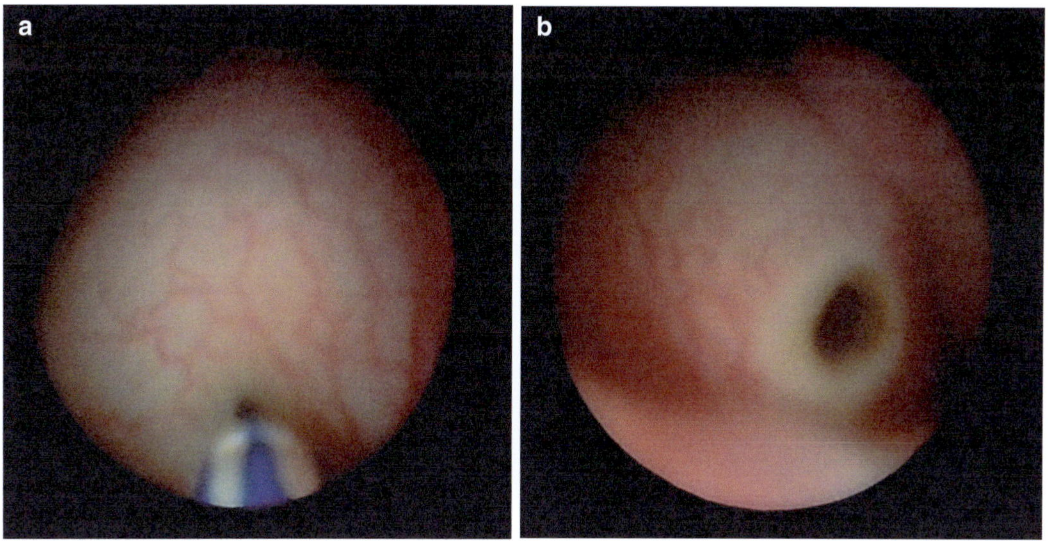

Fig. 43.5 Incision with the stylet wire of a 3 Fr ureteral catheter (**a**) and appearance of the hole after puncture (**b**)

43.5 Technique

The procedure starts with an endoscopic assessment of lower urinary tract anatomy. During this step, it is important to remind that the ureterocele tends to collapse while the bladder fills. This can be relevant for the assessment of ureterocele extension, which should be performed at low bladder volumes (Fig. 43.6). One should be aware that if a VCUG has been performed before the procedure, a discrepancy between the radiological and cystoscopic assessment of ureterocele extension, namely, intravesical vs. ectopic, can occur in about 25% of cases [2]. The contralateral or lower pole ureteral orifices, instead, can be easier to visualize with a collapsed ureterocele in a full bladder.

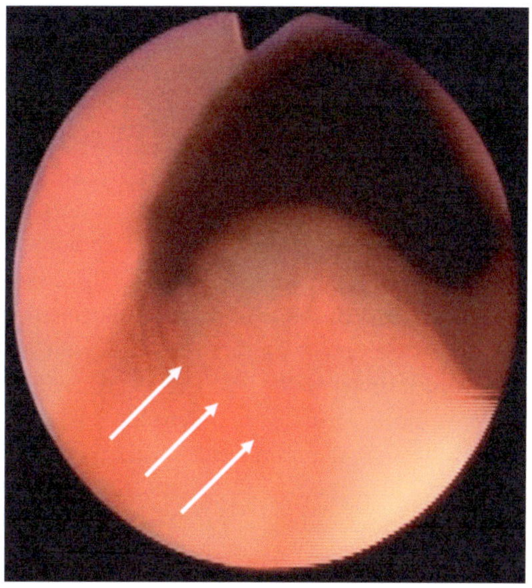

Fig. 43.6 Endoscopic appearance of a ureterocele protruding into the posterior urethra via the bladder neck

Before starting the endoscopic decompression, it is recommended to empty the bladder to 30–40% of maximum capacity to allow the ureterocele to re-expound.

The technique for endoscopic decompression of the ureterocele has substantially evolved over time. The first technique proposed was a wide uncapping of the ureterocele [2, 10]. This unavoidably causes a massive reflux in the ureterocele moiety with a high risk of UTI and need for secondary surgery. It has, therefore, become evident that a low opening of the ureterocele, as close as possible to the junction between the ureterocele wall and the bladder base allows to create an anti-reflux mechanism when the ureterocele collapses [2, 10]. In case of ectopic ureteroceles, early on, it was proposed that the ureterocele por-

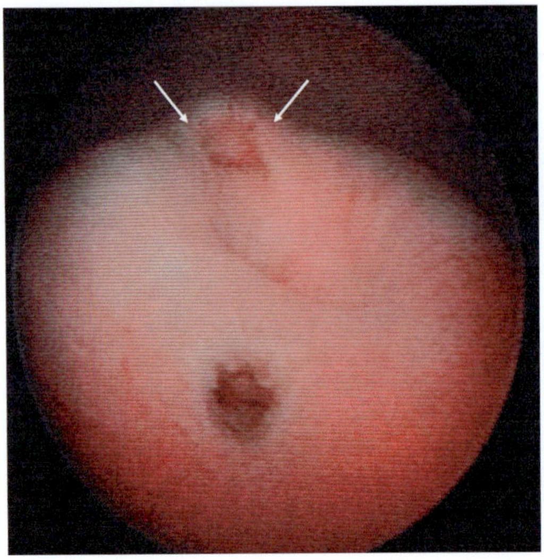

Fig. 43.7 Ureterocele collapsing after puncture. Note the lower pole ureteral orifice (arrows) sitting on top of the decompressed ureterocele

tion encroaching on the bladder neck or posterior urethra should be widely opened to avoid any urethral obstruction. It has, instead, become evident that the risk of BOO is small after ureterocele decompression also if the ectopic portion of the ureterocele is not opened, whereas its wide opening can increase the risk to end up with de novo VUR in the ureterocele moiety. This could actually be one of the major reasons accounting for the worse outcomes reported in ectopic vs. intravesical ureteroceles [2]. Therefore, opening the ureterocele medially, in a dependent position in its intravesical portion seems nowadays the technique of choice for all ureteroceles irrespective of their extension [11, 14]. The opening can either be a puncture (single or multiple) or an incision. There is no strong evidence in favor of one of the two techniques. In our practice, we rather prefer multiple small punctures to a single wide incision.

After puncture, ureterocele collapse is generally visible (Fig. 43.7 and Video 43.1). Another possible sign of an effective decompression is an increase in urine flow through the puncture site when pressure in applied on the ipsilateral flank. Intraoperative US is generally not helpful to assess the effectiveness of the decompression as the upper tract dilatation takes time to improve. Sometime, the lower pole orifice sitting on the ureterocele becomes visible after ureterocele decompression (Fig. 43.7). This can explain why the VUR status can change after ureterocele decompression. Under these circumstances, the distended ureterocele offered a backing to the lower pole ureter before ureterocele decompression that is lost thereafter.

43.6 Postoperative Care

Unless the presence of preoperative UTI, the procedure can generally be performed as a day care. Most surgeons, however, prefer to leave a transurethral catheter for bladder drainage for 24 to 48 h postoperatively.

We generally recommend a course of full dose oral antibiotics for 5 days postoperatively and, after that, to restart the patient on antibiotic prophylaxis until improvement in upper tract dilatation is documented on follow-up US.

Follow-up of these patients at the authors' centers typically involves clinical monitoring of UTI and serial US to assess upper urinary tract dilatation. As already mentioned, US findings should be interpreted cautiously. Improvement of upper tract dilatation can take time to occur, and the speedy is inversely correlated to the severity of the dilatation at the outset. In our practice, in an asymptomatic patient, we generally recommend the first reevaluation after 2 follow-up US performed at 2 and 4 months after endoscopic decompression. If the patient is well and the dilatation improves, we discontinue the prophylaxis and increase follow-up intervals. Later follow-ups should also allow to check the urinary continence status and the timely achievement of continence milestones.

Additional investigations such as VCUG, renal scintigraphy, or other imaging modalities are limited to selected patients with ongoing clinical issues, mainly postoperative UTI or lack of improvement of upper tract dilatation.

43.7 Results

The success of primary treatment of ureterocele strictly depends on the goals that surgery is expected to achieve. The general notion is that endoscopic treatment is more effective in single vs. duplex system ureteroceles and in intravesical vs. ectopic ureteroceles [7]. It should be noted, however, that the two things are often not independent risk factors, as 80% of duplex systems ureteroceles are ectopic. Therefore, the definition of ureterocele extension might not increase the risk for secondary surgery in a patient with duplex system ureterocele [15], and the latter is much easier to detect. Anyway, the different results reported for intravesical vs. ectopic ureteroceles can be misleading and have two possible explanations. One is, as mentioned before, the fact that different incision techniques were used in intravesical vs. ectopic cases increasing the risk to end up with a de novo reflux in the ureterocele moiety in ectopic cases. The second is that ectopic ureteroceles, due to their greater extension, might affect trigonal function more significantly than intravesical ones and, therefore, be more often associated with abnormalities in associated moieties (ipsilateral and contralateral), such as obstruction or VUR. The latter seldom completely disappear after endoscopic ureterocele decompression [2]. If one looks at the indications for secondary treatment in the different series, it is often clear that the secondary procedures most commonly performed were upper pole partial nephrectomies for nonfunctioning upper poles or ureteral reimplants for persistent/de novo VUR after endoscopic decompression irrespective of the presence of symptoms [11]. It is nowadays quite accepted that most of the ureterocele moieties are poorly functioning to begin with and function seldom improves significantly after endoscopic decompression [11]. Likewise, many patients, particularly those with DSU, have associated VUR preoperatively and this rarely ceases completely after surgery [2, 4, 11]. Therefore, expecting a significant function improvement or a complete VUR resolution after endoscopic decompression is just unrealistic, and it is more so in ectopic ureteroceles and in duplex systems. On the other side, however, accumulating evidences have clearly showed that poorly functioning upper poles can be left in situ if properly decompressed and seldom cause symptoms [16]; likewise, VUR in associated moieties can improve over time or anyway remain asymptomatic [17].

As mentioned before, the other important outcome is continence. Early series few years ago reported an increased risk for ureterocele patients to develop a large under-actieve bladder needing clean intermittent catheterization, or of bladder neck insufficiency potentially requiring subsequent surgery to improve bladder outlet resistances [2]. In contrast, recent reports, including some from the authors' institutions, suggest that continence problems are indeed quite exceptional in ureterocele patients [11, 18].

Tips and Tricks

- The authors have progressively moved from ureterocele incision to puncture in the attempt to make the smallest possible ureterocele opening allowing for satisfactory decompression as this seems to be the technique carrying the lowest risk of de novo VUR in the decompressed moiety [10, 11]. The counterpart of this is that the smaller the incision the higher the risk of reclosure and recurrence of the obstruction [11]. In the authors' opinion this untoward outcome is better prevented making multiple punctures than a single wider incision [11, 12]. Regarding the risk of failure of endoscopic decompression, it should be emphasized that one major feature differentiating ureteroceles is the thickness of the ureterocele wall [14]. Some ureteroceles are very thin and immediately decompress with a single puncture; others, instead, are thick-walled. Under these circumstances, multiple punctures or an incision might be necessary to achieve an effective and durable decompression. One possible trick in thick-walled ureteroceles could be to leave a stent in the puncture site for 48 h to keep open the hole while it heals. Others have also reported the use of a double J stent for a longer period for this purpose [19]. Admittedly, the assessment of ureterocele wall thickness remains somewhat subjective.

- Another important tip to consider during endoscopic decompression of a ureterocele is whether to perform a preemptive endoscopic treatment of VUR in associated moieties [19]. First of all, it should be noted that if one wants to consider this option, a preoperative VCUG is necessary to assess VUR status. This option is not generally offered at the authors' institutions if the treatment is performed in an asymptomatic infant as we tend to avoid any endoscopic treatment in the first 6–12 month of life in the absence of UTI. It might be reasonable, instead, in the older symptomatic patient.

43.8 Discussion

In many centers, endoscopic decompression is the initial management in the vast majority of ureterocele patients with an upper tract dilatation on US, based on the assumption that decompressing the upper tract reduces the risk of UTI. In keeping with this logic, as mentioned before, the preoperative workup could be limited to US only avoiding any preoperative VCUG or renal nuclear scan.

Nevertheless, while the need for treatment in the symptomatic patient or in patients with a history of UTI is generally agreed upon [7], the ideal management and timing for initial treatment in the asymptomatic neonate is controversial [2].

Under these circumstance, endoscopic decompression was considered at the beginning as an opportunity for a very early treatment before any UTI. Over time, however, it has become apparent that delaying treatment, at least by 3 to 6 months, does not increase significantly the risk of complications in these patients. Husmann et al. observed the same infection rates (8% vs. 9%) at 6 months of age in 32 DSU patients undergoing neonatal endoscopic decompression vs. 40 receiving only antibiotic prophylaxis [20]. Therefore, there is no need to rush into an early procedure in asymptomatic neonates and delayed treatment could be advantageous for anesthesiologic reasons and in order not to interfere with neonatal mother-to-child bonding.

Conservative management could be prolonged in some cases avoiding any need for surgery. Criteria for conservative management are not widely sheared but include the presence of no/poor function in the ureterocele moiety, the absence of high-grade VUR in any moiety, or evidence of BOO [2]. Including this treatment option in its own management algorithm clearly requires a full workup before starting any treatment. Reportedly, conservative management has been attempted also in ureterocele moieties with function but good upper tract drainage on diuretic renography. If conservative management is elected, antibiotic prophylaxis is generally recommended, but proposed protocols vary form the first year of life to until completion of toilet training or until the age of 5 years in cases of persistent VUR.

As mentioned, some reports suggest the use of an upper tract approach. Depending on moiety function and surgeon preference, it involves upper pole partial nephrectomy, upper to lower pole ureteropyelostomy, low ureteroureterostomy, or low ureteral clipping. Such approach has been proposed to be the most effective treatment modality particularly in patients with DSU and no associated VUR, where it is definitive treatment in more than 80% of cases [4]. Nevertheless, the evidence on the superiority of a treatment modality remains inconclusive [5]. We question that any of the mentioned procedures, also if performed using a minimally invasive approach, could be compared to an endoscopic decompression in terms of invasiveness.

Another important aspect related the follow-up of these patients is that if UTI occur, in most of the cases they happen during the toilet training process [11]. Moreover, in case of UTI associated with persistent/de novo VUR, the latter can be treated endoscopically in an all-endo approach which, even though may require multiple procedures, could be still considered less invasive than a single total reconstruction or even of a single upper pole partial nephrectomy performed using a minimally invasive approach [14, 17].

Take-Home Points

- Endoscopic decompression is an effective treatment option for ureterocele.
- One of multiple punctures should be performed in the intravesical portion of the ureterocele just above the junction between the ureterocele and the bladder base.
- Small punctures reduce the risk of de novo VUR but increase the risk of unsatisfactory ureterocele decompression.
- Poor function in the ureterocele moiety and persistent asymptomatic VUR in any moiety are not indications for secondary surgery.
- Long-term bladder function is generally normal in ureterocele patients.

References

1. Merguerian PA, Taenzer A, Knoerlein K, McQuiston L, Herz D. Variation in management of duplex system intravesical ureteroceles: a survey of pediatric urologists. J Urol. 2010;184(4 Suppl):1625–30. https://doi.org/10.1016/j.juro.2010.03.113.
2. Castagnetti M, El-Ghoneimi A. Management of duplex system ureteroceles in neonates and infants. Nat Rev Urol. 2009;6(6):307–15. https://doi.org/10.1038/nrurol.2009.82.
3. Meneghesso D, Castagnetti M, Della Vella M, et al. Clinico-pathological correlation in duplex system ectopic ureters and ureteroceles: can preoperative work-up predict renal histology? Pediatr Surg Int. 2012;28(3):309–14. https://doi.org/10.1007/s00383-011-3032-z.
4. DeFoor W, Minevich E, Tackett L, Yasar U, Wacksman J, Sheldon C. Ectopic ureterocele: clinical application of classification based on renal unit jeopardy. J Urol. 2003;169(3):1092–4. https://doi.org/10.1097/01.ju.0000049246.53911.04.
5. Cohen SA, Juwono T, Palazzi KL, Kaplan GW, Chiang G. Examining trends in the treatment of ureterocele yields no definitive solution. J Pediatr Urol. 2015;11(1):29.e1–29.e296. https://doi.org/10.1016/j.jpurol.2014.09.001.
6. Timberlake MD, Corbett ST. Minimally invasive techniques for management of the ureterocele and ectopic ureter: upper tract versus lower tract approach. Urol Clin North Am. 2015;42(1):61–76. https://doi.org/10.1016/j.ucl.2014.09.006.
7. Sander JC, Bilgutay AN, Stanasel I, et al. Outcomes of endoscopic incision for the treatment of ureterocele in children at a single institution. J Urol. 2015;193(2):662–6. https://doi.org/10.1016/j.juro.2014.08.095.
8. Castagnetti M, Cimador M, Esposito C, Rigamonti W. Antibiotic prophylaxis in antenatal nonrefluxing hydronephrosis, megaureter and ureterocele. Nat Rev Urol. 2012;9(6):321–9. https://doi.org/10.1038/nrurol.2012.89.
9. Ben Meir D, Silva CJ, Rao P, Chiang D, Dewan PA. Does the endoscopic technique of ureterocele incision matter? J Urol. 2004;172(2):684–6. https://doi.org/10.1097/01.ju.0000129228.92805.31.
10. Castagnetti M, Cimador M, Sergio M, de Grazia E. Transurethral incision of duplex system ureteroceles in neonates: does it increase the need for secondary surgery in intravesical and ectopic cases? BJU Int. 2004;93(9):1313–7. https://doi.org/10.1111/j.1464-410X.2004.04861.x.
11. Castagnetti M, Vidal E, Burei M, Zucchetta P, Murer L, Rigamonti W. Duplex system ureterocele in infants: should we reconsider the indications for secondary surgery after endoscopic puncture or partial nephrectomy? J Pediatr Urol. 2013;9(1):11–6. https://doi.org/10.1016/j.jpurol.2012.06.016.
12. Caione P, Gerocarni Nappo S, Collura G, et al. Minimally invasive laser treatment of ureterocele. Front Pediatr. 2019;7:106. https://doi.org/10.3389/fped.2019.00106.
13. Faure A, Boissier R. Optimal settings for the holmium: YAG laser in pediatric endourology: tips and tricks. J Pediatr Urol. 2020;16(2):244–50. https://doi.org/10.1016/j.jpurol.2020.03.002.
14. Hagg MJ, Mourachov PV, Snyder HM, et al. The modern endoscopic approach to ureterocele. J Urol. 2000;163(3):940–3.
15. Byun E, Merguerian PA. A meta-analysis of surgical practice patterns in the endoscopic management of ureteroceles. J Urol. 2006;176:1871–7.
16. Chertin B, Rabinowitz R, Pollack A, et al. Does prenatal diagnosis influence the morbidity associated with left in situ nonfunctioning or poorly functioning renal moiety after endoscopic puncture of ure-

terocele? J Urol. 2005;173(4):1349–52. https://doi.org/10.1097/01.ju.0000155439.68182.b4.
17. Jesus LE, Farhat WA, Amarante AC, et al. Clinical evolution of vesicoureteral reflux following endoscopic puncture in children with duplex system ureteroceles. J Urol. 2011;186(4):1455–8. https://doi.org/10.1016/j.juro.2011.05.057.
18. Paye-Jaouen A, Pistolesi F, Botto N, et al. Long-term bladder function after ureterocele decompression in children. J Urol. 2015;193(5 Suppl):1754–9. https://doi.org/10.1016/j.juro.2014.10.115.
19. Kajbafzadeh A, Salmasi AH, Payabvash S, Arshadi H, Akbari HR, Moosavi S. Evolution of endoscopic management of ectopic ureterocele: a new approach. J Urol. 2007;177(3):1118–23. https://doi.org/10.1016/j.juro.2006.11.001.
20. Husmann DA, Strand WR, Ewalt DH, Kramer SA. Is endoscopic decompression of the neonatal extravesical upper pole ureterocele necessary for prevention of urinary tract infections or bladder neck obstruction? J Urol. 2002;167(3):1440–2.

Minimally Invasive Treatment of Pediatric Bladder Tumors

44

Pascale Philippe Chomette, Alaa El-Ghoneimi, and Christine Grapin Dagorno

Learning Objectives

- Description of the pediatric bladder tumors which can benefit from minimally invasive treatment.
- Description of urothelial tumors.
- Review of papers on the treatment of bladder tumors in children and adolescents.
- Video of transurethral resection of fibroepithelial polyp and papillary urothelial tumor.
- Video of transperitoneal laparoscopy with atypical resection for urachal remnant.

44.1 Introduction

Pediatric bladder tumors are relatively rare [1]. Tumors come from different anatomical parts and different histological parts of the bladder.

Neoplasms in the pediatric population are mainly rhabdomyosarcoma [2] in those under 10 years old and papillary urothelial neoplasms [3] after 10 years old. Benign tumors include fibroblastic epithelial polyp, myofibroblastic tumor, and neurogenic tumor.

Minimally invasive treatment could be the only treatment for epithelial tumors or benign lesions of the bladder but could not be the treatment of choice for aggressive lesions such as rhabdomyosarcoma or urachal sarcoma.

The poor prognosis of bladder rhabdomyosarcoma needs acute treatment with a combination of surgery and brachytherapy [2], which is not the treatment of choice for urothelial tumors; we will not explain this treatment considering it is not a minimally invasive treatment.

Urachal sarcoma also needs a large resection and should not be resected through minimally invasive surgery [4].

Minimally invasive treatment will be the treatment of choice for papillary urothelial neoplasm which is a borderline tumor with an excellent prognosis in children [5] or the treatment for benign tumors which are very rare, such as fibrotic polyp tumor.

Minimally invasive treatment is essentially cystoscopic resection for intravesical lesions and partial cystectomy by laparoscopy in case of urachal remnant, myofibroblastic tumor, or neurogenic tumor [6].

Supplementary Information The online version contains supplementary material available at [https://doi.org/10.1007/978-3-030-99280-4_44].

P. P. Chomette (✉) · A. El-Ghoneimi · C. G. Dagorno
Children Cancer Unit/Pediatric Surgery Department, P. Philippe Chomette Robert Debré Hospital, Paris, France
e-mail: alaa.elghoneimi@rdb.aphp.fr

C. Esposito et al. (eds.), *Minimally Invasive Techniques in Pediatric Urology*,
https://doi.org/10.1007/978-3-030-99280-4_44

44.2 Types of Bladder Tumors in Children which Can Benefit from Minimally Invasive Treatment

44.2.1 Benign Lesions

44.2.1.1 Urothelial Papilloma Lesion

This lesion is rare and found accidentally after hematuria or pelvic pain [7]. Urothelial papillomas are benign polypoid lesions. Histologically, there is a broad vascular core covered by a normal urothelium and no atypia is found [7]. This lesion is treated by transurethral resection, recurrence is observed, and US and cystoscopy are needed upon follow-up [8].

44.2.1.2 Fibroepithelial Polyp

This is also a rare lesion, discovered after dysuria and hematuria. This pathology is solitary and benign without a risk of recurrence. Transurethral resection is the treatment of choice [8].

44.2.1.3 Inflammatory Myofibroblastic Bladder Tumors

These tumors are rare, arising from the wall of the bladder, and are characterized by a reactive proliferation of myofibroblasts. The etiology is poorly understood and is attributed to infectious or traumatic causes, and the presence of the lymphoma kinase gene ALK should be considered. Complete surgical resection is the treatment and transperitoneal laparoscopic partial cystectomy is proposed [6].

Others lesions such as neurofibroma and neurogenic tumors could benefit from atypical bladder resection through transperitoneal laparoscopy.

44.2.2 Malignant Lesions

Papillary urothelial neoplasms of low malignant potential are described as exuberant and exophytic tumors (Figs. 44.1, 44.2, 44.3, and 44.4).

This tumor is common in adolescents and children over 10 years old [9].

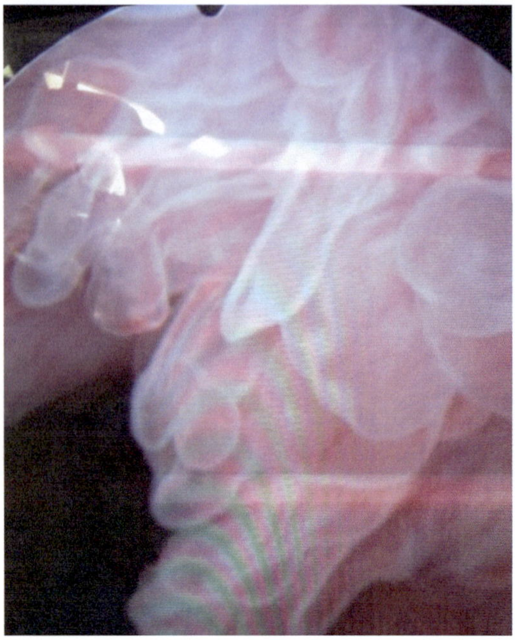

Fig. 44.1 Macroscopic aspect of a *papillary* urothelial tumor of low malignant potential

They are normally solitary and small. They occur at the posterior wall and ureteral orifices. These tumors are noninvasive and do not metastasize. Approximately 35% of *papillary* urothelial neoplasms can recur after complete resection. Therefore, follow-up is mandatory with US examination and regular cystoscopy within 5 years [10].

Urothelial carcinomas are rare in children, most of them have a low-grade morphology, but some occur in children with a predisposition for cancer such as Costello syndrome, hereditary nonpolyposis syndrome, or augmented bladder. They are frequently of high grade and have an aggressive and pejorative evolution [7].

44.2.2.1 Urachal Adenocarcinoma and Urachal Sarcoma

Urachal abnormalities are associated with a high risk of bladder carcinoma in adolescents or adults [4] (Fig. 44.5).

The poor prognosis of urachal cancer with the potential of a high risk of recurrence leads us to recommend prophylactic resection of incidental urachal remnants, and the urachal cyst can be

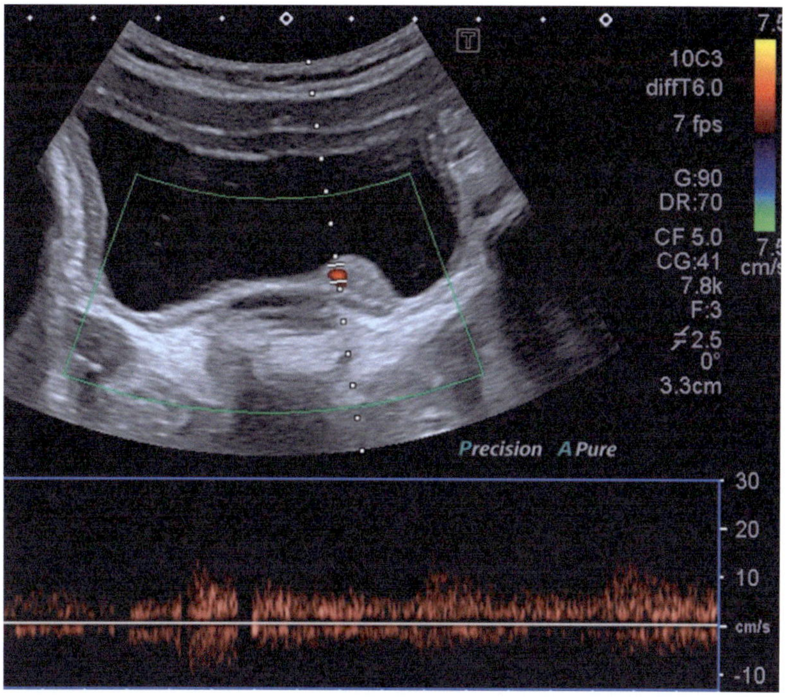

Fig. 44.2 Papillary urothelial neoplasm on ultrasound examination

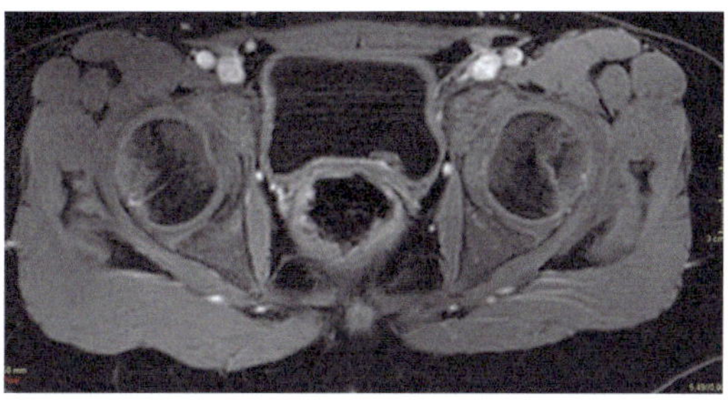

Fig. 44.3 Aspect of small papillary urothelial neoplasm on MRI

treated through transperitoneal laparoscopic partial cystectomy.

Benign or borderline tumors such as *papillary* urothelial neoplasms can benefit from endoscopic resection. Even in most patients with urothelial carcinomas, transurethral resection is the treatment of choice. There is no recommendation of adjuvant chemotherapy after resection, but partial cystectomy could be proposed for augmented bladder or other syndromic population because of a high risk of perforation during the procedure [7].

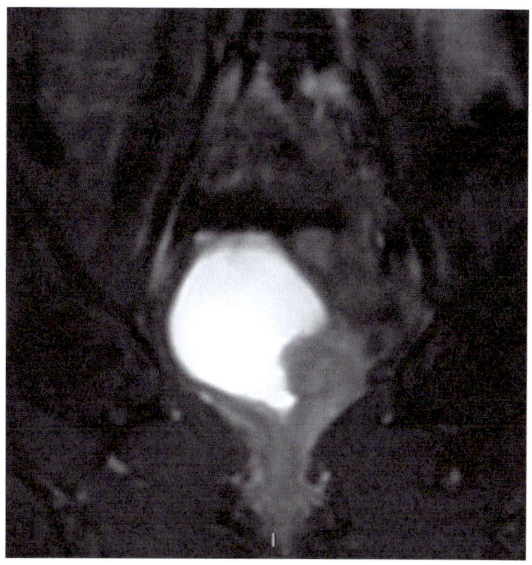

Fig. 44.4 Aspect of large papillary urothelial neoplasm on MRI

Urachal remnants and myofibroblastic tumors could be resected through laparoscopy not only with resection of the cyst but with partial cystectomy to have safe margins to avoid bladder carcinoma in children [7].

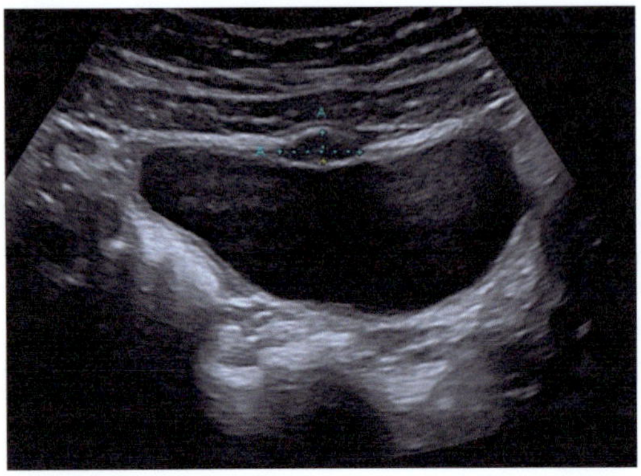

Fig. 44.5 Aspect of urachal cyst on ultrasound examination

44.3 Symptoms

Gross hematuria, dysuria, and pelvic pain are the main symptoms [10]. Hematuria after excluding urinary infection needs endoscopic exploration. Pelvic pain and dysuria in children necessitate imaging to detect eventual tumor or to detect urachal remnant.

44.4 Preoperative Imaging

- *Ultrasound examination* is the most common initial examination: a full bladder during the exam is a useful recommendation to avoid missing small lesions. The lesion is found in 90% of patients [11].
- The lesion is usually unique, and multiple lesions are rare in children.
- Computed tomography (CT) scan and magnetic resonance imaging (MRI) are performed for better characterization of the lesion and its extension to avoid transmural lesion. The exophytic aspect is the main radiologic definition of low-grade papilloma [11, 12].

44.5 Treatment

Gross hematuria or lesions detected by imaging necessitate exploration by endoscopy.

Transurethral cystoscopy is performed and the lesions are described.

Patients receive general anesthesia with orotracheal intubation and myorelaxation.

44.5.1 First Step: Biopsy

We usually use a 9.5-Fr operative cystoscope with a endoscopic biopsy forceps.

The lesions could be unique as a solitary or multiple polyp. Essential recommendation is to perform biopsy in case of rhabdomyosarcoma [2].

Papillary urothelial lesions have specific aspects but should benefit from biopsy.

In case of solitary and unique polyp, biopsy and resection could be authorized.

After histological examination, if the diagnosis of epithelial lesion is confirmed, endoscopic treatment is mandatory [7].

44.6 Transurethral Cystoscopic Resection

In case of urothelial lesions, an endoscopic resection using a diathermic or bipolar handle for cauterization is recommended.

Ureteral orifices are described and lesions are resected with the diathermic handle, the mucosae and submucosae are removed at the site of the lesion.

In case of a unique polyp, resection could be done using cold biopsy grasping forceps. Transurethral endoscopy permits exploration of the entire bladder, to identify the lesion and cut the lesion at the foot of the polyp. Cold section permits excellent histological examination of the margins of the polyp and eliminate rhabdomyosarcoma.

In case of positive margins in papillary urothelial neoplasms, resection should be repeated [5]. Instillation chemotherapy after resection is not recommended in children at this time but mitomycin instillation could be performed without complications at the time of resection [7].

No adjuvant chemotherapy is used for papillary urothelial tumors, but alternating endoscopy and ultrasound examination during follow-up is recommended.

44.6.1 Postoperative Care

A Foley catheter is kept for 24 h in order to evacuate hematuria and avoid vesical retention.

44.7 Treatment of Urachal Remnant or Other Mesenchymal Benign Lesion

Patients receive a general anesthesia and orotracheal intubation and myorelaxation.

A Foley catheter is positioned into the bladder before the surgery, and the access to the catheter must by allowed during the surgery.

44.7.1 Positioning

The child is placed in decubitus dorsal position, the screen is placed at the end of the table, and the surgeons are on both sides of the patient.

44.7.2 Procedure

We use a 10-mm trocar placed at the umbilical site and two other 5-mm trocars for instruments placed on the same line.

We use atraumatic fenestrated forceps and LigaSure™ Atlas to dissect the cyst or the urachal remnant. We follow the urachal tract and dissect from the wall, and at the end of the remnant or at the cyst, we precisely identify the limit of the bladder by filling it. We can clamp the Foley catheter or fill the bladder with serum at this step of the procedure. Then we can determine its limit and we use 5-mm Endo GIA automatic sutures for atypical resection of the bladder. We have to resect all the lesion to avoid urachal sarcoma or adenocarcinoma development.

The lesion is extracted in an Endo Bag and sent to the laboratory for histological examination.

The Foley catheter is kept in place for 48 h.

44.8 Discussion

The major initial presenting symptom of a bladder tumor is gross hematuria [7]. However, because of the rarity of bladder transitional cell carcinoma in children, rhabdomyosarcoma must be eliminated and cystoscopy and biopsy should be performed.

Ultrasound examination is reported as an excellent tool in detecting intravesical lesions [11]. MRI helps to determine the infiltration of the lesion. Most series report the excellent outcome of bladder carcinoma in children compared with that of older patients [8]. The treatment of choice is transurethral resection, and in case of papillary urothelial neoplasm, mitomycin instillation could be proposed at the time of resection; however, considering the indolent biologic behavior of these tumors in the pediatric population, this treatment is not necessary. Immunotherapy is used in recurrent neoplasms in adults and should not be proposed in the pediatric population [7].

Myofibroblastic or cystic tumors arising from the bladder wall are managed through minimally invasive treatment such as the transperitoneal laparoscopic approach with partial cystectomy [6].

44.9 Conclusion

Urothelial bladder tumors in children are essentially managed through minimally invasive treatment via transurethral endoscopic resection following the procedure in adults.

The risk of recurrence needs correct follow-up by alternating cystoscopy and ultrasound examination for a minimum of 3 years [1].

Transperitoneal laparoscopic resection is recommended for mesenchymal benign bladder tumors such as myofibroblastic tumors or urachal remnants, but urachal sarcoma or bladder adenocarcinoma needs radical procedures because of the risk of recurrence and the poor prognosis [4].

Take-Home Points

- Precisely define the histological type of bladder lesions through correct imaging and biopsy.
- Transurethral endoscopic resection could be repeated and urological endoscopic experience is required.
- Urachal remnants need to be removed and MIS is an excellent approach.
- MIS is not the technique for urachal sarcoma and urachal adenocarcinoma.
- Follow-up is essential to avoid massive recurrence.

References

1. Berrettini A, Castagnetti M, Salerno A, et al. Bladder urothelial neoplasms in pediatric age: experience at three tertiary centers. J Pediatr Urol. 2015;11(1):26.e1–5.
2. Leaphart C, Rodeberg D. Pediatric surgical oncology: management of rhabdomyosarcoma. Surg Oncol. 2007;16(3):173–85.
3. Saltsman JA, Malek MM, Reuter VE, et al. Urothelial neoplasms in pediatric and young adult patients: a large single center series. J Pediatr Surg. 2018;53(2):306–9.
4. Gleason JM, Bowlin PR, Bagli DJ, et al. A comprehensive review of pediatric urachal anomalies and predictive analysis for adult urachal adenocarcinoma. J Urol. 2015;193(2):632–6.
5. Di Carlo D, Ferrari A, Perruccio K, et al. Management and follow up of uroepithelial neoplasms of the bladder in children: a report from the TREP project. Pediatr Blood Cancer. 2015;62:1000–3.
6. Collin M, Charles A, Barker A, et al. Inflammatory myofibroblastic tumour of the bladder in children: a review. J Pediatr Urol. 2015;11(5):239–45.
7. Iglesias Lopes R, Figuereido Mello M, Lorenzo AJ. Recent advances in pediatric bladder malignancies. F1000 Res. 2020;9:147.
8. Alanee S, Shukla AR. Bladder malignancies in children aged < 18 years: results from the surveillance, Epidemiology and End Results database. BJU Int. 2010;106(4):557–60.
9. Keetch DW, Manley CB, Catalona WJ. Transitional cell carcinoma of bladder in children and adolescents. Urology. 1993;42(4):447–9.
10. Lerena J, Krauel L, Garcia-Aparicio L, Vallasciani S, Sunol M, Rodo J. Transitional cell carcinoma of the bladder in children and adolescents: six case series and review of the literature. J Pediatr Urol. 2010;6:481–5.
11. Shelmerdine SC, Lorenzo AJ, Gupta AA, et al. Pearls and pitfalls in diagnosing pediatric urinary bladder masses. Radiographics. 2017;37(6):1872–91.
12. Huang H, Li X, Jin J. Treatment of bladder transitional cell carcinoma: a single center experience of China. Arch Iran Med. 2015;18(4):250–2.

45 Minimally Invasive Techniques in Neurogenic Bladder

Emilio Merlini, Claudio Carlini, Ilaria Falconi, and Maria Grazia Faticato

Learning Objectives

- To learn about the risks related to an untreated neurogenic bladder and the physiopathological basis of its treatment.
- To learn about the endoscopic treatment of vesicoureteral reflux in neurogenic bladders using the same procedures employed in normal bladders.
- To learn about the treatment of incontinence aiming at reducing overactive bladder contractions and increasing bladder outlet resistance, either endoscopically or using laparoscopic or robotic-assisted laparoscopic procedures.

45.1 Introduction

The bladder is a unique organ in the human body because it receives a triple innervation from both the autonomic and somatic nervous system. The autonomic nervous system is represented by sympathetic (the hypogastric nerves) and parasympathetic (the pelvic nerves) innervation. Somatic innervation is carried by the pudendal nerves. During bladder storage, the viscoelastic properties of the bladder wall and the absence of an excitatory output from the parasympathetic nerves allow the bladder to store increasing volumes of urine, keeping the intravesical pressure low. In this phase the parasympathetic output is silenced, while the sympathetic nerves release neurotransmitters relaxing the detrusor muscle and increasing tension at the bladder neck and posterior urethral level. In late filling the somatic rhabdosphincter also increases its tone contributing to maintaining continence. Micturition starts with a relaxation of the bladder neck and sphincter muscle and at the same time inhibition of parasympathetic output stops, thus allowing a sustained contraction of the detrusor, while bladder neck and urethra are fully open. As a consequence, micturition takes place at a relatively low pressure. The interplay of autonomic and somatic innervation depends on the regulatory activity of the pontine micturition centre, which in turn receives inhibitory or excitatory inputs mainly from the prefrontal cortex, the preoptic region of the hypothalamus and the anterior cingulate gyrus, plus several other neural connections. Their balanced activity causes normal storage of urine at low pressure and complete voiding without undue resistance at the bladder neck and urethral level. Any damage to this complex interaction system can seriously disturb the blad-

E. Merlini (✉) · C. Carlini · I. Falconi · M. G. Faticato
Division of Paediatric Surgery, S.S. Antonio e Biagio e Cesare Arrigo Hospital, Alessandria, Italy
e-mail: ccarlini@ospedale.al.it; ilariafalconi1986@libero.it

C. Esposito et al. (eds.), *Minimally Invasive Techniques in Pediatric Urology*,
https://doi.org/10.1007/978-3-030-99280-4_45

Table 45.1 Practical classification of neurogenic bladder based on detrusor contractility and sphincter activity

Detrusor contractility	External sphincter activity
Normal	Normal (synergic or coordinated)
Overactive	Overactive (dyssynergic or uncoordinated)
Inactive	Inactive

der functions resulting in a neurogenic bladder. Causes of neurogenic bladder are, most frequently, congenital, including myelomeningocele and other spinal dysraphisms or cerebral palsy; less frequently, neurogenic bladder is acquired and secondary to a spinal or cerebral trauma or tumour. Neurogenic bladder can be simply classified according to two main factors, detrusor contractility and external sphincter activity (Table 45.1): Patients with incompetent bladder neck and external urethral sphincter are affected by complete urinary incontinence, irrespective of detrusor behaviour. Those patients with an overactive sphincter and hypoactive detrusor may show urinary retention which, in turn, causes overflow incontinence. The combination of an overactive detrusor and overactive sphincter includes approximately 55% of patients born with spina bifida, which is responsible for urinary incontinence and progressive detrusor deterioration; this combination is particularly dangerous for the upper urinary tract and the kidneys. Detrusor–sphincter dyssynergia generates bladder outlet obstruction leading to elevated intravesical pressures and incomplete emptying, with significant postvoiding residual urine, detrusor hypertrophy, reduction in bladder compliance, high-pressure vesicoureteral reflux (VUR) and frequent urinary tract infections (UTIs) causing progressive renal damage.

45.1.1 Preoperative Investigations

All patients affected by neurogenic bladder must be fully investigated before planning any therapeutic intervention, in order to decide the most appropriate procedures. Neurologic assessment and neuroradiologic evaluation with NMRI of the spine and, often, the brain are a necessary prerequisite to identify the neurologic condition. Videourodynamic is an essential tool to precisely diagnose patients affected by neurogenic bladder because similar symptoms may be caused by different pathophysiological situations. Urodynamic tests should be repeated every 2 or 3 years because functional features of the bladder change with time. The parameters and aspects investigated during videourodynamics are both anatomical and functional. Anatomical details of interest include the size and shape of the bladder, the opening of the bladder neck and, especially, the presence and grade of vesicoureteral reflux. Neurogenic bladder can be hypoactive, large and non-contractile, or, more frequently, overactive, showing inversion of diameters and assuming a "Christmas tree" appearance, with trabeculated walls and a non-relaxing external sphincter during micturition. Functional parameters are obtained during repeated bladder fillings: bladder capacity, pressure, compliance ($\Delta V/\Delta P$), EMG behaviour of perineal muscles (synergic or dyssynergic) during attempts at micturition and overactive bladder contractions. Registration of bladder pressure can also clarify if VUR occurs at low pressure or during a contraction; in the latter eventuality lowering bladder pressure is essential before attempting any correction of VUR. A reliable flowmetry coupled with perineal EMG is seldom obtainable because most children cannot void voluntarily, but in those children who are able to void, it is a useful and easily repeatable investigation. More sophisticated parameters are the leak point pressure (LPP) and the Valsalva leak point pressure (VLPP) that are an indirect measurement of bladder outlet resistance. Videourodynamic is essential to decide whether we need to lower the bladder pressure, inhibit contractions, augment the bladder and/or increase bladder neck resistance or bypass an obstructing sphincter.

45.1.2 Goals of Treatment

The main problems in children with neuropathic bladder are, most frequently, urinary incontinence and deteriorating renal function, which is less frequent, but of greater importance. The goal of treatment, therefore, is to have a child with normal renal function and continent; to accomplish these results, it is necessary to have a bladder of almost normal capacity, filling and emptying at low pressure (<30 cmH_2O) with no or minimal residual urine. Lastly, voiding or bladder emptying must be under voluntary control. A large number of patients can achieve these results by means of a conservative treatment only, but those who cannot achieve continence with a low-pressure bladder and stable upper tracts need a more aggressive approach. In recent years, the minimally invasive approach has gained a vast space also in the treatment of neurogenic bladder.

45.1.3 Conservative Treatment

The great majority of children affected by neurogenic bladder can be treated conservatively with a combination of intermittent clean self-catheterization (CIC) and dugs active on the bladder and/or urinary sphincter, most frequently anticholinergics. Not all patients affected by neurogenic bladder can achieve the proposed goals of treatment by means of conservative treatment only. Those with an inactive sphincter will be incontinent, and in these patients CIC is useless, as their bladder is usually always empty; children with a small fibrotic bladder do not respond to anticholinergic therapy, and both groups need a more aggressive operative approach to attain continence. Lastly, in patients with severe vesicoureteral reflux that does not disappear, lowering the bladder pressure, an operative approach to treat the VUR is needed.

45.2 Vesicoureteral Reflux in Neuropathic Bladder

VUR occurs in approximately 3–5% of newborns with neuropathic bladder secondary to myelomeningocele, which is usually associated with low compliance and detrusor sphincter dyssynergia. If untreated, the incidence of reflux increases with time in up to 30–50% at 5 years of age [1]. Low-grade refluxes in children who void spontaneously or have complete denervation of the external sphincter can be treated with low-dose antibiotic prophylaxis only. Children with high-grade reflux and a non-emptying bladder, in particular if they have detrusor overactivity and detrusor–sphincter dyssynergia, need to be treated promptly with CIC and anticholinergics; with this therapy, approximately 30–55% of refluxes disappear and the upper urinary tract is protected [2]. Indications for anti-reflux procedures are the same as for VUR in a normal bladder, namely, recurring pyelonephritis, appearance of new renal scars and persisting high-grade reflux despite maximal conservative management of bladder dysfunction.

45.2.1 Endoscopic Treatment of VUR in Neurogenic Bladder

Endoscopic treatment of VUR was popularized by O'Donnell and Puri in 1986 [3]. The treatment consists in the subureteric or, more recently, intra-ureteral submucosal injection of a bulking agent; this procedure allows elongation of the intravesical portion of the ureter, reduces the diameter of the ureter and causes a more solid fixation of the ureter to the trigone. A necessary prerequisite to any treatment of VUR in neurogenic bladder is a compliant, stable bladder, regularly emptied by means of clean intermittent catheterization.

45.2.1.1 Positioning and Technique of Injection

Any type of cystoscope with a working 4-Fr working channel may be used, but most authors, including us, prefer to use an offset lens 8- or 9-Fr cystoscope with a straight channel that allows the use of a metal needle. In our opinion, the semi-rigid metal needle is preferable to the flexible plastic one. Patient may be positioned in a lithotomy position or, as we prefer, can lie flat on the operating table, with both legs hanging outside the table border, suspended with straps.

This position avoids the rotation of the pelvis, keeping the trigone in the same plane as the posterior urethra.

The cystoscope is inserted inside the bladder and the ureteral orifices are identified; in neurogenic trabeculated bladders, the ureteral orifices may not be immediately visible; in such cases the use of a ureteral catheter to find the orifices and facilitate the injection may be extremely useful. The bladder must be only moderately distended to avoid extra-vesical injection of the bulking agent.

The needle is inserted at a 6 o'clock position, 3 mm distal to the ureteric orifice, and then advanced 5 mm in the subureteric space, as originally described by Puri and O'Donnell (STING procedure). If the orifice is wide and gaping, the hiatus can be hydrodistended using the irrigation system of the cystoscope and the injection is performed more proximally inside the ureteric orifice (HIT procedure) and the mound is created in the submucosal space. Cerwinka et al. [4] have described a further modification of the injection technique, associating a HIT to a more distal injection ("the double HIT") at the ureteric hiatus. They suggest a further more distal subureteric injection if, at the end of a double HIT, the ureteric orifice can still be hydrodistended.

45.2.1.2 Injectable Substances

Various substances are used as injectables; the polytetrafluoroethylene (Teflon ®) paste was the first one to be used, but it was later abandoned because of the risk of particle migration in various organs, including the lungs and brain. Teflon also elicits a vigorous inflammatory response with granuloma formation both in the local injection site and in other organs where particles migrate. Injectable collagen is a purified suspension of bovine collagen that is solubilized, subjected to enzymatic digestion to reduce its immunogenicity and to glutaraldehyde cross-linking to reduce reabsorption. Cross-linked collagen is still used as a bulking injectable agent, but it is not so popular as it used to be in the past, because concern has been raised on its possible immunogenicity and reabsorption after hydrolysis by collagenase, making results only temporary. In recent years, two agents have become more popular in the treatment of VUR and urinary incontinence, namely, polydimethylsiloxane (Macroplastique®) and hyaluronic acid–dextranomer (Dx-Ha, commercial names Deflux®, or Dexel®). Macroplastique® is a mixture of particulate silicone with povidone gel; the size of its particles is large enough to reduce the phenomenon of migration to other organs. Dx-Ha is a mixture of dextranomer and non-animal hyaluronic acid; it is currently the most frequently used substance for injection in children, mainly to correct VUR. Microspheres of Dx-Ha are non-immunogenic and do not migrate because of their size.

45.2.1.3 Results and Discussion

The results of endoscopic treatment of VUR in normal bladders depend on the grade of reflux – 78.5% in non-dilated ureters to 50.9% in grade V reflux – and on the substance injected.

Resolution of VUR (all grades) was achieved in 50% of patients using collagen; in 66.9% and 68.7% using PTFE (Teflon paste) and dextranomer, respectively; and finally, 76.5% using polydimethylsiloxane [5].

Endoscopic treatment of reflux in neurogenic bladder has been largely reported in the literature, with variable results, again depending on the reflux grade and the type of substance injected; in general, the overall results have been reported to be less favourable than in a normal bladder, with a success rate ranging from 53% to 86% [6]. Yokoyama et al. [7] employed cross-linked collagen with an initial success rate of 64%, which increased to 100% after a second treatment. Less favourable results were obtained by Haferkamp et al. [8] using collagen; in their patients, after 16 months of follow-up, VUR had disappeared in only 15% of treated ureters. Better results have been reported using Teflon® paste: Quinn et al. [9] obtained a satisfactory 90.2% success rate after two injections, and similar results (86%) have been reported by Puri et al. [10] in 1986. In 1996, Misra et al. [11] reported an initial 82% success rate, using Teflon® paste injections, but in four out of 57 ureters, VUR recurred and one patient suffered from bilateral vesicoureteric junction obstruction. In recent years, after stopping the use of Teflon paste, dextranomer/hyaluronic acid became the most popular substance employed in the endoscopic treatment of VUR. In 2004, Perez-Brayfield et al. [12] reported their experience in the endoscopic treatment of complex cases of VUR, including 11 ureters in patients with a neurogenic bladder. Their overall success rate was 68% after one implant, but in patients with a neurogenic bladder, positive results were obtained in 79% of cases. Granata et al. [13] and Engel et al. [14] have compared the resolution rate of VUR after endoscopic treatment using PTFE versus open surgical treatment. Granata has obtained a resolution rate of 72.5% endoscopically, versus 95.5% after transtrigonal ureteric reimplantation. Engel reported a 61% success rate after two injections as compared to 84.3% after ureteroneocystostomy. In recent years, a very promising experience using a totally endoscopic management of VUR in neurogenic bladder associating injection of botulinum toxin A (BoNT-A) in the detrusor with the subureteric injection of dextranomer/hyaluronic acid has been reported by Mosiello et al. [15] and Neel et al. [16] Mosiello et al. [15] reported an increase in maximum cystometric capacity and a decrease in maximum detrusor pressure in all seven patients. VUR disappeared in all 12 renal units, but relapsed in one patient (91.6% success rate). Neel [16] has obtained similar results with respect to bladder capacity and maximum bladder pressure, and 15 out of 16 refluxing ureters (93.75%) were cured.

Laparoscopic and robotic-assisted ureteroneocystostomies, both extra-vesical and vesicoscopic, have become more popular in recent years for the treatment of primary VUR, but despite their increasing popularity, to our knowledge, no specific report of their use to treat VUR secondary to neurogenic bladder has been published yet.

45.3 Urinary Incontinence

A child is defined continent if he/she has a dry interval equal or superior to 4 h and can attend to his/her activities without wearing diapers or other protections. Urinary incontinence in neurogenic bladders has different causes; it may depend on the inability of the bladder to store an adequate amount of urine at low pressure coupled with an overactive or inactive external sphincter or can be due to an inactive sphincter, irrespective of detrusor behaviour. Reduced bladder capacity and compliance may be due to an extensive fibrosis of the detrusor muscle, which loses its viscoelastic properties, or to an overactive detrusor.

45.3.1 Procedures on the Detrusor

When incontinence is secondary to a small or overactive bladder, the problem can be treated initially with drugs like anticholinergics; if these are ineffective, botulinum toxin A can be injected in the detrusor or, as a last resource, the bladder can be augmented with a loop of bowel.

45.3.1.1 Intravesical Botulinum Toxin Therapy

In a small number of patients, oral anticholinergics are ineffective or are not tolerated due to relevant side effects; in such cases, neurogenic detrusor overactivity (NDO) may be treated with intravesical injections of botulinum toxin type A (BoNT-A). BoNT-A has been approved for the treatment of NDO and OAB in adults, while its use in children is still off-label, despite the large number of studies showing positive results with minimal side effects in the paediatric population.

Material and Technique of Injection

Botulinum toxin (BoNT) is a potent neurotoxin synthesized by the Gram-positive bacterium *Clostridium botulinum*. There are seven immunologically distinct serotypes from type A to type G; the most commonly used type in intravesical therapy is serotype A, which is manufactured in two different commercial forms: onabotulinumtoxin A (ona-BoNT-A) (Botox®; Allergan Ltd., Irvine, CA, USA) and abobotulinumtoxinA (aboBoNT-A) (Dysport®, Ipsen Ltd., Slough, UK). These products, despite sharing similarities, are different drugs, with different molecular characteristics and dosage, and they must not be considered equivalents. Botox is injected using a cystoscope and a flexible needle; we prefer using an offset lens cystoscope with a straight working channel that makes insertion of the flexible plastic needle easier. Most authors, including us, use 10 units/Kg of body weight up to a maximum of 300 units of Botox, diluted in 30 mL of normal saline, which are injected all over the detrusor muscle, avoiding the trigone, for a total of 20–30 injections of 1 mL each.

Results and Discussion

The results of Botox injections for OAD in approximately 700 children starting from 2002 are reported in the literature, and most relevant data about the increase in maximum bladder capacity and compliance and reduction in maximum detrusor pressure are summarized in Table 45.2 (data and bibliography from a review by J.K. Badawi [17]). The effects of the injection last generally about 6 months and they can be repeated, but sometimes subsequent injections showed reduced efficacy and the interval between injections is shortened. There is a general agreement that the efficacy of Botox injections is maximal in overactive bladders, while they are ineffective in fibrotic bladders and extremely low compliance bladders; therefore, in both categories repeated injections are useless. Continence between catheterizations has been achieved in a percentage of patients varying from 45% to 88%. Greer et al. [18] have reported their experience with contemporary intradetrusorial and intrasphincteric injections of BTA with >90% reduction in urinary symptoms. Recently, Kajibafzadeh et al. [19] have proposed to deliver Botox to the bladder using electromotive drug administration (EMDA) with satisfactory results not only on detrusor overactivity, but also on bowel motility. EMDA is a combination of iontophoresis, electrophoresis and electroporation, applying an electrical current created between two electrodes, where the drug is uniformly delivered to the bladder wall. Experimental studies have shown a more diffuse and uniform distribution of Botox throughout the layers of the bladder as compared to the more heterogeneous distribution of the drug after injections. Clinically, an average 116% increase in MBC and 48% decrease in MDP were obtained, while incontinence improved in 80% of patients. The main disadvantage of Botox injections is the limited life span of their action, from 6 to 10 months on average, and, therefore, the need to repeat injections to lower bladder pressure; furthermore, they are inactive in fibrotic bladders.

A permanent method to decrease detrusor pressure and overactivity is to augment the bladder using detubularized bowel.

45.3.1.2 Bladder Augmentation and Appendicovesicostomy

Bladder augmentation can be performed with either the ileum or caecum or colon and generally causes an increase in bladder volume with a

Table 45.2 Review of the results of botulinum toxin A injection in the detrusor muscle to treat hyperactivity

Authors and year	MBC	MDP	Compliance	Duration of effect	No. of treatments	Continence
Schulte-Baukloh H et al. 2002	+27%		+45%			
Schulte-Baukloh et al. 2003	+35%	−40%		6 months		
Lusuardi et al. 2004	+118%	−45%	+183%			46%
Kajibafzadeh et al. 2006	+162%	−40%				88%
Altaweel et al. 2006	+56%	−48%	+156%	8.1 months	4	65%
Schulte-Baukloh et al. 2005	+72%	−39%	+109%	6 months	3–5	
Neel et al. 2008	+96%	−32%				83%
Horst et al. 2011	+33%	−17%				
La Nuè et al. 2012	+38%	−50%			3	
Khan et al. 2016	+46%	−43%	+104%	4.6 months	>2	45%

Data and bibliography modified from a review by J. K Badawi [17]
Abbreviations: *MBC* maximum bladder capacity, *MDP* maximum bladder pressure

reduction of storage pressure and detrusor overactivity. Its main disadvantage is the resulting voiding inefficiency that, in most patients, requires CIC to empty the bladder, but because most children with neurogenic bladder are already using CIC, bladder augmentation does not cause more assistance burden to both patients and caregivers.

Ileocystoplasty and Continent Catheterizable Channel: Robotic-Assisted Technique (RALIMA)

In recent years, bladder augmentation and appendicovesicostomy using either laparoscopy or a robotic-assisted procedure have been reported. The first case of complete laparoscopic intracorporeal paediatric ileocystoplasty was described in 2007, but the procedure did not gain much popularity due to the intrinsic difficulty of the technique. Robotic-assisted technology for urinary paediatric malformations has increased its role in the last years. The advantages over open surgery are improved cosmesis, limited blood loss, quicker recovery and less postoperative pain. When children with neurogenic bladders require bladder augmentation, robotic-assisted enterocystoplasty and appendicovesicostomy are, nowadays, a safe and feasible option. Despite the high cost, robotic-assisted laparoscopic procedures are well established in adult surgery and are becoming more and more popular in children, thanks to the 7 degrees of freedom of movement, three-dimensional vision, magnification and precision and, lastly, the availability of smaller instruments. In this section we report and describe the technique of robotic-assisted laparoscopic ileocystoplasty and Mitrofanoff appendicovesicostomy (RALIMA*) as it has been described and reported by Mohan Gundeti [20].

Preoperative Preparation

There are no specific precise selection criteria, but this approach is recommended for children aged over 6 years, with no previous major surgery and without severe kyphoscoliosis. In children with a ventriculoperitoneal shunt, a preoperative neurosurgical evaluation and protection of the shunt during the procedure are necessary. Bowel preparation is not mandatory. Antibiotic prophylaxis with cephalosporins and metronidazole and continuation of the therapy for at least 3 days are advisable. In older patients, prophylaxis of deep venous thrombosis is suggested.

Positioning

The patient is placed in a supine and 30° degrees Trendelenburg position, with legs in a low lithotomy position. Great care is observed in protecting all the pressure points with a silicone pillow. The robot is docked by bringing the surgical cart in between the legs of the patient, three arms are used, and the fourth is kept ready for eventual use. A bladder Foley catheter is placed in the sterile field, to be used for intraoperative inflation of the bladder and to test the ileocystoplasty at the end of the procedure. In addition, ureteric catheters may be used for easier identification of ureteric orifices.

Instrumentation

An optical 12-mm port is placed with an open technique in the umbilicus if the pubo-umbilical distance is equal or superior to 12 cm; otherwise, it is placed more cranially. Once the pneumoperitoneum (10–12 mmHg) is obtained, the other trocars are inserted: two 8-mm robotic trocars are inserted in the line of the camera port, 6 to 8 cm apart. A fourth 8-mm robotic port is placed in the left iliac fossa, on the anterior axillary line. These ports are sufficient for appendicovesicostomy, if ileocystoplasty is planned, an additional 12-mm assistant trocar is located in the right iliac fossa in the midclavicular line. Robotic instruments used are Prograsp forceps, needle and scissor; laparoscopic instruments used are suction device, Johannes forceps and LigaSure.

Surgical Technique

After exploration of the peritoneal cavity, the ileal loop that will be used to augment the bladder is identified; two stay sutures are inserted, 20 cm apart; the mesenteric length and mobility are tested; and the loop is isolated on its mesenteric pedicle. Bowel continuity is restored with an end-to-end anastomosis and the mesenteric window is closed. Then the appendix is isolated and separated from the caecum, and the caecal wall is closed in layers. The appendiceal mesentery is carefully isolated to obtain a sufficient length to reach the bladder wall without tension. The bladder is distended and detrusorotomy is performed along the right posterior wall to accommodate the appendix. The tip of the appendix is excised and spatulated, a small opening is created in the bladder mucosa, and an anastomosis between the appendix and the bladder is performed over an 8-Fr feeding tube. The detrusor is then imbricated over the appendix to create an anti-reflux tunnel.

The bladder is amply bivalved in the coronal plane to adapt to the detubularized ileal loop. The ileal loop is opened along its anti-mesenteric margin and the proximal and distal ends are sutured to the lateral apices of the cystotomy. Then the two long edges of the ileal loop are sutured to the margins of the cystotomy. Last, the caecal end of the appendix is passed through the abdominal wall and a cutaneous stoma is created. The new bladder is drained with a urethral and suprapubic catheter and another catheter is placed in the appendicovesicostomy. The size of the catheters must be appropriate to drain the abundant amount of mucus that is produced by the ileal loop, especially in the first postoperative period.

Postoperative Care

Patients are usually kept on antibiotic therapy for 3 days, and analgesia is performed using epidural catheter for 1–3 days; then paracetamol is used for 2–3 days after epidural catheter removal and feeding usually stars 2 days after surgery. The urethral catheter is removed after 5–7 days and patients can be discharged thereafter. The suprapubic catheter is used to cycle the bladder starting from the third postoperative week, and if there are no leaks or complications, patients can start to catheterize through the appendicovesicostomy after 4 weeks postoperatively.

Results

A total of 17 paediatric patients undergoing robotic-assisted laparoscopic ileocystoplasty (RALI) were reported in 2015 [21]. Overall, 15 underwent successful RALI, 11 also had appendicovesicostomy, six had antegrade colonic enema channel, and four had concomitant bladder neck closure. This group was compared with a similar group of 13 patients undergoing open ileocystoplasty. The median operative time was significantly longer for RALI (623 vs. 287), but they had a shorter median hospital stay (6 vs. 8). All other parameters – increase in bladder capacity, use of narcotic and complications – were similar.

45.3.2 Procedures on the Urethral Sphincter and Bladder Neck

Urinary incontinence may be secondary to a deficiency in the bladder outlet resistance alone or coupled with a low-compliance, overactive bladder. Sphincter insufficiency can be defined as a detrusor leak point pressure less than 25 cmH_2O or urinary leakage in the absence of a detrusor contraction. Many different operations have been devised for treating bladder outlet insufficiency: injection of bulking agents in the bladder neck; closure of the bladder neck; bladder neck reconfiguration such as the Young–Dees, Mitchell, Kropp or Pippi Salle procedures; and bladder neck and proximal urethra external compression using various types of slings or an artificial sphincter. The use of minimally invasive procedures to perform some of these procedures has been described in recent years. The less invasive procedure is injection of bulking agents in the submucosal layer of the proximal urethra and bladder neck.

45.3.2.1 Endoscopic Injection of Bulking Agents in the Bladder Neck and Proximal Urethra

This procedure was reported in 1982 by Politano [22] who was the first to inject a Polytef paste into the urethra to treat female incontinence, but as pointed out in the section on VUR, Teflon was later abandoned because of the risk of particle migration. The theory behind the use of bulking agents in the urethra depends on the concept that the urothelium lining the bladder neck and the urethra normally coapts and seals the lumen of the urethra contributing to maintain continence. When the walls of the bladder neck and proximal urethra are separated, this mechanism is ineffective; thus, injecting a bulking substance in the suburothelial space that elevates the urothelium and allows a better sealing of the urethral lumen may help re-establish contine.

Instruments and Injection Technique

Three methods to deliver the bulking substance are available: transurethral, using a cystoscope; periurethral, used only in females; and antegrade through a suprapubic cystotomy. The most commonly employed method is the transurethral route that is used in both sexes, via a cystoscope with a working channel of adequate size, at least 5 Fr, to accommodate the needle and a 0° or 6° lens; we prefer using a cystoscope with offset lens and a straight channel. In adult women, the bulking agent can be injected periurethrally with a needle inserted lateral to the urethral meatus and, under cystoscopic guidance, advanced to the proposed site for the injection.

In case of a very scarred bladder neck and a tortuous urethra, the substance can be delivered in an antegrade fashion via a suprapubic cystotomy. A second cystoscope placed in the urethra may help in choosing the appropriate place for delivery The injection must be performed very carefully, in the right position and in the right plane – submucosa – which may not be easy, especially in a reconfigured bladder neck, where scars and submucosal fibrosis may impede the creation of a coapting mound. Injections should be carried out at 4 and 8 o'clock positions at the level of the bladder neck, and the amount delivered should be sufficient to approximate the walls of the urethra. In males, it is essential to inject well above the veru montanum to prevent future epididymitis and retrograde ejaculations. In girls, we inject in the proximal third of the urethra including the bladder neck. In both sexes, it is advisable to avoid any instrumentation or catheterization of the urethra after injection, to avoid dislodgment or carving of the mound. In patients using CIC, it is wise to leave a suprapubic catheter for 2 or 3 weeks before starting regular catheterization.

Results

Reported results are variable in terms of success in treating incontinence; they are generally worse in neurogenic bladders than in the epispadias–exstrophy complex and in males in comparison to females. The use of bulking agents to achieve continence is reported either as a primary procedure or as a salvage procedure after a nonsuccessful surgical intervention like a sling or bladder neck reconfiguration, and in both groups, results are similar. Wan et al. [23] in 1992 reported very promising results using cross-linked collagen, after an average of 2.1 injections in eight children. After 13 months, 63% of patients were continent and 25% has shown improvement in their condition; after 4 years, continence persisted in 22% of cases. Worse results were reported by Kassouf [24] et al. in 2001, with only a 5% continence rate after an average of two injections. Using Macroplastique®, Guys et al. [25] reported that 33% of patients were continent and an additional 14% showed improvement after 6 years of follow-up; initial results deteriorated in the first 18 months after injection, but remained stable thereafter. Halachmi et al. [26] found Macroplastique® injections ineffective in the treatment of urethral incontinence. They had no complete success and only 42% improvement in continence. More favourable results have been reported by Lottman et al. [27] using Dx-Ha injections in children whose incontinence was secondary to neurogenic bladder or bladder–exstrophy complex. One month after the procedure, 73% of 33 children were dry or improved; this percentage decreased to 43% at 3 years and thereafter remained stable. Results were comparable in the two groups of patients. No significant difference in using either Teflon or De/Ha as the injectable substance to treat incontinence was found by Dyer et al. [28] After Teflon injection, 5% of cases were continent, and after De/Ha, the success rate was 14%, and an additional 14% showed improvement on their conditions. Similar results were reported by Godbole in 2002 [29], using collagen, Macroplastique or Teflon. Three out of 15 children (20%) were dry at a median follow-up period of 28 months, two after PTFE and one after collagen. Eight patients had some improvement, but later deteriorated to their original incontinence status.

We can conclude that endoscopic treatment of urinary incontinence has a very limited success; the great majority of patients deteriorating some months after treatment, because of various reasons, including reabsorption or displacement of the bulking substance or changes in detrusor compliance and activity. Therefore, more dependable procedures to make children continent should be employed, like bladder neck sling, bladder neck reconfiguration and artificial sphincter. Bladder neck slings and artificial urinary sphincter (AUS) increase urethral resistance exertion and external pressure, which is fixed in case of slings and variable in case of AUS. Despite an extensive experience with these procedures and their various combinations, there is not yet a general consensus on the best way to treat urinary incontinence secondary to sphincter insufficiency in children with neurogenic bladder. All these procedures have been carried out, recently, using minimally invasive techniques.

45.3.2.2 Artificial Urethral Sphincter (AUS)

An artificial urethral sphincter has the great advantage over slings and over most bladder neck reconfigurations by allowing spontaneous micturition in those patients who, preoperatively, were able to void without the aid of CIC. In a meta-analysis on 585 paediatric patients, volitional voiding occurred in 32% of cases, but this percentage tends to reduce with time. AUS can provide continence in the paediatric population in about 73% of cases, but, unfortunately, with a high rate of mechanical complications (53%) and the need for surgical revision (24%) or removal (23%) of the device [30]. The first case of robotic-assisted implantation of AUS (RALS-AUS) was reported in 2017 by Moscardi et al. [31] in a 6-year-old girl affected by neurogenic bladder and sphincter insufficiency.

Method and Surgical Technique

The procedure starts with port placement: first, an 8-mm camera port is placed a few millimetres above the umbilicus and the two additional 8-mm working ports are inserted 4 cm laterally at the umbilical level. Another assistant port is placed between the camera and the right port. The peritoneum is incised between the posterior bladder wall and the anterior vaginal wall, and dissection is carried out to reach the bladder neck. Next, the anterior aspect of the bladder is prepared as far as the anterior aspect of the bladder neck, the endopelvic fascia is incised on both sides of the urethra, the bladder neck is completely isolated, and after measurement of the length of the circumference, the cuff is inserted. The pressure-regulating balloon is inserted lateral to the bladder, and after closure of the peritoneum, through a small inguinal incision, the pump is positioned in the labia majora, or in the scrotum in males, and then deactivated for a 6- to 8-week period.

The RALS-AUS technique is similar to the open procedure, but offers the advantage of better visualization of the retrovesical space and a more accurate dissection and visualization of planes, especially in case of patients who had undergone multiple previous operations in the area.

45.3.2.3 Periurethral Slings

Bladder neck slings are a frequently used method, mainly in the treatment of female urinary incontinence. The original procedure consists in passing an isolated strip of rectus fascia between the bladder neck and anterior vaginal wall and re-attaching it to the anterior abdominal wall, thereby compressing and suspending the bladder neck. This procedure has become very popular in the adult female population affected by stress incontinence and, with time, has undergone many variations regarding both the material and the method of insertion. Slings have also been used in children, in particular in adolescent girls with neurogenic incontinence on intermittent catheterization. In this population, the success rate has been reported to be as high as 78% to 90%, but a lower success rate has been recorded in males. Sling placement is often associated with other procedures on the bladder neck, appendicovesicostomy and bladder augmentation; thus, it is difficult to evaluate the success rate of isolated sling placement. Snodgrass [32] has reported a 45% success rate with slings alone, compared to 82% continence rate when the sling was associated with bladder neck reconfiguration. The most common complications of bladder neck slings are erosion of the sling, which is more frequent when exogenous material was used and in patients with progressive deterioration of the bladder compliance and difficult bladder catheterization because of urethral angulation. In adult women, laparoscopic placement of periurethral slings has been reported very frequently, but this procedure has not become popular in children, probably because of the limited space in the abdomen and pelvis of children and adolescents affected by a myelomeningocele. Recently, few reports of robotically assisted placement of periurethral slings have been published. Storm et al. in 2008 [33] described a successful robotic-assisted laparoscopic approach for posterior bladder neck dissection and placement of a bladder neck sling in two paediatric patients.

45.3.2.4 Bladder Neck Reconfiguration

Bagrodia and Gargollo [34] reported about the first series of four paediatric patients affected by neurogenic incontinence who underwent robotic-assisted laparoscopic bladder neck reconfiguration, appendicovesicostomy and bladder neck sling placement.

Procedure and Surgical Technique

The procedure started with the development of the plane between the posterior bladder wall and anterior vaginal wall, and then the Retzius space was prepared. Further, a Leadbetter–Mitchell procedure was carried out, reconfiguring the urethra and bladder neck around a 5-Fr catheter; the upper limit of reconfiguration was the interureteric bar, and no ureteral reimplantation was necessary. Then the fascial sling was wrapped around the new bladder neck and suspended to the posterior pubic bone. Last, the appendix was harvested from the caecum and an appendicovesicostomy was created, placing the appendix in a trough created on the posterior wall of the bladder that was then closed around the appendix. The cutaneous stoma of the appendicovesicostomy was created at the umbilical level. In this first series of four patients, one required conversion and all patients achieved continence. In 2015, the same authors reported on a larger series of 38 patients who underwent the same procedures; conversion rate was 11% and continence was achieved in 82% of patients. Gundeti et al. [35] in 2016 published a multi-institutional series of 80 patients, of whom 31 underwent RALS-appendicovesicostomy only and 34 had additional bladder neck reconfiguration, with 15 also receiving bladder augmentation. The overall continence rate was 85.2% which raised up to 92% after additional surgery. The complication rate after RALS for neurogenic incontinence seems to be comparable with that reported after open surgery.

45.4 Conclusions

Minimally invasive procedures, both endoscopic and laparoscopic, have an increased role in the treatment of the most significant aspects of neurogenic bladder in children. Endoscopic treatment of VUR has given reliable and long-lasting results, while endoscopic treatment of incontinence is less satisfactory. Laparoscopic and, more recently, robotic-assisted procedures for complex reconstructions are promising, but technically demanding, and their use is not so popular due to the high cost of robotic-assisted procedures and their intrinsic difficulty. The advantages of using robotic-assisted procedures in the treatment of neurogenic bladders are not yet so evident as they are for other procedures like pyeloplasty.

References

1. Seki N, Akazawa K, Semoh K, et al. An analysis of risk factors for upper urinary tract. BJU Int. 1999;84:689.
2. Kass EJ, Koff SA. Diokno AC fate of vesicoureteral reflux in children with neuropathic bladders managed by intermittent catheterization. J Urol. 1981;125:63.
3. O'Donnell B, Puri P. Endoscopic correction of primary vesicoureteral reflux. Br J Urol. 1986;58:601.
4. Cerwinka WH, Scherz HC, Kirsch AJ. Dynamic hydrodistention classification of the ureter and the double hit method to correct vesicoureteral reflux. Arch Esp Urol. 2008;61(8):882.
5. Caldamone A. Injection therapy for vesicoureteral reflux. In: Docimo SG, editor. The Kelalis-king-Belman textbook of clinical pediatric urology. 6th ed. Boca Raton: CRC Press; 2017.
6. Charlotte QW, Franco I. Management of vesicoureteral reflux in neurogenic bladder. Investig Clin Urol. 2017;58(Suppl 1):554.
7. Yokoyama O, Ishiura Y, Seto C, et al. Endoscopic treatment of vesicoureteral reflux in patients with myelodysplasia. J Urol. 1996;155:1882.
8. Haferkamp A, Möhring K, Staehler G, et al. Long term efficacy of subureteral collagen injection for endoscopic treatment of vesicoureteral reflux in neurogenic bladder cases. J Urol. 2000;163:274.
9. Quinn FM, Diamond D, Boston VE. Endoscopic management of vesico-ureteric reflux in children with neuropathic bladder secondary to myelomeningocele. Z Kinderchir. 1988;43(Suppl 2):43.
10. Puri P, Guiney EG. Endoscopic correction of vesicoureteric reflux secondary to neuropathic bladder. Br J Urol. 1986;58:504.
11. Misra D, Potts SR, Brown S, Boston VE. Endoscopic treatment of vesico-ureteric reflux in neurogenic bladder. J Pediatr Surg. 1996;31:1262.
12. Perez-Brayfield M, Kirsch AJ, Hensle T, et al. Endoscopic treatment with dextranomer-hyaluronic acid for complex cases of vesicoureteral reflux. J Urol. 2004;172:1614.
13. Granata C, Buffa P, Di Rovasenda E, et al. Treatment of vesico-ureteric reflux in children with neuropathic bladder: a comparison of surgical and endoscopic correction. J Pediatr Surg. 1999;34:1836.
14. Engel JD, Palmer LS, Cheng EY, et al. Endoscopic correction of vesicoureteral reflux in children with neurogenic bladder dysfunction. J Urol. 1997;157:2291.
15. Mosiello G, Salsano M, Pascali M, et al. A minimally invasive approach in the treatment of vesicoureteral reflux in neurogenic bladder in children. Eur Urol. 2009;55:253.
16. Neel KF, Salem M, Soliman S. Total endoscopic management (TEM approach) of children with non compliant neuropathic bladder: a preliminary report. J Pediatr Urol. 2007;4:124.
17. Badawi JK. Botulinum toxin therapy in children with neurogenic detrusor overactivity *Turk*. J Urol. 2020;46:2.
18. Greer T, Abbot J, Breytenbach W, et al. Ten years of experience with intravesical and intrasphincteric onabotulinumtoxin a in children. J Pediatr Urol. 2016;12:94.
19. Kajbafzadeh AM, Ahmadi H, Montaser-Kouhsari I, et al. Intravesical electromotive botulinum toxin type a administration part II-clinical application. Urology. 2011;77:439.
20. Gundeti M, Acharia S, Zagaja G, et al. Paediatric robotic-assisted laparoscopic augmentation ileocystoplasty and Mitrofanoff appendicovesicostomy (RALIMA): feasibility od and initial experience with the University of Chicago technique. BJU Int. 2010;107:962.
21. Murthy P, Cohn J, Selig R, et al. Robot-assisted laparoscopic augmentation ileocystoplasty and Mitrofanoff appendicovesicostomy in children: updated interim report. Eur Urol. 2015;68:1069.
22. Politano VA. Periurethral Polytetrafluoroethylene injection for urinary incontinnece. J Urol. 1982;127:439.
23. Wan J, McGuire E, Bloom D, et al. The treatment of urinary incontinence in children using glutaraldehyde cross-linked collagen. J Urol. 1992;48:127.
24. Kassouf W, Capolicchio G, Berardinucci G, et al. Collagen injection for treatment of urinary incontinence in children. J Urol. 2001;165:1666.
25. Guys JM, Breaud J, Hery G, et al. Endoscopic injection with polydimethylsiloxane for treatment of pediatric urinary incontinence in the neurogenic bladder: long term results. J Urol. 2006;175:1106.
26. Halachimi S, Farhat W, Metcalfe P, et al. Efficacy of Polydimethylsiloxane injections to the bladder neck and leaking diverting stoma for urinary continence. J Urol. 2004;171:1287.
27. Lottman HB, Margaryan M, Bernuy M, et al. The effect of endoscopic injections of dextranomer based implants on continence and bladder capacity: a prospective study of 31 patients. J Urol. 2002;168:1863.
28. Dyer L, Franco I, Firlit C, et al. Endoscopic injection of bulking agents in children with incontinence: dextranomer/hyaluronic acid copolymer versus polytetrafluoroethylene. J Urol. 2007;178:1628.
29. Godbole P, Bryant R, Mackinnon AE, et al. Endourethral injection of bulking agents for urinary incontinence in children. BJU Int. 2003; 91:536.
30. Herndon C, Rink R, Shaw M. The Indiana experience with artificial urinary sphincters in children and young adults. J Urol. 2003;169:650.
31. Moscardi P, Ballesteros N, Abd-El-Barr A-E-R, et al. Robotic assisted laparoscopic artificial urinary sphincter and MACE procedure on a pediatric patient. J Pediatr Urol. 2017;13:527.

32. Snodgrass W, Barber T. Comparison of bladder outlet procedures without augmentation in children with neurogenic incontinence. J Urol. 2010;184:1775.
33. Storm DW, Fulmer BR, Sumfest JM. Robotic-assisted laparoscopic approach for posterior bladder neck dissection and placement of pediatric bladder neck sling: initial experience. Urology. 2008;75:1149.
34. Bagrodia A, Gargollo P. Robot-assisted bladder neck reconstruction, bladder neck sling and appendicovesicostomy in children: description of technique and initial results. J Endourol. 2011;8:1299.
35. Gundeti MS, Petravick ME, Pariser JJ, et al. A multi-institutional study of perioperative and functional outcomes for pediatric robot-assisted laparoscopic Mitrofanoff appendicovesicostomy. J Pediatr Urol. 2016;12:386.

Robotic Mitrofanoff Procedure

46

Alexander M. Turner, Salahuddin Syed, and Ramnath Subramaniam

Learning Objectives

- The role of the Mitrofanoff procedure in neuropathic bladder.
- Advantages of the robotic approach.

46.1 Introduction

Patients with neuropathic or non-neuropathic neuropathic bladders may, through bladder and/or sphincter dysfunction, suffer from upper tract compromise and incontinence. One common pattern occurs as a result of high pressure and infection from a poorly compliant, low-capacity bladder, with the kidneys taking multiple 'hits', leading to progressive renal failure and the need for renal replacement therapy. Another pattern results from bladder failure, where the detrusor muscle no longer relaxes to fill and contracts to void, instead filling passively and without sensation, leading to overflow incontinence and infection from urinary stasis. Dysfunction of the bladder neck, along with other causes such as posterior urethral valves and prune belly syndrome, can lead to the same final common pathways described above. Elegant pathways exist to account for the myriad dilemmas resulting from complex bladder problems [1], but the principles stay the same. Keeping the bladder empty reduces the chance of infection and helps dysfunction, and protecting the upper tracts from injury is paramount. The incontinence produced by the poorly compliant bladder is inconvenient but aids the reduction of upper tract pressure, so this should never be the prime or only focus of treatment. Clean intermittent urethral catheterisation (CIC) has revolutionised the management of neuropathic bladders, but if this is not possible due to anatomy, such as the ectatic urethra in prune belly syndrome, or technically, such as when a baby grows to be a strong-willed toddler, or pain in the growing male, an alternative must be sought. The open Mitrofanoff procedure, performed via a Pfannenstiel incision, revolutionised the treatment of the neuropathic bladder [2]. The procedure is used widely, with or without bladder augmentation procedures, to aid drainage of the bladder with intermittent catheter access, reducing infection and mitigating the effects of both the high-pressure, poorly compli-

Supplementary Information The online version contains supplementary material available at [https://doi.org/10.1007/978-3-030-99280-4_46].

A. M. Turner (✉) · S. Syed · R. Subramaniam
Paediatric Urology Department, Leeds General Infirmary, Leeds, UK
e-mail: alexander.turner@nhs.net; salahuddin.syed@nhs.net; ramnath.subramaniam@nhs.net

C. Esposito et al. (eds.), *Minimally Invasive Techniques in Pediatric Urology*,
https://doi.org/10.1007/978-3-030-99280-4_46

ant bladders and those which do not empty due to detrusor failure. CIC alone may reduce the incontinence produced by dysfunctional bladders, and methods to deal with the bladder neck for ongoing incontinence are outside the scope of this chapter, but if these are considered, urethral CIC or via Mitrofanoff should be established prior to any surgery, as the risk of increasing upper tract pressure is significant [1]. Important to mention is the concept of detrusorotomy, or autoaugmentation, which is performed robotically at the same time as the Mitrofanoff by the author in selected cases. This describes the procedure where incision of the detrusor muscle allows the urothelium to bulge and offset intravesical pressure and, since its inception for the tuberculous bladder in 1953, has received mixed reviews and periods in and out of favour [3]. Post-operative stretching of the urothelium, either actively with balloons or passively with increasing duration of catheter clamping post-operatively, may encourage increase in bladder capacity and compliance, but fibrosis and shrinkage remain as risks. A mini-detrusorotomy is of course required in the Mitrofanoff procedure to wrap the appendix in the bladder wall to prevent reflux. The external appearance of the Mitrofanoff stoma has also changed over time, with a skin-lined tunnel in the right iliac fossa replacing the visible mucosal lining often seen at the umbilicus, improving cosmesis.

46.2 Robotic Mitrofanoff

The first advantage of the robotic approach to the appendiculovesicostomy is the ability to assess whether the procedure is going to be feasible without causing significant morbidity to the patient. Thereafter, the advantages are legion, with the dexterity, optics and temporal efficiencies afforded by the device to achieve a swift, cosmetically pleasing result and, in our experience, a much-reduced hospital stay.

46.3 Patient Positioning and Planning

The patient is placed on the operating table in a supine position. The Trendelenburg position may be adopted to reduce small bowel interference in the field of view. The operative field is prepared from the nipples to the thighs, including the perineum, and drapes are applied. Once the area is sterile, a Foley catheter is placed transurethrally into the bladder with a bladder syringe attached, to allow intraoperative filling. Intraoperative analgesia can be achieved with epidural, TAP or local anaesthetic means, dependent upon local protocol.

46.4 Incision and Port Placement

In order to adequately visualise the pelvis and right iliac fossa, the camera port should be placed through an incision in a midline plane at a point between the umbilicus and xiphisternum (Fig. 46.1). Factors affecting this position include the patient's size and body habitus, but in children, our site of choice is in the epigastrium, as shown. The port is placed under direct vision, and insufflation is achieved with appropriate flow rate and pressure. The camera can then be inserted to

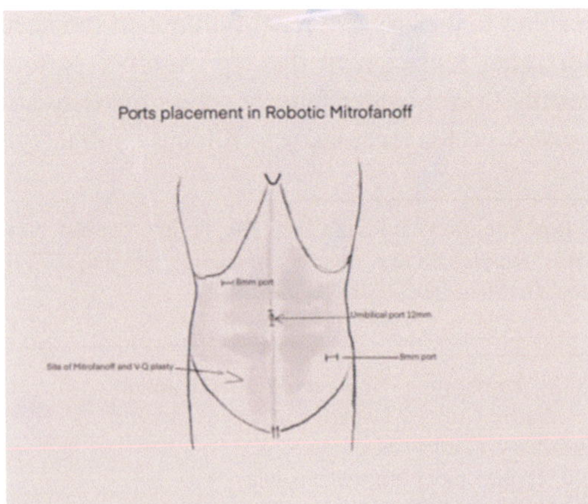

Fig. 46.1 Port placement

assess the anatomy. Should the procedure continue, the two working robotic ports should be placed as shown in the hypochondriac/lumbar regions to triangulate about the bladder/right iliac fossa.

A 5-mm accessory port is placed at the site of the mouth of the Mitrofanoff stoma, which is directly superficial to the base of the appendix and at the linea semilunaris. Through this port, disposable graspers can stabilise the caecum and appendix during the procedure.

Note: An absent, short or difficult appendix position, combined with very contracted bladder, may lead to abandonment of the MIS procedure, and this can be assessed by direct vision or with a grasper via an additional port (usually the accessory port). Remember to allow for the distension of the insufflated abdomen when assessing appendix adequacy.

46.5 Robot Positioning

This procedure requires an extreme side-docking position (Fig. 46.2). In adult patients for pelvic procedures, the robot can be often placed between the legs in lithotomy position, but this is near universally impossible in children. The cart should be advanced at a 5- to 10-degree angle to the operating table to the right of the patient, so the arms point backwards towards the pelvis, triangulating towards a position midway between the bladder and right iliac fossa.

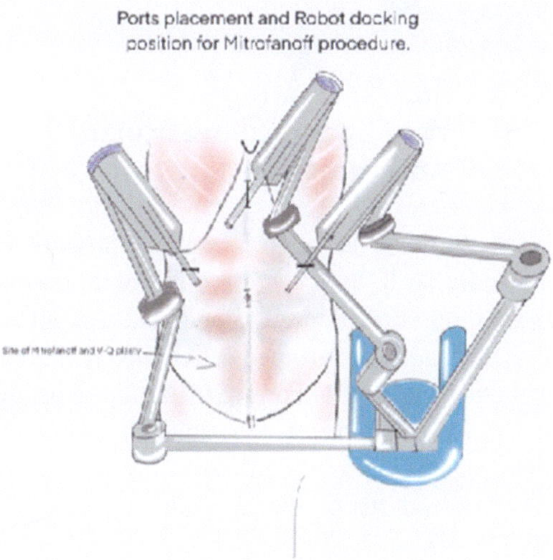

Fig. 46.2 Extreme side dock robot position

46.6 Robotic Mitrofanoff Procedure Steps

46.6.1 Step 1: Prepare the Appendix

With the assistant stabilising the caecum, the appendix mesentery is approached and dissected in a plane close to the caecum. Some small vessels here may need to be sacrificed, given adequate branching onto the appendix, to allow for mobilisation. Dissection proximally towards the root of the mesentery and skeletonisation of the mesenteric vessels may be required to achieve additional mobilisation of the appendix towards the bladder.

A 3/0 PDS suture is delivered to the abdomen to transfix the base of the appendix, leaving a good length of suture when cutting. The appendix base is then divided. A 2/0 PDS endoloop device is then passed through the accessory port, with the robotic forceps passing through the loop to pick up the long ends of the transfixion suture. The endoloop can then be snugged down onto the caecum at the appendix base, proximal to the transfixion, while the caecum is lifted carefully (Fig. 46.3). All sutures can be trimmed to length once the defect in the caecum is secure.

The assistant then grasps the open end of the appendix with the locking ratchet engaged. As the appendix enters the port, the port should be slid over the grasper so that the appendix is delivered to the skin surface. This is one of the more challenging parts of the procedure and preparation with an experienced assistant is vital to ensure everyone knows what is to be done. Release of the pneumoperitoneum may

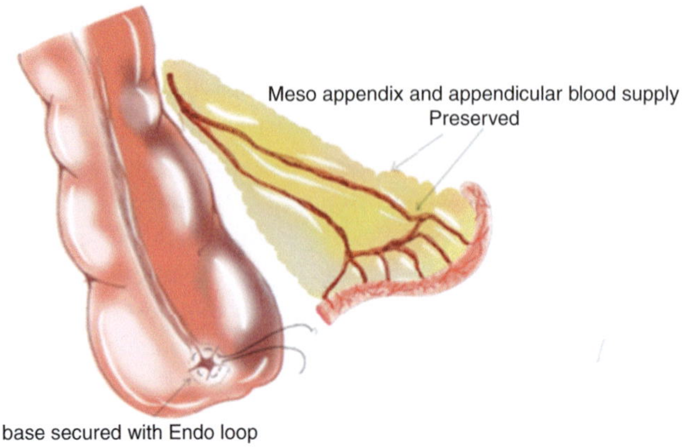

Fig. 46.3 Isolation of the appendix on its mesentery

be required for this step. Once the appendix appears at the skin, the assistant passes a suture through it to stop it from passing back inside the abdomen. At this stage, the appendix can be flushed with saline to remove debris, so that the effluent is safely removed away from the wound.

46.6.2 Step 2: Prepare the Bladder

Using plasmakinetic forceps or bipolar scissors, the peritoneum overlying the superior third of the bladder is opened. Extracorporeal stay sutures (e.g., 3/0 Prolene) can be used to hitch the bladder forward to reveal the posterior surface of the bladder. To ease dissection, the bladder can be partially filled with saline. The dissection plane is scored onto the bladder to mark its direction. Bear in mind the position of the appendix and bladder without stay sutures and insufflation, to remove the possibility of a kink; the path from the skin to the bladder must lie in a direct line.

A detrusorotomy is performed so that the urothelium bulges and the cut edges should be undermined to widen it. The detrusorotomy should be of an appropriate length to ensure a good detrusor tunnel and wide enough to easily wrap around the appendix, typically at least 2 cm long and 1 cm wide. Care must be taken not to breach the urothelium and any such injury should be repaired with 6/0 PDS suture.

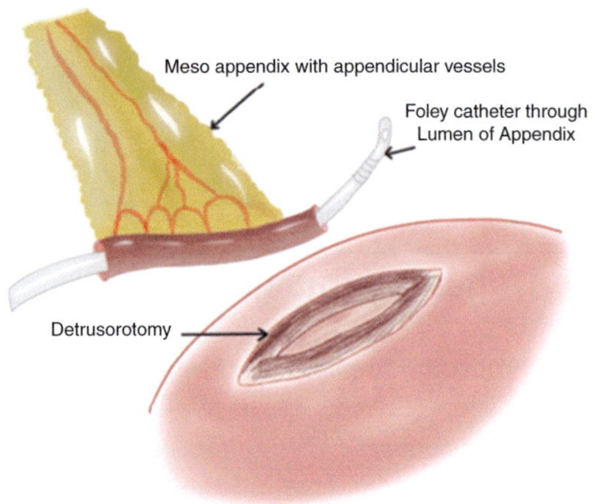

Fig. 46.4 Preparation of the appendix and detrusorotomy

46.6.3 Step 3: Creating the Appendiculovesicular Anastomosis

A Ch12 Foley catheter is passed through the appendix so it stretches the blind end and diathermy scissors are used to open the end, allowing the catheter to emerge. At this point, the catheter should be withdrawn to the mid-appendix position. The open end of the appendix is brought to the distal end of the detrusorotomy and the orientation and lie of the appendix are assessed (Fig. 46.4).

A 5/0 PDS suture is passed through the full-thickness inferior leaflet of the appendix and

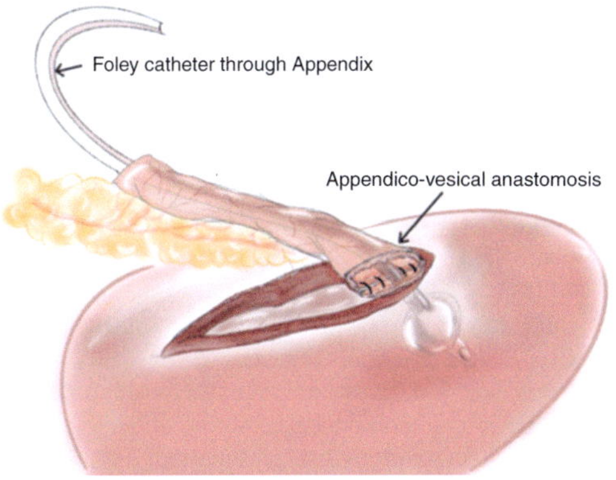

Fig. 46.5 Catheter placement in the bladder

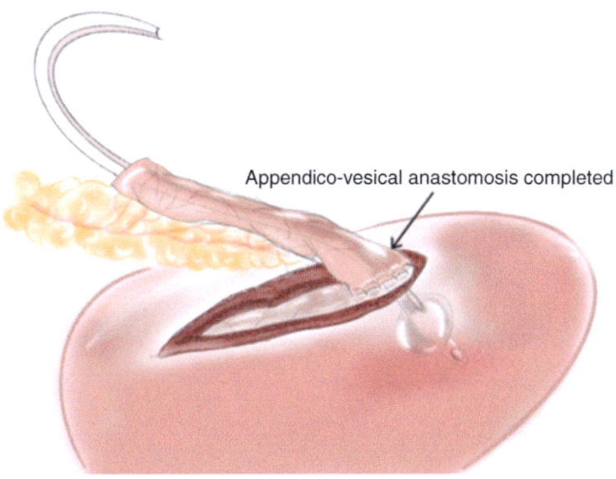

Fig. 46.6 Appendiculovesicular anastomosis

anastomosed to the urothelium. Two to three more sutures are placed along the infero-lateral side to secure half the appendix.

The urothelium is opened with a small incision and the assistant immediately advances the catheter into the bladder, filling the balloon (Fig. 46.5).

The anastomosis to the superomedial appendix is completed (Fig. 46.6). A 5/0 PDS is used to join the detrusor edges over the appendix, including the wall of the appendix for two sutures, to prevent shearing. The wrap should comfortably accept the appendix with the catheter within. The urethral catheter can now be placed on free drainage (Fig. 46.7).

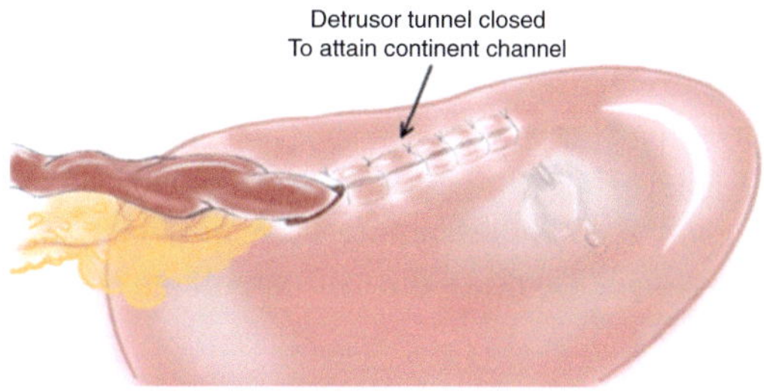

Fig. 46.7 Detrusor wrap

46.6.4 Step 4: Final Intra-Abdominal Steps

The peritoneum is closed around the appendix with 5/0 PDS and any fluid spillage in the pelvis can be aspirated via one of the working robotic ports. The undocking procedure can then take place and the three robotic port sites closed with sutures of choice.

46.6.5 Step 5: Creating the Skin-Lined Appendiculocutaneous Anastomosis

The loss of pneumoperitoneum allows for a tension-free anastomosis. At the site of the accessory port, the skin is marked to perform a VQ plasty as previously described [4]. The skin 'V' flap is laid into a spatulation of the appendix and anastomosed with 5/0 PDS to prevent stricture. The Q flap is raised and inverted to reach over the mouth of the stoma and the superior free edge of the appendix is sutured to the inverted medial free edge of the flap. The skin is then fashioned to close the wound to cover the flap.

46.7 Post-Operative Actions

The patient can eat and drink when they feel well enough to do so. The urethral catheter can be removed on the first post-operative day, with the Mitrofanoff catheter remaining on free drainage for 6 weeks. If combined with an autoaugmentation procedure, clamping of this catheter should take place to allow the bladder to stretch, according to local protocols.

The patient is normally well enough to go home the day after surgery. After 6 weeks, CIC can commence down the Mitrofanoff channel.

46.8 Conclusion

The robotic Mitrofanoff procedure is relatively new and outcome data are minimal. Complications regarding stenosis at the stoma still exist but have improved and are less of a function of the robotic approach and more of the improved appendiculo-cutaneous anastomosis. Functional complications are also similar in nature and frequency to the open techniques, but the benefit lies predominantly in the much reduced operative morbidity, faster recovery times and cosmesis, when performed by experienced robotic surgeons [5].

References

1. Stein R, Bogaert G, Dogan HS, Hoen L, Kocvara R, Nijman RJM, et al. EAU/ESPU guidelines on the management of neurogenic bladder in children and adolescent part II operative management. Neurourol Urodyn. 2020;39:498–506. https://doi.org/10.1002/nau.24248.
2. Mitrofanoff P. Trans-appendicular continent cystostomy in the management of the neurogenic bladder. Chir Pediatr. 1980;21:297–305.
3. González R, Ludwikowski BM. Alternatives to conventional enterocystoplasty in children: a critical review of urodynamic outcomes. Front Pediatr. 2013;1:1–9. https://doi.org/10.3389/fped.2013.00025.
4. England RJ, Subramaniam R. Functional and cosmetic outcome of the VQ Plasty for Mitrofanoff stomas. J Urol. 2007;178:2607–10. https://doi.org/10.1016/j.juro.2007.08.030.
5. Cohen A, Pariser J, Anderson B, Pearce S, Gundeti M. The robotic appendicovesicostomy and bladder augmentation: the next frontier in robotics, are we there? Urol Clin North Am. 2015;42:121–30.

Robotic Management of Bladder Stones in Children

47

Ciro Esposito, Maria Escolino, Fulvia Del Conte, Vincenzo Coppola, Mariapina Cerulo, Giuseppe Autorino, Felice Crocetto, and Alessandro Settimi

Learning Objectives

- To describe the step-by-step techniques of robotic management of BS.
- To present long-term outcomes of the robotic management of BS.
- To report the latest results of the major international papers about BS.
- To show a video with robotics management of BS.
- To describe tips and tricks in the management of BS and to show all the new technologies available in pediatric urology that can be adopted to treat BS.

47.1 Introduction

Urolithiasis in childhood is rare in the developed world, and BS represent 1% to 5% of all urinary tract stones [1, 2]. In developed countries, the main component of BS is struvite or calcium oxalate dihydrate, while in the developing countries the main component is ammonium acid urate [1]. In the last few decades, transurethral lithotripsy has become an alternative method to open cystolithotomy. However, this approach is restricted in children by the narrow caliber of the urethra in children. With increasing use of percutaneous techniques, an alternative solution to remove BS could be performing a percutaneous suprapubic bladder stone removal in children [3, 4]. Percutaneous cystolithotomy (PCCL) has been demonstrated to be adequate, safe, and rapid in managing vesical stones in children. In the recent years, in case of large BS, robotic surgery seems an excellent solution to safely remove BS [5, 6].

This chapter is focused on the operative technique of robotic-assisted bladder stone removal.

47.2 Preoperative Preparation

Preoperative examinations should focus on the anatomical malformations of the entire urinary tract and their functional implications. Investigations have to include ultrasonography and plain abdomen x-ray to measure the stone size. Rarely a computer tomography is indicated [3, 7].

Supplementary Information The online version contains supplementary material available at [https://doi.org/10.1007/978-3-030-99280-4_47].

C. Esposito (✉) · M. Escolino · F. Del Conte
V. Coppola · M. Cerulo · G. Autorino · A. Settimi
Pediatric Surgery Unit, Federico II University of Naples, Naples, Italy
e-mail: ciroespo@unina.it; maria.escolino@unina.it; fulvia.delconte@unina.it; vincenzocoppola1992@gmail.com; mariapina.cerulo@unina.it; autorino.giuseppe@gmail.com; settimi@unina.it

F. Crocetto
Urology Unit, Federico II University of Naples, Naples, Italy
e-mail: felice.crocetto@unina.it

C. Esposito et al. (eds.), *Minimally Invasive Techniques in Pediatric Urology*,
https://doi.org/10.1007/978-3-030-99280-4_47

Cystoscopy can be performed preoperatively. An intestinal preparation with simethicone, enema, and liquid diet is desirable especially in young children.

Preoperative antibiotic prophylaxis should be administered either with a broad-spectrum medication or according to the child's specific urine testing [5, 8].

All patients and their parents have to sign a specifically formulated informed consent before the procedure. Patients receive general anesthesia with orotracheal intubation and myorelaxation. A Foley catheter is positioned into the bladder using sterile precautions just before surgery and a nasogastric tube is placed in order to keep the stomach empty during the procedure [8, 9].

47.3 Positioning

In case of robotic bladder stone removal, the patient should be placed in a supine decubitus position, with the table in a 15° Trendelenburg position. This approach uses the gravity for the retraction of the intestinal loops. Two surgeons and a nurse start the procedure at the operative table; then after trocars and robot docking, the console surgeon moves to the console and the bedside surgeon remains at the operative table with the nurse (Fig. 47.1). The monitor for the bedside surgeon and the nurse is positioned at patient's feet. We always adopt three robotic trocars of 8 mm and a 5 mm for the bedside surgeon. The trocars are positioned in triangulation with the optic in order to achieve a better ergonomics (Fig. 47.2) [10, 11].

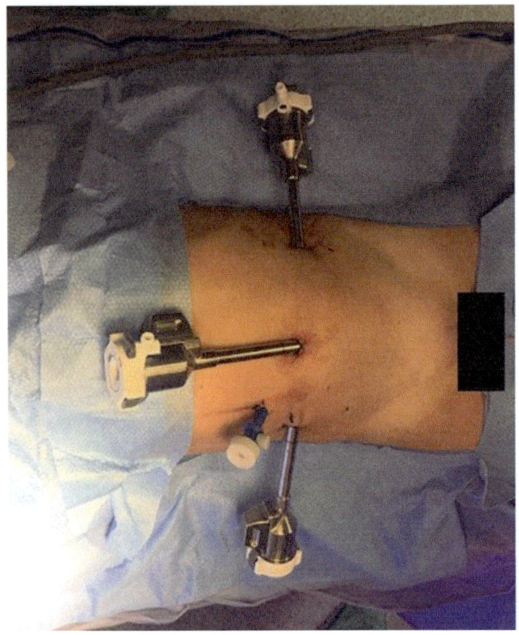

Fig. 47.2 Trocar positioning

Fig. 47.1 Team positioning

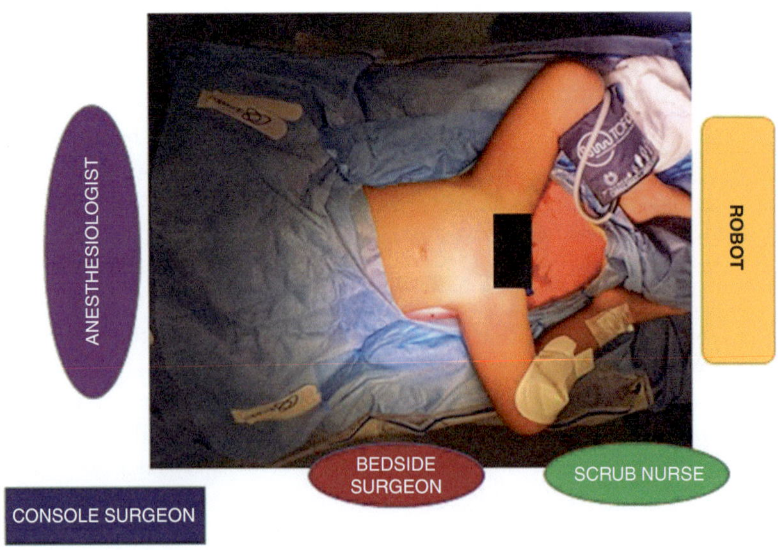

47.4 Instrumentation

Regarding the robotic procedure, we adopt an 8-mm 30-degree optic, two other robotic 8-mm instruments (needle holder, scissors, curve Maryland and fenestrated forceps). We also adopt a 5-mm trocar for the bedside surgeon to introduce and remove the needles, to cut the suture, and to expose or retract tissues. We adopt an endobag introduced into the abdomen through the umbilicus to remove the stones. In general, we leave an indwelling Foley catheter into the bladder for a couple of days. We also need a long straight needle at the beginning of the procedure to fix the bladder to the abdominal wall [12, 13].

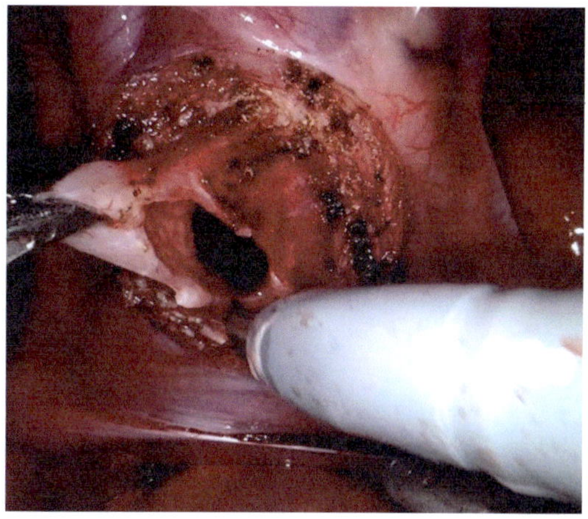

Fig. 47.4 Bladder opening

47.5 Technique

All the procedures are performed under general anesthesia with orotracheal intubation.

The technique is divided in two phases: cystoscopy and robotic surgery. Cystoscopy is performed as the first step of the procedure to check the bladder anatomy and the location of the stone [6, 8].

The patient is placed in the Trendelenburg position and the da Vinci robot is docked over the patient's feet.

Using a big straight needle and a 2/0 absorbable suture, two sutures may be placed to lift up the bladder to the abdominal wall and to enhance visualization of the posterior bladder wall (Fig. 47.3) [5, 14]. The bladder is filled with saline solution and a 2.5–3 cm detrusor incision is made longitudinally to the level of the mucosa for about 2 cm. The detrusor muscle is then separated from the mucosa laterally, the mucosa is opened longitudinally, and the bladder is opened (Fig. 47.4).

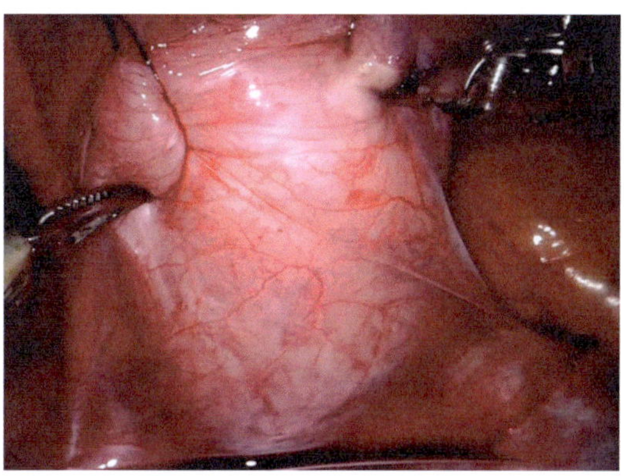

Fig. 47.3 Bladder suspension

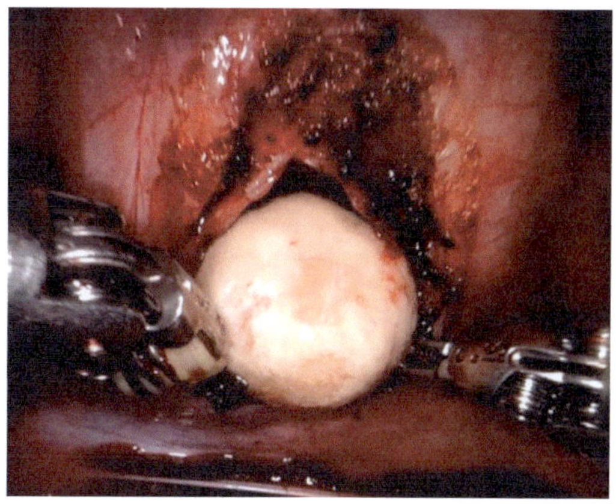

Fig. 47.5 Stone removal

The endobag is introduced into the abdomen through the navel and opened and positioned near the bladder. The big stone is retrieved using robotic instruments (Fig. 47.5) and then positioned into the endobag (Fig. 47.6) [14].

The bladder is closed in two layers: firstly, the mucosa and thereafter the detrusor muscle, both with a running 2-3/0 absorbable suture. At the end, the bladder is filled to check the quality of

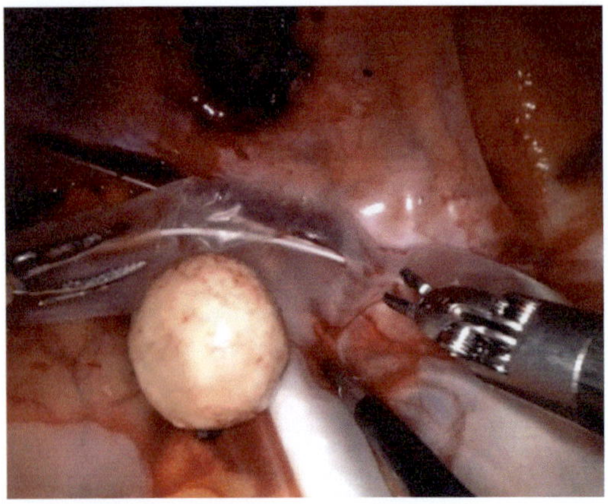

Fig. 47.6 Stone extraction through endobag

suture. The endobag containing the stone is finally removed thorough the navel.

The working ports are removed and the trocar's orifices are closed using separates stitches.

A bladder catheter is left in place postoperatively in all cases. No other drains are left after surgery [10, 14].

47.6 Postoperative Care

Patients start oral feeding a few hours postoperatively. Analgesic therapy is rarely necessary;

Paracetamol (dosage 15 mg/kg at an 8-h interval) is usually administered in the first 12–24 h postoperatively. A short-term antibiotic therapy is performed for 48–72 h postoperatively [5, 15]. Patients are discharged on 2^{nd}or third postoperative day (POD). Postoperative clinical controls are scheduled on 7th and 30th POD and thereafter annually [7, 8].

47.7 Results

The median duration of surgery in our experience is 60 min (range 40–85), including docking time. The indications for surgery include bladder stones larger than 15 mm, especially in boys whose narrow sized urethra restricts endoscopic removal of the stones [15, 16].

We had no complications in our series.

Stone-free rate was 100% in the postoperative period, and at 1 year all patients were observed to be stone-free on ultrasound and abdominal x-ray.

The composition of the removed stones was always analyzed after surgery, and the patients were referred for postoperative controls to the nephrologist for the long-term follow-up [8, 9].

Tips and Tricks

- Regarding the patient position, a 15° Trendelenburg position is a crucial point for the success of this procedure; in fact, using this patient's positioning, the intestinal loops slide down and you have an excellent exposure of the bladder [5, 14].
- It is important to fix the bladder to the abdominal wall using two big straight needles to have a good exposure of the bladder during the procedure.
- It is important to open the bladder longitudinally, firstly the detrusor muscle and then the mucosa for about 2 cm. It is also important to open the endobag under the bladder before removing the stone to avoid losing the stone or part of it in the abdominal cavity [14].
- It is also important to train the robotic team (surgeons and nurses) to reduce docking time.
- The role of bedside surgeon is crucial to introduce and remove needles, to cut sutures, and to help the surgeon during the procedure.
- We always prepare a laparoscopic kit in case of conversion from robotics to laparoscopy.

47.8 Discussion

Bladder stones in pediatric population is a rare pathology.

In analyzing the international literature, there are several techniques to treat BS using open cystolithotomy, endoscopic techniques, or, in the last few years, robotic surgery [13, 17].

In the last few decades, transurethral lithotripsy has become an alternative method to open cystolithotomy [12, 18]. However, this approach is restricted in children by the narrow caliber of the urethra. In fact, after the fragmentation of the stone, it is difficult to remove the stone's fragment through the urethra above all in small children.

With increasing use of percutaneous techniques, a plausible simple solution in children should be percutaneous suprapubic bladder stone removal [19].

PCCL has been demonstrated to be adequate and rapid in managing bladder stones in children [12, 20].

However, PCCL, in children, has a high complication rate, for instance, leakage of urine, fistula formations, or acute abdomen, during postoperative period, for an intraperitoneal bladder perforation. The problem with PCCL is that, using this technique, it is not easy to close the bladder through a 3–4 cm incision and sometimes there are leaks or fistula formation.

Moreover, there are complications linked to the technique itself, such as bladder perforation or bleeding [15].

In the last 5 years, due to the huge development of robotic surgery, thanks to the 6° of freedom of robotic instruments and the 3D vision for the surgeon and the accuracy of suturing, robotic removal of bladder stones seems to be ideal in patients with a stone bigger than 15 mm or smaller but in patients with a narrow urethra or in patients with a neurogenic bladder [13, 14].

The main advantage of robotic BS removal is that you can perform a true minimally invasive procedure and you have no risk to damage the urethra, which happens when you remove the stone fragments through it as it happens via endoscopy [13].

In addition, thanks to the perfect suture of the bladder using robotics instruments, you have no bladder leaks or perforations, as it happens for PCCL, and we had no postoperative complications in our series.

However, before starting robotic procedure, it is important to perform cystoscopy to check bladder anatomy and stone location [14].

Key points of the procedure are fixing the bladder to the abdominal wall with two stitches, using an endobag to remove the stone and closing the bladder in two layers [10].

It is important to remember that urolithiasis is a complex pathology and it is important that these patients have to be followed in pre- and postoperative period by a multidisciplinary team of pediatric nephrologists and pediatric urologists.

In conclusions, there are several techniques for the treatment of solitary bladder calculi in children: open cystolithotomy, transurethral endoscopic stone removal, and percutaneous cystolithotomy, and all these techniques have a high rate of complications.

Robotic BS removal is an elegant and safe technique to adopt to remove large bladder stones in pediatric population [13].

This technique is easy to perform and with a low rate of complication compared to the other techniques, and the disadvantages of robotic procedure are the high costs and the need of a dedicated team trained in robotic surgery.

Take-Home Points

- Before starting BS robotic removal, it is preferable to have a strong experience in robotics.
- A team (surgeons and nurses) training in robotic surgery is essential before starting robotic procedures.
- During the learning curve period, it is preferable to work with an expert surgeon on the second robotic console.
- The role of bedside surgeon is crucial for the success of the procedure.
- A bladder suspension with two stitches and the use of an endobag are important points for the success of the procedure.

References

1. Lopez M, Hoppe B. History, epidemiology and regional diversities of urolithiasis. Pediatr Nephrol. 2010;25:49–59.
2. Shah J, Whitfield HN. Urolithiasis through the ages. BJU Int. 2002;89:801–10.

3. Schwartz BF, Stoller ML. The vesical calculus. Urol Clin N Am. 2000;27:333–46.
4. Papatsoris AG, Varkarakis I, Dellis A, Deliveliotis C. Bladder lithiasis: from open surgery to lithotripsy. Urol Res. 2006;34:163–7.
5. Phillippou P, Massod MK, Junaid J, Buchholz IN. The Management of Bladder Lithiasis in the modern era of Endourology. Urology. 2012;79:980–6.
6. Gangkak G, Yadav SS, Tomar V, Vyas N, Jain D. Pneumatic cystolithotripsy versus holmium: yag laser cystolithotripsy in the treatment of pediatric bladder stones: a prospective randomized study. Pediatr Surg Int. 2016;32:609–14.
7. Naqvi SA, Rizvi SA, Shahjehan S. Bladder stone disease in children: clinical studies. J Pak Med Assoc. 1984;34:94–101.
8. Deswanto IA, Basukarno A, Birowo P, Rasyid N. Management of 1 bladder stones: the move towards non-invasive treatment. Med J Indones. 2017;26:128–33.
9. Liu G, Deng Y, Zhang S, Zhao X, Yao D, Zhang Q, et al. Minimally invasive percutaneous suprapubic cystolithotripsy: an effective treatment for bladder stones with urethral strictures. Int J Clin Exp Med. 2016;9:19907–12.
10. Sultan S, Umer SA, Ahmed B, Naqvi SAA, Rizvi SAH. Update on surgical management of pediatric urolithiasis. Front Pediatr. 2019;2:252. https://doi.org/10.3389/fped.2019.00252.
11. Silay MS, Ellison JS, Tailly T, Caione P. Update on urinary stones in children: current and future concepts in surgical treatment and shockwave lithotripsy. Eur Urol Focus. 2017;3:164–71. https://doi.org/10.1016/j.euf.2017.07.005.
12. Bansal A, Kumar M, Sankhwar S, Goel S, Patodia M, Aeron R, et al. Prospective randomized comparison of three endoscopic modalities used in treatment of bladder stones. Urologia. 2016;83:87–92.
13. Sarica K, Sahin C. Contemporary minimally invasive surgical management of urinary stones in children. Eur Urol Suppl. 2017;16:2–7.
14. Humphreys MR. The emerging role of robotics and laparoscopy in stone disease. Urol Clin North Am. 2013;40:115–28.
15. Donaldson JF, Ruhayel Y, Skolarikos A, MacLennan S, Yuan Y, Shepherd R, Thomas K, Seitz C, Petrik A, Türk C, Neisius A. Treatment of Bladder Stones in Adults and Children: A Systematic Review and Meta-analysis on Behalf of the European Association of Urology Urolithiasis Guideline Panel. Eur Urol. 2019;76(3):352–67.
16. Bhatia V, Biyani CS. A comparative study of cystolithotripsy and extracorporeal shock wave therapy for bladder stones. Int Urol Nephrol. 1994;26:27–31.
17. Singh KJ, Kaur J. Comparison of three different endoscopic technique in management of bladder calculi. Indian J Urol. 2011;27:10–3.
18. Ener K, Agras K, Aldemir M, Okulu E, Kayigil O. The randomized comparison of two different endoscopic techniques in the management of large bladder stones: transurethral use of nephroscope or cystoscope? J Endourol. 2009;23:1151–5.
19. Agrawal MS, Aron M. Experience with percutaneous bladder and urethral surgery in children. Asian J Surg. 1999;22:223–6.
20. Tugcu V, Polat H, Ozbay B, Gurbuz N, Eren GA, Tasci AI. Percutaneous versus transurethral cystolithotripsy. J Endourol. 2009;23:237–41.

48 Robotic Bladder Neck Construction for Voiding Continence

Alfredo Berrettini, Dario Guido Minoli, Michele Gnech, and Gianantonio Manzoni

Learning Objectives

- To describe step-by-step techniques of robotic-assisted bladder neck construction/plication to achieve voiding continence.
- To show a video with the techniques.
- To discuss appropriate patient selection for the techniques.

48.1 Introduction

The application of minimally invasive techniques in pediatric urology has evolved rapidly over the last 15 years. Increasingly more complex reconstructive procedures can be performed in the pediatric population either laparoscopically or with robotic assistance including Mitrofanoff appendicovesicostomy and enterocystoplasty.

Supplementary Information The online version contains supplementary material available at [https://doi.org/10.1007/978-3-030-99280-4_48].

A. Berrettini · D. G. Minoli · M. Gnech · G. Manzoni (✉)
Department of Pediatric Urology, Fondazione IRCCS Cà Granda Ospedale Maggiore Policlinico Milan, Milan, Italy
e-mail: alfredo.berrettini@policlinico.mi.it; darioguido.minoli@policlinico.mi.it; michele.gnech@policlinico.mi.it; gianantonio.manzoni@policlinico.mi.it

Urinary incontinence secondary to an absent or incompetent bladder neck/sphincteric mechanism is a challenging area. A philosophical decision is required whether to aim for voiding continence or simply secure dryness which will require lifelong intermittent catheterization. This chapter is concerned only with the former, i.e., constructing a functional bladder neck for voiding continence and not with the many alternatives such as slings, artificial urinary sphincters, and bladder neck closures and continent diversion which are dealt with elsewhere. This type of functional bladder neck reconstruction is largely confined to the exstrophy/epispadias complex and cloaca/urogenital sinus groups of abnormalities. The patients selected for this approach should have the outflow weakness documented video-urodynamically and have a compliant bladder capacity of the order of 50% of the expected capacity for age (Fig. 48.1).

The excellent 3D robotic exposure of the bladder neck region has evolved through the vast experience gained by adult urologists performing radical cysto-prostatectomy. This new approach to *pediatric* bladder neck reconstructive urology opens new fascinating horizons and stimulating perspectives compared to the traditional frustrating and very demanding open surgery.

The aim of this chapter is to describe our preliminary experience in robotic bladder neck construction techniques for voiding continence in children.

C. Esposito et al. (eds.), *Minimally Invasive Techniques in Pediatric Urology*,
https://doi.org/10.1007/978-3-030-99280-4_48

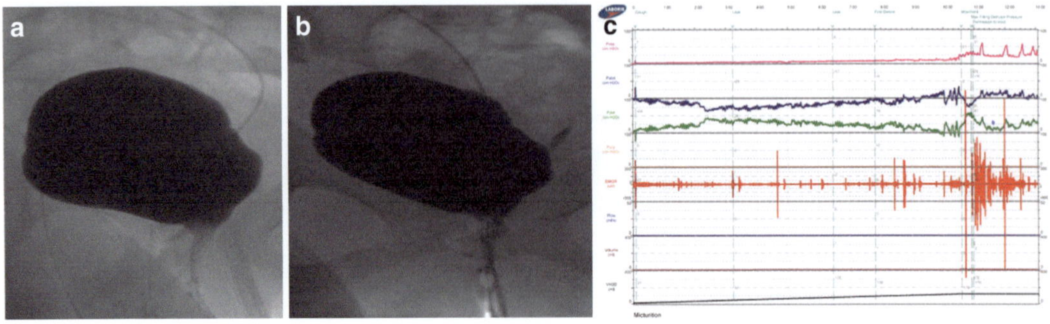

Fig. 48.1 Video-Urodynamic study

48.2 Preoperative Preparation

A standard extensive intestinal preparation is not necessary but a simple enema should be given the evening before the surgery. Perioperative antibacterial prophylaxis (usually with a cephalosporin) should be administered.

Patients receive a general anesthesia with endotracheal intubation and muscle relaxation.

When the "keel" bladder neck construction (KBNC) procedure is planned, a preliminary cystoscopy is performed and JJ stent ureteral catheters are placed bilaterally to allow secure identification of the ureteral orifices during the procedure.

A Foley catheter is positioned into the bladder but is not draped into the operative sterile field. A nasogastric tube is placed in order to keep empty the stomach during the procedure.

48.3 Positioning

The patient is placed in a supine position with the legs wide open. The patient is secured to the bed with wide adhesive tape and strips. All pressure points, including the heels, must be carefully padded and protected to prevent pressure lesions. We generally use a depression mattress in order to move the patient into the desired position easily and for transfer onto the operating table.

The patient is then prepped and draped. During the robotic procedure for bladder neck plication (BNP), it is necessary to simultaneously access the urethra and bladder neck endoscopically to confirm and to monitor the progression of the reconstructive procedure.

The operating table is inclined in the Trendelenburg position moving the bowel cranially by gravity and facilitating exposure of the bladder and the pelvic region.

48.4 Instrumentation

The *DaVinci Si* robot is positioned between the patient's open legs, as commonly used for pelvic procedures such as vesicoureteric reimplant or prostatectomy.

A 12 mm trocar is placed for the camera in the midline, through an umbilical or supraumbilical incision. The trocar is positioned with an open access and direct view of the peritoneum to reduce the risk of bowel lesion.

After an initial overview of the abdominal cavity, the 8 mm robotic ports are positioned. Depending on the type of procedures, two or three trocars are positioned: one to two in the left and one in the right. A three-arm configuration is used for KBNC, while two arms could be enough for BNP. The 5 mm assistant port is finally placed in the right side. A distance of approximately 8 cm is respected between the robotic ports.

The robot can now be docked and the instrumentation placed: we use a 30° down camera in 12 mm port, monopolar scissors, and needle holder on the right arm while a bipolar Maryland

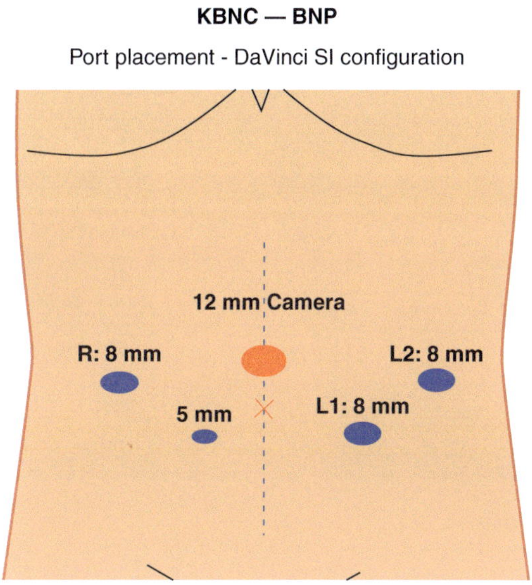

Fig. 48.2 KBNC—BNP ports placement

forceps is connected to the left. When the third robotic arm is active, a Maryland or a needle driver is used. The final configuration is showed in Fig. 48.2.

When using the *DaVinci Xi* device, the port siting changes due to its different peculiarities. An angled linear port configuration is used to align the ports from the right lower quadrant toward the left costal margin with the 5 mm assistant port placed in the left lower quadrant and the robot is side docked on the patient's right side.

48.5 Technique

In our institute we generally use two different surgical techniques for the construction of a voiding bladder neck: BNP and KBNC.

Once docking and instrument insertion into the abdomen are completed, the procedure is started with the opening of the pelvic peritoneum using a wide transverse incision. Movement of the catheter and visualization of the balloon or combined endoscopic-robotic maneuvers can help to identify the bladder neck region. Preliminary dissection is performed retropubically and laterally with special care in order to avoid venous bleeding in the male and vaginal injury in the female. Complete posterior urethral dissection, as for a sling placement, is not necessary.

In BNP, after isolation of the bladder neck, without bladder opening, a progressive plication of the proximal urethra is achieved with multiple interrupted braided polyester (polyethylene terephthalate) 2/0 sutures. Simultaneous endoscopic control with direct vision of the lumen caliber reduction is very helpful (Video 48.1) [1].

In KBNC, the bladder neck is prepared and the anterior bladder wall is opened in the midline. Two holding stitches may help to better expose and stabilize the bladder neck region. The Foley catheter is removed and the position of the new bladder neck is identified as the point halfway between the verumontanum and the ureteric orifices (male) or halfway from the external urethral meatus to the ureteric orifices (female). Starting from this point and extending caudally, two mucosal triangles are outlined and the mucosa excised leaving only a midline mucosal strip of adequate width/ depending on the age of the patient which will constitute the "new" posterior urethra and bladder neck. Only the mucosal layer is excised without damaging or incising the muscular component (Fig. 48.3a, b).

The intact midline mucosal strip is measured and folded over a Nelaton catheter of adequate size (usually 8 FG) tubularized with interrupted 5/0 Maxon sutures. A second and a third layer, above the neoconstructed bladder neck, are obtained by detrusor approximation with interrupted 4/0 or 3/0 Vicryl stitches. The anatomical reconstruction will provide a funnel with a "keel" reconfiguration (Fig. 48.4; Video 48.2) [2].

A percutaneous suprapubic cystostomy and a transurethral catheter are mandatory to assure postoperative optimal bladder drainage. All instruments and ports are removed and the fascia is closed with 2–0 Vicryl. Skin is closed with a subcuticular suture with 5–0 Monocryl. Skin adhesives are used to cover the incisions.

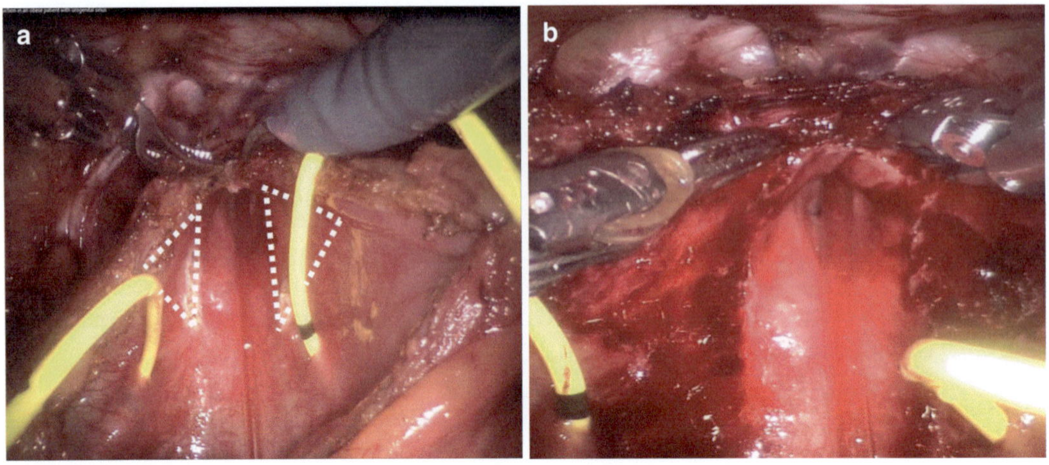

Fig. 48.3 KBNC. (**a**) Outline of mucosal triangles. (**b**) Post-excision

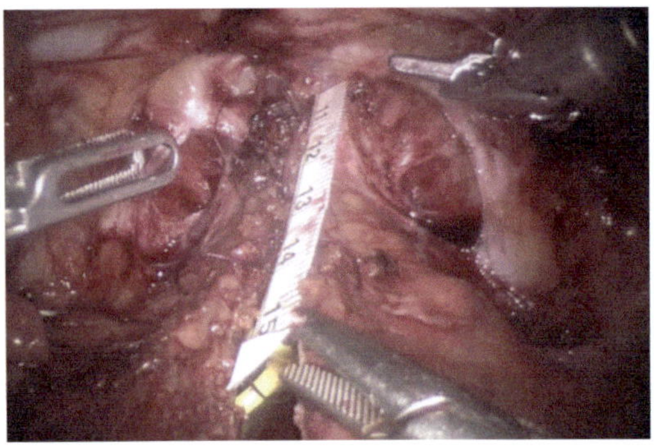

Fig. 48.4 KBNC final appearance

48.6 Postoperative Care

Patients start oral feeding a few hours postoperatively. Analgesic therapy is based on Paracetamol (dosage 15 mg/kg at 8 h intervals) and ketorolac (dosage 0.3 mg/kg at 8 h intervals, if necessary) usually administered in the first 12–24 h postoperatively. Antibiotic therapy is maintained for 72 h postoperatively. Patients are usually discharged from hospital on the 4th/5th postoperative day with both the transurethral and suprapubic catheters on constant free drainage (day and night). The first postoperative clinical control is scheduled after 1 week. After 4 weeks, the transurethral catheter is removed and the first suprapubic MCUG is performed: depending on the outcome, a safe suprapubic cystostomy removal can be performed. If the patient is not fully ready for regular spontaneous micturition, the suprapubic cystostomy is maintained with a clamp, void, release training program. After removal of the suprapubic catheter, regular renal/bladder US is scheduled to check both the upper urinary tracts and postvoid residuals.

Tips and Tricks

- It is mandatory to perform a preliminary cystoscopy in order to have all the information about the urethral length, ureteral orifices, and the position of the verumontanum. This is a crucial step to understand the anatomy in order to correctly position the newly constructed bladder neck and posterior urethra.
- -During cystoscopy, if KBNC is planned, bilateral ureteric stents should always be placed to have complete control of the ureteral orifices during the intravesical surgery.
- A transurethral Foley catheter with the balloon inflated is useful to identify the bladder neck.
- During BNP procedure, a simultaneous endoscopic view is very helpful and important to confirm the correct position of the plication sutures.

- During KBNC procedure, the use of a Nelaton catheter (8 FG) is preferable to a Foley catheter. If a Foley is used, the balloon should be deflated at the end in order to avoid any subsequent risk of bladder neck breakdown. It is important to suture the urethral strip close to its edges to ensure that the lumen remains uniform in caliber and to use interrupted sutures for security. The transurethral catheter is left in place and fixed both internally and externally.
- The use of a suprapubic diversion is mandatory to guarantee complete bladder drainage and to keep total control until regular and safe bladder emptying, with spontaneous voiding, is eventually achieved.

48.7 Discussion

Robotic-assisted laparoscopic bladder surgery in children has gained widespread acceptance for complex reconstructive procedure over the last two decades. The use of the robot is particularly advantageous for procedures that necessitate suturing in an area with limited access such as bladder neck construction techniques for voiding continence.

Patient selection is crucial, and our main indications for voiding continence procedures have been quite rigid and limited only to the epispadias or cloaca/urogenital sinus anomalies.

Even for this limited group of patients, many surgical techniques for bladder neck repair have been presented but there is no consensus on which is the best option and there are no standardized protocols [3, 4]. An adequate bladder capacity with normal compliance is mandatory prerequisites to consider a robotic procedure aiming at voiding continence.

As already confirmed in the literature, laparoscopic bladder neck plication is successful [5–7]. Therefore robotic-assisted BNP seems a very logical option to achieve voiding continence, and preliminary experience is very encouraging.

In addition to the benefit of working in a small space with excellent and 3D vision, other significant advantages of the robotic versus an open reconstruction are:

- A minimally invasive approach with better cosmetic results
- Lower intraoperative blood loss with a more precise dissection
- Decreased postoperative narcotic use and hospital stays

Take-Home Points

- Robotic-assisted laparoscopic surgery represents a minimally invasive solution for some of the most severe reconstructive challenges in pediatric urology.
- Robotic-assisted laparoscopic surgery allows excellent vision within the pelvis and the retropubic region, facilitating any type of bladder neck repair.
- Preliminary experience with KBNC or BNP performed robotically is encouraging and opening new horizons.

References

1. Minoli DG, Albo G, De Marco EA, Gnech M, Montanari E, Manzoni GA, Berrettini A. Robotic bladder neck plication for incontinence treatment. Cent European J Urol. 2021;74(2):274–5.
2. Minoli DG, De Marco EA, Gnech M, Rocco B, Manzoni G, Berrettini A. Laparoscopic robotic-assisted “keel” bladder neck construction. Presented 28th Congress of the European Society for Pediatric Urology (ESPU) Barcelona. J Pediatr Urol. 2020;16:e857–8.
3. Gargollo PC, Manzoni G, Rocco B. Robotic bladder outlet procedures. In: Mattioli G, Petralia P, editors. Pediatric robotic surgery. Springer International Publishing Switzerland; 2017. p. 109–20.
4. Bagrodia A, Gargollo P. Robot-assisted bladder neck reconstruction, bladder neck sling and appendico-vesicostomy in children: description of technique and initial results. J Endourol. 2011;25(8):1299–305.

5. Kajabfzadeh AM, Talab SS, Elmi A, et al. Single-stage subsymphyseal cystoscopic-guided bladder neck plication and urethra-genitoplasty in female epispadias: presentation of long-term follow-up. BJU Int. 2011;108(7):1200–7.
6. Lazarus J, Van Den Heever A, Kotekaas B, et al. Female epispadias management by bladder neck plication via a perineal approach. J Pediatr Urol. 2012;8:244–8.
7. Yadav SS, Agarwal N, Kumar S, et al. Single-stage female epispadias repair by combined infra-symphyseal bladder neck plication and urethrogenitoplasty: a novel technique. Urology. 2017;100:240–5.

Part V

Urethra

Management of Posterior Urethral Valves

49

V. Di Benedetto, C. Arena, R. Patti, and M. G. Scuderi

Learning Objectives

- To describe the technique of endoscopic resection of posterior urethral valves (PUV).
- To show a video with the technique.
- To describe tips and tricks of endoscopic resection.

49.1 Introduction

Posterior urethral valves (PUVs) occur in 1/5000–25,000 live births and constitute 10% of urinary obstruction diagnosed in utero [1–4]. PUVs are associated with high fetal and neonatal mortality (30%) and considerable lifelong morbidity. The morbidity is related to the congenital obstruction of the urinary tract at the critical time in organogenesis which may have a profound and lifelong effect on kidney, ureter, and bladder function [4]. In severe cases, the disorder can lead to anhydramnios and pulmonary dysplasia during the canalicular phase of lung development. Mortality is related to ongoing renal damage in children. The gold standard for postnatal diagnosis is voiding cystourethrography (VCUG), while prenatal diagnosis is dependent on routine screening ultrasonography. The diagnosis of PUV is sometimes difficult because of its wide spectrum in terms of severity and morphology. The most typical PUV is presented in neonates with history of prenatal bilateral hydronephrosis or in infants with acute pyelonephritis associated with massive vesicoureteral reflux (VUR). This group of PUV is easy to be diagnosed by typical findings in VCUG. More than half of the patients with PUV will have VUR at the time of diagnosis (Fig. 49.1) [2]. Secondary VUR may be difficult to detect in ordinary imaging studies because it does not present with conventional findings, such as dilatation of posterior urethra (Fig. 49.2). Dilatation of posterior urethra is often observed during the voiding phase of

Supplementary Information The online version contains supplementary material available at [https://doi.org/10.1007/978-3-030-99280-4_49].

V. Di Benedetto (✉) · C. Arena · R. Patti
M. G. Scuderi
Pediatric Surgery Unit, University of Catania, Catania, Italy

Pediatric Surgery Unit, NICU Policlinico-San Marco Hospital, Catania, Italy
e-mail: vdb@chirpedunict.it; carmela.arena@policlinico.unict.it; mg.scuderi@policlinico.unict.it

C. Esposito et al. (eds.), *Minimally Invasive Techniques in Pediatric Urology*,
https://doi.org/10.1007/978-3-030-99280-4_49

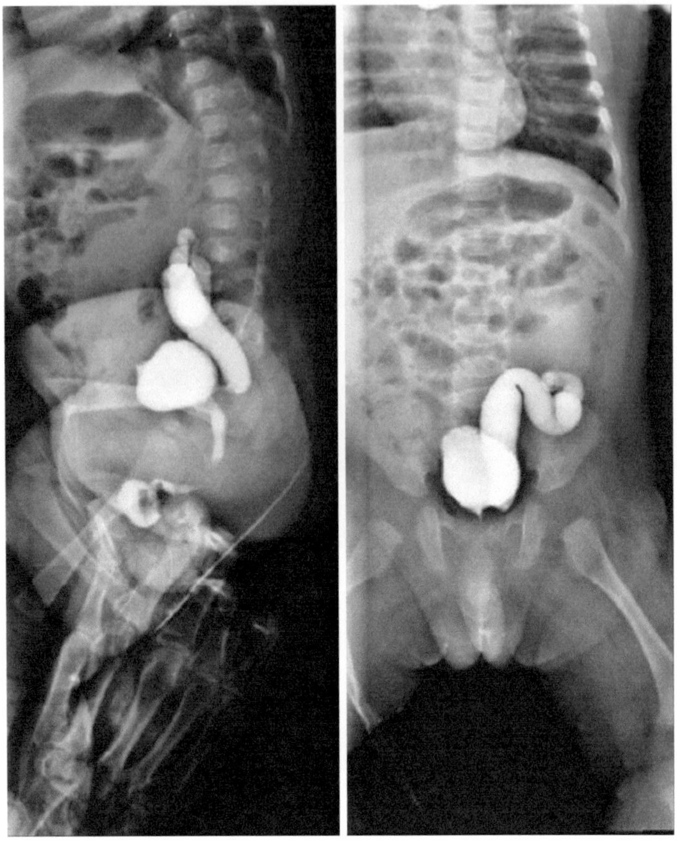

Fig. 49.1 Massive RVU in VCUG

VCUG but segmental narrowing of the bulbomembranous urethra could be a single abnormality. Other abnormal urethral findings are transient urethral kink or angulation of the membranous urethra. It is crucial to take serial photographs during voiding to make an accurate diagnosis. Until recently there has been no reference standard based on findings in VCUG and endoscopy [5]. Although Young's classification of PUV is well known, Douglas Stephens added a more precise explication for each type of Young's classification in 1996. Stephens' detailed explanation is considered to be the most useful and easily understood with regard to structural characteristics based on embryology. There are two main types of PUV: type 1 and type 3. Type 2 was originally defined by Young in 1919 but was later considered an overclassification. Type 4 is rare [5].

49.2 Preoperative Preparation

In a full-term baby, the standard of care for PUV is cystoscopic valve incision. The current methods of incision include electrocautery incision, cold knife incision, and laser fulguration [3, 4]. In infants with extremely low birth weight, the urethra might be too small to admit cystoscopy equipment safely. Long-term catheter drainage is inadvisable because of the risk of candidemia. Rather than risking stricture with cystoscopic instrumentation, these babies should either undergo percutaneous cystostomy and rarely open vesicostomy or the use of Fogarty balloon valve ablation under fluoroscopic guidance [3]. Patients with severe disease often require multiple surgical intervention and may develop long-term complication, including urinary incontinence and important loss of renal function [4]. All parents have to sign a specifically

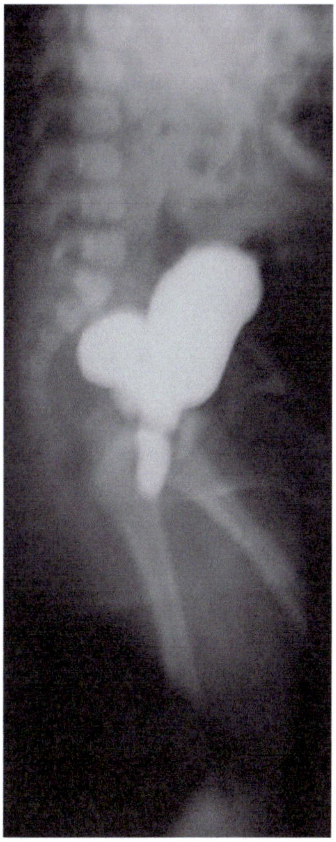

Fig. 49.2 Dilation of posterior urethra

informed consent before the procedure. Anesthesia is general but it is possible to do valve resection in spinal anesthesia. All patients receive antibiotic prophylaxis with i.v. ceftriaxone and gentamicin.

49.3 Positioning

The patient is placed in gynecological position. Surgeon's position is at the feet of the patient and the monitor is on the left of the surgeon.

49.4 Instrumentation

We use a 9,5 Fr pediatric cystoscope (Storz). We performed valve resection using a point electrocautery via a 3 Fr ureteric catheter with metal stylet passed through the cystoscope (Fig. 49.3).

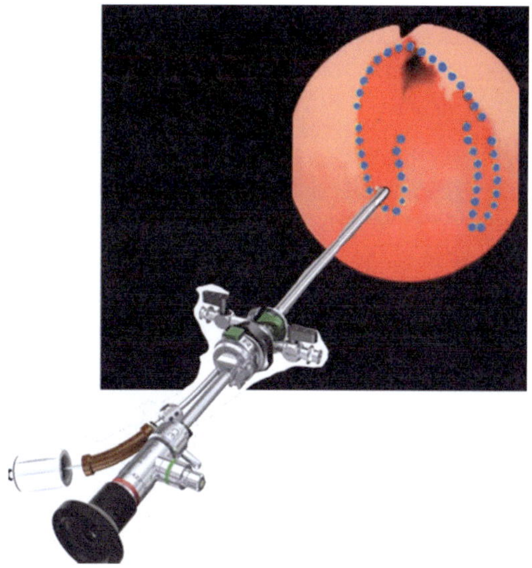

Fig. 49.3 9.5 Fr pediatric cystoscope. 3 Fr ureteric catheter with metal stylet passed through the cystoscope

49.5 Technique

After filling the bladder with saline solution, we perform the urethrocystoscopy using a 9,5 Fr cystoscope. After identifying the valves, a 3 Fr ureteric catheter is passed through the channel of the cystoscope and electrofulguration is performed. Fulguration is done mainly at 5, 7 and 12 o'clock position. For type 1 PUV, a major incision is made on the membranous lesion at the 12 o'clock position, and an additional incision was made if necessary on any valvular lesion in the 5 or 7 o'clock position (Figs. 49.4 and 49.5). For type 3, an incision is made on the membranous lesion in the 12 o'clock position. For both types, the incision on the membranous lesion in the 12 o'clock position is long and deep enough for complete excision. The adequacy of the fulguration is confirmed intraoperatively by gentle pressure on the bladder with cystoscope positioned just distal to the verumontanum to look for absence of valvular obstruction. Another method to check for adequacy of fulguration may be to observe the urinary stream by Crede maneuver with patient under anesthesia. The urethral catheter is left in place after procedure for 14 days.

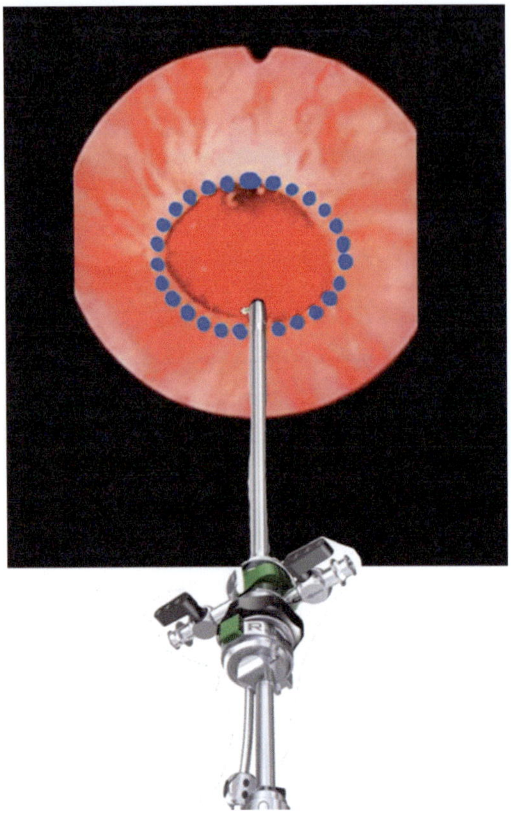

Fig. 49.4 A major incision is made on the membranous lesion at the 12 o'clock position, and an additional incision was made if necessary on any valvular lesion in the 5 or 7 o'clock position.

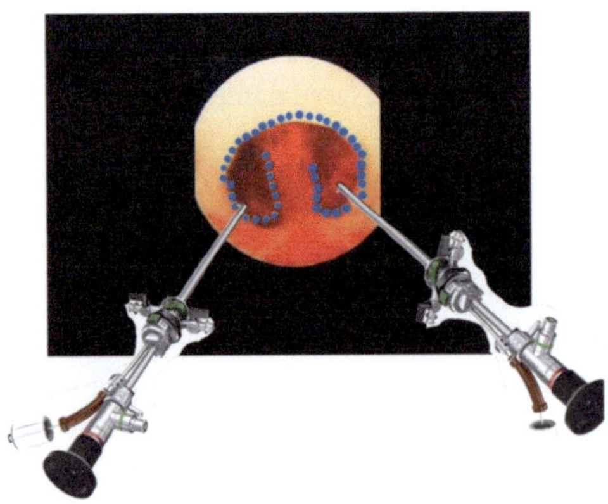

Fig. 49.5 An additional incision is made if necessary on any valvular lesion in the 5 or 7 o'clock position

49.6 Postoperative Care

The postoperative therapy included i.v. antibiotics (ceftriaxone and gentamicin) and Paracetamol.

A small-size Foley urethral catheter is left in situ. Patients are discharged with an indwelling catheter the day after procedure, and they return 14 days after discharge to have a VCUG and remove catheter.

49.7 Results

The timing of valve ablation varies according to age at presentation. Successful voiding and improvement of stream are considered as the criteria of successful treatment. Follow-up includes ultrasonography (US) to look for resolution of hydroureteronephrosis (HUN) at 2 weeks and 3 months after treatment, VCUG to look for the resolution of VUR and valve remnants at 1 and 6 months after treatment, and DTPA renal scan to evaluate renal function at 12 months. Urodynamic study is performed in selected patients. Repeat cystourethroscopy is performed in patients who continue to have obstructive voiding at VCUG, persistence or deterioration of bilateral HUN, no decrease in posterior urethral dilatation, presence of valve remnants, nonresolution of bilateral VUR, and no improvement in renal function or new onset renal insufficiency. Refulguration is performed in boys with valve remnants. Complications after valve ablation reported literature are in 5% to 25% of cases. Stricture formation occurs infrequently ranging from 0% to 25% and can be treated successfully with visual internal urethrotomy (VIU). Up to 60% of VUR will resolve after valve ablation [3, 6]. Downgrading or resolving VUR and/or improvement in upper tract dilatation may be considered as indirect signs of urinary tract decompression. However, despite successful valve ablation, VUR and HUN may persist. Hence, VUR is expected to resolve after the release of urethral obstruction. Spontaneous resolution rates range between 27% and 79% at 2 weeks to more than 1 year following valve ablation. Some reflux can take as long as 3 years [2]. Those children with persistent upper tract dilation may have bladder emptying problems related to valve bladder syndrome or have a large urine output as a result of renal tubular damage, residual infravesical obstruction, or, rarely, ureterovesical junction obstruction [2]. Notwithstanding surgical relief of urethral obstruction, ongoing bladder dysfunction is a cause of morbidity and a potential threat to upper tract function. The prevalence of bladder dysfunction has been estimated to be 75–80% in boys studied urodynamically after PUV ablation [7]. A small, contracted bladder in infancy that progresses to a large-capacity, poorly compliant bladder, often found in the presence of persistent upper tract dilatation and nephrogenic diabetes insipidus, has been termed valve bladder. This can create a self-injurious cycle, with persistent dilatation leading to a renal concentrating defect and blood increase in creatine. Regular urodynamic monitoring is crucial in the management of these patients. Abnormal renal development persists into childhood and adolescence: 30–42% of patients develop end-stage renal failure, making VUP the most common cause for pediatric renal transplantation [3].

Tips and Tricks

- Early endoscopic resection of the valves has advantage, regarding bladder function, over long-term diversion. Small instruments are used to avoid urethral damage. We try to minimize fulguration time and to avoid excessive deep fulguration for the risk of current injury to surrounding corpus spongiosum. We do not use loop resectoscope for risk of urethral strictures.

49.8 Discussion

The major goals in treatment of PUV are restoration of bladder voiding function, control of infections, preservation of renal function, maintenance of continence, and elimination of obstruction and VUR. Several opinions for surgical management of infants with PUVs are available and the mainstay of treatment is primary valve ablation [8–10]. Currently, surgeons have better instruments to treat valves endoscopically using different modality under direct vision, with minimal incidence of complications [8, 11]. Various techniques of valve ablation were used: hot loop resectoscopy, cold knife urethrotome, hook diathermy electrode, Bugbee electrode, and Fogarty catheter. Prevention of urethral stricture after valve ablation depends on many factors. These include gentle surgical technique, avoidance of oversized instrumentation in a small caliber urethra, fulguration time minimization, excessive and deep fulguration avoidance, fulguration under direct vision, shorten the duration of preoperative catheterization, and use of nonreactive small-sized catheters [8]. Bladder and renal functions are often unstable and usually change during life, requiring lifelong monitoring. It was found that neonatal valve ablation would protect the bladder functions and allow normal bladder cycling and healing. This underscores the importance of routine prenatal screening and early intervention for the valves. These findings suggest that the long-term prognosis of PUV might be improved by prenatal diagnosis [12, 13]. VUR and UTIs are not associated with worse renal outcomes, although these parameters remain vital in guiding treatment and may influence the number of surgeries in patient life. Further investigation and longer follow-up are needed to identify patients at risk for late progression to CKD or end-stage renal disease (ESRD) [4]. Large retrospective studies of people with posterior urethral valves (PUVs) have reported chronic renal insufficiency (CRI) in up to one third of the participants and end-stage renal failure in up to one quarter of them. Nadir creatinine (lowest creatinine during the first year following diagnosis) is the recognized prognostic indicator for renal outcome in PUV. Elevated nadir creatinine is the only independent risk factor for poor renal outcome as reported in literature [14]. The management of children with PUV is a continuous process that starts with the antenatal detection and early fulguration of the valves. The identification of the bladder dysfunction and its appropriate management will prevent the deleterious effects on the upper tracts and improves the long-term survival.

Take-Home Points

- Importance of prenatal diagnosis for baby birth in pediatric urologic center.
- Early resection of urethral valves and evaluation of renal status.
- Very strict follow-up to minimize the poor renal outcome in older life.

References

1. Oktar T, Acar O, Sancaktutar A, Sanli O, Tefik T, Ziylan O. Endoscopic treatment of vesicoureteral reflux in children with posterior urethral valves. Int Urol Nephrol. 2012;44:1305–9.
2. Oktar T, Salabas E, Acar O, Atar A, Nane I, Ander H, Ziylan O. Residual valve and stricture after posterior urethral valve ablation: how to evaluate? J Pediatr Urol. 2013;9:184–7.
3. Diamond DA, Chan IHY, Holland AJA, Kurtz MP, Nelson C, Estrada CR Jr, Bauer S, Tam PKH. Advances in paediatric urology. Lancet. 2017;390:1061–71.
4. Bilgutay AN, Roth D, Gonzales ET Jr, Janzen N, Zhang W, Koh CJ, Gargollo P, Seth A. Posterior urethral valves: risk factors for progression to renal failure. J Pediatr Urol. 2016;12:179.e1–7.
5. Nakai H, Hyga T, Kawai S, Kubo T, Nakamura S. Aggressive diagnosis and treatment for posterior urethral valves as an etiology for vesicoureteral reflux or urge incontinence in children. Investig Clin Urol. 2017;58(Suppl 1):46–53.
6. Priti K, Rao KL, Menon P, et al. Posterior urethral valves: incidence and progress of vesicoureteral reflux after primary fulguration. Pediatr Surg Int. 2004;20:136–9.
7. Sarin YK, Sinha S. Efficacy of bladder neck incision on urodynamic abnormalities in patients with posterior urethral valves. Pediatr Surg Int. 2013;29:387–92.
8. Sarhan O, El-Ghoeneimi A, Hafez A, Dawaba M, Ghali A, Ibrahiem E. Surgical complications of posterior urethral valve ablation. 20 years of experience. J Pediatr Surg. 2010;45:2222–6.
9. Chertin B, Cozzi D, Puri P. Long-term results of primary avulsion of posterior urethral valves using a Fogarty balloon catheter. J Urol. 2002;168:1841–3.
10. Farhat W, Mc Lorie G, Capolicchhio G, et al. Outcome of primary valve ablation versus urinary tract diversion in patients with posterior urethral valves. Urology. 2000;56:653–7.
11. Yohannes P, Hanna M. Current trends in the management of posterior urethral valves in the pediatric population. Urology. 2002;60:947–53.
12. Kilby MD, Morris RK. Fetal therapy for the treatment of congenital bladder neck obstruction. Nat Rev Urol. 2014;11:412–9.
13. Kousidis G, Thomas DF, Morgan H, Haider N, Subramaniam R, Feather S. The long-term outcome of prenatally detected posterior urethral valves: a 10 to 23-year follow-up study. BJU Int. 2008;102:1020–4.
14. Coleman R, King T, Nicoara CD, Bader M, McCarthy L, Chandran H, Parashar K. Nadir creatinine in posterior urethral valves: how high is low enough? J Pediatr Urol. 2015;11(6):356.e1–5. https://doi.org/10.1016/j.jpurol.2015.06.008.

50 Minimally Invasive Management of Urethral Stenosis and Stricture

Rafal Chrzan

Learning Objectives

- To list the causes of urethral stenosis and stricture.
- To get familiar with various treatment options and tools for endourological ablation.
- To learn the steps of urethroscopy.
- To be able to get the patient through the procedure.

50.1 Introduction

Although the lack of a precise definition, the term stenosis refers to any kind of narrowing of a tubular organ, whereas stricture is commonly used for the acquired pathological scar tissue occluding the lumen. Obstruction is even a more general term describing any pathology that disturbs passage, and it could be external (e.g., compression) as well as internal from the origin (e.g., thickening of the wall, foreign bodies).

Table 50.1 Examples of urethral stenosis and stricture

Stenosis	Stricture
Primary and secondary bladder neck hypertrophy	Iatrogenic after surgery, e.g., hypospadias repair, anorectal malformations (Fig. 50.2)
Posterior urethral valves (Video 50.1)	Posttraumatic—Straddle injury, pelvic fracture
Cobb's collar/ Moormann's ring (Video 50.2)	Iatrogenic after catheterization (false route)
Syringocoele (Fig. 50.1)	Postinfectious (Fig. 50.3)
Congenital distal urethral valve	
External meatus stenosis	

Stenosis and stricture can occur along the whole urethra which must be kept in mind during cysto-urethroscopy (Table 50.1). Congenital stenosis can have a huge impact on function of the urinary tract leading to kidney function impairment early in life. Lower urinary tract symptoms (LUTSs) and recurrent urinary tract infections (UTIs) might be the first signs of the urethral anomalies in children and adults. Furthermore, any urethral instrumentation and/or surgical procedures involving urethra can also cause a iatrogenic stricture. For practical reasons one term—urethral stenosis (US)—will be used in this chapter.

US is predominantly found in males. Congenital anomalies are probably quite common. The incidence of posterior urethral valves is

Supplementary Information The online version contains supplementary material available at [https://doi.org/10.1007/978-3-030-99280-4_50].

R. Chrzan (✉)
Department of Paediatric Urology, Jagiellonian University Medical College and University Children's Hospital, Kraków, Poland
e-mail: rafal.chrzan@uj.edu.pl

C. Esposito et al. (eds.), *Minimally Invasive Techniques in Pediatric Urology*,
https://doi.org/10.1007/978-3-030-99280-4_50

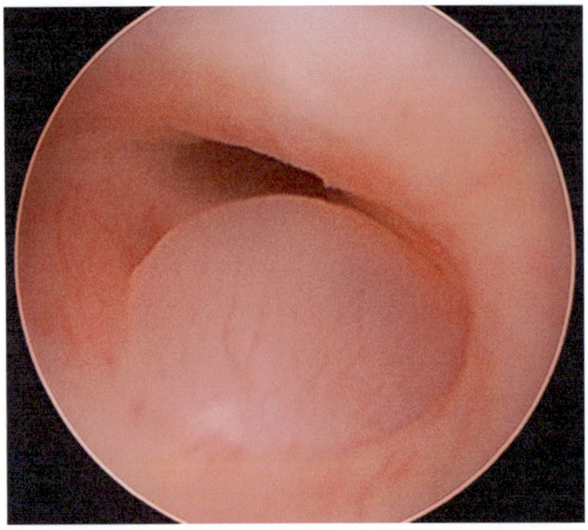

Fig. 50.1 Syringocoele

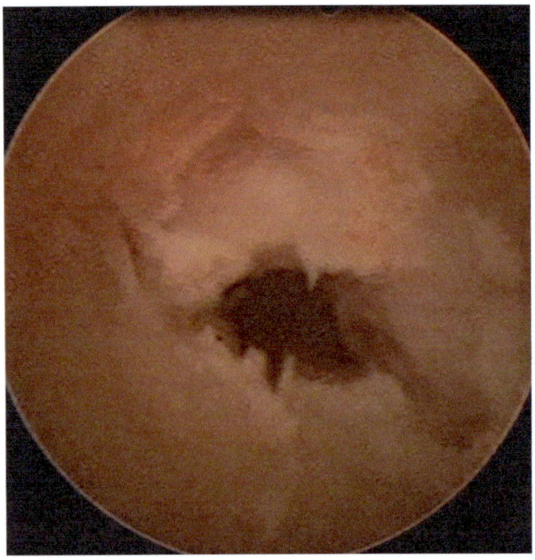

Fig. 50.2 Iatrogenic stenosis after hypospadias repair

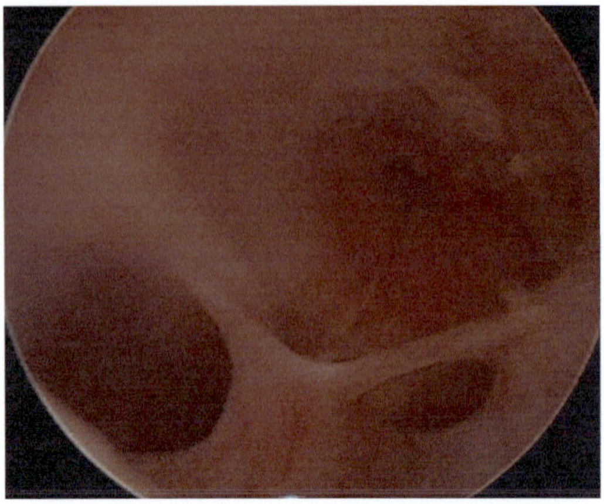

Fig. 50.3 Postinfectious changes in the distal urethra

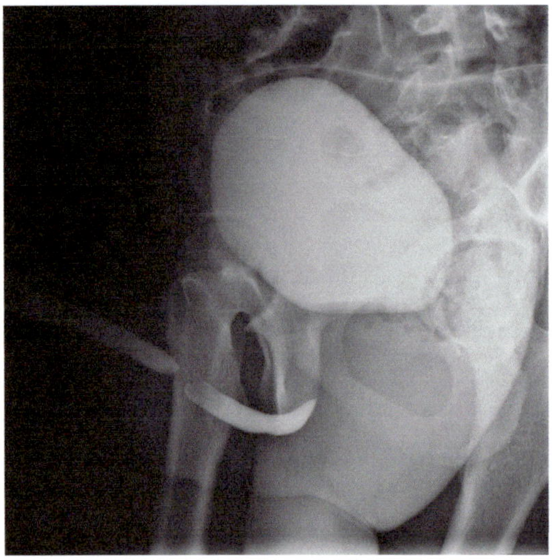

Fig. 50.4 Posttraumatic stenosis—simultaneous retrograde urethrography and voiding urethrocystography

estimated at 1:5000–8000 of births. However, this refers only to the most severe cases diagnosed due to deterioration of the upper urinary tract. The mini-valves, Cobb's collar, syringocoele, external meatus stenosis, etc. leading to LUTS can become symptomatic rather late and the real epidemiology is not really known [1–7]. Hypospadias repair might be follwed by a US but the incidence can vary enormously depending on the method and the definition of failure [8]. The prevalence of bulbar urethra posttraumatic stricture in adult is 229–627 per 100,000 in the United States but there is no reliable data for the pediatric population on that [9–11].

Diagnostic tools and pathways are out of the scope of this chapter. Anyhow, in every child suspected for a US, the standardized protocols must be followed. Thorough assessment of the lower urinary tract function must be done including bladder/bowel diary, ultrasound, and uroflowmetry. Invasive urodynamics (pressure-flow study) and imaging (urethrography, voiding-cystourethrography) must be scheduled in selected cases depending on the underlying pathology and medical history (Fig. 50.4) [10, 12].

Cystourethroscopy is performed for making the final diagnosis. After direct visualization of the lumen of the urethra, minimally invasive treatment can be performed at the same time. Incision of the stenotic part should be considered depending on the intraoperative finding (location and length). Various tools have been explored for that through decades. Cold knife and laser depending on surgeon's experience are used [11, 13, 14]. Some others may prefer a monopolar cautery [15]. The goal is to widen the stenotic part and to reduce the risk of recurrence. Repeated dilation can be offered to some patients. However, in the young population, open surgical approach might be the best option [10, 16, 17].

50.2 Preoperative Preparation

The local protocols must be followed to schedule a patient for the cystoscopy and minimally invasive intervention. Urinalysis must be done in all and urine culture in those with a risk for a urinary tract infection. Antibiotics should be given circa 30 min before endoscopy. The patient and/or the caregivers must be counseled on the risks related to the procedure, including the need for a suprapubic diversion.

50.3 Positioning

The procedure is done in the lithotomy position with buttocks at the edge of the table. This to avoid collision between the handle of the cystoscope and the table when introducing the instrument into proximal part of the urethra. The monitor must be put at the right level for the proper ergonomic position. C-arm should be available in selected cases (Figs. 50.5 and 50.6).

50.4 Instrumentation

The basic equipment consists of a monitor, a light source and cable, a camera, a telescope, and an irrigation system. The head of the camera should

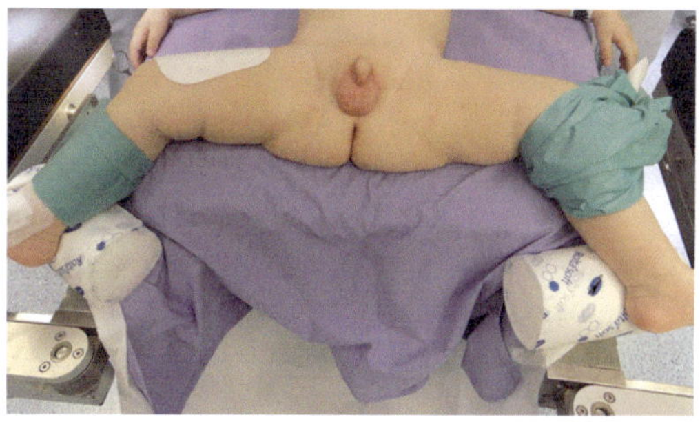

Fig. 50.5 Positioning of the patient

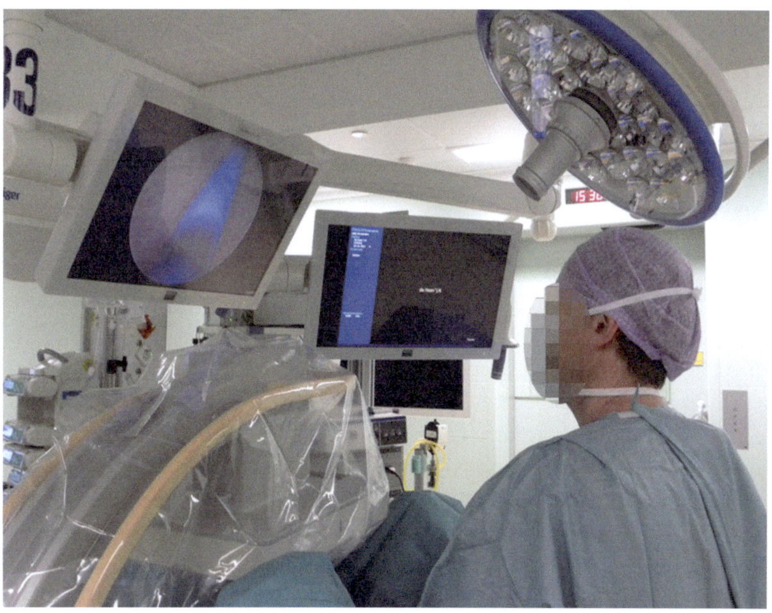

Fig. 50.6 Ergonomic position during endoscopy

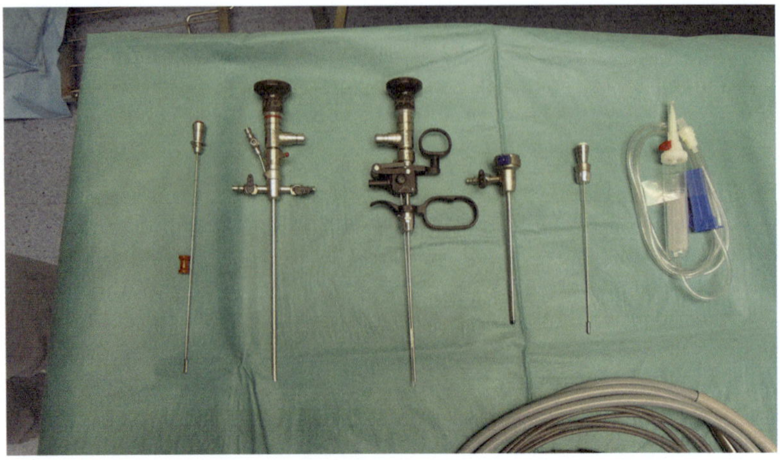

Fig. 50.7 Instrumentation

be as light as possible. For irrigation 0.9% NaCl is used for the diagnostic endoscopy and when a cold knife or a laser are used for incision. Monopolar cautery requires nonconductive (nonelectrolyte-containing) fluids [18].

The telescopes vary in size and length depending on the age of the patients. In neonates and older children, a telescope with a 30-degree optical angle is used for the primary assessment. For newborns, a very fine 5-degree compact telescopes with a 3 Fr working channel are available. For handling (making incision), 0- or 5-degree telescopes are used depending on the age to enable a straight visualization and optimal approach (Fig. 50.7).

The size of the sheath must be reasonably chosen. The bigger the instrument the better the visualization and manipulation but also the higher the risk of iatrogenic injury. Rigid resectoscopes from 8.5 Fr through 11 Fr to 14.5 Fr are available for children. A compact 5-degree cystoscope in various size with a working channel can be used for introduction on a laser fiber.

A cold knife, a holmium/YAG laser as well as a monopolar cautery can be used for incising of the stenotic part. Every tool has its pros and cons that the operating urologist must be familiar with. A different sheath is dedicated for the cold knife and the monopolar cautery. The setting of the energy source must be carefully chosen to provide sufficient tissue penetration but to minimize side effects related to high temperature (Videos 50.3 and 50.4).

Stents and guide wires must be used to ensure safety and limit the risk of complications in some cases. Depending on the intraoperative findings and the procedure, a bladder catheter should be left to stent the urethra. The safest way is to introduce an open-end catheter over a guide wire.

50.5 Technique (Videos 50.3 and 50.4)

There is no gold standard technique and the local protocols must be followed. The patient is put in the lithotomy position and the field is being prepared including the suprapubic region. Lubricant is used directly into the urethra which might limit visibility and also put on the sheath of the endoscope. The penis is straightened upward and a 30-degree cystoscope is introduced into the distal urethra. During the whole procedure, the lumen of the urethra must be visible and followed. As soon as the stenosis is identified and depending on its location and the origin, it could be gently passed through but primary dilation should be avoided. If the stenotic part is to narrow, then a guide wire should be introduced. Then, the 30 system is replaced by a 0- or 5-degree one with a tool that has be chosen for making the incision. In a case of bleeding that might limit visibility, the procedure should be aborted and a bladder catheter is introduced over a guide wire.

50.6 Postoperative Care

The local protocols must be followed. Antibiotics can be considered postoperatively in selected cases. The patient can be discharge on the same day. Depending on the invasiveness and the prognosis, a bladder catheter might be considered. However, there is no evidence that prolonged stenting can improve the outcome. In many cases, no catheter is needed for the bladder emptying but might be required to decompress the upper urinary tract.

50.7 Results

Success of the endoscopic treatment of the US can be assessed in many ways. The goal is to eliminate the narrowing. In patients with congenital anomalies, a single incision is very effective. In some, the "second look" procedure might be required to remove the remaining infravesical obstruction (Video 50.5). However, when taking into consideration LUTS and renal function, the long-term outcome can be unsatisfactory due to progressive bladder dysfunction, e.g., up to 20% of the PUV patients end up with the end-stage renal disease [15, 19, 20]. The literature on the results of the endoscopic treatment of the less common anomalies (Cobb's collar, syringocoele) as well as iatrogenic and posttraumatic strictures in children is sparse.

In the adult population, directly visualized urethrotomy (DVIU) is commonly used to treat US. According to the literature, the success rate varies enormously, between 8% and 80%. Location of the US and the length of the segment are important factors that influence the outcome. The prognosis is better for the newly diagnosed US. There is a tendency to the progressive recurrence over time [10, 16].

Tip and Tricks

- Positioning of the patient at the edge of the table.
- Double check all parameters (light source, laser, and cautery settings).
- Frequent emptying of the bladder during the procedure improves the fluid flow and visualization.
- Lumen of the urethra must be visible or a guide wire must be used.
- Do not rush, use lubricants, and stay gentle.
- Stop on time in case of a lack of visibility, ensure the urine outflow, and reschedule.
- Ergonomic position might reduce tiredness.

50.8 Discussion

DVIU has been proposed by Sachse in 1972. This technique has evolved over the decades as many different tools for making an incision have been introduced. Nowadays, holmium/YAG laser and cold knife are commonly used for this purpose by the majority of urologists. Monopolar cautery can also be useful under strict conditions. In experienced hands, it is a safe and effective instrument. The most common concern is scaring tissue and local recurrence. When using any tool, the urologist must be familiar with its properties to minimize the risk for complications [9, 11, 15].

Urethra narrowing can occur at any level and in the pediatric population the congenital anomalies are the most common. Those can be successfully solved by means of a DVIU. Nevertheless, the long-term outcome in terms of maintaining renal function and resolving LUTS depends mainly on the bladder function/dysfunction. The most common cause of an iatrogenic stenosis in children is hypospadias surgery. Children with anorectal malformations (ARM) and fistula draining into the urinary tract can also require urological management. In case of US, endoscopic management can be considered following the same rules as for the posttraumatic narrowing. However, one must keep in mind that patients with ARM are at risk for developing neurogenic lower urinary tract dysfunction that must be treated accordingly.

Simple dilation of UI is seldom effective and therefore should not be recommended in the pediatric population. It might be offered as an additional maneuver after DVIU. Local applications of steroids and mitomycin C have been proposed, but there is no evidence on their effectiveness.

Following the recommendations for the adult population, the incision can be done in those with a short-segment (< 1.5–2 cm) narrowing in the distal urethra. Prolonged stenting (> 72 h) probably does not improve the results. In case of a long-segment stenosis of the distal urethra and when proximal urethra is involved, an end-to-end anastomosis or urethra augmenting surgery should be done as the long-term outcome of DVIU is rather poor [10, 16]. Those rules can probably be also applied to the treatment of a failed hypospadias repair in children.

Take-Home Points

- Stenosis can occur along the whole urethra.
- Imaging is important but direct visualization of the stenosis in necessary in any suspected case.
- Urethroscopy requires proper training.
- Minimally invasive procedures are not suitable for all patients and open procedures in children might be the best option.
- Long-term follow-up is mandatory.

References

1. Ansari MS, Yadav P, Srivastava A, Kapoor R, Ashwin SP. Etiology and characteristics of pediatric urethral strictures in a developing country in the 21st century. J Pediatr Urol. 2019;15(4):403.e1–8. Available from: http://www.jpurol.com/article/S1477513118303905/fulltext
2. Brownlee E, Wragg R, Robb A, Chandran H, Knight M, McCarthy L. Current epidemiology and antenatal presentation of posterior urethral valves: outcome of BAPS CASS National Audit. J Pediatr Surg. 2019;54(2):318–21. Available from: http://www.jpedsurg.org/article/S0022346818307516/fulltext
3. Cranston D, Davies AH, Smith JC. Cobb's collar–a forgotten entity. Br J Urol. 1990;66(3):294–6. Available from: https://pubmed.ncbi.nlm.nih.gov/2207545/
4. Hennus PML, Hoenjet E, Kieft JH, de Jong TPVM, de Kort LMO. The long-term effect of superficial bladder neck incision on ejaculation and incontinence in boys with primary and secondary bladder neck obstruction. Front Pediatr. 2017;5:152. Available from: http://www.ncbi.nlm.nih.gov/pubmed/28752084
5. Joudi M, Fathi M, Hiradfar M. Incidence of asymptomatic meatal stenosis in children following neonatal circumcision. J Pediatr Urol. 2011;7(5):526–8. Available from: http://www.jpurol.com/article/S1477513110004341/fulltext
6. Kaplan GW. Urethral strictures in children. Curr Opin Urol. 2012;22(6):462–6. Available from: http://journals.lww.com/00042307-201211000-00006
7. Thakkar D, Deshpande AV, Kennedy SE. Epidemiology and demography of recently diagnosed cases of posterior urethral valves. Pediatr Res. 2014;76(6):560–3. Available from: https://www.nature.com/articles/pr2014134
8. Winberg H, Arnbjörnsson E, Anderberg M, Stenström P. Postoperative outcomes in distal hypospadias: a meta-analysis of the Mathieu and tubularized incised plate repair methods for development of urethrocutaneous fistula and urethral stricture. Pediatr Surg Int. 2019;35(11):1301–8. Available from: https://pubmed.ncbi.nlm.nih.gov/31372729/
9. Kaplan GW, Brock JW, Fisch M, Koraitim MM, Snyder HM. SIU/ICUD consultation on urethral strictures: urethral strictures in children. Urology. 2014;83(3 Suppl):S71–3. Available from: http://www.goldjournal.net/article/S0090429513011680/fulltext
10. Lumen N, Kuehhas FE, Djakovic N, Kitrey ND, Serafetinidis E, Sharma DM, et al. Review of the current management of lower urinary tract injuries by the EAU trauma guidelines panel. Eur Urol. 2015;67(5):925–9. Available from: http://www.europeanurology.com/article/S0302283814013918/fulltext
11. Torres Castellanos L, Moreno Bencardino MC, Bravo-Balado A, García Mayorga CA, Vargas Manrique I, Fernández N. Evaluation of the efficacy and safety of laser versus cold knife urethrotomy in the management of patients with urethral strictures: a systematic review and meta-analysis of randomized clinical trials. Urol Int. 2017;99(4):453–9. Available from: https://pubmed.ncbi.nlm.nih.gov/28697506/
12. Chang S-J, Van Laecke E, Bauer SB, von Gontard A, Bagli D, Bower WF, et al. Treatment of daytime urinary incontinence: a standardization document from the International Children's Continence Society. Neurourol Urodyn. 2017;36(1):43–50. https://doi.org/10.1002/nau.22911.
13. Shoukry AI, Abouela WN, Elsheemy MS, Shouman AM, Daw K, Hussein AA, et al. Use of holmium laser for urethral strictures in pediatrics: a prospective study. J Pediatr Urol. 2016;12(1):42.e1–6. Available from: http://www.jpurol.com/article/S1477513115002971/fulltext
14. Sun F, Wentong Z, Yan Z, Qingyu D, Aiwu L. Application of endoscopic Ho:YAG laser inci-

sion technique treating urethral strictures and urethral atresias in pediatric patients. Pediatr Surg Int. 2006;22(6):514–8. Available from: https://link.springer.com/article/10.1007/s00383-006-1692-x
15. de Jong TPVM, Kuijper CF, Chrzan R, Dik P, Klijn AJ, Vijverberg MA. Efficacy and safety of urethral de-obstruction in boys with overactive bladder complaints. J Pediatr Urol. 2013;9(6 Pt B):1072–6. Available from: http://www.sciencedirect.com/science/article/pii/S1477513113000740
16. Shaw NM, Venkatesan K. Endoscopic management of urethral stricture: review and practice algorithm for management of male urethral stricture disease. Curr Urol Rep. 2018;19(3):19. Available from: https://pubmed.ncbi.nlm.nih.gov/29479640/
17. Waterloos M, Verla W, Spinoit AF, Oosterlinck W, Van Laecke E, Hoebeke P, et al. Urethroplasty for urethral injuries and trauma-related strictures in children and adolescents: a single-institution experience. J Pediatr Urol. 2019;15(2):176.e1–7. Available from: https://pubmed.ncbi.nlm.nih.gov/30581060/
18. Gielchinsky I, Pode D, Duvdevani M, Yutkin V, Landau EH, Hidas G, et al. The transparency of irrigation fluids used in endoscopic surgery. J Endourol. 2017;31(7):701–4. Available from: https://pubmed.ncbi.nlm.nih.gov/28385032/
19. Kajbafzadeh A. Congenital urethral anomalies in boys. Part I: posterior urethral valves. Urol J. 1997;2(2):59–78. Available from: https://pubmed.ncbi.nlm.nih.gov/17602414/
20. Sarhan O, El-Ghoneimi A, Hafez A, Dawaba M, Ghali A, Ibrahiem E-H. Surgical complications of posterior urethral valve ablation: 20 years experience. J Pediatr Surg. 2010;45(11):2222–6. Available from: http://www.ncbi.nlm.nih.gov/pubmed/21034948

Part VI

Miscellaneous

Prenatal Minimally Invasive Procedures for Fetal Lower Urinary Tract Obstruction

51

Rodrigo Ruano, Ayssa Teles Abrao Trad, and Jose L. Peiro

51.1 Introduction

Fetal lower urinary tract obstruction (LUTO) is a bladder outlet obstruction resultant from congenital renal outflow tract anomalies. It represents a spectrum of pathologies characterized by dilated fetal bladder and bilateral hydronephrosis that can occur as an isolated defect (isolated LUTO) or be accompanied by other congenital abnormalities in approximately 20% of cases (complex LUTO) [1].

LUTO is associated with high degree of perinatal mortality and long-term morbidity. The severity of obstruction is highly variable and dependent on the underlying mechanism; posterior urethral valve (PUV) is the most common cause of LUTO, representing up to 63% of cases in male fetuses. Other causes include urethral atresia, urethral stenosis, and prune belly syndrome [2].

Cloacal malformation and obstructive ureterocele impacted in the bladder neck are the most common causes of LUTO in females. In cloaca, due to the urine outlet obstruction and the reflux to the vaginal cavity, there will be a progressive vaginal enlargement (hydrocolpos) that is observed in 30% of the patients, which eventually compress the adjacent structures, such as the ureterovesical junction [3].

Mild forms of the disease in LUTO can have favorable outcomes but, when more severe, usually formed early in gestation, it leads to dysplastic kidney changes and eventually oligohydramnios or anhydramnios that may result in secondary pulmonary hypoplasia and renal failure [4].

Supplementary Information The online version contains supplementary material available at [https://doi.org/10.1007/978-3-030-99280-4_51].

R. Ruano
Maternal-Fetal Medicine Division, Department of Obstetrics and Gynecology, Mayo Clinic, Rochester, MN, USA

Obstetrics & Gynecology and Pediatrics, Mayo Clinic College of Medicine, Rochester, MN, USA

Fetal Diagnostic and Therapeutic Section, Department of Obstetrics and Gynecology, Mayo Clinic, Rochester, MN, USA
e-mail: Ruano.Rodrigo@mayo.edu

A. T. A. Trad
Maternal-Fetal Medicine Division, Department of Obstetrics and Gynecology, Mayo Clinic, Rochester, MN, USA
e-mail: TelesAbraoTrad.Ayssa@mayo.edu

J. L. Peiro (✉)
University of Cincinnati Medical College, Cincinnati, OH, USA

Cincinnati Children's Fetal Care Center, Pediatric General and Thoracic Surgery Division, Cincinnati Children's Hospital Medical Center (CCHMC), Cincinnati, OH, USA
e-mail: Jose.Peiro@cchmc.org

C. Esposito et al. (eds.), *Minimally Invasive Techniques in Pediatric Urology*,
https://doi.org/10.1007/978-3-030-99280-4_51

51.2 Epidemiology

LUTO affects two to three infants per 10,000 live births. A higher incidence is expected when including elective termination and intrauterine fetal death. It is more common in male fetuses and no risk factors have been identified for non-syndromic cases of LUTO. Mortality rates vary but can be as high as 80% to 90% [3]; LUTO is responsible for 15% to 20% of pediatric end-stage renal failure [5] as well as 10 to 60% of pediatric renal transplants [2].

51.3 Prenatal Diagnosis

LUTO is diagnosed antenatally with ultrasound (US) examination demonstrating consequences of outlet obstruction (Fig. 51.1) such as distended bladder with thickened wall, ureteral dilation, renal hyper-echogenicity, bilateral hydronephrosis, subcortical renal cysts, renal dysplasia, or severe oligohydramnios (amniotic fluid index <5 cm or maximum vertical pocket <2 cm). More severe forms of the disease can be perceived in the first trimester, but the majority is diagnosed at the time of routine anatomic survey in the second trimester. Fetal anatomic ultrasound screening has improved prenatal detection of the disease with a 29% increase in diagnosis demonstrated over the course of 14 years [5].

The sensitivity of US diagnosis of LUTO has been set by two large studies between 50% and 59% [1, 5]. However, when looking at specific parameters, such as renal hyper-echogenicity, sensitivity has been shown to reach numbers as high as 95% [5]. According to a retrospective cohort study, dilated bladder and thickened bladder wall were the best indicators of LUTO, with sensitivities of 96.8% and 93.5%, respectively [6].

Comprehensive fetal anatomic survey is warranted to rule out complex LUTO; fetal echocardiography, genetic counseling, chorionic villous sampling, and amniocentesis are all components of the investigation depending on initial presentation and clinical suspicion. Recent studies suggest diagnostic benefit from adding magnetic resonance imaging (MRI) to the workup of fetuses with LUTO (Fig. 51.2), reasoning that whereas US evaluation may be difficult with reduction in amniotic fluid, MRI is not affected and may confirm the diagnosis as well as provide additional information [7].

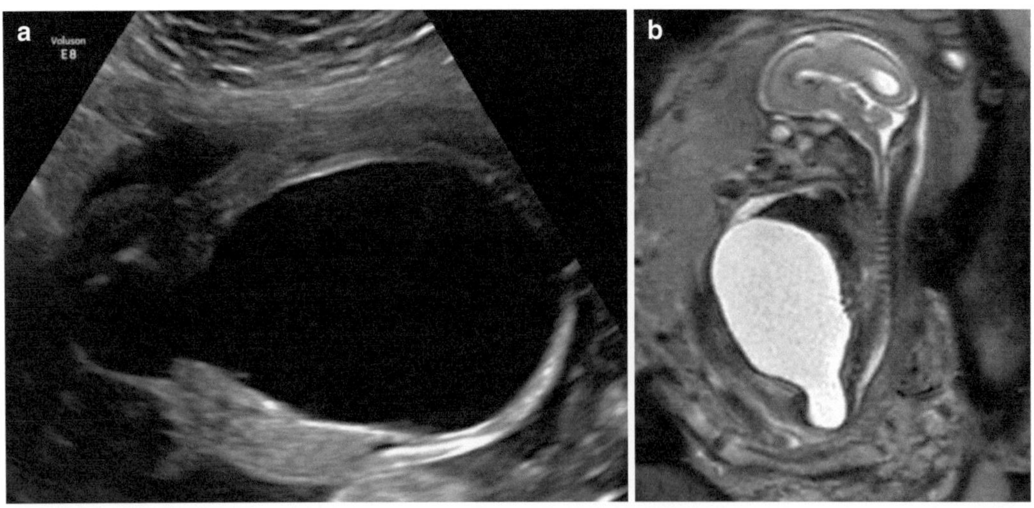

Fig. 51.1 Prenatal ultrasounds (**a**) and fetal MRI (**b**) at 22 weeks' gestation. Posterior urethral valves (PUV) showing distended bladder and posterior urethra (keyhole sign) with anhydramnios. (Images from Cincinnati Fetal Care Center)

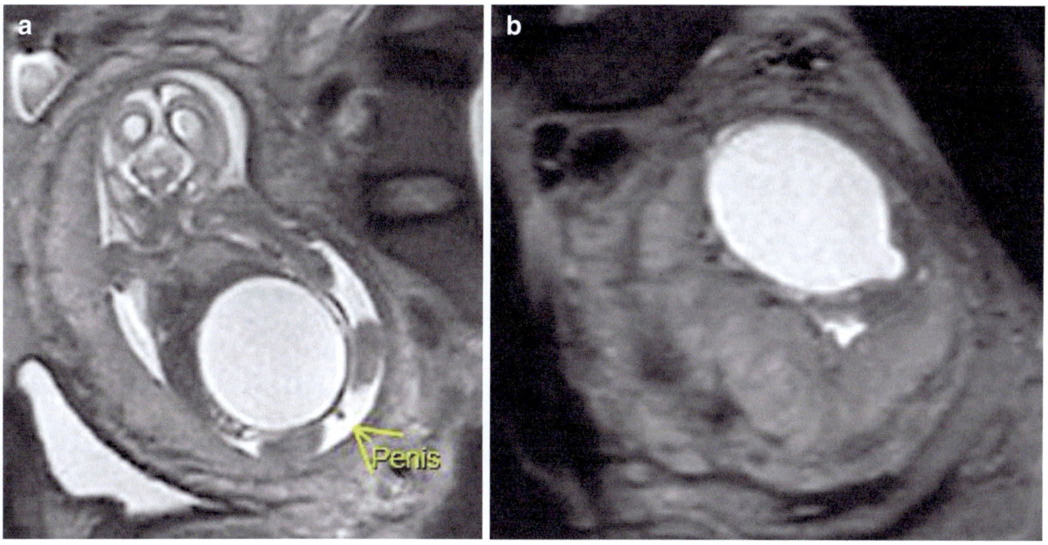

Fig. 51.2 Fetal MRI coronal (**a**) and axial (**b**) sections. Urethral atresia showing distended bladder and posterior urethra (keyhole sign) with oligohydramnios. Amnioinfusion before US and MRI can improve imaging resolution and diagnosis. (Images from Cincinnati Fetal Care Center)

51.4 Prognosis

Several markers have been studied to possibly aid the practitioner in providing prognostic information to the prospective parents. Sonographic findings of megacystis greater than 12 mm that only resolve after the 23rd week of pregnancy have been associated with very poor prognosis [8]. Other sonographic indicators of poor prognosis include hyper-echogenicity of the kidneys, presence of cortical cysts, and absence of amniotic fluid during the critical canalicular phase of fetal lung development [9], between the 16th and 25th week of gestation.

Prognostic indicators for fetal renal function should be used in combination with sonographic findings. Favorable renal function is characterized by fetal urine with electrolyte biochemistry within the parameters of sodium <100 mEq/L, chloride <90 mEq/L, osmolality <200 mOsm/L, and Beta-2-microglobulin <6 mg/L [10]. In addition, it has been demonstrated that fetal bladder refilling of <27% in 48 h after vesicocentesis is correlated to high probability of progression to intrauterine renal failure and the need for dialysis shortly after birth [11].

51.5 Treatment

51.5.1 Rationale for Fetal Intervention

The correct selection of candidates for fetal intervention is important to avoid unnecessary procedures and related complications in those who are likely to survive without any intervention. The rationale for fetal intervention is based on the understanding of the natural course and detrimental outcomes of LUTO. By permitting restoration of the amniotic fluid volume, fetal therapy has the potential to ameliorate pulmonary hypoplasia and possibly prevent end-stage renal disease [2].

It is accepted that patients most likely to benefit from invasive procedures have a normal karyotype, lack other developmental abnormalities, and have oligohydramnios/anhydramnios as well as a favorable urinary biochemistry.

51.5.2 Treatment Based on Prenatal Classification

After a diagnosis of LUTO, physicians must determine who would benefit from fetal therapy.

In addition to the expected risks inherent to any fetal intervention, the outcomes presented in the literature are conflicted, likely because of lack of standardization in candidate selection, uncovering the need for a staging tool.

In 2012, there was an attempt to standardize LUTO prenatal evaluation and develop a classification system to better define subsets of patients that would benefit from fetal intervention. The proposed classification, according to severity, defines three stages: I (mild LUTO), II (severe LUTO with prenatal findings suggestive of preserved fetal renal function), and III (severe LUTO with prenatal findings suggestive of fetal abnormal renal function). It takes into consideration variables of amount of amniotic fluid, echogenicity of fetal kidneys, renal cortical cysts, renal dysplasia, and fetal urinary biochemistry. According to this classification, fetal intervention is indicated in stage II patients to prevent pulmonary hypoplasia and severe renal impairment. Stage III patients would require further studies to determine the potential benefit [12] and as there is no fetal urine production to fill the amniotic cavity with any bladder drainage or diversion. The only way to obtain a pulmonary survivor is to replace amniotic fluid from an external source by serial percutaneous ultrasound-guided amnioinfusions or amnioport placement.

In 2017, a staging system that stratifies disease severity by structural abnormalities identified with US and sequential fetal biochemistry measurements at 18–30 weeks was introduced by Ruano et al. [13]. With the aim of determining appropriate interventions, the characteristic features of the Ruano staging system are as follows: stage I LUTO is a mild form, with normal fetal renal anatomy (normal echogenicity, no cysts or dysplasia), normal amniotic fluid index, and favorable fetal urinary biochemistry at 18–30 weeks; bladder dilation or hydronephrosis may be present. These patients have an overall good prognosis and can have a conservative management with weekly US monitoring.

Stage II LUTO is characterized by oligohydramnios (or anhydramnios), fetal renal hyperechogenicity but without cysts or dysplasia, and favorable fetal biochemistry after a maximum of three sequential samplings. The prognosis of these patients is uncertain, but they are candidates for fetal intervention (vesicoamniotic shunting or fetal cystoscopy) to prevent secondary pulmonary hypoplasia due to oligohydramnios.

Fetuses with stage III LUTO have severe obstruction, fetal renal hyper-echogenicity with cysts or dysplasia, anhydramnios, and an unfavorable urinary biochemistry. These patients are also candidates for fetal intervention (vesicoamniotic shunting with or without serial amnioinfusion) but they have a poor prognosis, and there is still a need for additional evidence supporting the benefit of intervention.

Stage IV LUTO is a progression of stage III which occurs spontaneously or after fetal vesicoamniotic shunt placement. It is associated with end-stage renal disease even before birth. US findings show renal hyper-echogenicity with cysts and dysplasia, anhydramnios, and fetal anuria (bladder filling rate $\leq$ 27% after initial vesicocentesis). The prognosis of stage IV LUTO is extremely poor, and there are no viable prenatal treatment options for these patients. Management usually involves palliative care; serial amnioinfusion from an external source may also be useful for intrauterine fetal renal failure but this warrants further study.

51.5.3 Therapeutic Options

There are five potential prenatal interventions for LUTO in addition to termination of pregnancy: fetal vesicoamniotic shunt (VAS) placement and/or fetal cystoscopy, and less likely fetal vesicostomy, when fetal urine production is still present, and serial amnioinfusion or amnioport, when there is not fetal urine production to supply fluid for the amniotic cavity. Benefit in postnatal survival has been demonstrated with VAS and fetal cystoscopy [12] but preserved renal function in 2 years is a proven benefit of only the latter [14, 15].

Vesicoamniotic shunting aims for sustained bladder decompression with the help of a bladder catheter that allows continuous bladder drainage. Due to the small caliber and long length of the catheter, complete decompression may not be seen in all cases. Complications related to bladder shunts occur in up to 45% of cases which include shunt blockage (25%) and shunt migration (20%) as well as urinary ascites, preterm labor, chorioamnionitis, and iatrogenic gastroschisis. The most serious maternal complication related to vesicoamniotic shunting is infection which increases the risk for fetal death. Shunt displacement from the bladder may cause urine ascites, massive fetal abdomen distention, diaphragmatic elevation, intra-abdominal and intrathoracic hemodynamic changes, and even fetal hydrops [4].

Open fetal surgery for vesicostomy requires the fetal abdomen to be opened below the umbilical cord insertion. The bladder is opened and sutured to the fetal skin, allowing urine to outflow [16]. This procedure was offered by some fetal surgeons in highly selected cases to achieve a permanent and complete bladder decompression to restore the amniotic fluid and prevent pulmonary hypoplasia at birth. The goal is to achieve bladder drainage without the inconvenient of clotting or dislodgement that happens with VAS. Nowadays, it is considered experimental and should balance the risk/benefit ratio, as the hysterotomy required to perform the fetal vesicostomy carries the risks of open fetal surgery in general such as prematurity and dehiscence of the uterine scar.

Fetal cystoscopy involves direct visualization of the urinary outflow tract for etiological diagnosis and specific treatment. The longer procedure duration and need for minimal maternal movement generates the need for regional anesthesia. Fetal cystoscopy provides visual diagnosis of the cause of obstruction, differentiating PUV from complete urethral atresia. When visualization and angle is appropriate, laser ablation of the valves is probably the best choice, but if not, the placement of a double-J transurethral catheter remains a good alternative. To obtain a better visualization entering from the dome of the bladder, some surgeons prefer a maternal minilaparotomy to mobilize the fetus and the uterus before insertion of the trocar. PUV ablation is a challenging procedure associated with technical limitations that can lead to complications such as urological fistulas (in approximately 10% of the cases) and prematurity with a mean gestational age at delivery of 34.6 ± 2.5 weeks [17]. Other possible origin of bladder neck obstruction is prolapsed ureterocele, which can be incised and decompressed by laser through fetal cystoscopy or fetoscopy [18].

Serial amnioinfusion has been indicated under experimental bases in cases of patients with LUTO with a poor prognostic profile such as stage IV, who are not candidates for the previously established fetal interventions. This procedure involves repeated infusion of sterile warm saline or lactated Ringer's solution to restore amniotic fluid for oligohydramnios until 28–30 weeks with the intent to prevent severe pulmonary hypoplasia and perinatal demise. If pulmonary development is sufficient after birth, neonates will require renal replacement therapy with chronic dialysis and kidney transplant. Ethical and clinical questions persist on its benefits and safety particularly because renal transplantation cannot usually be offered to children under 2 years of age [19].

Amnioport is an innovative technique used experimentally since 2010 which allows instillation of crystalloid solutions, without repetitively puncturing the amniotic sac [20] by subcutaneous insertion of a port venous access system connected to a permanent intrauterine silicone catheter. This procedure is still offered when vesicoamniotic shunt or fetoscopic ablation for suspected posterior urethral valves fails to restore amniotic fluid volume (AFV) but also offered primarily in cases of renal dysplasia with no or inadequate fetal urine production, defined as fetal urine production unable to maintain a deepest vertical pocket >2 cm in the second trimester. The parents should be counseled that this is still considered an unproven therapeutic innovation performed specifically to help prevent lethal pulmonary hypoplasia and not to treat the fetal urinary system.

51.6 Preoperative Preparation

After extensive counseling, the patient elects to proceed with fetal intervention in hope to release or bypass the obstruction to improve the outcome of the fetus. We always discuss all potential therapeutic options including transuterine fetal cystoscopy, possible laser ablation or disruption of the posterior urethral valves, and transurethral catheter placement if possible, with a fall back plan of vesicoamniotic shunt placement. Informed consent should be obtained and all of patient and her family's questions answered.

Patients are screened at admission and placed in an NPO diet. Vitals including blood pressure, heart rate, temperature, as well as pain score and urine are checked at regular intervals. Preoperative prophylaxis includes intravenous antibiotics (e.g., cefazolin 2 g + metronidazole in NaCl 500 mg) and tocolysis (magnesium sulfate 6 g bolus followed by 2 g/h or indomethacin 25 mg Q8 for 24 h or nifedipine 10 mg Q8 for 24 h).

51.7 Maternal and Fetal Positioning

The patient is taken to the operating room after informed consent is obtained. Maternal anesthesia varies depending on the service from a combination of local skin anesthesia with maternal sedation to a combination of epidural analgesia and general anesthesia. The mother is placed in the supine position with a left uterine tilt.

Once the mother is anesthetized, patient is prepped in a sterile fashion and ultrasound probe is placed in a sterile sheath. Fetal position is carefully evaluated as well as the scope or shunt trocar entry in the uterus is meticulously planned, using color-Doppler to verify the absence of vasculature.

51.8 Fetal Surgical Techniques and Instruments

51.8.1 Vesicoamniotic Shunting

There are basically two types of VAS catheters, the Rodeck and the Harrison, both based on a multi-perforated double pigtail tube. The shunts themselves are constructed differently in terms of material and size, and in addition their insertion techniques slightly differ (Fig. 51.3). Recently, appeared in the market a new auto-expandable shunt, which VAS apparently is associated with a lower rate of early dislocation and feasible for the first trimester [21].

For this procedure, fetal anesthesia using fentanyl (15 μgL/kg) and pancuronium (0.5 to 2 mg/kg) is administered either via intramuscular using

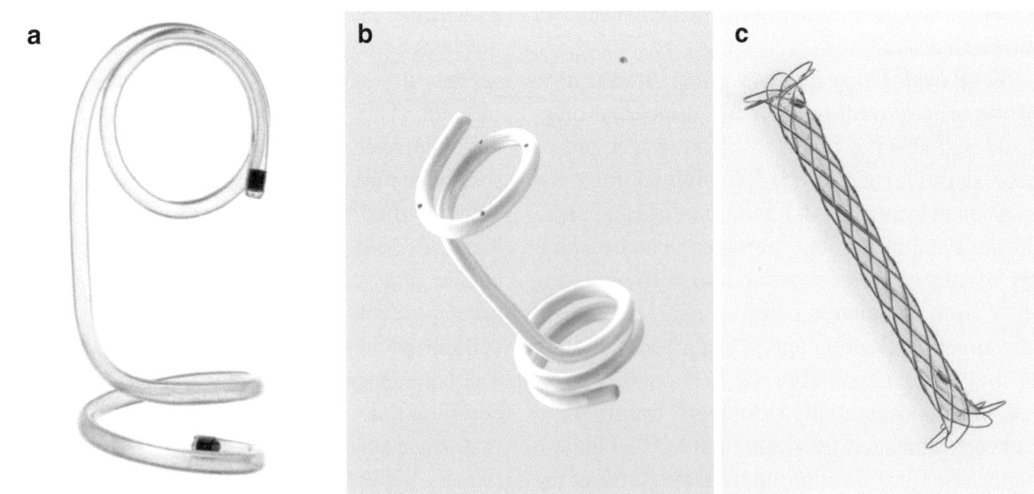

Fig. 51.3 Different types of vesicoamniotic shunts. (**a**) Rodeck. (**b**) Harrison. (**c**) Somatex

an ultrasound-guided 22-gauge needle or through an umbilical vein injection. An entry site for the shunt trocar (a double pig tailed catheter) is selected by using color-Doppler ultrasonography to check for vascularity, and the skin is then entered by stab incision with a #11 scalpel. Under continuous ultrasound guidance, the fetal shunt needle and trocar are introduced into the amniotic cavity and carefully advanced into the bladder of the fetus. The sharp needle is then removed, and the shunt is introduced down the shaft of the needle using the pusher; the distal loop of the shunt must be seen by ultrasound in the fetal bladder before withdrawing the trocar through the fetal abdominal wall until the distal coils of the shunt are deployed into the amniotic cavity. After double-checking the correct position of the shunt using ultrasounds, the needle is removed from the maternal abdomen.

Severe oligohydramnios and anhydramnios represent the main technical difficulty to place a catheter in those patients; therefore, amnioinfusion immediately before placing the vesicoamniotic shunt is necessary. Please see the description of the procedure below (serial amnioinfusion). It is also important to place the shunt as low as possible in the bladder, in order to prevent catheter displacement after bladder decompression. The trocar needs to be carefully manipulated inside the amniotic cavity to avoid misplacing the shunt into the fetal abdomen or maternal uterine wall, and sometimes a gentle manipulation of the fetus away from the maternal uterine wall is required.

51.8.2 Fetal Cystoscopy

51.8.2.1 Percutaneous Ultrasound-Guided Fetal Cystoscopy

Fetal anesthesia should also be administered for this intervention. Under conventional two-dimensional ultrasound guidance, a curved trocar for the fetoscope is introduced percutaneously into the distended fetal bladder through the maternal abdomen, uterine wall, and amniotic cavity. Once inside the fetal bladder, the fetoscope with at least 70° field of view is inserted into the trocar sheath and directed toward the bladder neck with dilated proximal urethra [22, 23].

If fetal PUVs are identified, it can be treated using hydro-ablation, guide wire, or laser fulguration of occluding membranes by introducing a laser fiber into the upper channel and emitting shots of pulsed neodymium-doped yttrium aluminum garnet (Nd:YAG) or diode, laser using low power (maximum 30 W) setting, and 100 Joules; the procedure is concluded when the bladder is found to be empty and Doppler ultrasound confirms passage of fluid through the patent urethra into the amniotic cavity. If a nonmembrane-like obstructive structure is found, then the diagnosis is likely urethral atresia and no attempt to perforate this structure should be undertaken. The procedure should then be converted to VAS placement.

51.8.2.2 Maternal Mini-Laparotomy-Assisted Fetal Cystoscopy

A vertical infra-umbilical midline incision is performed before dissecting down to the fascia level using electrocautery. The fascia is split at the midline to expose the uterus. At this point, anesthesia team should titrate to relax the uterine tone with inhalation anesthetic agents. Ultrasound is then used to confirm the position of the fetus, the location of the posterior urethra, and the distended bladder. It is also recommended to mark out the external edges of the placenta if it lays anterior to avoid entering in proximity. Amniocentesis needle is then kindly introduced in the amniotic cavity with US guidance, followed by amnioinfusion before the fetus can be positioned for the best fetal rigid cystoscopic approach.

We use the insertion of two transuterine T-fasteners (about 1 cm apart) into the fetal bladder dome (Fig. 51.4) under ultrasound guidance before inserting a 10-French Cook Check-Flo cannula, originally designed for vascular access, by Seldinger technique, or using a sharp trocar, also under ultrasound guidance (Fig. 51.5). The fetal intravesical T-fasteners allow the bladder wall to be on traction and in contact with the fetal abdominal wall to prevent ascites and orientate better the rigid cystoscope from the dome to the

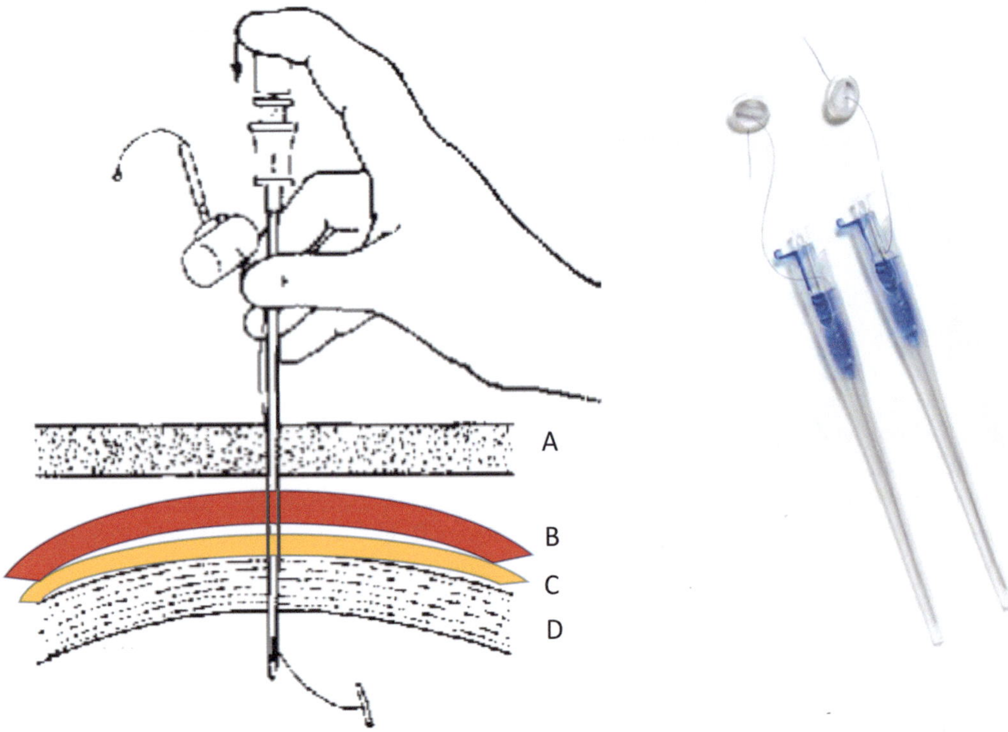

Fig. 51.4 T-fasteners to prepare the fetal bladder for access with rigid cystoscopy. Anchorage of the layers: (**a**) Maternal abdominal wall, (**b**) uterine wall, (**c**) fetal abdominal wall, and (**d**) fetal vesical wall

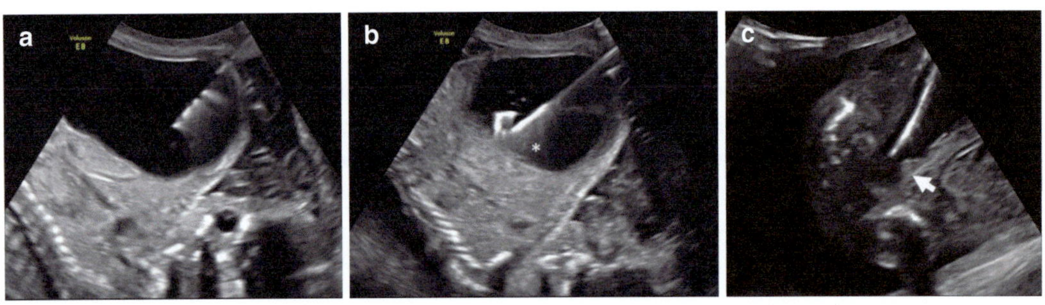

Fig. 51.5 Ultrasound guidance during fetal rigid cystoscopy at 22 weeks' gestation for PUV. (**a**) Intravesical needle, after T-fasteners placed. (**b**) Wire introduction for Seldinger insertion of 10-Fr cannula. (**c**) Intravesical rigid cystoscope facing posterior urethra. (Images from Cincinnati Fetal Care Center)

bladder neck and the distended posterior urethra. At this point, we can advance the 2.7 mm sheath fetoscope that contains the 2 mm telescope into the distended bladder and posterior urethra. A visual diagnosis of the obstructed fetal urethra is performed, identifying either posterior urethral valves or a blind end corresponding to a urethral atresia (Fig. 51.6). By inserting a wire through the fetoscope and attempt to pass it beyond the posterior urethra, we can assess the nature of the obstruction. In case of atresia, we can place a vesicoamniotic shunt through the same passage of the fetoscope (Fig. 51.7). Usually, we insert a Rocket shunt through the Cook cannula into the fetal bladder without problems under ultrasound guidance. The shunt can be completely deployed using the fetoscope with the second end of the shunt positioned well in the amniotic space.

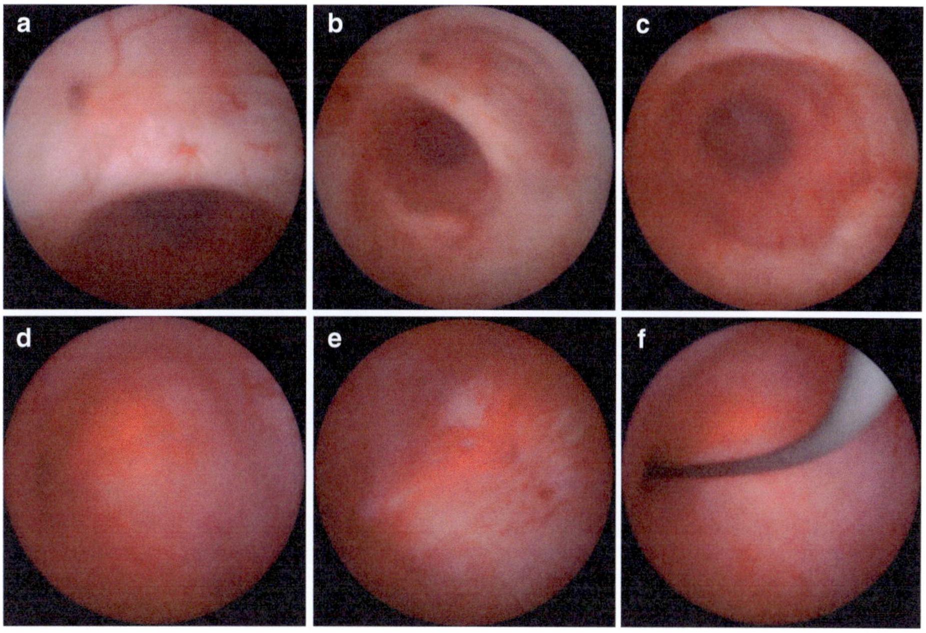

Fig. 51.6 Fetal cystoscopy for urethral atresia. (**a**) Fetal bladder with ureteral orifices. (**b**) Bladder neck. (**c**) A closer view of bladder neck. (**d**) Looking for possible PUV. (**e**) Identification of obstruction with thick tissue. (**f**) Insertion of a wire through the fetoscope in an attempt to pass it beyond the posterior urethra but unable to. These findings suggested urethral atresia as the cause of the BOO. We decided to place a vesicoamniotic Rocket shunt through the same passage of the fetoscope through the Cook introducer into the fetal bladder without problem under ultrasound guidance. (Images from Cincinnati Fetal Care Center)

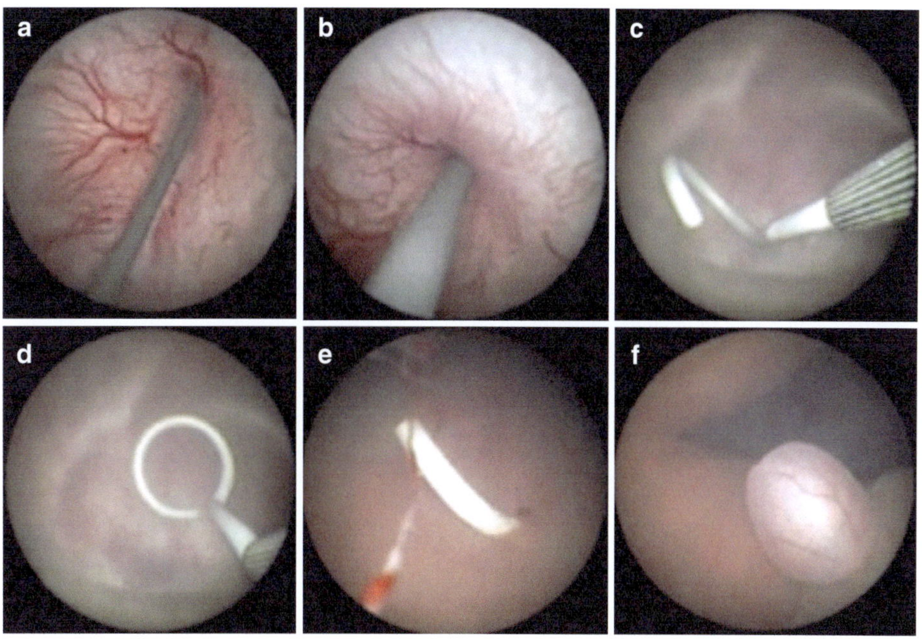

Fig. 51.7 Fetal cystoscopy for urethral atresia and VAS. (**a**) Fetal bladder with probe glide wire. (**b**) Identification of obstruction with thick tissue of urethral atresia. (**c** and **d**) Insertion of a Harrison-type vesicoamniotic shunt through a different passage of the fetoscope under ultrasound guidance and direct visualization. (**e**) Cystoscopic view of the intravesical end of the shunt. (**e**) Fetoscopic intra-amniotic view of the abdominal wall end of the shunt. (**f**) Fetoscopic view of the male genitalia. (Images courtesy from Dr. Marcio L. Miranda)

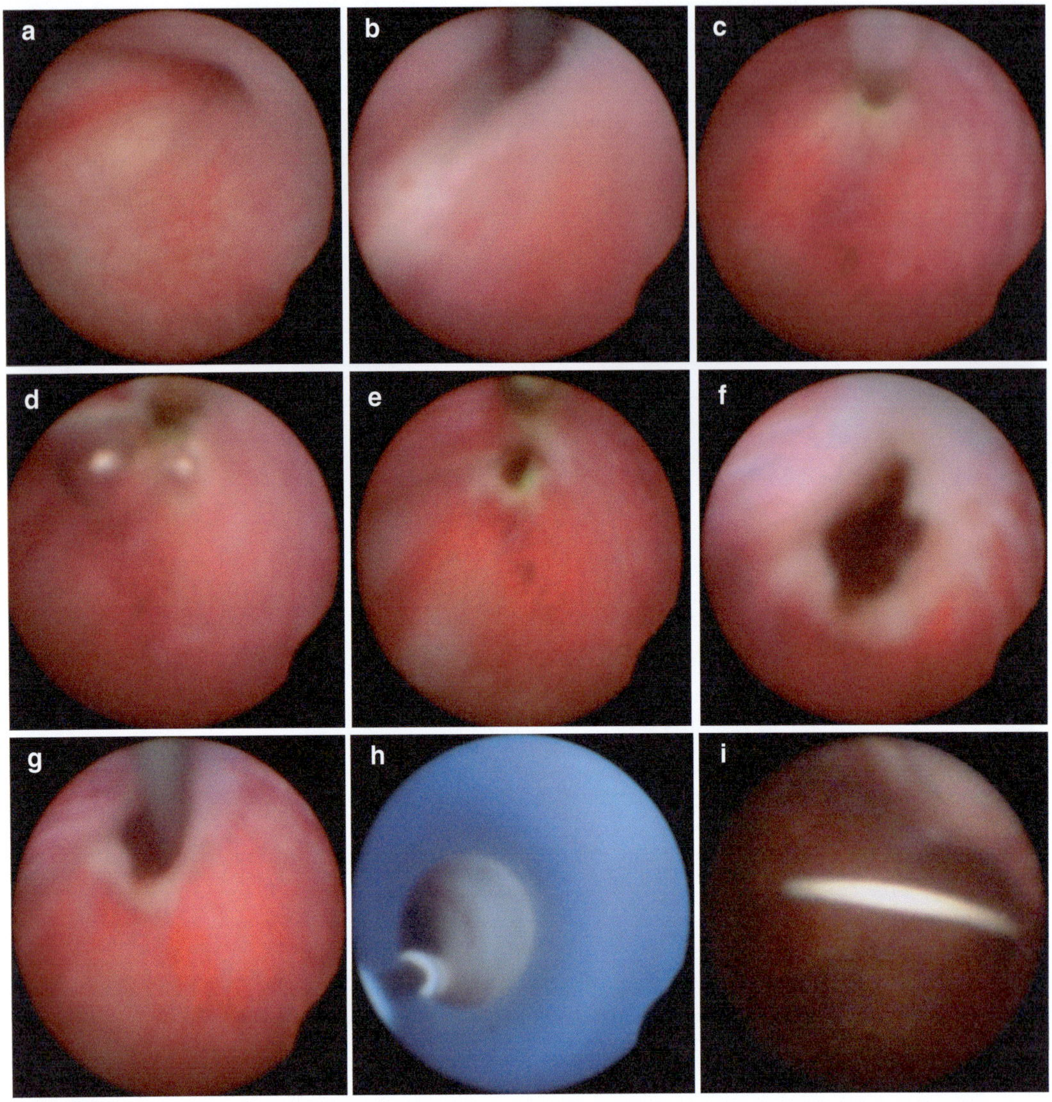

Fig. 51.8 Fetal cystoscopy for PUV. (**a**) Fetal bladder neck. (**b**) Insertion of a wire through the fetoscope in an attempt to pass obstruction on the posterior urethra. These findings suggested the **presence of PUV** as the cause of the BOO. (**c**) Laser fiber at the level of PUV. (**d**) Laser energy with bubbling for valves ablation. (**e**) Already perforated the thickened tissue using 10 watts of laser power. (**f**) Detailed view of perforation and patent urethra. (**g**) Glided wire probing urethral patency through the penis. (**h**) Then, placed a double-J catheter over the transurethral glide wire. (**i**) One end of it remains in the amniotic space while the other end is left inside of the fetal bladder. (Images from Cincinnati Fetal Care Center)

In case we clearly identify posterior urethral valves, we need to pass a glide wire through the fetoscope into the fetal bladder to probe the posterior urethra before **PUV ablation** (Fig. 51.8). Then, the diode 600-micron laser fiber replaces the wire to ablate and perforate the valve tissue using 10–20 watts of laser power. When reinserted the glide wire, we should be able to advance it through the urethra into the amniotic cavity. At this point, optionally, or in the case laser was not used for unsafe angulation or visualization of the valves, a **double J trans-urethral catheter** can be placed (Fig. 51.9). To accomplish that, advance a double-J catheter over the

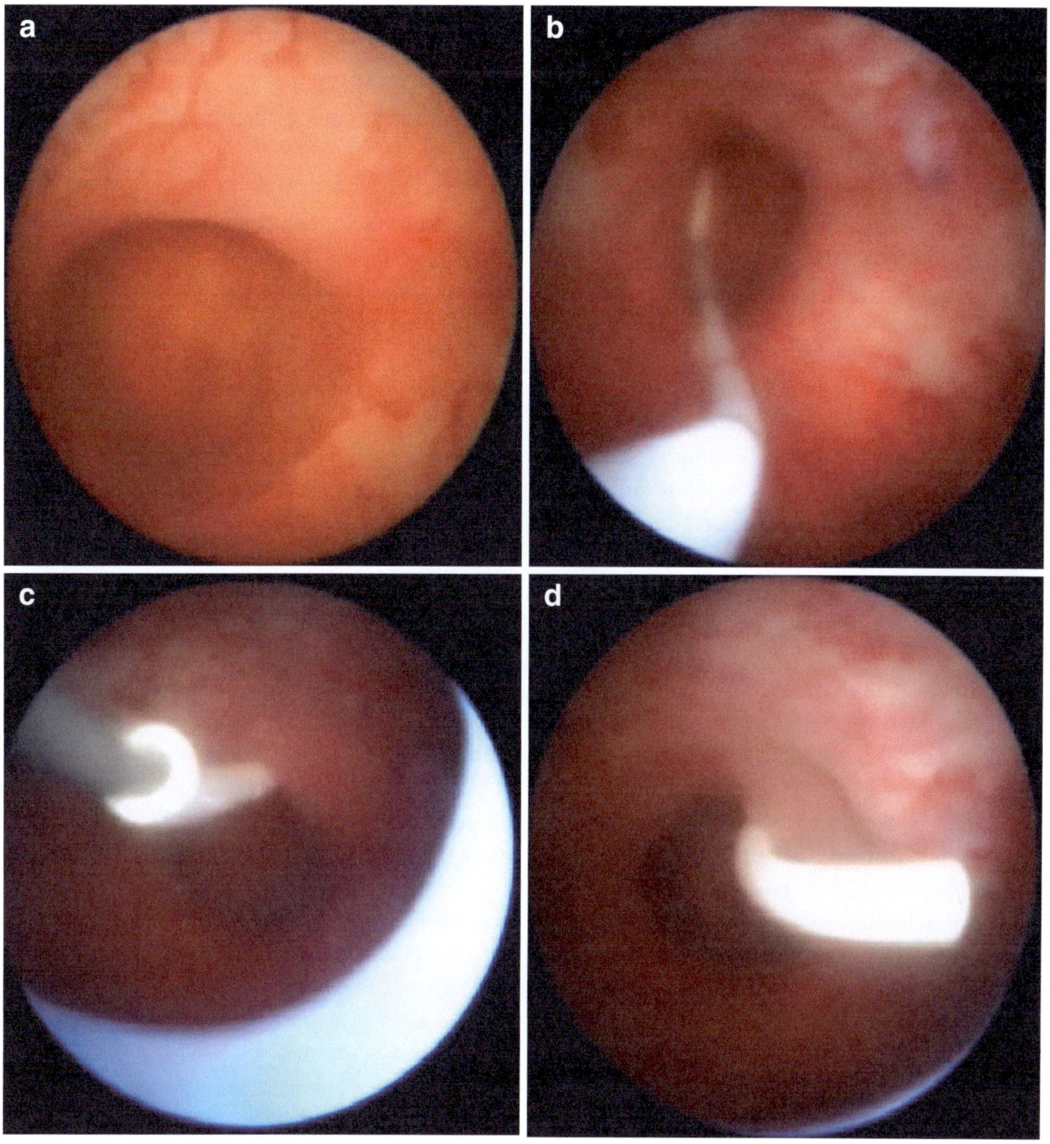

Fig. 51.9 Cystoscopic fetal transurethral catheterization for PUV. (**a**) Fetal bladder neck with enlarged posterior urethra. (**b**) Insertion of a wire through the fetoscope to pass obstruction on the posterior urethra when valves are not well visualized. (**c**) Inserted double-J catheter over the transurethral glide wire. (**d**) Transurethral catheter with view of the end inside the fetal bladder. (Images from Cincinnati Fetal Care Center)

transurethral glide wire until one end of it is in the amniotic space while the other end was left inside of the fetal bladder. Before the double-J catheter is completely deployed, the fetoscope can be inserted in parallel without its outer sheath through the Check-Flo cannula alongside the glide wire to visualize and control the catheter. Rechecking with the complete fetoscope is always possible to confirm the proper position of the catheter and eventually to pull a few centimeters of the catheter back into the bladder under direct fetoscopic vision using 1-mm graspers. We can check the other end of the catheter in the amniotic cavity through the penis exiting the urethral meatus in good position by ultrasound imaging or direct visualization with the fetoscope. We usually instill antibiotics into the fetal bladder and the amniotic cavity. Then, carefully, the fetoscope and the introducer should be removed completely. A simple or figure-of-eight stitch is placed around the Cook cannula before the trocar and the fetoscope are removed. The previously placed figure-of-eight suture is then tied down to form watertight closure of the fetoscopic insertion site. Next, the uterus is repositioned and the peritoneal cavity irrigated. Once hemostasis is reassured, the fascia can be closed using running continuous #1 looped PDS suture. The subcutaneous tissues are closed in layers using interrupted absorbable sutures. The skin incision is then closed using a suture in running subcuticular fashion. Mother and fetus usually tolerate the procedure well, and we need to check periodically that the fetal cardiac rhythm, rate, and function are normal throughout the entire procedure.

51.8.3 Serial Amnioinfusion

51.8.3.1 Percutaneous Ultrasound-Guided Amnioinfusion

This procedure involves repeated infusion of sterile warm saline or lactated Ringer's solution to restore amniotic fluid for oligohydramnios between 20 and 36 weeks' gestation with the intention of preventing severe pulmonary hypoplasia and perinatal demise and promoting a bridge to renal dialysis and transplant. An entry site for the needle is selected by using color-Doppler ultrasonography to check for vascularity. Then, under ultrasound guidance, a 20- or 22-gauge needle is introduced in the amniotic cavity to infuse sterile warm lactate ringer until a normal amount of amniotic fluid is observed (main vertical pocket of 5 or amniotic fluid index of 8 cm). This procedure is repeated subsequently whenever severe oligohydramnios is observed again [19].

51.8.3.2 Serial Amnioinfusion through Amnioport

A maternal small laparotomy is required to partially expose the gravid uterus. Under ultrasound guidance, a 20-gauge EchoTip needle is inserted into the amniotic sac to infuse warm saline to restore a minimum intra-amniotic fluid volume to achieve a normal pocket of amniotic fluid >2 cm and < 8 cm. This can be done during the operation or percutaneously the day before. The introducer needle can then be placed into the created pocket to allow placement of the sheath and introducer via Seldinger. A 6.6-Fr catheter is then placed using the Seldinger technique under ultrasound guidance using the peel-away sheath and introducer inserted into the amniotic space; intra-amniotic antibiotics are instilled at this point. Significant catheter length (more than 30 cm) is threaded through the introducer into the amniotic space under ultrasound guidance. The portion exterior to the uterus is secured by an absorbable purse-string suture at the insertion site and covered by imbricating the uterine serosa over the catheter for 5 cm using a Witzel tunnel technique in order to prevent catheter dislodgement. The catheter is cut to enough length, after passing through the fascia at one side of the laparotomy and then tunneled subcutaneously to a pocket created by another incision usually over the maternal lower costal margin. The reservoir or port venous access system (Cook Medical, Vandergrift, Pa., USA) is secured to the fascia at three points with 3-0 Prolene sutures, leaving the silicon membrane facing up to allow easy percutaneous access using a 20- to 22-gauge needle designed for the port system (Fig. 51.10). The laparotomy and small incisions are closed routinely. Postoperative infusions of normal saline can be done serially, as many times we need, under ultrasound guidance, to maintain the AFV in a normal range. At delivery, the small chest wall incision is reopened to remove the reservoir directly. Then, with gentle traction on the catheter, this can be removed entirely through the chest incision (refer to Video 51.1).

51.9 Postoperative Care

Postoperative care may vary according to the chosen intervention. Commonly, patients are kept in prophylactic antibiotics and prophylactic tocolysis for a maximum 24 h after surgery and

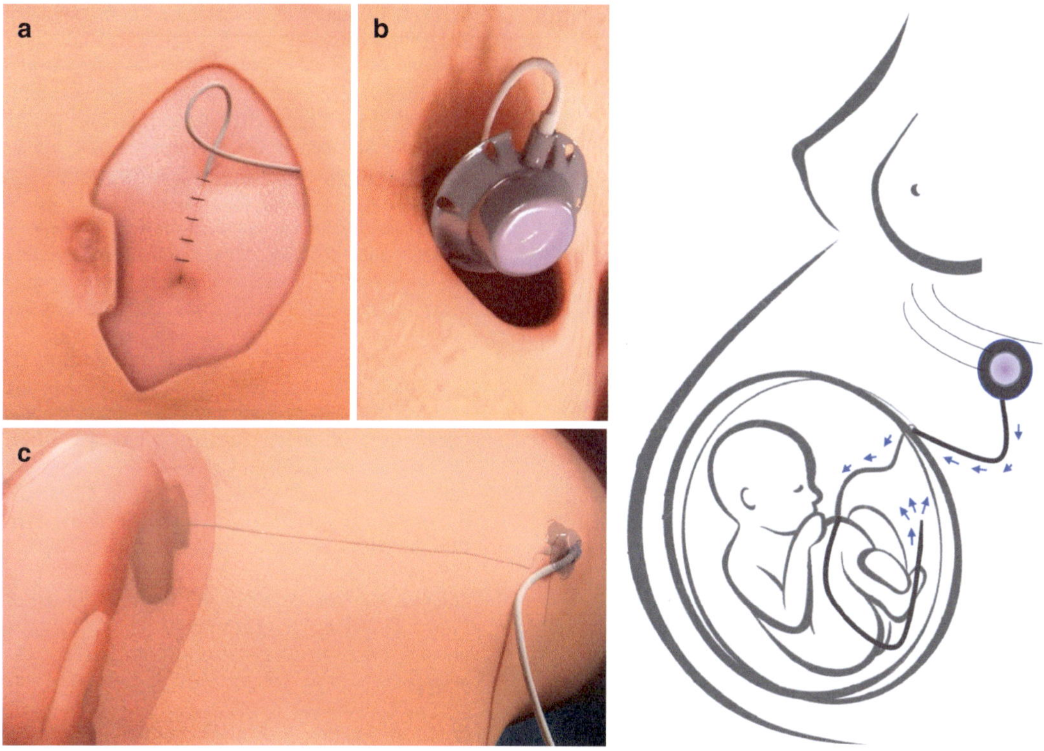

Fig. 51.10 Amnioport placement. (**a**) Intrauterine catheter. (**b**) Costal subcutaneous port system. (**c**) Accessed implanted port with connected subcutaneous and intrauterine catheter ready for amnioinfusion. (Images from Cincinnati Fetal Care Center)

then discharged home within 24 h if no complications arise. A follow-up ultrasound is performed on the first postoperative day before verifying fetal status, bladder condition, and amount of amniotic fluid. Weekly ultrasound follow-up evaluations may be indicated to evaluate fetal shunt dislodgements or re-obstruction of the fetal urethra. A multidisciplinary evaluation and follow-up are necessary for delivery plan and postnatal management.

51.10 Future Directions

Studies with standardized patient populations and long-term follow-up are needed for better establishing the benefits of fetal interventions and to compare both surgical methods based on better classification of the severity of the disease prenatally. Ideally, a randomized controlled trial should be performed with an appropriate urinary obstruction cohort to compare VAS and cystoscopy, with case stratification based on US, fetal urine biochemistry, and the etiology of obstruction.

Amnioinfusion is still an experimental procedure that must be further investigated as a possible treatment for stage IV disease, and a new innovation for neonatal/pediatric technology and treatment to allow for fetal transition to transplantation will contribute.

Take-Home Points

- Fetal lower urinary tract obstruction (LUTO) is a bladder outlet obstruction in the fetuses caused by different congenital anomalies.
- Prenatal diagnosis is mainly based on ultrasound examination.

- Fetal cystoscopy is the only method to visually diagnose prenatally the cause of the LUTO.
- There are different stages of severity of LUTO.
- Specific fetal intervention can be indicated for different stages of the disease.
- Fetal vesicoamniotic shunt placement, fetal cystoscopy, and serial amnioinfusion are current in utero therapeutic options for LUTO.
- The ultimate goal of fetal urological therapy is mostly to obtain a pulmonary survivor by restoring amniotic fluid amount rather than improve renal function as kidney damage happens early in gestation before we can offer any treatment.

References

1. Malin G, Tonks AM, Morris RK, Gardosi J, Kilby MD. Congenital lower urinary tract obstruction: a population-based epidemiological study. BJOG. 2012;119(12):1455–64.
2. Ruano R. Prenatal regenerative fetoscopic interventions for congenital anomalies. BMJ. 2020;370:m1624.
3. Peiro JL, Scorletti F, Sbragia L. Prenatal diagnosis of cloacal malformation. Semin Pediatr Surg. 2016;25(2):71–5.
4. Ruano R. Fetal surgery for severe lower urinary tract obstruction. Prenat Diagn. 2011;31(7):667–74.
5. Anumba DO, Scott JE, Plant ND, Robson SC. Diagnosis and outcome of fetal lower urinary tract obstruction in the northern region of England. Prenat Diagn. 2005;25(1):7–13.
6. Bernardes LS, Aksnes G, Saada J, Masse V, Elie C, Dumez Y, et al. Keyhole sign: how specific is it for the diagnosis of posterior urethral valves? Ultrasound Obstet Gynecol. 2009;34(4):419–23.
7. Pico H, Dabadie A, Bourliere-Najean B, Philip N, Capelle M, Aschero A, et al. Contribution of the foetal uro-MRI in the prenatal diagnosis of uronephropathies. Diagn Interv Imaging. 2014;95(6):573–8.
8. Fontanella F, Duin L, Adama van Scheltema PN, Cohen-Overbeek TE, Pajkrt E, Bekker M, et al. Fetal megacystis: prediction of spontaneous resolution and outcome. Ultrasound Obstet Gynecol. 2017;50(4):458–63.
9. Ibirogba ER, Haeri S, Ruano R. Fetal lower urinary tract obstruction: what should we tell the prospective parents? Prenat Diagn. 2020;40(6):661–8.
10. Enninga EA, Ruano R. Fetal surgery for lower urinary tract obstruction: the importance of staging prior to intervention. Minerva Pediatr. 2018;70(3):263–9.
11. Ruano R, Safdar A, Au J, Koh CJ, Gargollo P, Shamshirsaz AA, et al. Defining and predicting 'intrauterine fetal renal failure' in congenital lower urinary tract obstruction. Pediatr Nephrol. 2016;31(4):605–12.
12. Ruano R, Sananes N, Wilson C, Au J, Koh CJ, Gargollo P, et al. Fetal lower urinary tract obstruction: proposal for standardized multidisciplinary prenatal management based on disease severity. Ultrasound Obstet Gynecol. 2016;48(4):476–82.
13. Ruano R, Dunn T, Braun MC, Angelo JR, Safdar A. Lower urinary tract obstruction: fetal intervention based on prenatal staging. Pediatr Nephrol. 2017;32(10):1871–8.
14. Sananes N, Cruz-Martinez R, Favre R, Ordorica-Flores R, Moog R, Zaloszy A, et al. Two-year outcomes after diagnostic and therapeutic fetal cystoscopy for lower urinary tract obstruction. Prenat Diagn. 2016;36(4):297–303.
15. Nassr AA, Shazly SAM, Abdelmagied AM, Araujo Júnior E, Tonni G, Kilby MD, et al. Effectiveness of vesicoamniotic shunt in fetuses with congenital lower urinary tract obstruction: an updated systematic review and meta-analysis. Ultrasound Obstet Gynecol. 2017;49(6):696–703.
16. Crombleholme TM, Harrison MR, Langer JC, et al. Early experience with open fetal surgery for congenital hydronephrosis. J Pediatr Surg. 1988;23(12):1114–21.
17. Sananes N, Favre R, Koh CJ, Zaloszyc A, Braun MC, Roth DR, et al. Urological fistulas after fetal cystoscopic laser ablation of posterior urethral valves: surgical technical aspects. Ultrasound Obstet Gynecol. 2015;45(2):183–9.
18. Chalouhi GE, Morency AM, De Vlieger R, et al. Prenatal incision of ureterocele causing bladder outlet obstruction: a multicenter case series. Prenat Diagn. 2017;37(10):968–74.
19. O'Hare EM, Jelin AC, Miller JL, Ruano R, Atkinson MA, Baschat AA, et al. Amnioinfusions to treat early onset Anhydramnios caused by renal anomalies: background and rationale for the renal Anhydramnios fetal therapy trial. Fetal Diagn Ther. 2019;45(6):365–72.
20. Polzin WJ, Lim FY, Habli M, Van Hook J, Minges M, Jaekle R, et al. Use of an Amnioport to maintain amniotic fluid volume in fetuses with Oligohydramnios secondary to lower urinary tract obstruction or fetal renal anomalies. Fetal Diagn Ther. 2017;41(1):51–7.
21. Strizek B, Gottschalk I, Recker F, et al. Vesicoamniotic shunting for fetal megacystis in the first trimester with

a Somatex® intrauterine shunt. Arch Gynecol Obstet. 2020;302(1):133–40.
22. Ruano R, Duarte S, Bunduki V, Giron AM, Srougi M, Zugaib M. Fetal cystoscopy for severe lower urinary tract obstruction—initial experience of a single center. Prenat Diagn. 2010;30(1):30–9.
23. Kurtz MP, Koh CJ, Jamail GA, Sangi-Haghpeykar H, Shamshirsaz AA, Espinoza J, et al. Factors associated with fetal shunt dislodgement in lower urinary tract obstruction. Prenat Diagn. 2016;36(8):720–5.

Robot-Assisted Laparoscopy in Differences of Sexual Development: Resection of Embryological Remnants

52

Céline Sinatti, Piet Hoebeke, and Anne-Françoise Spinoit

Learning Objectives

- To describe the different steps of robot-assisted laparoscopic resection of embryological remnants associated with differences of sexual development conditions.
- To present the outcomes of robot-assisted resection of embryological remnants.
- To show a video with the technique of robot-assisted resection of embryological remnants.

52.1 Introduction

Differences of sexual development (DSD) are congenital conditions based on chromosomal and/or gonadal differences leading to a variety of atypical internal and external anatomical sex development. DSD affects approximately 1 in 1000 individuals [1]. Diagnosis, treatment, and follow-up of patients with DSD are performed by a multidisciplinary team of pediatric endocrinologists, pediatric gynecologists, gynecologists, and pediatric urologists, together with psychologists, pathologists, and geneticists. When surgical treatment is needed, it may include reconstruction of the external genitalia and open or laparoscopic investigation of the internal genitalia, the gonads, and the presence of embryological remnants.

Multiple techniques for genital reconstructions are described while surgery of the internal gonadal structures is limited to diagnosis, biopsy, and if applicable removal. The surgery of the internal gonadal structures or Müllerian/Wolffian remnants might benefit from a minimally invasive approach like robot-assisted laparoscopy.

The initial embryo is multipotent, and during evolution, some structures are meant to evolve, while others are meant to disappear in the normal differentiation into male or female embryo.

Table 52.1 provides an overview of the urogenital structures and their normal evolution.

The embryological remnants in men result from incomplete regression of the Müllerian duct, which develops to form the uterine tubes, uterus, and upper part of the vagina in the female. This duct normally regresses at the tenth week of fetal life in in the male under the influence of anti-Müllerian hormone [2] (Fig. 52.1).

In some rare conditions, some ducts do not completely disappear.

Supplementary Information The online version contains supplementary material available at [https://doi.org/10.1007/978-3-030-99280-4_52].

C. Sinatti · P. Hoebeke · A.-F. Spinoit (✉)
Department of Pediatric Urology, Ghent University Hospital, Ghent, Belgium
e-mail: Celine.sinatti@ugent.be; Piet.hoebeke@ugent.be; anne-francoise.spinoit@uzgent.be

C. Esposito et al. (eds.), *Minimally Invasive Techniques in Pediatric Urology*,
https://doi.org/10.1007/978-3-030-99280-4_52

Table 52.1 Overview of urogenital structures and their normal evolution

Paramesonephric ducts	Mesonephric ducts
Also known as Müllerian ducts	Also known as Wolffian ducts
Paired ducts of embryo	
Run down sides of urogenital ridge and terminate in sinus tubercle in primitive urogenital sinus	
In ♀: Fallopian tubes, uterus, cervix, and vagina	In ♀: Urinary system
In ♂: Disappear	In ♂: Urinary system + ductus deferens
Mesodermal origin	

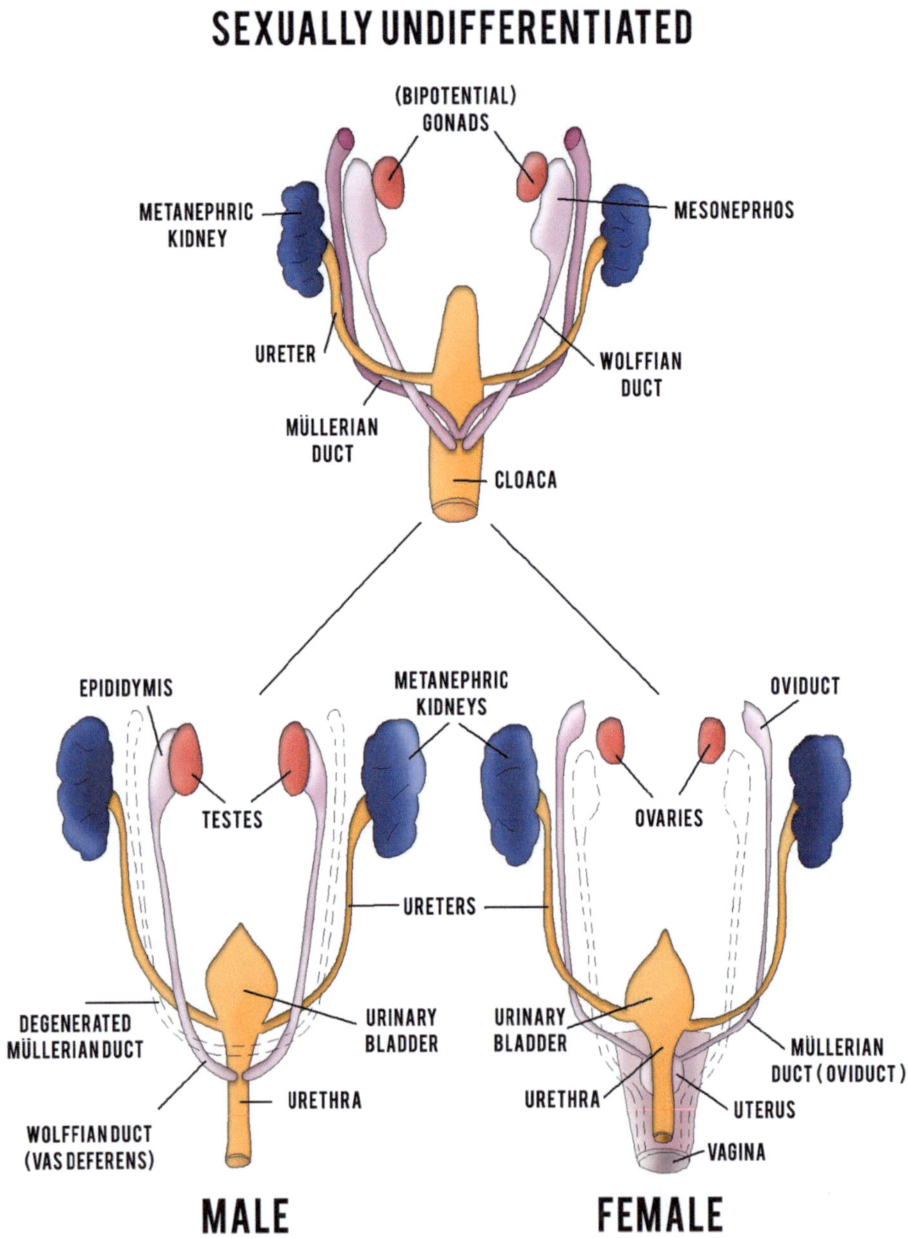

Fig. 52.1 Provides an overview or the primary urogenital system and its evolution. Note the persistence of the Müllerian ducts in female and the persistence of Wolffian ducts in males. (© Illustration by Bram Nevejans)

Various Remnants from Müllerian ducts in boys:

- Hemi-uterus.
- Utricle cyst.

Ectopic kidney in females with aberrant ureteric insertion:

- In uterus.
- In cervix.
- In urethra.

52.1.1 Actual Trends in DSD Surgery

Surgery for DSD was performed early in life and with a sex binary approach striving at maximal feminization in female-assigned individuals and maximal virilization in male-assigned individuals. Recent evolution is that the surgery is often delayed till later age and genital reconstruction is done with more caution.

An important concept related to this evolution is that surgery tends to be as minimalistic as possible and delayed where possible. This minimalistic approach follows the general evolution in technology, allowing mini-invasive surgery when possible.

52.1.2 Background of Minimally Invasive Surgery in Children: The Robotic Platform

Over the last few years, robotic-assisted laparoscopy in pediatric urology has been increasingly embraced, with the pyeloplasty considered as the first and most frequent indication. Two large multicentric comparisons of open pyeloplasty, conventional laparoscopic pyeloplasty, and robot-assisted laparoscopic pyeloplasty showed a high success rate and a significant shorter hospital stay for the robotic approach [3, 4]. Besides pyeloplasty, other reconstructive pediatric urologic cases are described in literature, such as ureteral reimplantation, ureteroureterostomy, Mitrofanoff, and other reconstructive bladder and bladder neck surgery. In our center, robot-assisted laparoscopy is also performed for resection of pelvic embryological remnants in DSD patients when indicated. In Ghent University Hospital, the experience started in 2013 with the Si platform before we merged in 2018 to having two available platforms with dual console, one X and one Xi. All platforms are used in children. The da Vinci Xi® (Intuitive Surgical, Sunnyvale, CA, USA) platform was released in 2014 with several advantages compared to its previous version released in 2006, the da Vinci Si®. These advantages include easier docking, a wider range of motion, an ability to attach the endoscope to any arm, and a better anatomical access in multiquadrant surgeries. Moreover, the camera fits on all 8 millimeters ports, which confers an advantage compared to the 12 mm camera port of the Si system.

52.2 Indications for Minimally Invasive Surgery

Symptomatic embryological remnants and undifferentiated gonads represent the bulk of the surgical indications. In many cases, an initial laparoscopic assessment of the internal gonadal and reproductive structures can be necessary at a young age as part of the diagnostic workup. It is usually a classical diagnostic laparoscopy, for which the robotic platform is not mandatory, even if biopsies need to be harvested.

Resection of a dysgenetic gonad is necessary when it has a high risk for malignancy, even at a young age [5]. Recently there is much more understanding in which conditions dysgenetic gonads are at risk for malignant development [6]. It can be challenging in some cases if those gonads are not in a typical location, and the robotic platform might be a good help.

The robotic platforms offer, with no doubt, a huge advantage for patient and surgeon in case of resection of symptomatic remnants which are often located in deep pelvic positions between other structures.

This chapter is focused on the operative technique of robot-assisted laparoscopic surgery in

DSD with Müllerian remnants in boys and ectopic kidneys with an aberrant ureter in girls.

52.2.1 The Utricle Cyst

The utricle cyst is an embryological remnant of the distal portion of the Müllerian duct system and is a bag-like structure situated between the bladder and the rectum, with an orifice at the prostatic urethra in the seminal colliculus. Utricle cysts are most commonly found in males under 20 years of age and they reportedly occur in 1–5% of the general population [7]. They are often associated with hypospadias; 14% of patients with hypospadias have a concomitant utricle cyst [8]. The utricle cyst is only symptomatic in 5% of the cases causing obstructive and irritative urinary tract symptoms, post-void dripping, and hematuria [7]. As the diagnosis is not always obvious, some patients undergo multiple diagnostic procedures for recurrent urinary tract infections before a utricle cyst is suspected.

A utricle cyst is initially suspected on cystoscopy, where a sacculation with a dorsal opening at the level of the seminal colliculus is seen. A cystography will enforce the presumption by showing an important contrast collection at the proximal urethra. A MRI helps ideally to be performed to allow a detailed anatomical assessment and plan the correct surgical strategy. Figure 52.2 shows a preoperative uroflow is performed to evaluate the urinary flow curve before and after surgery. Typically, an obstructive plateau-shaped curve is seen before surgery due to compression of the urethra through a urine-filled utricle during voiding. In these cases, after surgery a normal clock-shaped curve is observed.

52.2.2 Hemi-Uterus

Persistence of the proximal portion of the Müllerian duct results in the development of the uterus, fallopian tubes, and/or broad ligament at the side of a dysgenetic gonad, as seen in patients with mixed gonadal dysgenesis (MGD). MGD is defined in individuals who typically have a differentiated gonad on one side and a streak gonad (usually intra-abdominal) on the other side [2]. It is also possible that both gonads are dysgenetic and need to be removed. It is a rare clinical entity with a worldwide incidence of 1.5:10000 live births [9]. Sex chromosome mosaicism (45, X/ 46 XY) is the most common karyotype expressed in MGD and often associated with the presence of a (hemi-)uterus [10]. In male-assigned individuals, these female structures are not sex conform and can be removed.

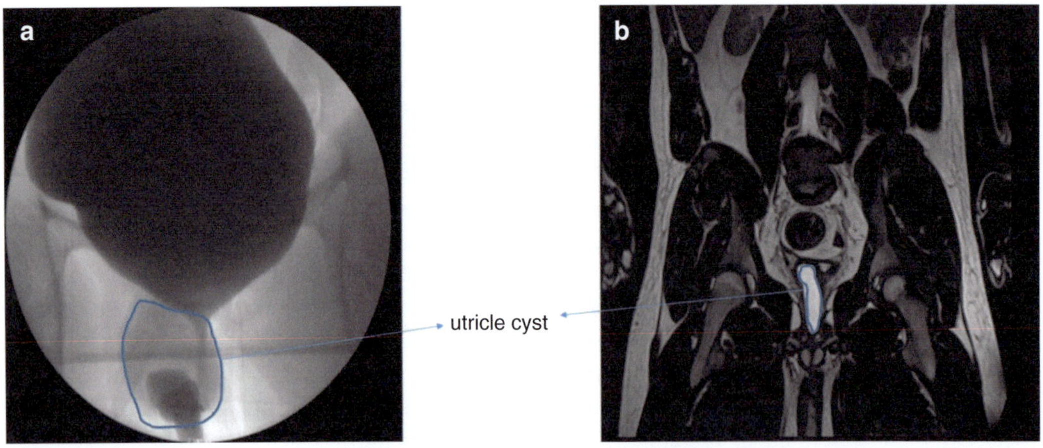

Fig. 52.2 (**a**) Preoperative cystography showing important contrast collecting starting at the proximal urethra. (**b**) Preoperative MRI confirming the diagnosis of a utricle cyst and allowing good anatomical definition of the structure

During clinical examination undescended testis and/or hypospadias may be found. Ultrasound can suggest a uterus-like structure with an intra-abdominal gonad, but visualization might be difficult.

52.2.3 Ectopic Kidney with Aberrant Ureter

Failure of kidney migration during embryonic life results in an ectopic kidney, which can present in several forms: pelvic kidney, ectopic thoracic kidney, and cross-fused renal ectopia. The incidence of a pelvic kidney varies between 1:500 and 1:1200 [11]. The pelvic kidney can be a rare cause of recurrent urinary tract infection (UTI), warranting nephrectomy in some cases, if the kidney is nonfunctional. Most cases of ectopic kidney might remain asymptomatic throughout life, and the clinical recognition is estimated to be only 1:500 to 1:1200 [11]. Pelvic kidneys draining into the vagina in girls cause vaginal discharge and/or incontinence.

When a pelvic kidney with aberrant ureter is suspected, a cystography needs to be performed to exclude vesicoureteral reflux. An ultrasound will show a unique orthotopic kidney on one side and no kidney on the other side. In most cases, it is also possible to locate the ectopic kidney with ultrasound, but it can be really cumbersome. However, to know the precise location of the kidney and the drainage of the ureter, a MRI needs to be conducted. Figure 52.3 shows a DMSA scan is performed to show if the ectopic kidney is functional. In case of a nonfunctional kidney, a nephrectomy needs to be executed. In case of a functional kidney, the ureter needs to be reimplanted.

52.3 Preoperative Preparation

After obtaining consent from the parents and when possible from the child, patient undergoes a general anesthesia with orotracheal intubation, myorelaxation, and antibiotic prophylaxis according to the local hospital's policies.

Patient is brought into a modified lithotomy position with legs in the stirrups. Disinfection and classical draping are realized. If cystoscopy is not planned during the same surgery session, a bladder catheter is placed.

52.4 Positioning

Depending on the system used, the position of the robot will defer. With the Si systems, a classical side-docking position will allow cystoscopy during the procedure (Fig. 52.4). With the X system, a classical side-docking is also pre-

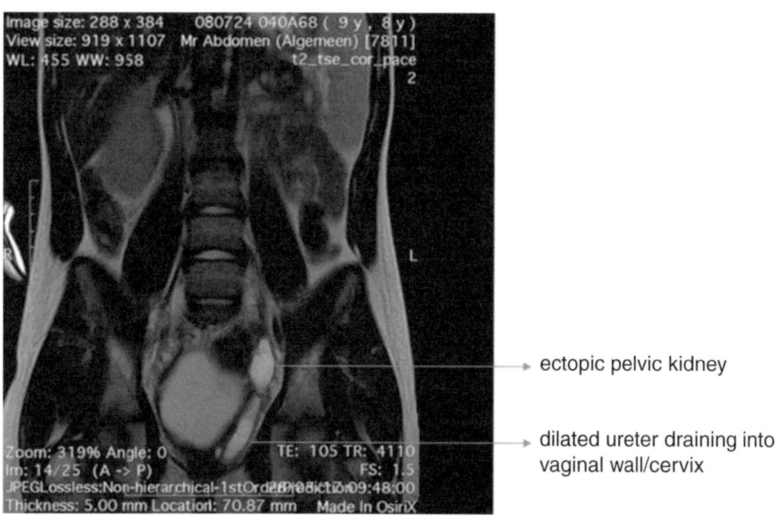

Fig. 52.3 Preoperative MRI shows a dysplastic ectopic kidney located in the pelvis, with dilated ureter draining into the vaginal wall or in the cervix

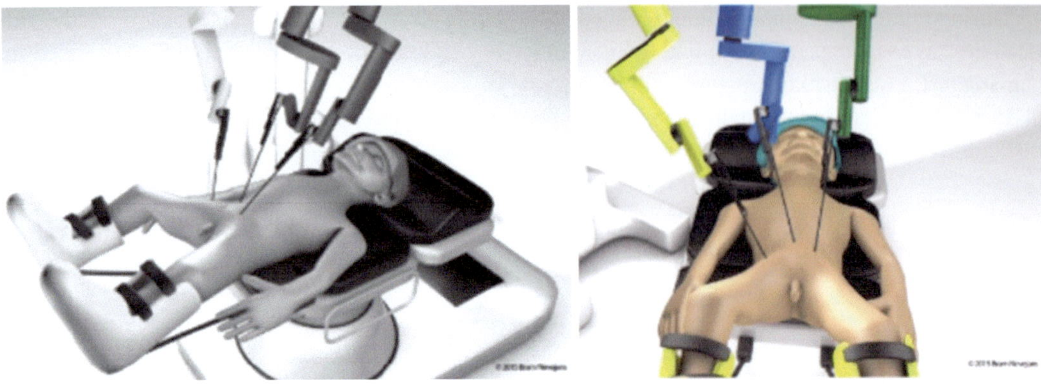

Fig. 52.4 The patient is positioned in a robot adapted lithotomy position with side-docking. (© Illustration by Bram Nevejans)

ferred, while with the Xi, the robot can be positioned anywhere as long it does not stand in the way for possible cystoscopy. Only three robotic arms are used, and in some cases one additional assistant port is used. The camera-trocar is placed in the umbilicus using the Hasson technique [12]. The robotic trocars are placed under sight on the midclavicular line at the level of the umbilicus. The assistant port, when used is placed left (Fig. 52.5). Correct position of the robot while side-docking is essential to allow movement of the instruments in the Si and X systems (Fig. 52.6). Techniques are illustrated in this chapter video (Video 52.1).

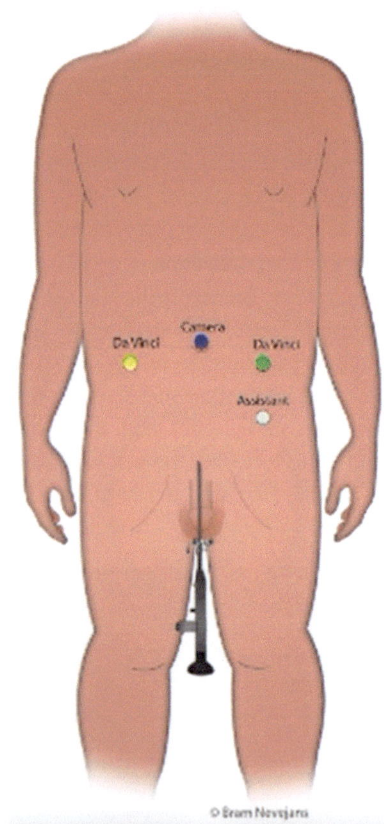

Fig. 52.5 We prefer to use three or four trocars: the optic trocar 8 or 12 mm depending on the system) in the umbilicus, two 8-mm working trocars at the midclavicular line, and eventually a 5-mm assistant trocar placed. (© Illustration by Bram Nevejans)

52.5 Instrumentation

In our center, the Da Vinci Xi® robotic surgical system is used for this procedure. As mentioned above, only three robotic arms and one assistant port are used. We adopt an 8-mm 0-degree camera, two 8-mm instruments, and one 5-mm instrument. We use nontraumatic EndoWrist™ Fenestrated Bipolar Forceps, EndoWrist™ Maryland Bipolar Forceps, EndoWrist™ Large Needle Driver, and EndoWrist™ Monopolar Curved Scissors.

During resection of the utricle cyst, cystoscopy is performed with a 9.5 Fr operative cystoscope.

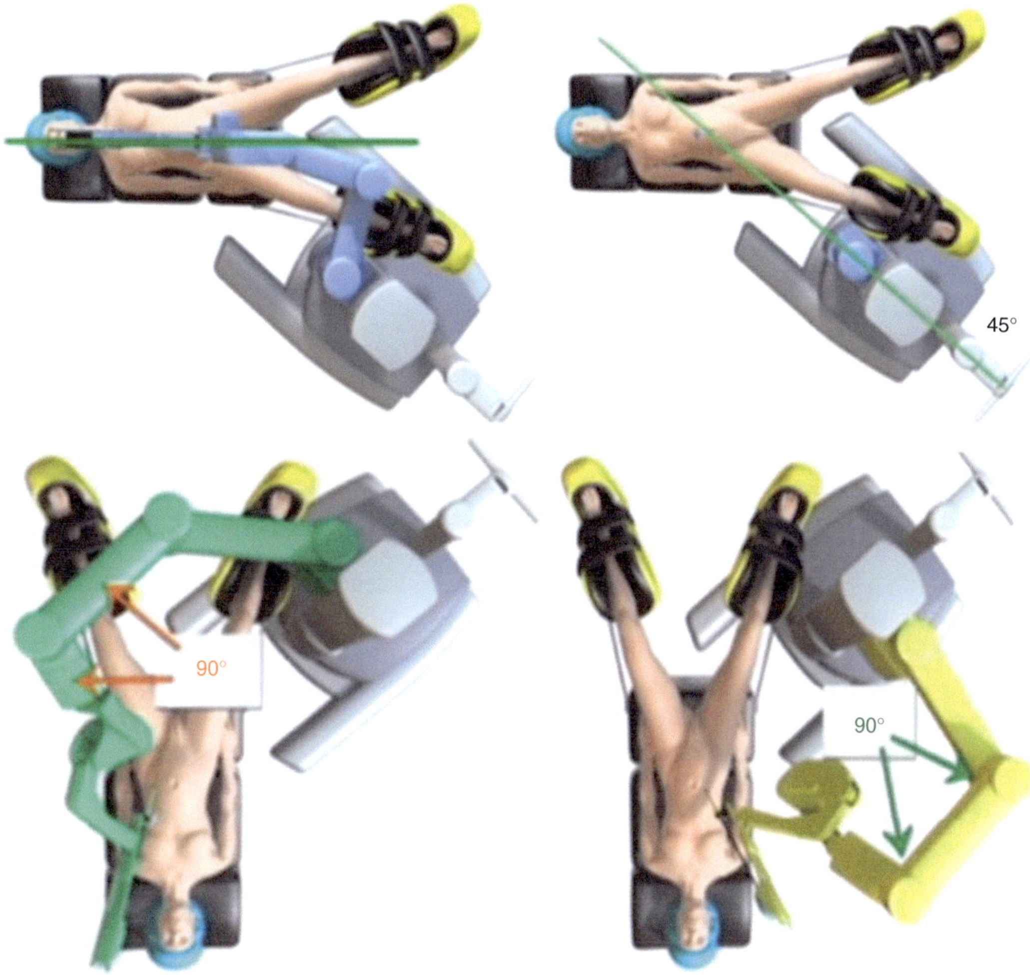

Fig. 52.6 Side-docking of the robotic cart in case of use of the Si and X system. (© Illustration by Bram Nevejans)

52.6 Technique

52.6.1 Utricle Cyst

After opening of the peritoneum, the cyst is progressively dissected from the bladder wall anteriorly and the rectum posteriorly. The vas deferens are identified laterally and left aside. Cystoscopy during the dissection improves identification of the structure while preserving the vas deferens laterally. A traction suture is placed at the proximal end before complete resection is performed. After identification of the cyst neck at the level of the urethra, the cyst is transected leaving a small stump in order to preserve the vas opening into the colliculus. After resection the defect is closed with a barbed wire and the endopelvic fascia is closed. At last, the peritoneum is closed.

52.6.2 The Hemi-Uterus

After opening the peritoneum, diagnostic exploration is performed to identify the uterus-like structure which is located at the side of the dysgenetic gonad. In most cases, the dysgenetic gonad can be found at the internal inguinal ring and is connected to the uterus-like structure by the round ligament. The (hemi-) uterus often ends blindly on the bladder. After identifying the structures, they are selectively resected with mono- and bipolar coagulation. The distal part of uterus-like structure ending on to the bladder is cauterized. The defect of the peritoneum is closed.

52.6.3 The Ectopic Kidney with Aberrant Ureter

After identifying the ectopic kidney, a stay suture is placed in order to retract the ipsilateral ovary from the surgical field. Opening of the peritoneum is performed just over the ectopic kidney. The iliac vessels are identified. The dilated ureter is dissected from the surrounding tissues toward its drainage in the vaginal wall. After placing a stay suture to the distal part of the ureter, the ureter is fully excised. The distal part is cauterized. At last, the defect of the vagina and the peritoneum are closed. A drain is placed in the pelvis in case of large purulent evaluation.

52.7 Postoperative Care

When no postoperative complications occur, the patient can leave the hospital 1 day after surgery. In case of utricle cyst, a bladder catheter should be left in situ for 1 week, and a cystography should be performed at removal to evaluate if the cyst was completely resected. If after 1-year follow-up no new problems occurred and the urinary complaints are resolved, then the patient may be discharged of further follow-up.

52.8 Results

In our center, six patients were treated with a robot-assisted resection of pelvic embryological remnants between 2015 and 2019. Three of them, all male XY patients, had a symptomatic utricle cyst. The fourth patient, a 1-year-old male 45, X/46, XY DSD patient, had a uterus-like structure and an intra-abdominal gonad on ultrasound. Two young girls, 7- and 8-year-olds, had a dysplastic pelvic kidney with ureter draining in the vaginal wall.

52.8.1 Utricle Cyst

For the three patients undergoing a utricle cyst resection, console time was respectively 95, 80, and 85 min. Total surgery time was respectively 135, 120, and 130 min. Estimated blood loss (EBL) was less than 5 mL in all three patients. No intra- or postoperative complications were recorded. The bladder catheter was left in situ for 1 week, and postoperative cystography at removal of the catheter showed complete resection of the cyst. At 1-year follow-up, all three patients showed no further problems and reported complete resolution of the urinary symptoms. Afterward, they were discharged from further follow-up.

52.8.2 Hemi-Uterus

For the patient with the hemi-uterus and the dysgenetic gonad, console time was 35 min and total surgical time was 65 min. EBL was less than 5 mL. No intraoperative complication occurred. The postoperative period was marked by a urinary retention which was successfully treated by clean intermittent catheterization during 1 week. Pathology report showed tuba, corpus uteri, vagina, and streak gonad with some organization of Sertoli-like cells in primitive sex cords. The patient is doing well and underwent a successful two-staged hypospadias repair 2 years after surgery.

52.8.3 The Ectopic Kidney with Aberrant Ureter

For the two patients with the pelvic kidney and aberrant ureter, console time was 65 and 70 min and total surgical time was 90 and 100 min, respectively. EBL was less than 5 mL in both patients. Pathological study showed atrophic nephrogenic structures and inflamed ureteric structures. No intraoperative or postoperative complications were registered. At 1-year follow-up, both patients were satisfied and symptom free. Afterward, they were discharged from further follow-up.

Tips and Tricks

- As the most difficult part of the surgery is to gain space, care must be taken to maximize the available working space. Using the tensile strengths of the skin to gain more room by making a "tent" effect is a very useful trick.
- Placing the initial trocar into the umbilicus is a very good trick in children: as the umbilicus is a scar in itself, it maximizes the cosmetics but is also technically easier; in children, the peritoneum is sticky to the umbilical scar, making it way much easier to access the abdomen.
- The abdominal wall in children is very elastic. Placement of trocars is the most difficult part of the surgery and should always be done under vision. A puncture of the peritoneum usually helps getting easier into the pediatric abdominal wall.

52.9 Discussion

Until a few decades ago, decisions regarding surgery were essentially made by the surgeon, seldom in a multidisciplinary team, and usually without much discussion with the parents about treatment possibilities. Nowadays, more attention is given to the parents and the child, while a multidisciplinary approach is mandatory. When possible, a conservative approach is adopted until the patient is able to participate with his parents to the decision-making and eventual even in state of being in demand for surgery.

The removal of Müllerian remnants is aimed at relieving symptoms when present, preserving fertility, and preventing neoplastic degeneration. In an open surgery, several ways of approach have been advocated to access the retrovesical space and to remove the remnants, going from retrovesical to transvesical approaches causing a lot of damage to otherwise healthy tissues. These open procedures are often technically challenging and require prolonged hospitalization. Furthermore, they have the potential risk of infection and injury of the vas deferens, ureters, rectum, and bladder neck. For these reasons, endoscopic treatment was introduced with encouraging results but with several limitations such as a high recurrence rate [13]. Laparoscopy has become the gold standard treatment in the last two decades since the first intervention described by McDouglas et al. in 1994. Laparoscopy obviates the abovementioned disadvantages by providing an optimal anatomical visualization and by permitting fine dissection of the embryological remnants with excellent exposure of the surrounding structures and without damaging healthy tissues. Furthermore, it is associated with a low incidence of postoperative complications [13]. A few cases are described of Müllerian remnant resection with the robotic platform [13–15]. They confirm our findings that robot-assisted laparoscopy enhances the advantages of conventional laparoscopy by improving anatomical visualization and surgical precision.

Laparoscopic nephrectomy has become the standard of care for removal of benign nonfunctional kidneys [16]. Many studies have also demonstrated its safety in children [11]. Removal of pelvic kidneys, draining into the vagina in girls or into the urethra in boys, might be a surgical challenge in conventional laparoscopy. Only a few cases of robot-assisted nephrectomy of a pelvic kidney with aberrant ureter have been described [11]. In our experience, the robotic platform offers a good dexterity and facilitates a complete resection of the structure which, avoiding to leave a ureteric stump into the vaginal or urethral wall, might be the case in conventional laparoscopy. Furthermore, the side-docking position permits concurrent cystoscopic and vaginoscopic/hysteroscopic exploration if needed [11].

In conclusion, we believe that robot-assisted surgical management of DSD in a pediatric is safe and feasible in a specialized hospital with multidisciplinary team. However, large case series and randomized controlled trials should be performed to confirm this finding.

52.10 Future

Several series have showed that bladder neck reconstruction and closure with robot-assisted laparoscopy are feasible and safe in pediatric patients with incontinence [17, 18]. Over 65% of patients with the exstrophy-epispadias complex (EEC), a DSD consisting of an abdominal midline malformation, need a bladder neck procedure at one time during their childhood [19]. We think the minimally invasive technique, with the Da Vinci® robot system or any platform that hopefully come to be available, is the way to future improvements in outcomes for in EEC patients. However, fluent mobilization of the instruments may be inhibited due to scar tissue following primary bladder closure.

Take-Home Points

- Robot-assisted resection of Müllerian remnants and ectopic kidneys is feasible and safe.
- The robotic platform enables a good visualization of pelvic structures and its surrounding tissues.
- The robotic platform offers a good dexterity and facilitates a complete resection of the pelvic embryological remnants, which might be challenging in conventional laparoscopy.

References

1. Ostrer H. Disorders of sex development (DSDs): an update. J Clin Endocrinol Metab. 2014. https://doi.org/10.1210/jc.2013-3690.
2. Yu TJ. The character of variant persistent müllerian-duct structures. Pediatr Surg Int. 2002. https://doi.org/10.1007/s00383-002-0718-2.
3. Silay MS, Spinoit AF, Undre S, et al. Global minimally invasive pyeloplasty study in children: results from the pediatric urology expert Group of the European Association of urology young academic urologists working party. J Pediatr Urol. 2016. https://doi.org/10.1016/j.jpurol.2016.04.007.
4. Chan YY, Durbin-Johnson B, Sturm RM, Kurzrock EA. Outcomes after pediatric open, laparoscopic, and robotic pyeloplasty at academic institutions. J Pediatr Urol. 2017. https://doi.org/10.1016/j.jpurol.2016.08.029.
5. Morin J, Peard L, Vanadurongvan T, Walker J, Dönmez Mİ, Saltzman AF. Oncologic outcomes of pre-malignant and invasive germ cell tumors in patients with differences in sex development—a systematic review. J Pediatr Urol. 2020. https://doi.org/10.1016/j.jpurol.2020.05.002.
6. Cools M, Looijenga LHJ, Wolffenbuttel KP, T'Sjoen G. Managing the risk of germ cell tumourigenesis in disorders of sex development patients. Endocr Dev. 2014. https://doi.org/10.1159/000363642.
7. Shebel HM, Farg HM, Kolokythas O, El-Diasty T. Cysts of the lower male genitourinary tract: embryologic and anatomic considerations and differential diagnosis. Radiographics. 2013. https://doi.org/10.1148/rg.334125129.
8. Priyadarshi V, Singh JP, Mishra S, Vijay MK, Pal DK, Kundu AK. Prostatic utricle cyst: a clinical dilemma. APSP J Case Rep. 2013. https://doi.org/10.21699/ajcr.v4i2.53.
9. Mouafo Tambo FF, Dahoun S, Kamadjou C, et al. Mixed gonadal dysgenesis in Yaoundé: a preliminary experience about three cases. Afr J Paediatr Surg. 2016. https://doi.org/10.4103/0189-6725.187822.
10. Soheilipour F, Abed O, Behnam B, Abdolhosseini M, Alibeigi P, Pazouki A. A rare case of mixed gonadal dysgenesis with mosaicism 45, X/46, X, +mar. Int J Surg Case Rep. 2015. https://doi.org/10.1016/j.ijscr.2014.12.011.
11. Waterloos M, Ploumidis A, Pappas A, et al. Robot-assisted resection of ectopic kidney in children: an anatomical illustration. J Pediatr Urol. 2019. https://doi.org/10.1016/j.jpurol.2018.10.018.

12. Lafullarde T, Van Hee R, Gys T. A safe and simple method for routine open access in laparoscopic procedures. Surg Endosc. 1999. https://doi.org/10.1007/s004649901095.
13. Hong YK, Onal B, Diamond DA, Retik AB, Cendron M, Nguyen HT. Robot-assisted laparoscopic excision of symptomatic retrovesical cysts in boys and young adults. J Urol. 2011. https://doi.org/10.1016/j.juro.2011.07.113.
14. Wu JA, Hsieh MH. Robot-assisted laparoscopic hysterectomy, gonadal biopsy, and orchiopexies in an infant with persistent mullerian duct syndrome. Urology. 2014. https://doi.org/10.1016/j.urology.2013.10.006.
15. Lima M, Maffi M, Di Salvo N, et al. Robotic removal of Müllerian duct remnants in pediatric patients: our experience and a review of the literature. Pediatr Med Chir. 2018. https://doi.org/10.4081/pmc.2018.182.
16. Hamilton BD, Gatti JM, Cartwright PC, Snow BW. Comparison of laparoscopic versus open nephrectomy in the pediatric population. J Urol. 2000. https://doi.org/10.1016/S0022-5347(05)67856-1.
17. Gargollo PC. Robotic-assisted bladder neck repair: feasibility and outcomes. Urol Clin North Am. 2015. https://doi.org/10.1016/j.ucl.2014.09.013.
18. Storm DW, Fulmer BR, Sumfest JM. Robotic-assisted laparoscopic approach for posterior bladder neck dissection and placement of pediatric bladder neck sling: initial experience. Urology. 2008. https://doi.org/10.1016/j.urology.2008.07.005.
19. Sinatti C, Waterschoot M, Roth J, Van Laecke E, Hoebeke P, Spinoit AF. Long-term sexual outcomes in patients with exstrophy-epispadias complex. Int J Impot Res. 2020. https://doi.org/10.1038/s41443-020-0248-2.

Laparoscopic Treatment of Prostatic Utricle in Children

53

Aurélien Scalabre, Matthieu Peycelon, Alaa El-Ghoneimi, and François Varlet

Learning Objectives

- To present quick diagnosis of prostatic utricle (clinics, imaging).
- To describe step-by-step techniques of laparoscopic excision of prostatic utricle, using peroperative cystoscopy.
- To report the updated results of the review of literature.
- To show a video with the technique of prostatic utricle excision.

53.1 Introduction

Described by Morgagni in 1742 (De Sedibus XLIV 19), the prostatic utricle is a constant Müllerian duct remnant in man. But large and pathologic utricles are uncommon and Felderman found only 120 reported cases in 1987 [1]. A dual origin seems to be admitted from endodermal urogenital sinus and mesodermal Müllerian and Wolffian ducts. A prostatic utricle may result from incomplete regression of Müllerian duct or incomplete androgen-mediated closure of the urogenital sinus, explaining the common association between prostatic utricle and disorders of sexual development (DSD), hypospadias, and cryptorchidism [2–5]. In patients with normal genitalia, a huge prostatic utricle may be encountered, sometimes with renal agenesis (Fig. 53.1).

Many prostatic utricles are asymptomatic, especially when associated with hypospadias. Lower urinary tract symptoms, post-void dribbling, or urethral discharge may reveal the lesion. Dribbling incontinence, epididymitis, and urinary retention occur more commonly in patients with an enlarged prostatic utricle. Renal and bladder ultrasonography (RBUS), voiding cystourethrogram (VCUG), and MRI allow the diagnosis. The most common sign is the midline position of a "cyst" behind the bladder like a Müllerian duct cyst. It is thus different from a seminal vesicle cyst which is located in a lateral position.

When prostatic utricles are symptomatic, various techniques have been advocated for removal of enlarged utricles, including suprapubic, transvesical, posterior, or even perineal approaches but resulting in incomplete excision in 58% [2]. The first pediatric laparoscopic excision of a prostatic utricle was described by Yeung

Supplementary Information The online version contains supplementary material available at [https://doi.org/10.1007/978-3-030-99280-4_53].

A. Scalabre · F. Varlet (✉)
Pediatric Surgery Department, University Hospital, Saint-Etienne, France
e-mail: aurelien.scalabre@chu-st-etienne.fr; francois.varlet@chu-st-etienne.fr

M. Peycelon · A. El-Ghoneimi
Pediatric Urology Department, Robert Debre University Hospital, Paris, France
e-mail: matthieu.peycelon@aphp.fr; alaa.elghoneimi@aphp.fr

C. Esposito et al. (eds.), *Minimally Invasive Techniques in Pediatric Urology*,
https://doi.org/10.1007/978-3-030-99280-4_53

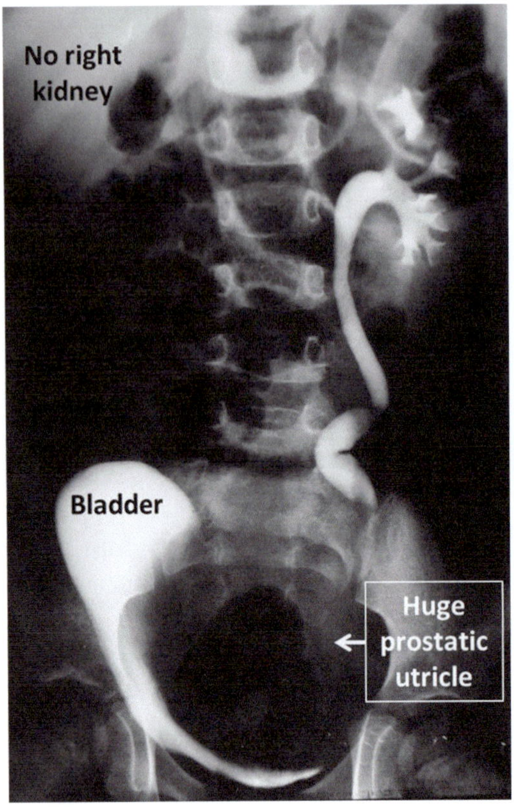

Fig. 53.1 Huge prostatic utricle shifting right the bladder and no right renal function

et al. in 2001 with the aim of removing the entire lesion and sparing the vas deferens, seminal vesicles, and bladder [6].

53.2 Preoperative Preparation

RBUS and MRI are appropriate imaging studies for the diagnosis in case of symptomatic patients. VCUG shows usually a communication between the urethra and prostatic utricle. This is particularly interesting to know because a telescope may be inserted inside the utricle during the surgical procedure to guide the utricular dissection and excision. The different techniques available for the surgical treatment of prostatic utricle and their potential complications are explained to the patients and their parents before surgery. A urine culture is performed a few days before surgery to ensure that urine is sterile. A broad-spectrum antibiotic is routinely administered intravenously on induction of general anesthesia.

53.3 Positioning

The child is placed in a dorsolithotomy position. The abdomen and perineum are prepped. The first step is doing a cystourethroscopy in order to see the utricular orifice on the verumontanum before going inside the utricle. Once cannulated, the cystoscope will guide the surgeon during the laparoscopic procedure. If the opening is too narrow, a ureteral stent can be left in the utricle before filling it. A Fogarty* stent with inflated balloon can also be inserted. Rarely, any cannulation can be done because of a very narrow duct, but in this case prostatic utricle is usually large and easy to see (Fig. 53.2).

Then the laparoscopy can begin, and the surgeon stands at the head when the child is younger than 10 years old. This best position is modified when the patient is more than 10 years old and the surgeon must stand laterally. The assistant and the nurse stand on each side. The video column is placed at the feet of the patient.

53.4 Instrumentation

An urethrocystoscope is required to begin the procedure and its caliber depends on the child's age and size. A 30° lens is mandatory to have a better view of the posterior wall of the bladder. The size and length of telescope and instruments depend on the child: 5 or 10 mm lens, 3 or 5 mm instruments according to the child's size. No specific instrument is required: scissors, atraumatic forceps, dissector, monopolar hook, bipolar forceps, needle holder, and suction.

53.5 Technique

A transumbilical incision is done to place the first trocar according to the Hasson technique. Two 3-mm diameter ports are inserted under direct

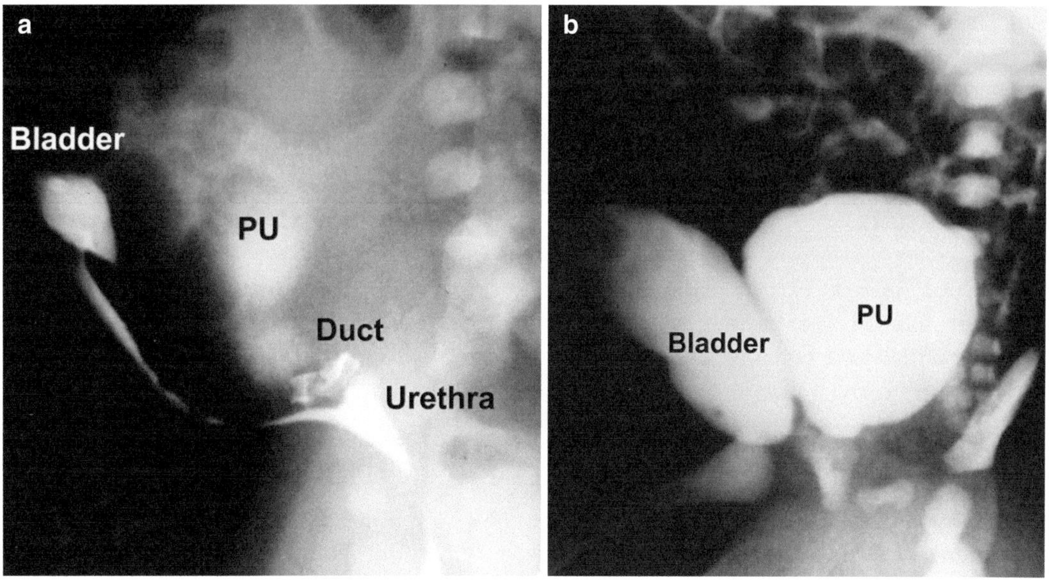

Fig. 53.2 Narrow duct between the urethra and prostatic utricle (PU) and shifted bladder (**a**). Huge prostatic utricle (**b**)

vision, one in each flank to act as operating instrument ports, more or less high according to the child. A Trendelenburg position is required for freeing the pelvic cavity. To have a good exposure of the posterior wall of the bladder, 1 or 2 transparietal suprapubic stitches can be used before opening the peritoneum at the level of prostatic utricle, guided by the cystoscope light in the utricle. The vas deferens are often close to the utricle and must be released as the two ureters. Then the top of the utricle is grasped and dissected very close until the lower part of the utricle, with monopolar hook or scissors, bipolar forceps, or a sealing device.

The plan between the bladder and the utricle is usually thin. We have to keep in mind to be close to the utricle to avoid opening the bladder. If it is too adhesive to the bladder, you must open the utricle and dissect safely with a good vision. During the lower dissection, we recommend using blunt dissection from the utricle base with minimal traction on the nearby neurovascular bundles to preserve normal erectile and ejaculatory function after surgery. Moreover special attention should also be given to protect the blood supply around the ureter. When you arrive to the low and narrow part of the utricle, you cut it transversally, leaving a small piece of distal utricle, and you burn the mucosa of this remaining part with a monopolar hook before closing it by 2 or 3 stitches.

Sometimes, one or both vas can enter into the utricle. In order to spare them, the way is to leave a strip of utricular wall attached to the vas, sometimes with a strip of bladder, and to dissect all the way down to its confluence with the utricle. The utricle is finally resected around this point of confluence and any resulting defect occurs afterward.

At the end of procedure, the peritoneum can be closed by a running absorbable suture. The specimen is pulled out through the umbilicus. A bladder catheter is left at the end of procedure for a few days, especially in case of bladder opening and suture.

53.6 Postoperative Care

Antibiotic treatment is administered during the procedure and may be continued with regard to intraoperative findings. Oral feeding may be allowed the same day. Analgesics are required during 1 or 2 days. According to the quality of the utricular opening suture, the Foley* catheter will be removed after a few days. The patient may be discharged with a catheter and will come back in clinics for its removal.

53.7 Results

Since 2001, in case of patients younger than 18 years old, 33 laparoscopic treatments of prostatic utricle have been collected in the literature [8–15] of which five are by robot-assisted laparoscopy. Robotics certainly allow a best 3D view for excising the utricle and sparing the surrounding structures [16–18]. One conversion was mentioned for bleeding [13]. Sparing the vas deferens was possible in 67.8% by laparoscopy and robot-assisted laparoscopy (19/28 cases). No difference for number of ligated vas between laparoscopy and open surgery was noted. Laparoscopy allows shorter operative time, lower estimated blood loss, and shorter hospital stay [6, 11, 15]. Only one epididymitis occurred 3 months after the surgery. A small utricular stump was identified without complication in one case.

53.8 Complications

An unknown bladder perforation can occur leading to abdominal pain, vomiting, low diuresis, tenderness, and effusion on RBUS. A new bladder catheter must be placed. If no improvement is noted, a redo laparoscopy must be done to suture the bladder. A huge urinoma will require drainage. Urinary tract infection can occur and must be treated with antibiotics. In the long-term follow-up, complications are uncommon, but there is a risk of infertility, especially if vas deferens were ligated or injured. Tumor risk should be considered because of a current evidence of 3% of malignancy in the Müllerian duct remnants with a peak of incidence around the fourth decade of life [2].

Tips and Tricks

- Transparietal suspension of the bladder is very useful to have a good exposure, to allow a good stabilization, and to avoid inserting another trocar. It is then easier to find the plan between the bladder and the prostatic utricle.
- Nevertheless, the plan between the bladder and the cyst can be difficult to identify, and sometimes the cyst must be opened to complete the dissection safely and to avoid any bladder, vas, or nerve injury.
- But the most important trick is to use indwelling cystoscope inside the utricle during laparoscopy.

53.9 Discussion

The incidence of prostatic utricle is between 11 and 14% in the literature, in association with hypospadias or disorders of sexual development and up to 50% in case of perineal hypospadias [7]. From a wide but non exhaustive literature review, 33 pediatric patients were identified and underwent a laparoscopic excision of prostatic utricle from 2001. About 24/33 (72.7%) had a penoscrotal or perineal hypospadias and only two had a distal hypospadias [6, 8–18]. Among other associated malformations, renal agenesis was noted in 2/7 children without hypospadias, but in each operated case a dysplastic kidney was found. Then it is better to avoid the term "renal agenesis" and to use "dysplastic kidney" when it is not seen by RBUS or MRI.

Prenatal diagnosis is sometimes possible. Two cases of prostatic utricle associated with hypospadias [19, 20] and two cases with dysplastic kidney without hypospadias [5, 20] were reported.

Most of prostatic utricles are asymptomatic, especially when small. If large, symptoms typically consist of urinary tract infections, epididymitis, urinary retention, post-void dribbling, and sometimes pain or abdominal mass. Imaging allows doing diagnosis with RBUS, VCUG, and MRI, the latter being helpful to evaluate cystic pelvic masses since it can provide improved soft tissue contrast to study the different organs behind and below the bladder. The differential diagnosis for such pelvic masses in males includes considerations of other "cysts" than prostatic utricle, such as urachal cyst and bladder diverticulum, but especially as Müllerian duct cyst (MDC) or seminal vesicle dilatation. Prostatic utricle and MDC are located midline and seminal vesicle dilation is located lateral to midline and usually unilateral. MDC has normal external genitalia and no communication with the urethra.

In symptomatic patients, complete excision is recommended to prevent recurrence of symptoms or future neoplastic changes, and many different surgical approaches have been proposed. The suprapubic extravesical approach allows an easy exploration of other pelvic organs but offers a poor exposure, particularly when dissecting the lower part of the prostatic utricle. The transvesical transtrigonal approach was described in children with good exposure and uneventful postoperative course, but vesicoureteral reflux was reported in 25% of the patients in the long-term follow-up [3]. This author speculated that splitting the posterior bladder wall might transiently interfere with the function of the trigonal musculature. The perineal approach was also used with a low risk of injury of the rectum, external sphincter, and pudendal nerves, but the success rate of the procedure was low [2, 3]. Posterior trans- or pararectal approaches were described with a risk of rectal fistula and injury of pelvic nerves. To avoid these complications, endoscopic treatment was proposed by using electrofulguration of the utricular wall, causing obliteration by scarification. The success rate of 66% after a single treatment and 83% after repeated treatments leads to stop this kind of procedure [21]. Finally in 1977 Schurke et al. showed that suprapubic, retrovesical, and transvesical approach for excising of the prostatic utricle resulted in incomplete excision in 58% of the cases; the perineal approach was successful in only 43%; transperineal or transrectal cyst aspiration and endoscopic procedure resulted in a 35% recurrence rate [2].

According to these complications and results, McDougall described the first laparoscopic excision of Müllerian duct remnant in 1994 in a 48-year-old patient with good result for continence and erectile function [22]. In children, Yeung et al. reported the first laparoscopic approach for excising the prostatic utricles in 2001. They described four cases with the use of cystoscope to help the dissection, leaving the telescope in situ inside the utricle during the laparoscopic procedure to facilitate its subsequent identification and mobilization [6]. Sometimes the duct between urethra and prostatic utricle was too narrow to be cannulated and only a ureteral or Fogarty* stent could be introduced. This is better than nothing because in a few cases no stent can be placed through the duct as shown in Fig. 53.2.

Since 2001 in patients younger than 18 years old, 33 laparoscopic treatments of prostatic utricle were reported in the literature [8–15] of which five were by robot-assisted laparoscopy [16–18]. Beside the great advantage of transillumination from the indwelling cystoscope, other tricks were described, especially transparietal bladder dome suspension to get a good exposure of the posterior bladder wall or to leave a small part of utricular wall to spare a vas entering into the prostatic utricle [6, 15]. Robot-assisted laparoscopy certainly allows the best 3D view for excising the utricle and sparing the surrounding structures.

When compared to open surgery, laparoscopic approach offers a minimally invasive access to retrovesical space, provides a clean view of the deep pelvic structures, and reduces the incidence of injury to the bladder, the rectum, the ureters, the vessels, and the nerves. In laparoscopic cases, the excision was complete without significant difference for age and utricular size or complications. About sparing of the vas deferens, when noted in publication, the number was 19/28 cases (67.8%) by laparoscopy and robot-assisted laparoscopy, the same rate than in open surgery. There was also no difference for number of ligated vas between laparoscopy and open surgery. Probably, each surgeon decided according to his/her philosophy, independently of the type of approach. The best way seems to be conservative, but leaving a small strip of utricular wall might lead to a tumor risk.

It is difficult to miss the report of a rare complication in which the bladder was accidentally removed instead of prostatic utricle during laparoscopic excision in a 24-year-old man [23].

Laparoscopy allows shorter operative time, lower estimated blood loss, and shorter hospital stay [6, 11, 15]. In the follow-up, UTIs occurred after open surgery and minimal residual utricular stump can remain [15]. From the 33 selected laparoscopic cases in the literature, one conversion was reported for bleeding and one epididymitis occurred 3 months after surgery.

While enlarged prostatic utricles are most commonly benign, Schuhrke et al. reported a 3% incidence of malignancy in a case series of 88 patients with this condition [2]. From the 33 reviewed pediatric patients, Gualco et al. reported a 16-year-old boy who presented with a primary clear cell adenocarcinoma of the prostatic utricle after a 6-month history of intermittent hematuria and an associated right renal agenesis [24]. Other reported malignancies in the prostatic utricle include urothelial carcinoma, endometrial carcinoma, and squamous cell carcinoma [25]. Thus, it seems to be very important to do a total excision of prostatic utricle, and today laparoscopic approach provides the best way to avoid this risk of malignancy. A longer follow-up is however required.

53.10 Conclusion

Prostatic utricles are not common but should be considered in boys with proximal hypospadias. Sometimes an enlarged prostatic utricle can occur in childhood leading to urinary retention, abdominal mass, or epididymitis. Nowadays the laparoscopic approach or the robot-assisted laparoscopy seem to be the best approach to remove prostatic utricles and to allow preservation of surrounding structures, especially vas deferens, ureters, and neurovascular bundles.

Take-Home Points

- The diagnosis is not always easy and you have to discuss with your radiologist because several differential diagnoses are possible among ureterocele, seminal vesicle cyst, Müllerian duct cyst, and ejaculatory duct cyst.
- Asymptomatic prostatic utricle must be supervised.
- Before starting a prostatic utricle excision, a cystoscopy allows to cannulate it in order to facilitate its identification during laparoscopy.
- During surgical treatment, keep in mind to avoid any injury of the bladder, ureter, vas deferens, pelvic vessels, and nerves.

References

1. Felderman T, Schellhammer PF, Devine CJ, Stecker JF. Müllerian duct cyst: conservative management. Urology. 1987;29:31–4.
2. Schuhrke TD, Kaplan GW. Prostatic utricle cysts (mullerian duct cysts). J Urol. 1978;119:765–7.
3. Ikoma F, Shima H, Yabumoto H. Classification of enlarged prostatic utricle in patients with hypospadias. Br J Urol. 1985;57:334–7.
4. Ritchey ML, Benson RC, Kramer SA, Kelalis PP. Management of müllerian duct remnants in the male patient. J Urol. 1988;140:795–9.
5. Varlet F, Coupris L, Laumonier F, Duverne C. La dilatation congénitale de l'utricule prostatique. Ann Urol (Paris). 1992;26:39–48.
6. Yeung CK, Sihoe JDY, Tam YH, Lee KH. Laparoscopic excision of prostatic utricles in children. BJU Int. 2001;87:505–8.
7. Coppens L, Bonnet P, Andrianne R, DE Leval J. Adult Mullerian duct or utricle cyst: clinical significance and therapeutic management of 65 cases. J Urol. 2002;167:1740–4.

8. Willetts IE, Roberts JP, MacKinnon AE. Laparoscopic excision of a prostatic utricle in a child. Pediatr Surg Int. 2003;19:557–8.
9. Nanni L, D'Urzo C, Pintus C, Riccipetitoni G, Perrelli G. Laparoscopic approach to müllerian derivatives in a male with mixed gonadal dysgenesis. Surg Laparosc Endosc Percutan Tech. 2003;13:128–32.
10. Lima M, Aquino A, Domini M, Ruggeri G, Libri M, Cimador M, Pelusi G. Laparoscopic removal of Müllerian duct remnants in boys. J Urol. 2004;171:364–8.
11. Luo JH, Chen W, Sun JJ, Xie D, Mo JC, Zhou L, Lu J. Laparoscopic management of Müllerian duct remnants: four case reports and review of the literature. J Androl. 2008;29:638–42.
12. Jiwane A, Soundappan SVS, Pitkin J, Cass DT. Successful treatment of recurrent epididymo-orchitis: laparoscopic excision of the prostatic utricle. J Indian Assoc Pediatr Surg. 2009;14:29–30.
13. Barrena S, Aguilar R, Olivares P, Lobato R, López Pereira P, Martínez Urrutia MJ, Jaureguizar E. Laparoscopic resection of the prostatic utricle in children. Cir Pediatr. 2010;23:15–8.
14. Hong YK, Onal B, Diamond DA, Retik AB, Cendron M, Nguyen HT. Robot-assisted laparoscopic excision of symptomatic retrovesical cysts in boys and young adults. J Urol. 2011;186:2372–8.
15. Aminsharifi A, Afsar F, Pakbaz S. Laparoscopic management of müllerian duct cysts in infants. J Pediatr Surg. 2011;46:1859–64.
16. Jia W, Liu GC, Zhang LY, Wen YQ, Fu W, Hu JH, Xia HM. Comparison of laparoscopic excision versus open transvesical excision for symptomatic prostatic utricle in children. J Pediatr Surg. 2016;51:1597–601.
17. Lima M, Maffi M, Di Salvo N, Ruggeri G, Libri M, Gargano T, Lardy H. Robotic removal of Müllerian duct remnants in pediatric patients: our experience and a review of the literature. Pediatr Med Chir. 2018;40:27–30.
18. Nguyen A, Arora H, Reese J, Kaouk J, Rhee A. Robot-assisted laparoscopic excision of prostatic utricle in a 3-year old. J Pediatr Urol. 2018;14:343–4.
19. Johal NS, Kraklau D, Deniz K, Mushtaq I. An unusual case of a prenatally detected large Müllerian duct remnant. Pediatr Surg Int. 2005;21:764–6.
20. Le Vaillant C, Podevin G, Quere MP, Talmant C, Heloury Y, Boog G. Prenatal diagnosis of enlarged prostatic utricle by ultrasonography and magnetic resonance imaging. Ultrasound Obstet Gynecol. 2008;31:588–91.
21. Husmann DA, Allen TD. Endoscopic management of infected enlarged prostatic utricles and remnants of rectourethral fistula tracts of high imperforate anus. J Urol. 1997;157:1902–6.
22. McDougall EM, Clayman RV, Bowles WT. Laparoscopic excision of müllerian duct remnant. J Urol. 1994;152:482–4.
23. Kumar V, Punatar C, Jadhav K, Sagade S. Accidental cystectomy during laparoscopic excision of prostatic utricle cyst—a rare complication. Int Braz J Urol. 2018;44:826–30.
24. Gualco G, Ortega V, Ardao G, Cravioto F. Clear cell adenocarcinoma of the prostatic utricle in an adolescent. Ann Diagn Pathol. 2005;9:153–6.
25. Zhang C, Li X, He Z, Xiao Y, Li S, Zhou L. Squamous cell carcinoma of the enlarged prostatic utricle in an adult. Urology. 2012;79:23–4.

Laparoscopic Treatment of Seminal Vesicle Cyst

54

François Varlet, Aurélien Scalabre, S. Vermersch, and N. Diraduryan

Learning Objectives
- To present quick diagnosis of SVC (clinics, imaging).
- To describe the step-by-step techniques of laparoscopic excision of SVC.
- To report the latest results of the review of literature.
- To show a video with the technique of SVC excision.

54.1 Introduction

Seminal vesicle cysts are very rare with a prevalence of 0.004% or 1 case in 24,000 males [1]. The mesonephric duct induces both reproductive and renal systems between the 4th and 12th weeks of gestation, explaining common associations of renal and genital malformations. Seminal vesicle cysts can be associated with dysplastic kidney, especially in a congenital syndrome first described by Zinner in 1914, characterized by the coexistence of ejaculatory duct stenosis, renal agenesis or dysplasia, and ectopic ureter orifice in the seminal vesicle [2]. Seminal vesicle cysts are sometimes isolated. Stenosis of the ejaculatory duct may occur rather during the second through third decades of life, resulting in a seminal vesicle dilatation rather than a real cyst.

The seminal vesicle cysts can remain asymptomatic and can be diagnosed incidentally by ultrasonography (US). Otherwise patients experience symptoms as dysuria, urinary frequency or dribbling, hematuria, perineal, scrotal, suprapubic, rectal or abdominal pain, ejaculatory pain, or epididymitis. The initial imaging method is currently US showing a lateralized retrovesical cyst and potential ipsilateral renal malformations. MRI helps to assess the relationship between the cyst and the surrounding organs, especially with the bladder and the ureters (Fig. 54.1). It can also help to identify a small or ectopic kidney, sometimes more difficult to see with US [3].

Conservative follow-up is the usual management for asymptomatic or minimally symptomatic seminal vesicle cysts. Surgical treatment is considered in case of recurrent pain, dysuria, or hematuria. Cysts larger than 5 cm are indications for surgery for a few authors [4, 5]. Transrectal, transabdominal or transperineal aspiration and transurethral unroofing were reported to give temporary results, recurrence, and infection, and thus they were abandoned. Several open surgery

Supplementary Information The online version contains supplementary material available at [https://doi.org/10.1007/978-3-030-99280-4_54].

F. Varlet (✉) · A. Scalabre · S. Vermersch · N. Diraduryan
Pediatric Surgery Department, Hôpital Nord, CHU de Saint-Etienne, Saint-Etienne, France
e-mail: francois.varlet@chu-st-etienne.fr; aurelien.scalabre@chu-st-etienne.fr; sophie.vermersch@chu-st-etienne.fr; norayk.diraduryan@chu-st-etienne.fr

C. Esposito et al. (eds.), *Minimally Invasive Techniques in Pediatric Urology*, https://doi.org/10.1007/978-3-030-99280-4_54

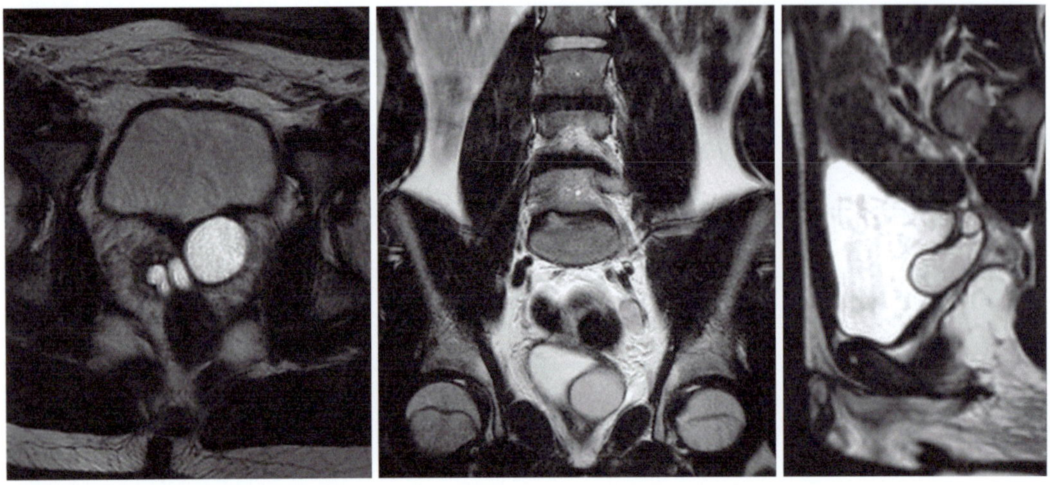

Fig. 54.1 MRI of seminal vesicle cyst

techniques were described, mostly with a transvesical approach because of the location of the seminal vesicles, deep in the pelvic cavity. There are now multiple reports supporting the safety and effectiveness of laparoscopic excision of seminal vesicle cysts because of an easier approach of the posterior wall of the bladder and seminal vesicles than in open procedures, even in infants or child [6, 7].

54.2 Preoperative Preparation

US and MRI imaging are usually sufficient in symptomatic cases. Renal isotope study, although not mandatory, can be used to assess the relative renal function in case of renal agenesis or parenchymal anomalies. The different techniques available for the surgical treatment of seminal vesicle cysts and their potential complications are explained to the patients and their parents before surgery. After puberty, a sperm analysis seems to be very important before surgery to assess the future results of cyst excision [8]. A bacteriologic urine exam is performed a few days before surgery to ensure that urine is sterile. Cystoscopy is always interesting to study the urethra, the verumontanum, and the bladder and can help to eliminate differential diagnosis. A broad-spectrum antibiotic is routinely administered intravenously on induction of general anesthesia.

54.3 Positioning

The child is placed in a supine position. When he is younger than 10 years old, the surgeon stands at the head and the video column is at the child's feet. This best position is modified for children older than 10 years old, and the surgeon has to stand on the patient's side. The assistant and nurse stand on one side, usually opposite to the seminal vesicle cyst. A transurethral catheter is inserted to empty the bladder in order to have a good view of the posterior wall and the cyst.

54.4 Instrumentation

A 30° lens is mandatory to ensure a good vision of the posterior wall of the bladder. A 10 mm lens telescope and 5 mm instruments can be used, although a 5 mm lens and 3 mm instruments are better suited for younger patients. No specific instrument is required: scissors, atraumatic forceps, dissector, monopolar hook, bipolar forceps, needle holder, and suction.

54.5 Technique

A transumbilical incision is done to place the first trocar according to the Hasson technique. Two trocars are inserted in the iliac fossae or flanks, according to the child's size. A Trendelenburg position is required to free the pelvic cavity. To have a good exposure of the posterior wall of the bladder, one or two transparietal suprapubic stitches can be done before opening the peritoneum at the level of the seminal vesicle cyst. The vas deferens is often close to the cyst and must be dissected and reclined in order to spare it. Then the cyst is grasped and dissected with monopolar hook, scissors, or bipolar forceps toward the lower part of the seminal vesicle. In case of Zinner syndrome, the lower ureter is dissected first until its connection with the vesicle is localized. The plane between the bladder and the cyst is usually very thin, therefore, the dissection must stay close to the cyst to avoid bladder opening. The cyst can be opened to complete dissection if necessary. We recommend using blunt dissection around the cyst base with minimal traction on the nearby neurovascular bundles for the sake of preserving normal erectile and ejaculatory function after surgery. Moreover special attention should be given to protect the blood supply around the ureter [4]. Once dissection of the seminal vesicle is complete, it is transected transversally. The mucosa inside the remaining part of the vesicle is burned using monopolar hook, and the vesicle is closed by two or three stitches. In Zinner syndrome, the procedure is completed by a nephrectomy of the dysplastic kidney, usually very adhesive to the surrounding tissues. The peritoneum can be closed afterward by a running suture. The specimen is pulled out through the umbilicus incision. The bladder catheter is removed at the end of the procedure, except in case of bladder injury and suture.

54.6 Postoperative Care

The hospital stay is usually short, after assessing correct voiding and pain control. Most patients are discharged after 24 to 48 h.

54.7 Complications

An unnoticed bladder perforation can lead to abdominal pain, vomiting, oliguria, tenderness, and effusion on US. A bladder catheter must be inserted and a redo laparoscopy has to be considered to suture the bladder and stop the urine leakage. Urinary tract infections are another potential complication, treated by antibiotics. Infertility is a long-term concern, although surgery can result in semen quality improvement as reported by Benyó [8]. For this author, laparoscopy offers real advantages over other treatment options probably because of sparing of the surrounding vessels, nerves, and vas deferens.

54.8 Results

Only 13 children were operated on by laparoscopy with our three personal cases [6, 7, 9, 10, 12, 13] of whom four children by robot-assisted laparoscopy [14, 15]. The postoperative course was uneventful, except one with pelvic hematoma requiring a redo laparoscopy at day 1. Every symptoms disappeared after surgery with good results at 34, 5 months of follow-up.

Tips and Tricks

- Transparietal suspension of bladder is very useful to have a good exposure allowing good stabilization and avoiding placing another trocar.
- In case of Zinner syndrome, the first dissection of ureter facilitates the seminal vesicle identification. After that it is easier to find the plan between bladder and vesicle. Nevertheless the plan between the bladder and the cyst can be difficult to identify. If it is too adhesive, the cyst can be opened to complete dissection safely, avoiding bladder, vas, or nerve injury.

54.9 Discussion

Seminal vesicle cyst can be acquired and isolated (without renal malformation) or congenital and commonly associated with ipsilateral renal agenesis or dysplastic kidney due to maldevelopment of the mesonephric duct in embryo. Schukfeh et al. demonstrated that dysplastic or multicystic kidneys are anomalies commonly associated with seminal vesicle cyst. Because these dysplastic kidneys become very small and cannot be seen by imaging, even by CT scan or MRI [9], they are often mistaken for renal agenesia. Merrot et al. reported ten seminal vesicle cysts among 52 boys with dysplastic kidney (19.2%) suggesting that follow-up of these children should be performed even after puberty to detect genitourinary malformations [10].

Prenatal diagnosis was reported only by Valla et al. in 2003 with left renal agenesis and pelvic cystic mass, 12 mm in diameter and retrovesical, at 22 weeks of gestation [6].

Seminal vesicle cysts are often asymptomatic. With our three personal cases, we identified 64 patients younger than 18 years old reported in the literature and 32 (50%) presented no symptoms. Dysuria, urgency, urinary retention, urinary tract infections, epididymitis, hematuria, and pain were the common symptoms in 32 (50%) children [3, 5–7, 9, 11–31], of which one 2-month-old boy presented a seminal vesicle abscess [31]. US, CT scan, and MRI easily showed the seminal vesicle cyst [3, 22], and renal malformations were demonstrated in 59 children (92.2%). Differential diagnosis has to be discussed because other genital malformations can produce a pelvic cystic mass, especially prostatic utricle and Müllerian duct cyst, but these lesions are always located in the midline [32]. The seminal vesicle cyst can bulge into the bladder and look like an ureterocele as in this child we treated for a duplex system, but we found only one ureter during nephroureterectomy and finally the cyst depended from an ipsilateral seminal vesicle cyst. The bilobar appearance should draw attention (Fig. 54.2). A cyst of the ejaculatory duct is a rarer anomaly than seminal vesicle cyst but also have the aspect of a lateralized retrovesical cyst on US [33, 34].

In case of asymptomatic seminal vesicle cyst, conservative management is indicated. Among the 64 reviewed patients, the chosen treatment was reported in 55 and 31 had a conservative management (56.3%). The parents and the adolescents should be informed of potential future symptoms that should lead to consultation with a pediatric surgeon or an urologist, in order to assess the new situation and discuss a surgical treatment.

When the seminal vesicle cyst is or becomes symptomatic, a surgical excision is needed,

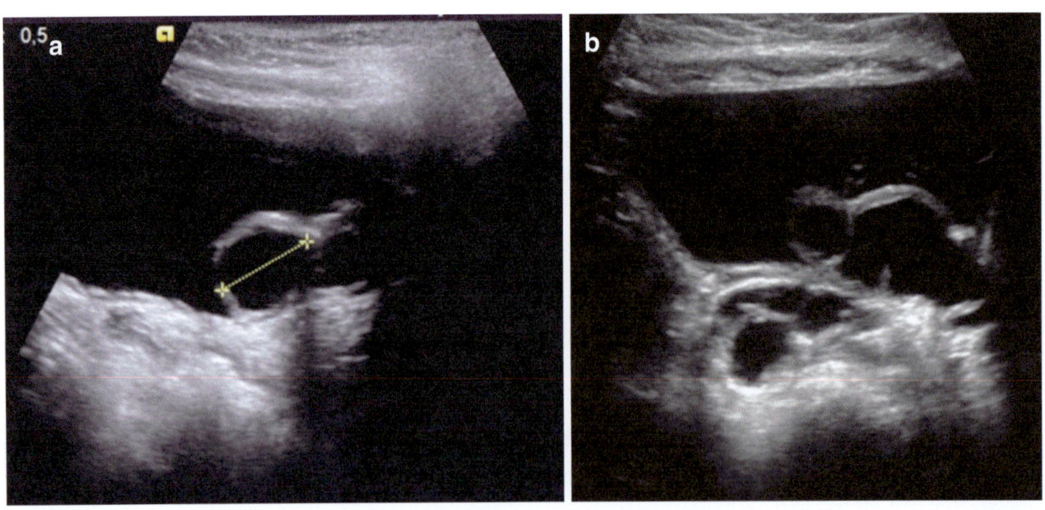

Fig. 54.2 Seminal vesicle cyst mimicking an ureterocele (**a**) but the bilobar appearance should draw attention (**b**)

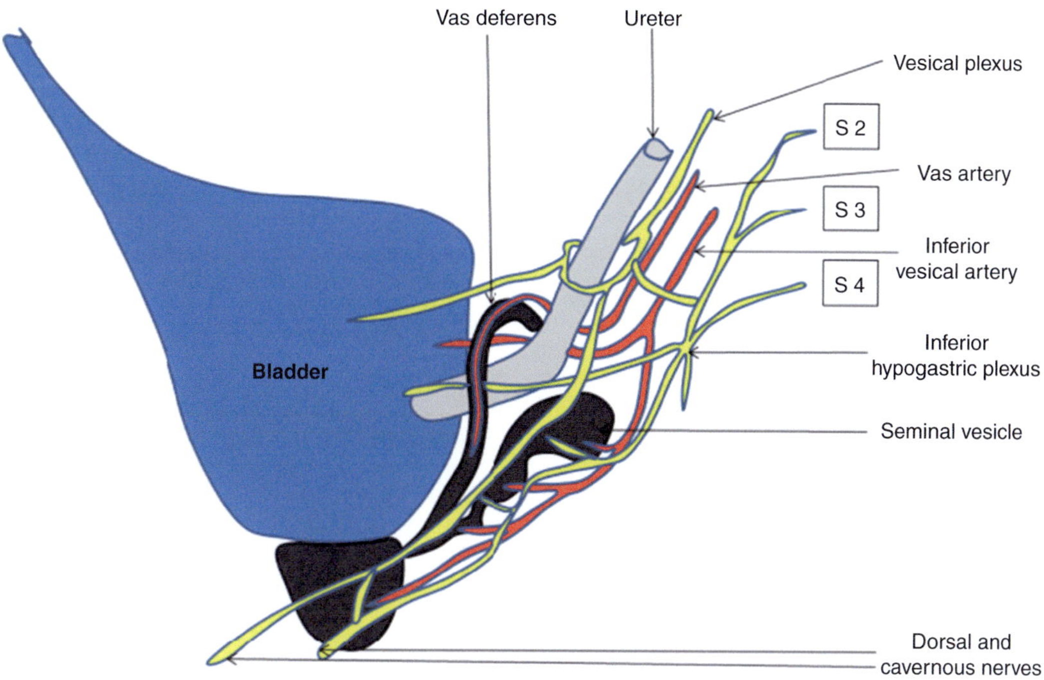

Fig. 54.3 Anatomy around seminal vesicle

because puncture of the cyst or transurethral unroofing is usually ineffective [35]. In open surgery, suprapubic transvesical and perineal approaches were reported with good outcomes. However, potential morbidity includes rectal and bladder laceration, erectile neurovascular bundle injury, and pelvic urinoma because of the deep location of the cyst in the pelvic cavity and poor visualization [4]. Transperitoneal laparoscopic approach provides an excellent access and view on the posterior wall of the bladder and seminal vesicle cyst. The dissection can be close to the cyst to avoid injury of the vas deferens, ureter, ejaculatory duct, and lateral vascular pedicles of the prostate (Fig. 54.3). Robot-assisted laparoscopic excision now affords a natural extension of conventional laparoscopy to achieve less traumatic dissection with 3D vision and easy manipulation of instruments.

From the 64 pediatric cases reported in literature, 24 underwent a seminal vesicle cyst excision, 11 by open surgery, and 13 by laparoscopy [6, 7, 17, 23, 26, 30] or robot-assisted laparoscopy [25, 27].

Although symptoms disappear after cyst excision in the majority of patients, they should be followed in the long term to assess their fertility potential. Benyó et al. reported that the sperm analysis is not often studied before and after surgery in postpubertal patients. Only 4 out of 40 adult patients treated for seminal vesicle cyst had available data regarding sperm quality. Preoperative and postoperative sperm analysis seems to be very important to do in adolescents to assess the outcomes of surgery and to give prognosis factors for future fertility. Quality of erections should also be evaluated before and after surgery [8].

54.10 Conclusion

Seminal vesicle cysts are often associated with ipsilateral dysplastic kidney. A small kidney is always found and resected during surgery and should not be mistaken with renal agenesia. When the seminal vesicle cyst is symptomatic, surgical excision is required. Nowadays, endo-surgery provides a good approach by laparoscopy or robot-assisted laparoscopy.

References

1. Sheih CP, Hung CS, Wei CF, Lin CY. Cystic dilatations within the pelvis in patients with ipsilateral renal agenesis or dysplasia. J Urol. 1990;144:324–7.
2. Zinner A. Ein fall von intravesikaler samenblaszyste. Wein Med Wochenschr. 1914;64:605–9.
3. Chen HW, Huang SC, Li YW, Chen SJ, Sheih CP. Magnetic resonance imaging of seminal vesicle cyst associated with ipsilateral urinary anomalies. J Formos Med Assoc. 2006;105:125–31.
4. Zhang DX, Li XG, Gao Y, Liu YS, Wang JK, Chen J, Chen L, Wang K, Cui XG, Xu DF. Transperitoneal laparoscopic excision of seminal vesicle cyst: a single-center experience. J Endourol. 2012;26: 1153–9.
5. Kanavaki A, Vidal I, Merlini L, Hanquinet S. Congenital seminal vesicle cyst and ipsilateral renal agenesis (Zinner syndrome): a rare association and its evolution from early childhood to adolescence. Eur J Pediatr Surg Reports. 2015;3:98–101.
6. Valla JS, Carfagna L, Tursini S, Mohaidi MAL, Bosson N, Steyaert H. Congenital seminal vesicle cyst: prenatal diagnosis and postnatal laparoscopic excision with an attempt to preserve fertility. BJU Int. 2003;91:891–2.
7. Basillote JB, Shanberg AM, Woo D, Perer E, Rajpoot D, Clayman RV. Laparoscopic excision of a seminal vesicle cyst in a child. J Urol. 2004;171:369–71.
8. Benyó M, Berczi C, Jozsa T, Csanadi G, Varga A, Flasko T. Fertility preservation in cases of laparoscopic treatment of seminal vesicle cysts. Cent European J Urol. 2012;65:144–5.
9. Schukfeh N, Kuebler JF, Schirg E, Petersen C, Ure BM, Glüer S. Dysplastic kidney and not renal agenesis is the commonly associated anomaly in infants with seminal vesicle cyst. BJU Int. 2008;103:816–9.
10. Merrot T, Lumenta DB, Tercier S, Morisson-Lacombes G, Guys JM, Alessandrini P. Multicystic dysplastic kidney with ipsilateral abnormalities of genitourinary tract: experience in children. Urology. 2006;67:603–7.
11. Denes FT, Montellato NI, Lopes RN, Barbosa Filho CM, Cabral AD. Seminal vesicle cyst and ipsilateral renal agenesis. Urology. 1986;28:313–5.
12. Zaontz MR, Kass EJ. Ectopic ureter opening into seminal vesicle cyst associated with ipsilateral renal agenesis. Urology. 1987;29:523–5.
13. King BF, Hattery RR, Lieber MM, Berquist TH, Williamson B Jr, Hartman GW. Congenital cystic disease of the seminal vesicle. Radiology. 1991;178:207–11.
14. Sheih CP, Liao YJ, Li YW, Yang LY. Seminal vesicle cyst associated with ipsilateral renal malformation and hemivertebra: report of 2 cases. J Urol. 1993;150:1214–5.
15. Terai A, Tsuji Y, Terachi T, Yoshida O. Ectopic ureter opening into the seminal vesicle in an infant: a case report and review of the Japanese literature. Int J Urol. 1995;2:128–31.
16. Sheih CP, Li YW, Liao YJ, Hung CS. Bilateral congenital cysts of the seminal vesicle with bilateral duplex kidneys. J Urol. 1998;160:184–5.
17. Ikari O, Castilho LN, Lucena R, D'Ancona CA, Netto NR Jr. Laparoscopic excision of seminal vesicle cysts. J Urol. 1999;162:498–9.
18. Phillis TM Jr, Teague JL. Seminal vesicle cyst in a child with a contralateral upper urinary tract abnormality. BJU Int. 1999;83:359–60.
19. Jones J, Dahms SE, Fichtner J, Hohenfellner M, Thüroff JW. An unusual case of ureteral ectopia in the seminal vesicle: diagnosis and surgical management. Urol Int. 1999;62:130–2.
20. Steffens J, Oberschulte-Beckmann D, Siller V, Röttger P, Polsky MS. Ectopic refluxing ureter entering a seminal vesicle cyst associated with ipsilateral renal dysplasia. World J Urol. 2000;18:232–4.
21. Livingston L, Larsen CR. Seminal vesicle cyst with ipsilateral renal agenesis. AJR Am J Roentgenol. 2000;175:177–80.
22. Murphy JO, Power RE, Akhtar M, Torreggiani WC, McDermott TE, Thornhill JA. Magnetic resonance imaging in the diagnosis of seminal vesicle cysts and associated anomalies. J Urol. 2003;170(6 Pt 1):2386.
23. Hoschke B, May M, Seehafer M, Helke C. Mündung eines Megaureters mit aplastischer Niere in eine Samenblasenzyste. Fallbericht einer laparoskopischen Intervention. Urologe A. 2003;42:1092–6.
24. Van Meegen MA, Kokke F, Dik P, Fockens P, Benninga MA. A seminal vesicle cyst palpable in the rectum. Endoscopy. 2006;38:E7.
25. Moore CD, Erhard MJ, Dahm P. Robot-assisted excision of seminal vesicle cyst associated with ipsilateral renal agenesis. J Endourol. 2007;21:776–9.
26. Hong YK, Onal B, Diamond DA, Retik AB, Cendron M, Nguyen HT. Robot-assisted laparoscopic excision of symptomatic retrovesical cysts in boys and young adults. J Urol. 2011;186:2372–8.
27. Ahallal Y, Tazi MF, Khallouk A, Elammari J, Elfassi MJ, Farih MH. Conservative management of a congenital seminal vesicle cyst associated with ipsilateral renal agenesis revealed by cystitis: one case report. Case Rep Urol. 2011;2011:125753.
28. Dudek-Warchoł T, Szmigielska A, Krzemień G, Warchoł S. Ectopic ureter, renal dysplasia, and recurrent epididymitis in an infant: case report and review of the literature. Clin Case Rep. 2014;2:7–9.
29. Farrelly JS, Cleary MA, Weiss RM, Morotti R, Stitelman DH. Acquired seminal vesicle cyst in a teenager with a urethral stricture of unknown etiology. J Pediatr Surg Case Rep. 2016;7:8–12.
30. Cascini V, Di Renzo D, Guerriero V, Lauriti G, Lelli CP. Zinner syndrome in pediatric age: issues in the

diagnosis and treatment of a rare malformation complex. Front Pediatr. 2019;7:129.
31. Fujinaga S, Hirano D, Hara S, Uchida H, Kitano Y, Kobayashi K, Tada M, Someya T, Ohtomo Y, Shimizu T. Seminal vesicle abscesses associated with ipsilateral multicystic dysplastic kidney in an infant. Pediatr Nephrol. 2008;23:1551–4.
32. Furuya R, Furuya S, Kato H, Saitoh N, Takahash S, Tsukamoto T. New classification of midline cysts of the prostate in adults via a transrectal ultrasonography-guided opacification and dye-injection study. BJU Int. 2008;102:475–8.
33. Pimpalwar A, Chowdhary S, Huskisson J, Corkery JJ. Cysts of the ejaculatory system--a treatable cause of recurrent epididymo-orchitis in children. Eur J Pediatr Surg. 2002;12:281–5.
34. Yanai T, Okazaki T, Yamataka A, Urao M, Kobayashi H, Kato Y, Lane GJ, Miyano T. Cysts of the ejaculatory system: a report of two cases. Pediatr Surg Int. 2005;21:939–42.
35. Gözen AS, Alagöl B. Endoscopic management of seminal-vesical cyst with right renal agenesis causing acute urinary retention: case report. J Endourol. 2006;20:919–22.

Laparoscopic Lymphatic Sparing Palomo Varicocelectomy in Children Using Indocyanine Green (ICG) Fluorescence Lymphography

55

Ciro Esposito, Maria Escolino, Fulvia Del Conte, Giuseppe Autorino, Vincenzo Coppola, Mariapina Cerulo, Rachele Borgogni, and Alessandro Settimi

Learning Objectives

- To describe the step-by-step techniques of laparoscopic Palomo varicocele repair.
- To present long-term outcomes of laparoscopic lymphatic sparing Palomo varicocelectomy.
- To report the latest results of the major international papers about varicocele repair using MIS.
- To show a video with the technique of laparoscopic lymphatic sparing Palomo varicocelectomy.
- To describe tips and tricks of laparoscopic lymphatic sparing Palomo varicocelectomy using ICG fluorescence technology.

Supplementary Information The online version contains supplementary material available at [https://doi.org/10.1007/978-3-030-99280-4_55].

C. Esposito (✉) · M. Escolino · F. Del Conte · G. Autorino
V. Coppola · M. Cerulo · R. Borgogni · A. Settimi
Pediatric Surgery Unit, Federico II University of Naples, Naples, Italy
e-mail: ciroespo@unina.it; maria.escolino@unina.it; fulvia.delconte@unina.it; autorino.giuseppe@gmail.com; vincenzocoppola1992@gmail.com; mariapina.cerulo@unina.it; rachele.borgogni@gmail.com; settimi@unina.it

55.1 Introduction

Laparoscopic Palomo varicocelectomy is one the most common approaches adopted to treat pediatric varicocele. Palomo technique, according to the reports of the literature [1, 2], gives excellent results in children, with success rates of >95% but with a 20–30% incidence of postoperative hydrocele, requiring redo surgery in most cases. For this reason, in recent years, lymphatic sparing procedures have been applied for varicocele repair to decrease the incidence of secondary hydrocele and ensure a better andrological outcome for children [3–5].

Indocyanine green (ICG) has traditionally been used to assess liver function. In recent years, ICG fluorescence has been adopted in adults to perform angiography in case of tumors and to check the anomalies of biliary tract during laparoscopic cholecystectomy.

More recently, a novel method to measure human lymphatic pumping using a solution of ICG with fluorescence video control has been described [13, 14].

This chapter is focused on the operative technique of laparoscopic Palomo varicocele repair using ICG fluorescence technology to spare lymphatic vessels.

C. Esposito et al. (eds.), *Minimally Invasive Techniques in Pediatric Urology*,
https://doi.org/10.1007/978-3-030-99280-4_55

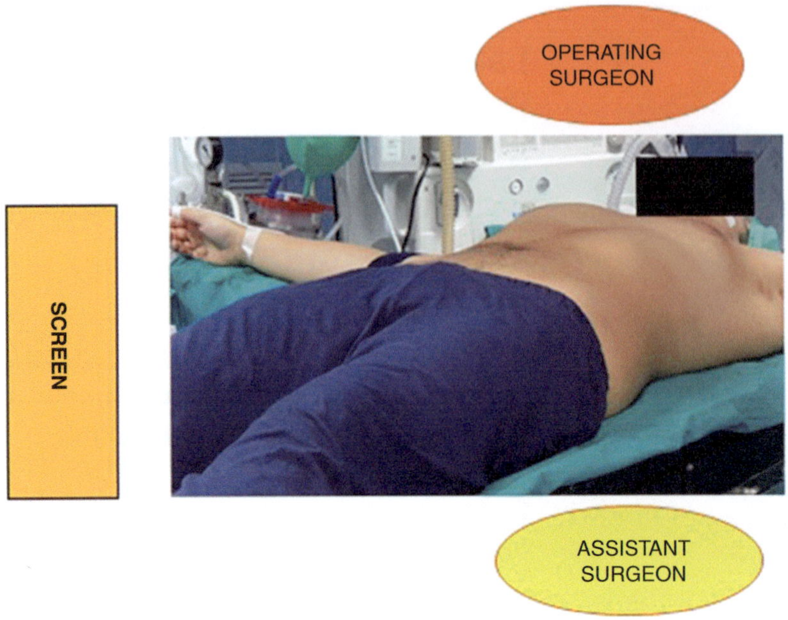

Fig. 55.1 The patient is positioned in supine decubitus on the operative table with the screen at his feet, the surgeon on his side contralateral to the pathology, and the assistant in front of him

55.2 Preoperative Preparation

Preoperative clinical examinations should focus to grade the varicocele according to Dublin Amelar scale. Investigations have to include testis ultrasonography with echo-color Doppler study to measure testis volume in comparison with the other side and to grade the varicocele using the echo color Doppler study [1].

In patient older than 16 years, we prefer to perform also a sperm analysis.

All patients and their parents have to sign a specifically formulated informed consent before the procedure. Patients receive a general anesthesia with orotracheal intubation and myorelaxation. A Nelaton catheter is adopted to empty the bladder using sterile precautions just before surgery.

55.3 Positioning

The patient should be placed in a supine position with the table with 15° of Trendelenburg position. The surgeon is positioned on the patient side contralateral to the pathology and the assistant stand on the contralateral side, and the monitor is positioned at the feet of the patient (Fig. 55.1). We always adopt a 5- or a 10-mm 0-degree optic and two other trocars of 5 mm for operative instruments. In general, we prefer to adopt 5-mm working trocars so as to use intraoperatively a clip applier for vessel control. The trocars are positioned in triangulation with the optic in order to achieve a better ergonomics (Fig. 55.2) [6].

55.4 Instrumentation

Regarding the laparoscopic procedure, we adopt a 5-/10-mm 0-degree optic and all 5-mm instruments. We use an atraumatic fenestrated grasping forceps to manage tissues, one curved dissector to isolate vessels, a hook cautery to perform dissection, and scissors to cut. The spermatic vessel control is usually performed using 5-mm titanium clips or if you want you can ligate them with a suture [6]. In the last 4 years, we adopted ICG-enhanced fluorescence technology in order to easily identify the lymphatic vessels and to spare them during the procedure to avoid hydrocele formation postoperatively. To use ICG technology, you need a special equipment represented

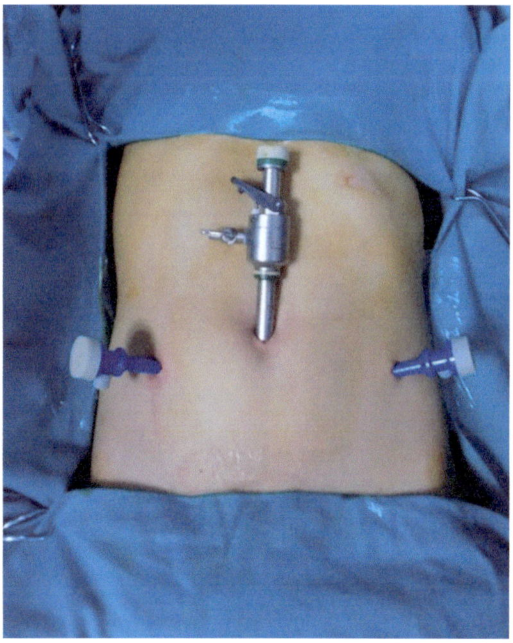

Fig. 55.2 We prefer to use three trocars: one 5–10-mm optic trocar in the umbilicus and two 5-mm working for operative instruments

by a special camera system and a special laparoscope equipped with a specific filter for near-infrared (NIR) light detection and obviously a vial of ICG dye (5 mg/mL) to be injected intratesticularly perioperatively [6–8, 10].

55.5 Technique

All the procedures were performed under general anesthesia with orotracheal intubation.

The first 5- or 10-mm trocar for the 0° optic was placed at umbilical level using open technique, and thereafter other two 5-mm working trocars were placed under vision in triangulation with the optic port. After pneumoperitoneum induction, the posterior peritoneum covering the inner spermatic vessels (ISV) was opened performing a 2-cm T-shaped incision with the monopolar hook, at a distance of about 3–4 cm from the internal inguinal ring [6] (Fig. 55.3).

After this step, a vial of ICG (5 mg/dL) was diluted with 10 mL of distilled water, and only

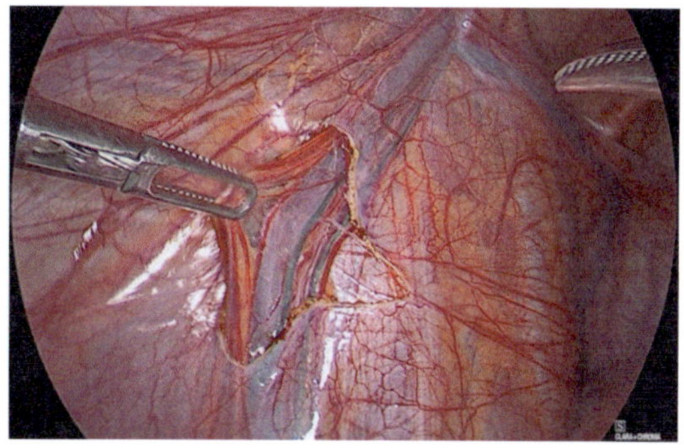

Fig. 55.3 The posterior perioneum is opened to identify the inner spermatic vessels (ISV)

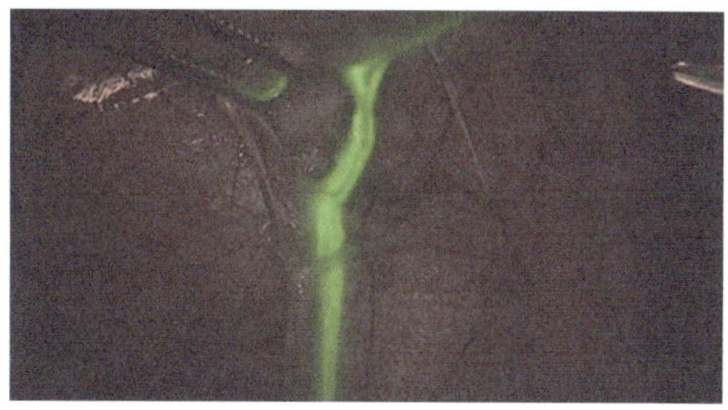

Fig. 55.4 Using ICG-enhanced fluorescence, the ISV appear green colored

2 mL of this solution was directly injected into the body of the left testicle using a 23G needle. Using the near-infrared mode, the lymphatic vessels appeared fluorescent and were clearly identified and spared; then the entire spermatic bundle was clipped and divided according to Palomo's principle (Figs. 55.4 and 55.5) [13, 14]. Also using the standard white light mode, the lymphatics were clearly visible because they appeared green. The ICG is commonly metabolized by the liver; for this reason, the patients' urine was normally colored after surgery and also the injection site on the scrotum presented no sign of the dye. The trocar orifices were closed using resorbable sutures, steri-strips, or glue.

55.6 Postoperative Care

Patients start oral feeding few hours postoperatively. Analgesic therapy is rarely necessary; Paracetamol (dosage 15 mg/kg at 8-h interval)

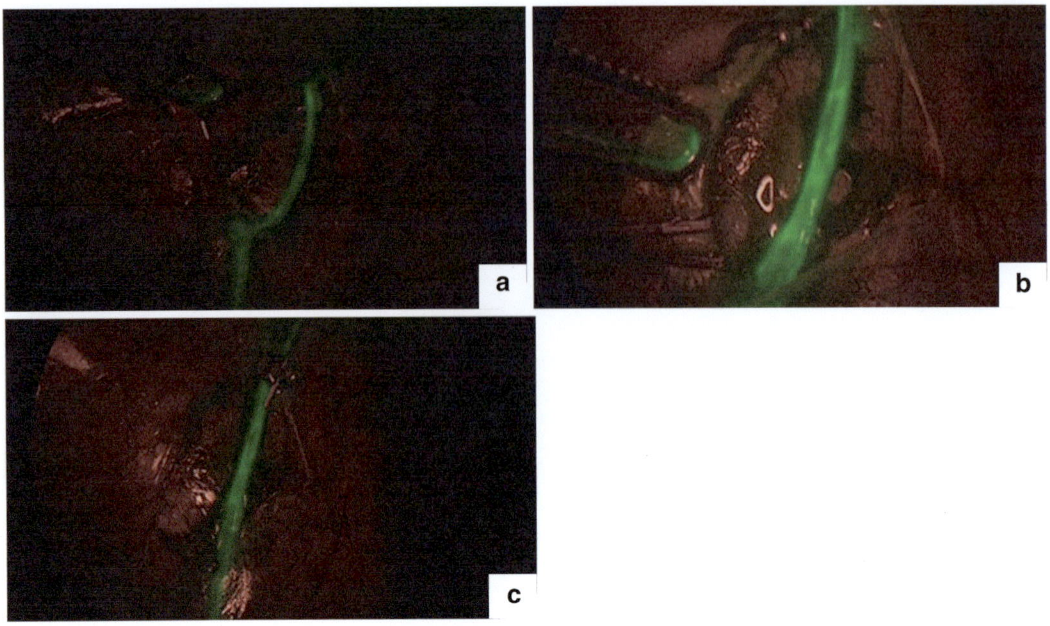

Fig. 55.5 The lymphatic vessels green colored are spared (**a**) and the spermatic bundle is clipped (**b**) and sectioned (**c**)

is usually administered in the first 12–24 h postoperatively. Patients are discharged from hospital the same evening in a day surgery setting or the day after surgery. Postoperative clinical controls are scheduled on 7th and 30th POD and thereafter annually for the first 2 years after surgery to search for a persistence of varicocele or to check the hydrocele formation. No US exam is performed after surgery. In children older than 16 years, a sperm analysis is performed 6–12 months after surgery [4, 16].

55.7 Results

In our experience, all the procedures were completed in laparoscopy with no conversion to open surgery or intraoperative complications.

In about 10–15% of patients, a lysis of adhesions of colon covering the ISV was performed as additional procedure during the same surgery. The average operative time was 18 min (range 10–25 min).

About 20–60 s after the intratesticular injection of ICG, the fluorescence of the lymphatics was clearly detected in 100% of the patients [14]. The lymphatic vessels appeared fluorescent using the near-infrared mode and green using the standard white light mode. In some patients, after a time interval of about 2–5 min from lymphatic visualization, also gonadal veins were observed using ICG fluorescence, although somewhat dully. In all patients, about two to three lymphatic vessels were identified and spared during the procedure. All patients restarted full oral feeding mean 2 h postoperatively and the average analgesic requirement was 12 h (range 8–24 h). The average length of hospital stay was 24 h (range 12–48 h). No allergy or other adverse events induced by ICG were observed in our series. No patients in our series experienced any testicular pain secondary to the intratesticular injection, either early or late after surgery. At a maximum follow-up of 72 months, no recurrence or persistence of varicocele was recorded and no postoperative hydrocele was observed. Two patients presented postoperatively umbilical port-site infection,

Tips and Tricks

- Regarding the patient's position, a 15° Trendelenburg position is a crucial point for the success of the procedure; in fact, using this patient's positioning, the loops slide down and you have an excellent exposure of the inner inguinal ring and of the ISV. In case of intestinal adhesions on the ISV, it is fundamental to perform a lysis of adhesions to have a good view on the ISV [16].
- Regarding the management of ISV, we believe that it is safe to ligate hilar vessels using endoscopic 5-mm clips. It is important to remember that 5-mm clips available on the market are medium size clips (8 mm of length). For this reason in children older than 15 years, sometimes 5-mm clips are too small to close the entire spermatic bundle. For this reason you have two possibilities: to ligate the spermatic bundle with a suture or to use bigger clips of large size but in this case you have to change a 5-mm trocar with a 10–12-mm trocar. It is also important to remember that if you use clips to close vessels, it is forbidden to use monopolar energy or sealing devices to seal the vessels between clips, in order to avoid the risk of clips dislodgement, which may occur immediately or later in the postoperative period [1, 2, 4].
- As for the ICG injection, you have to perform it directly inside the testicle and you have in a 100% of cases a good view of the lymphatics in about 60 s after the injection [14–16].
- At the end of the procedure, it is not necessary to close the peritoneum onto the spermatic vessels.

treated with oral antibiotics and local therapy (II Clavien). All patients were highly satisfied with the postoperative cosmetic appearance of the umbilicus [15, 16].

55.8 Discussion

Varicocele is a frequent pathology in pediatric population, with an incidence of 15–20%, and it is associated with testicular damage and subsequent testicular hypotrophy [5, 9].

Several reports stated that varicocele is related to sperm DNA disorders and male infertility, which are improved by surgical repair.

Laparoscopic Palomo technique is the most common approach adopted in children.

According to the reports of the international literature, the laparoscopic Palomo procedure resulted in a significant decrease of the operative failure rate compared with the artery sparing procedures, with no increase in the incidence of testicular hypotrophy/atrophy [9].

The main disadvantage reported with Palomo procedure was the high rate of postoperative hydrocele (10–30%) since during this technique no attempt is made to preserve the lymphatic vessels that are difficult to identify, because they are similar to small veins [1, 2].

Therefore, lymphatic sparing procedures have been applied for varicocele repair to decrease the incidence of postoperative hydrocele. Different vital dyes have been applied to perform lymphography during lymphatic sparing varicocelectomy, including patent V or its isomer isosulfan blue [11, 12].

In a recent article, we reported the standardization of lymphatic sparing Palomo technique using preoperative intradartoic/intratesticular injection of isosulfan blue. This procedure reported excellent results with a 0% rate of postoperative hydrocele. No adverse event related to isosulfan blue injection such as orchitis, allergy, or anaphylactic shock was reported in our series [4].

In recent years, ICG-enhanced fluorescence has been introduced in laparoscopic surgery to improve visualization and provide detailed anatomical information during surgery.

The ICG dye can be injected into the human blood stream with practically no adverse effects.

ICG becomes fluorescent once excited with light of a specific wavelength in the near-infrared spectrum delivered by a Xenon light source. After intravenous injection, ICG is rapidly bound to plasma proteins, especially lipoproteins. ICG is rapidly extracted unaltered through the liver and almost completely excreted without conjugation in bile about 8 min after injection [14, 15]. Fluorescence can be detected using specific scopes and cameras and then transmitted to a video screen, thus enabling the observer to visualize areas of anatomical interest where the dye has accumulated (biliary ducts, vessels, and lymph nodes) [10, 11].

To date, a few data about the use of ICG to perform lymphography in pediatric patients affected by varicocele have been reported.

We also standardized the technique of injection of ICG, as we already reported for isosulfan blue and we outlined the differences between the two vital dyes [6, 14].

The main difference is that isosulfan blue is metabolized by the kidney and consequently the urines appear blue for 1–2 days after surgery, whereas ICG is metabolized by the liver and the urines remain normal after surgery. Isosulfan blue injection leaves a blue slick on the scrotum for about 1–2 weeks postoperatively, whereas the scrotum appears normally colored after ICG injection [6, 7].

After ICG injection, there are two modalities of visualization of lymphatics: they appear fluorescent using the near-infrared mode whereas they appear green at the standard white light mode.

Switching from standard white light mode to near-infrared mode is simply done through foot-pedal control. The onset of fluorescence of lymphatics is about 20–60 s after ICG injection, and the duration of fluorescence is about 15 min. In this way, it is sufficient a single injection to allow completion of the entire procedure with no loss of the fluorescence.

In addition, the modality of administration of ICG, which is directly injected into the testicular parenchyma, is technically easier compared with the intradartoic/intratesticular injection previously described for isosulfan blue.

As for disadvantages related to the use of ICG, special equipment, including a camera system that can be operated in dual mode for both white light and fluorescence imaging and an ICG laparoscope equipped with a special filter for optimal reproduction during INC-enhanced fluorescence and standard white light imaging, are needed in the operative theater [14, 15].

In conclusion, lymphatic sparing laparoscopic Palomo varicocelectomy using ICG fluorescence lymphography is a feasible and versatile technique to adopt for treatment of children and adolescents with varicocele. The intratesticular injection of ICG and use of fluorescence vision resulted in a safe and effective method, allowing identification of lymphatic vessels in 100% of cases in our series. In addition, no allergy to ICG or postoperative hydrocele was reported after a midterm follow-up [13, 15].

Take-Home Points

- Laparoscopic Palomo procedure is a basic laparoscopic procedure. However, to perform it you need special camera and special optic to use ICG fluorescence technology and a vial of ICG.
- Before starting Palomo varicocele repair, you have to empty the bladder using a Nelaton catheter.
- You need three trocars with an optic of 5–10-mm 0-degree, plus two 5-mm trocars.
- The easiest way to close the spermatic bundle is a 5-mm clip applier.
- A long-term outcome is important to check the persistence/recurrence of varicocele and the hydrocele appearance.

References

1. Parrilli A, Roberti A, Escolino M, Esposito C. Surgical approaches for varicocele in pediatric patient. Transl Pediatr. 2016;5:227–32.
2. Borruto FA, Impellizzeri P, Antonuccio P, Finocchiaro A, Scalfari G, Arena F, Esposito C, Romeo C. Laparoscopic vs open varicocelectomy in children and adolescents: review of the recent literature and meta-analysis. J Pediatr Surg. 2010;45:2464–9.

3. Esposito C, Valla JS, Najmaldin A, Shier F, Mattioli G, Savanelli A, Castagnetti M, McKinley G, Stayaert H, Settimi A, Jasonni V, Guys JM. Incidence and management of hydrocele following varicocele surgery in children. J Urol. 2004;171:1271–3.
4. Esposito C, Monguzzi G, Gonzalez-Sabin MA, Rubino R, Montinaro L, Papparella A, Esposito G, Settimi A, Mastroianni L, Zamparelli M, Sacco R, Amici G, Damiano R, Innaro N. Results and complications of laparoscopic surgery for pediatric varicocele. J Pediatr Surg. 2001;36:767–9.
5. Liang Z, Guo J, Zhang H, Yang C, Pu J, Mei H, Zheng L, Tong Q. Lymphatic sparing versus lymphatic non-sparing laparoscopic varicocelectomy in children and adolescents: a systematic review and meta-analysis. Eur J Pediatr Surg. 2011;21:147–53.
6. Esposito C, Iaquinto M, Escolino M, Cortese G, De PT, Chiarenza F, Cerulo M, Settimi A. Technical standardization of laparoscopic lymphatic sparing varicocelectomy in children using isosulfan blue. J Pediatr Surg. 2014;49:660–3.
7. Groenlund JH, Telinius N, Skov SN, Hjortdal V. A validation study of near-infrared fluorescence imaging of lymphatic vessels in humans. Lymphat Res Biol. 2017;15:227–34.
8. Unno N, Nishiyama M, Suzuki M, Tanaka H, Yamamoto N, Sagara D, Mano Y, Konno H. A novel method of measuring human lymphatic pumping using indocyanine green fluorescence lymphography. J Vasc Surg. 2010;52:946–52.
9. La Vignera S, Condorelli R, Vicari E, D'Agata R, Calogero AE. Effects of varicocelectomy on sperm DNA fragmentation, mitochondrial function, chromatin condensation, and apoptosis. J Androl. 2012;33:389–96.
10. Capolicchio JP, El-Sherbiny M, Brzezinski A, Eassa W, Jednak R. Dye-assisted lymphatic-sparing laparoscopic varicocelectomy in children. J Pediatr Urol. 2013;9:33–7.
11. Golebiewski A, Krolak M, Komasara L, Czauderna P. Dye assisted lymph vessels sparing laparoscopic varicocelectomy. J Laparoendosc Adv Surg Tech A. 2007;17:360–3.
12. Chiarenza SF, Giurin I, Costa L, Alicchio F, Carabaich A, De Pascale T, Settimi A, Esposito C. Blue patent lymphography prevents hydrocele after laparoscopic varicocelectomy: 10 years of experience. J Laparoendosc Adv Surg Tech A. 2012;22:930–3.
13. Esposito C, Settimi A, Del Conte F, Cerulo M, Coppola V, Farina A, Crocetto F, Ricciardi E, Esposito G, Escolino M. Image-guided pediatric surgery using Indocyanine green (ICG) fluorescence in laparoscopic and robotic surgery. Front Pediatr. 2020;8:314.
14. Esposito C, Del Conte F, Cerulo M, Gargiulo F, Izzo S, Esposito G, Spagnuolo MI, Escolino M. Clinical application and technical standardization of indocyanine green (ICG) fluorescence imaging in pediatric minimally invasive surgery. Pediatr Surg Int. 2019 Oct;35(10):1043–50.
15. Esposito C, Turrà F, Del Conte F, Izzo S, Gargiulo F, Farina A, Severino G, Cerulo M, Escolino M. Indocyanine green fluorescence Lymphography: a new technique to perform lymphatic sparing laparoscopic Palomo Varicocelectomy in children. J Laparoendosc Adv Surg Tech A. 2019 Apr;29(4):564–7.
16. Esposito C, Escolino M, Castagnetti M, Cerulo M, Settimi A, Cortese G, Turrà F, Iannazzone M, Izzo S, Servillo G. Two decades of experience with laparoscopic varicocele repair in children: standardizing the technique. J Pediatr Urol. 2018;14(1):10.e1–7.

Management of Impalpable Testis 56

Thomas Middleton, Syed Salahuddin, and Ramnath Subramaniam

Learning Objectives
- To explain the rationale behind management of impalpable undescended testis.
- To understand the techniques to evaluate the presence and position of the impalpable testis by laparoscopy and proceed to definitive procedures.
- To lay out the decision-making process for what procedure a child with an undescended testicle actually needs.

56.1 Introduction

56.1.1 Etiology

In normal embryological development, the testes develop in the retroperitoneum and descend to the deep inguinal ring and then through the inguinal canal across the third trimester. The testes may still descend in the first couple of months after birth which is one of the reasons why it is not advocated to surgically intervene on undescended testes in the first few months of life. Undescended testes (also referred to as cryptorchidism) occur in about 1% of boys [1] and the testicle can position itself anywhere along the path of its descent. A testicle may even be outside of the normal path of development altogether (an ectopic testicle) but this is rare and beyond the scope of this chapter. The reasons why the testicular descent arrests abnormally are multifactorial and not fully understood.

56.1.2 Malignancy Risk

The risk of testicular malignancy is raised in boys with undescended testes estimated at around three times that of the general population [2]. Although the actual risk remains low [3, 4], there is some evidence that an early orchidopexy may reduce the rate [5]. Moreover, a testicle in the scrotum may be self-examined allowing testicular malignancies to be picked up earlier than if they remain in an undescended position.

56.1.3 Fertility

Fertility can be affected by cryptorchidism. In men with a unilateral undescended testicle, paternity rates are essentially normal at around 90% but in men with bilateral undescended testes, paternity rates are much lower at around 50% [6].

Supplementary Information The online version contains supplementary material available at [https://doi.org/10.1007/978-3-030-99280-4_56].

T. Middleton · S. Salahuddin · R. Subramaniam (✉)
Paediatric Urology Department, Leeds General Infirmary, Leeds, UK
e-mail: thomas.middleton@nhs.net; salahuddin.syed@nhs.net; R.Subramaniam@leeds.ac.uk

C. Esposito et al. (eds.), *Minimally Invasive Techniques in Pediatric Urology*,
https://doi.org/10.1007/978-3-030-99280-4_56

It is hard to know exactly to what extent an orchidopexy improves paternity rates but when undescended testes are not corrected early, there is evidence showing the development of the testicle is impaired [7].

56.1.4 Other Adverse Sequelae of Cryptorchidism

Testes that are undescended and palpable in the groin and thus are external cannot swing if knocked and therefore may be more vulnerable to trauma; anecdotally it is not infrequent for boys with undescended testes to get discomfort from them (although note that these partly descended testes are the ones that would be approached by an open procedure). Furthermore, boys with undescended testes are more at risk of testicular torsion [8].

56.2 Preoperative Preparation

The diagnosis of undescended testes is made by clinical examination. It should not be underestimated that it may be difficult particularly in boys who are uncooperative to examination or in children with a lot of overlying fat. It is important to try to establish not only the absence of the testicle from the scrotum but whether the testicle is palpable at all as this will change the surgical approach.

Ultrasound is not a routine part of our practice in diagnosing undescended testes. An intra-abdominal testicle may not be visible on scan and essentially always require an evaluation by laparoscopy.

In keeping with UK guidance [9], we would aim to operate on undescended testes at around 1 year of life although it is not infrequent for boys to present much later. In cases of bilateral impalpable testes, it would be advisable to not routinely operate on both at the same time, but we recognize this practice is variable between surgeons and centers [10]. Neonates with bilateral impalpable testes require special consideration as these children may in fact have an underlying abnormality of sexual differentiation and discussion with a pediatric endocrinologist early is advisable [11].

56.3 Procedure

56.3.1 Examination under Anesthetics (EUAs)

If the testicle is impalpable, the procedure starts with an examination under anesthetics as it will sometimes be palpable with the child relaxed. The testes are examined in the anesthetic room with the child asleep. This may help the anesthetist to decide whether to intubate the child (which they may be more inclined to do for laparoscopy if the testicle is impalpable) or whether a laryngeal mask airway is appropriate.

56.3.2 Palpable Testicle

If the testis is palpable on EUA, an open orchidopexy is performed with the child in a supine position. For technical details which is beyond the scope of this chapter, please refer to BJUI Knowledge [12] series on UDT by the same authors.

56.3.3 Impalpable Testicle

If the testis remains impalpable, the next step would be to establish pneumoperitoneum and evaluate the position of the testis in the abdomen. It is worthwhile emphasizing at this point, in cases of bilateral impalpable testes, we would only advocate operating on one side at a time, as alluded to earlier. The operating surgeon stands at the cranial end of the bed on the opposite side of the testicle being operated on; the assistant stands opposite to the operating surgeon. The screen will need to be on the opposite side of the table toward the caudal end as shown in Fig. 56.1.

If the anesthetic machine is at the cranial end of the bed, the surgeons may be very close to the anesthetist and some anesthetists will prefer to have the bed turned so that the head is away from the anesthetic machine: it is worth discussing this preoperatively.

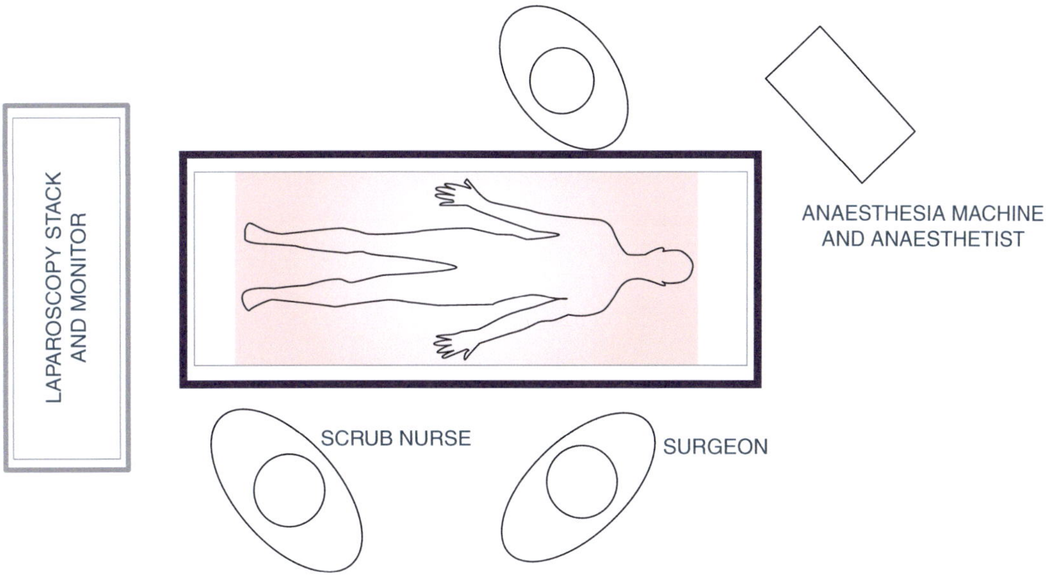

Fig. 56.1 Theatre layout for laparoscopy in a case of impalpable testis

56.4 Instrumentation

The size of instruments vary according to the size of the child and the exact laparoscopic equipment used will depend on the center where you work. In vast majority, there is usually a camera port and two working instrument ports. The instruments should triangulate toward the corresponding groin as area of interest. In the smallest children it may be feasible to simply place the instruments through and incision in the abdominal wall without a port to minimize scar size. A grasping instrument and a dissecting instrument will be required. Options for the dissecting instruments include diathermy hook, diathermy enabled scissors, and endoscopic clips.

To allow the mobilized testicle is brought into the scrotum, two options are available. You may choose to first reroute the mobilized testicle into the groin via a crease incision and then bring it down to the scrotum like open orchidopexy. The other option is to directly place the mobilized testicle into the scrotum and here a step port will be required either at the second stage of a traditional two-staged (Fowler-Stephen) FS procedure or occasionally a single-stage laparoscopic procedure.

56.5 Technique

Decision-making algorithm is presented in Fig. 56.2.

56.5.1 Open Procedure

If a testicle is palpable, this would be the only operation they should need; if laparoscopy is performed for an impalpable testicle and the cord structures are seen to enter the deep ring, then a groin exploration is the next step with a view to open orchidopexy.

56.5.2 Laparoscopy

An umbilical camera port is placed to evaluate the deep inguinal ring from inside to see if the testicle is present next to it or if cord structures pass through the ring. Two instrument ports are placed on either side of the abdomen triangulating toward the side being operated on. At this point, it is worthwhile to mention the evaluation should begin with the contralateral normal side in case of unilateral pathology to allow comparison.

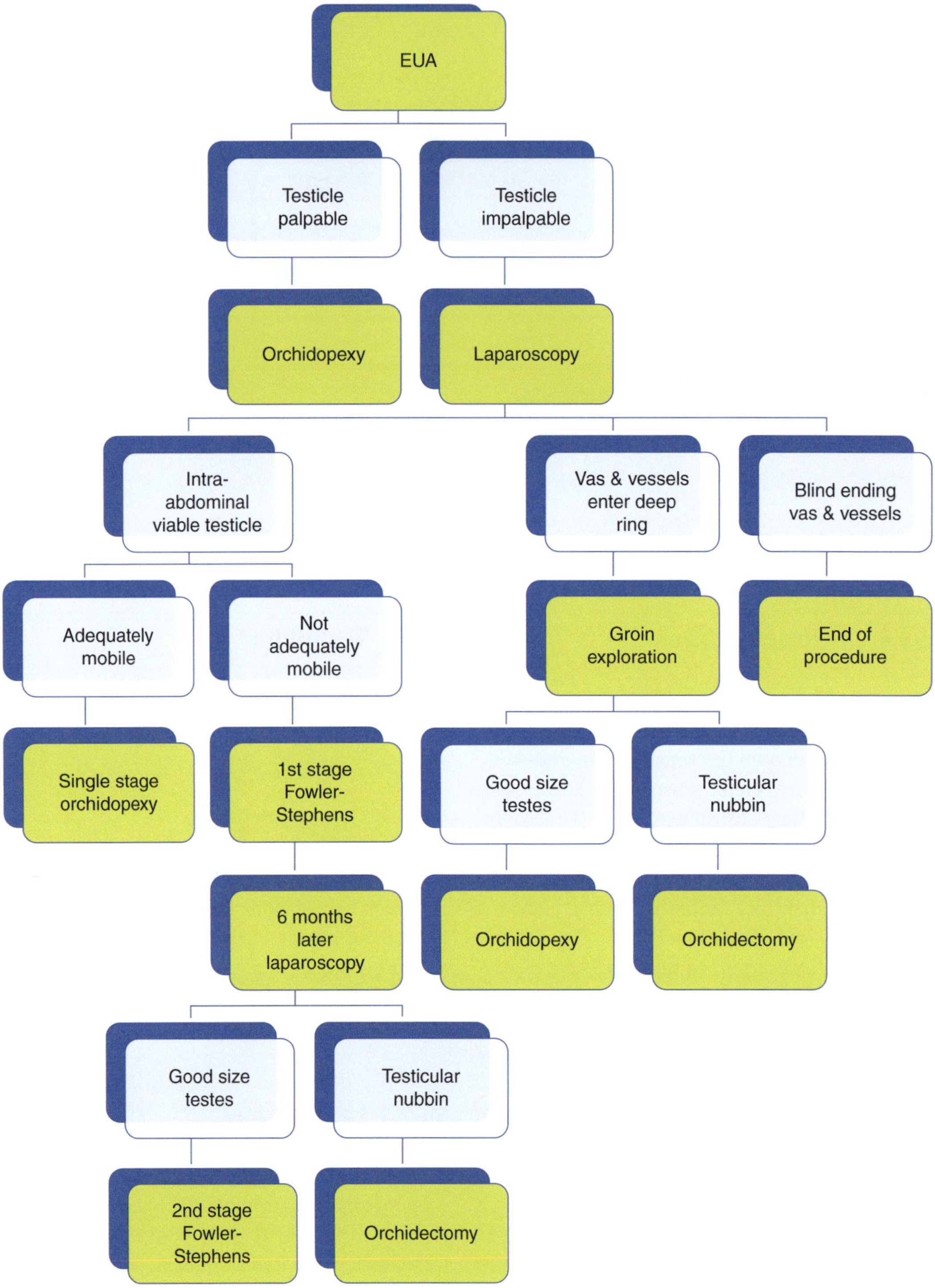

Fig. 56.2 Decision-making algorithm for management when a unilateral testicle was impalpable on the child in clinic

The possible scenarios one may encounter are an intra-abdominal testis, blind ending vas and vessels, or vas and vessels entering the internal ring which are demonstrated in Fig. 56.3.

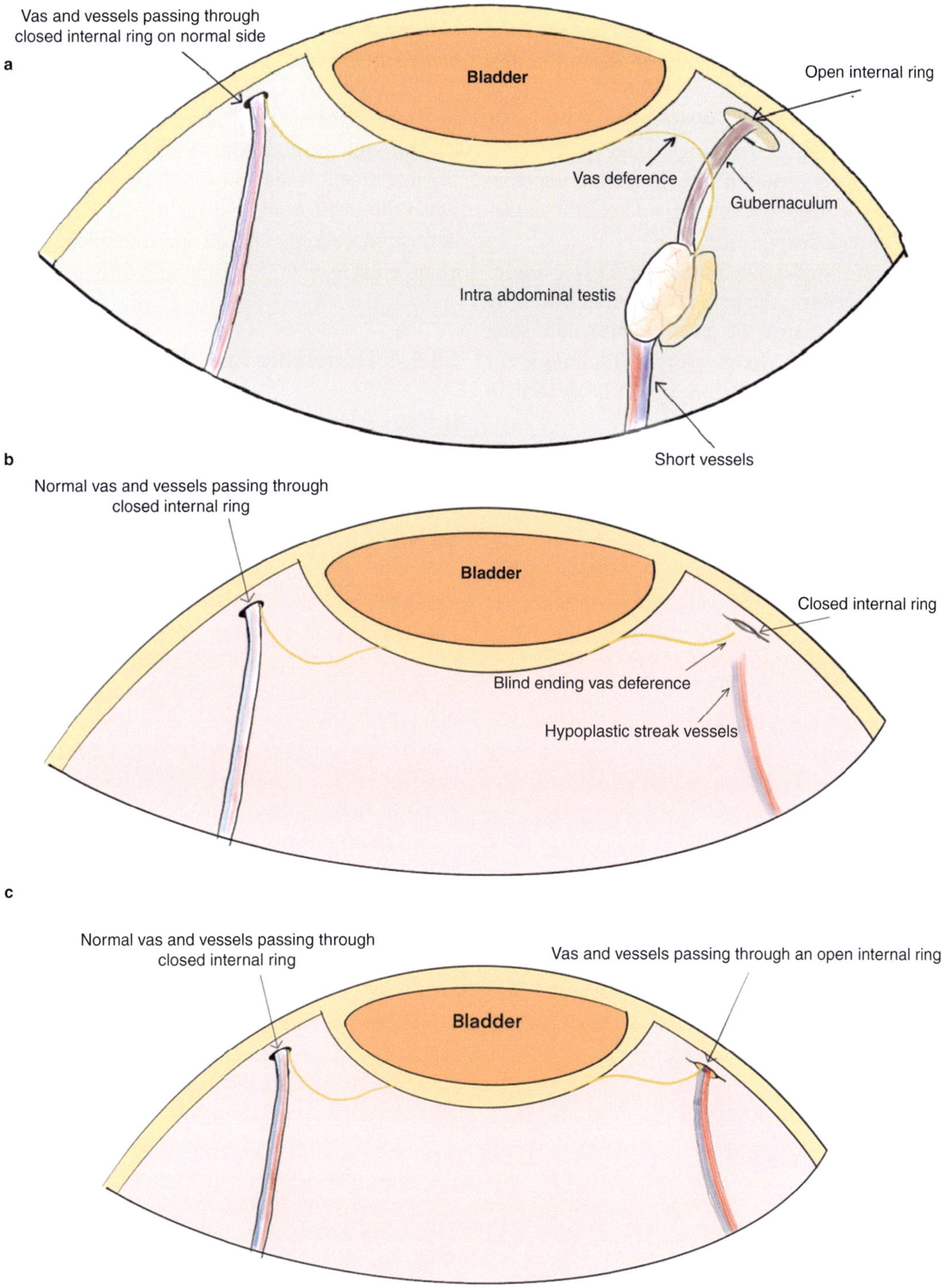

Fig. 56.3 Possible scenarios on laparoscopy in a case of impalpable testis

56.5.3 Viable Intra-Abdominal Testicle

If there is a viable testicle in the abdomen, an assessment is made if it can be stretched across to the opposite internal ring and evaluate if it has adequate length on its vas and vessels for a single-stage procedure. While rates of testicular atrophy are higher for single-stage procedures, this risk is very small if only low-lying impalpable testes with good length are selected for single-stage orchidopexy [13].

If there is adequate cord length for a single-stage procedure, the testis is mobilized well by dissecting it free of attachments and then delivered into the hemiscrotum. Technique for delivering the mobilized testis is described later.

If there is not adequate length on the cord, a first-stage Fowler-Stephens procedure is undertaken. The principle of this procedure is to ligate the main testicular vessels to gain adequate length of the cord but allow the collateral supply from the artery of the vas and the cremasteric artery to develop to their full potential before bringing the testicle down and putting them under pressure.

After assessing the length on the vessels and determining it is inadequate for a single-stage procedure, the vessels are either interrupted with a ligature or clips. Some divide the vessels after interrupting but that is not mandatory and can be left until second stage. That concludes the first stage of the procedure.

The second-stage procedure is performed in 4–6 months' time to give the collateral vessels opportunity to develop. Again, the child would have a central camera port placed in the umbilicus and the testicle assessed for viability. If the testicle was viable, two working ports would be placed through the previous incisions. The testicle would then be mobilized further by releasing any peritoneal attachments with dissection as far lateral as possible to preserve the best possible collateral blood supply.

56.5.3.1 Technique for Delivering Mobilized Testis into Scrotum

This is achieved by inserting a step port either directly through an incision in the scrotum, be passed up through the inguinal canal and into the abdominal cavity, or some prefer to make a groin incision as for an open procedure and pass the port through the deep ring. A laparoscopic grasping instrument is then passed through the port to grasp the testicle and deliver it into the wound before proceeding as per an open orchidopexy for an inguinal testicle.

56.5.4 Nonviable Testicle

If at any stage a nonviable testicle was found, the remnant tissue is excised.

56.5.5 Alternative Techniques

One emerging alternative treatment proposed for impalpable testes is stretching the impalpable testicle across the peritoneal cavity and fixing it on the contralateral side under tension [14]. The theoretical advantage is the preservation of the vessels but with the possible risks of the fixed cord acting as a band for bowel volvulus as well as the testicle atrophying from the stretch.

Another considered idea is that of microvascular anastomosis whereby the testicular vessels are divided and then undergo micro-anastomosis to the inferior epigastric vessels as an autotransplantation [15]. This requires microscopic equipment and may not be practical in most centers.

Finally in gubernacular sparing techniques, boys who have undergone first-stage Fowler-Stephens do not have their gubernaculum divided but instead the peritoneum is lifted a flap and mobilized with the testicle down through the inguinal canal (again with the hope of minimizing atrophy from further vessel loss). This is the subject on an ongoing clinical trial [16] (refer to Video 56.1).

56.5.6 Postoperative Care

All the above procedures for cryptorchidism can be done as a day case if the child has no specific comorbidity affecting anesthesia and they can often return to full activity within a couple of days. We use steri-strips or glue as dressing and usually advise the parents to protect the area from getting wet for 2–3 days. We advocate the avoidance of strenuous physical activity (such as sports) for 2 weeks post-op.

56.6 Outcomes

Orchidopexy is one of the most common pediatric surgical procedures and about 20% of undescended testes are impalpable for which the two-staged Fowler-Stephens procedure or occasionally single-stage laparoscopic approach is the mainstay of treatment.

The majority of boys with cryptorchidism have good outcomes. In the short-term, post-op complications such as bleeding are rare. Rates of success are quoted as around 95% for palpable testes and 85% for impalpable testes [17]. Follow-up for boys who undergo orchidopexy is recommended initially at 6 weeks to 3 months post-op and then at 6 months so that any scarring and testicular ascent have time to occur.

Paternity in men who have had unilateral cryptorchidism is essentially normal even in cases where the testicle has either not developed at all or is excised. In cases of bilateral cryptorchidism, paternity rates after bilateral orchidopexies are about 50% [6] and are essential which is discussed pre- and postoperatively.

As mentioned above, testicular malignancy remains higher in men who have undergone orchidopexy than those that have not and while formal screening is not usually required, we would encourage all boys to self-examine once a month from the start of puberty.

Take-Home Points

- Most boys with cryptorchidism do well, even with an impalpable testis but fertility and malignancy risk are affected.
- Operating on undescended testis may mitigate some of the impairment of testicular function and malignancy risk but they are not normalized, and this should be clear in-patient counseling.
- For reasons pertaining to both the anesthetic and the surgery, impalpable testes should be managed in tertiary pediatric surgery units.
- When embarking on an operation for an impalpable testicle, there are multiple possibilities on what procedure the child will require, and these are summarized in the flow chart below.

References

1. Sistermans K, Hack WWM, Meijer RW, Van der Voort-Doedens LM. The frequency of undescended testis from birth to adulthood: a review. Int J Androl. 2007;31(1):1–11.
2. Lip SZ, Murchison LE, Cullis PS, Govan L, Carachi R. A meta-analysis of the risk of boys with isolated cryptorchidism developing testicular cancer in later life. Arch Dis Child. 2013;98(1):20–6.
3. Pettersson A, Richiardi L, Nordenskjold A, Kaijser M, Akre O. Age at surgery for undescended testis and risk of testicular cancer. N Engl J Med. 2007;356(18):1835–41.
4. Higgins E, Smith DE, Gao D, Wilcox D, Cost NG, Saltzman AF. The impact of age at orchiopexy on testicular cancer outcomes. World J Urol. 2019;38:2531–6.
5. Walsh TJ, Dall'Era MA, Croughan MS, Carroll PR, Turek PJ. Prepubertal orchidopexy for cryptorchidism may be associated with lower risk of testicular cancer. J Urol. 2007;178:1440–6.
6. Fertility guidelines. European association of urology. Cryptorchidism. 2017. http://uroweb.org/guideline/male-infertility/#5_6.
7. Kollin C, Stukenborg JB, Nurimo M, Sudqvist E, Gustafsso T, Soder O, Toppari J, Nordenskjold A, Ritzen EM. Boys with undescended testes: endo-

crine, volumetric and morphometric studies on testicular function before and after orchidopexy at nine months or three years of age. Endocr Res. 2012;97(12):4588–95.
8. Clinical knowledge summary. NICE. Undescended testes. 2020. https://cks.nice.org.uk/undescended-testes#!topicSummary.
9. British Association of Paediatric Surgeons, British Association of Paediatric Urologists, Association of Paediatric Anaesthetists, UK National Screening Committee. Commissioning guide: paediatric orchidopexy for undescended testis. 2015. http://www.bapu.org.uk/documents/consensus.
10. Mostafa IA, Shalaby MS, Woodward MN. Bilateral orchidopexies: synchronous or metachronous? Survey of BAPS and BAPU members and single-Centre comparison. J Pediatr Surg. 2019;54(2):310–2.
11. Ahmed SF, Achermann JC, Arlt W, Balen A, Conway G, Edwards Z, Elford S, Hughes IA, Izatt L, Krone N, Miles H, O'Toole S, Perry L, Sanders C, Simmonds M, Watt A, Willis D. Society for endocrinology UK guidance on the initial evaluation of an infant or an adolescent with a suspected disorder of sex development. Clin Endocrinol. 2015;84(5):771–88.
12. BJUI. Surgery for undescended testes: open and laparoscopic. 2019. https://doi.org/10.18591/BJUIK.0241.
13. Shehata SM, Shehata SMK, Baky Fahmy MA. The intra-abdominal testis: lessons from the past, and ideas for the future. Pediatr Surg Int. 2013;29:1039–45.
14. Shehata S, Shalaby R, Ismail M, Abouheba M, Elrouby A. Staged laparoscopic traction-orchidopexy for intraabdominal testis (Shehata technique): stretching the limits for preservation of testicular vasculature. J Pediatr Surg. 2016;51(2):211–5.
15. Okur H, Alkan Y, Karakaya AE, Guzel M. Microvascular orchidopexy. J Pediatr Urol. 2007;3(1):88.
16. Macmaster University. One vs two stage gubernacular sparing laparoscopic orchidopexy (GSLO). Clinical Trial Identifier NCT02936024 Expected completion. 2021.
17. Roy C, Cullis PS, Clark C, Munro FD. Retrospective analysis of testicular outcomes following laparoscopic two-stage fowler Stephens orchidopexy. J Pediatr Surg. 2020;55(2):300–3.

Application of 3D Reconstruction in Pediatric Urology

57

Amane Allah Lachkar, Luc Soler, and François Becmeur

Learning Objectives

- To describe the use of 3D reconstruction.
- To emphasize the importance of using 3D preoperative planning for better risk management.
- To prepare a surgical procedure for each new patient and learn this new process.
- To show a video presenting the many possibilities offered by one of these software programs.

57.1 Introduction

Before going to the operative room with the patient, the surgeon needs to come forward with an appropriate indication: is it really necessary to operate the patient? Is there another way to treat this patient? The surgeon decides on the best advantage/disadvantage balance for the patient. It depends on the severity of the pathology. Some procedures are benign and can ensure recovery with a low morbidity rate but may be inadequate due to either social reasons or to the severity of the pathology. The surgical answer has to be gradually adapted to the seriousness of the illness.

In addition, many other questions remain for each patient: what may be dangerous in this specific anatomy and pathological condition? What is the probability to come across any adverse (unpredictable) event? In case of complication, how serious is it according to the Clavien-Dindo classification? And considering the illness, the tumor, the malformation, is it acceptable?

Until recent times at the beginning of this century, we only knew about "surgery for everyone" with general principles for each procedure. Naturally, we could mentally prepare for our surgical procedure. Images had become increasingly precise since the 1970s. However, even with a serious preoperative workup using various CT scans or MRIs, preparing different surgical approaches and strategies, we failed to obtain real knowledge and to be confident with the patient. We discovered a part of the patient only once surgery was being performed. Some technical difficulties arose and occurred unexpectedly. That could be the origin of mistakes, errors, and complications.

Supplementary Information The online version contains supplementary material available at [https://doi.org/10.1007/978-3-030-99280-4_57].

A. A. Lachkar · F. Becmeur (✉)
Department of Paediatric Surgery, Hôpital de Hautepierre, Strasbourg, France
e-mail: AmaneAllah.LACHKAR@chru-strasbourg.fr; Francois.Becmeur@chru-strasbourg.fr

L. Soler
IRCAD, Strasbourg, France
e-mail: luc.soler@visiblepatient.com

C. Esposito et al. (eds.), *Minimally Invasive Techniques in Pediatric Urology*,
https://doi.org/10.1007/978-3-030-99280-4_57

Until now, the best risk management in pediatric surgery is probably the use of 3D preoperative planning. It allows the surgeon to be perfectly confident with the patient and with difficulties that may be encountered. Thanks to this new tool, surgeons became capable of doing and redoing the procedure many times in their own brain.

We will get the opportunity to add 3D printing more and more often. Preoperative simulation will be available to improve basic skills, and more particularly so with the improvement of 3D printing and the development of new materials.

And most importantly, during laparoscopic procedures or robot-assisted procedures, it became possible to add and overlay the 3D reconstruction of the patient onto the same screen. As a result, the surgeon can be perfectly guided during the procedure and anticipate risks. What has been planned will be performed. The elements of surprise will disappear. They are a source of incidents and trouble, complications, morbidity, and mortality.

57.2 How Does it Work?

3D reconstruction, classically provided by radiologist from CT scan or MRI, are based on direct volume rendering (Fig. 57.1). This tool, freely accessible in every workstation, is very useful and does not require any preprocessing. Every initial voxel gray level is replaced by an associated voxel color and transparency allowing a better distinction between anatomical and pathological structures even when they are not delineated in reality. Hence, this technique offers a good visualization of anatomical and pathological structures. Nevertheless, as organs are not delineated, accurate dimensions and volumes cannot be provided. Equally, providing a volume after resection, or cutting a section of these structures without cutting neighboring structure, is impossible.

Thus, to solve this issue, many teams have developed software using surface rendering based on organ segmentation. It can be performed with a standard medical imaging workstation (Syngo™ from Siemens Healthineers, AW™ from GE Healthcare, IntelliSpace™ from Philips, Vitrea™ from Canon Medical System), with a more specific workstation (Myrian™ from Intrasense, Synapse™ from Fuji), or with a distant online service that can be compared to a medical analysis laboratory (Visible Patient Solution™) (Table 57.1).

Those medical devices software provide a 3D patient modeling. Three tools are then available:

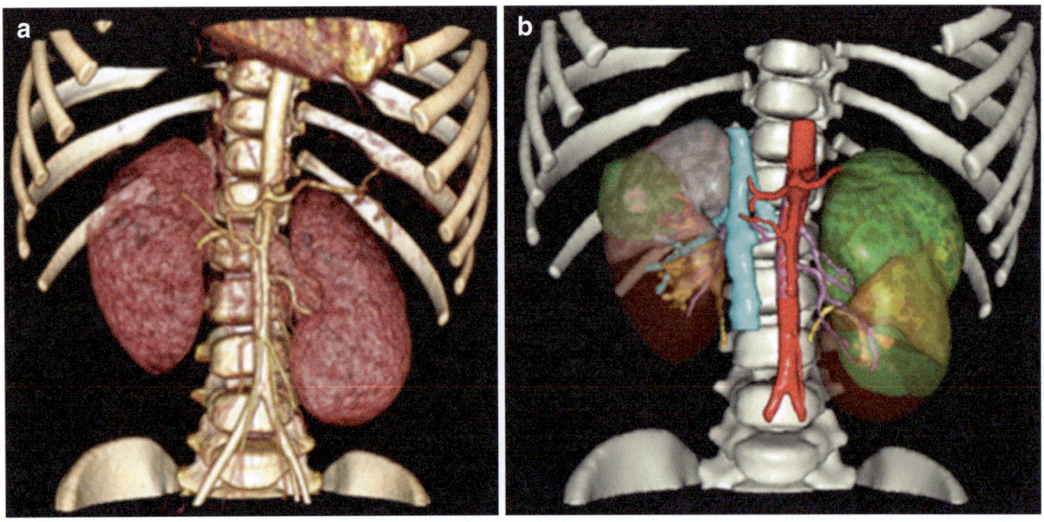

Fig. 57.1 (**a**) Direct volume rendering 3D reconstruction (**b**) Surface rendering 3D reconstruction

Table 57.1 Comparison between different 3D reconstruction options

DVR	SR	
-Free -Available on every workstation -Topographic data -Normal and pathological anatomy -No clip applying system -No volume calculation -No virtual resection	-Payment -Segmentation -Virtual Clone -Accuracy -Clip applying system -Volume calculation -Virtual resection	
	Workstation	**Online service**
	-Time consuming -Radiologist or surgeon -Available only on computer	-Less time consuming -Imaging experts with double checking -Available on computer, phone and tablet

- An anatomical atlas directly derived from the CT scan images of the patient (Fig. 57.2b).
- A 3D virtual model of the patient (Fig. 57.2c).
- A clip applying system (video in supplements).

57.2.1 The Anatomical Atlas

The anatomical atlas is defined by CT scan or MRI slices after delineation and coloring. This is the first step of the process. The surgeon must recognize the pathology, identify which malformation or which tumor has to be treated, and what can be the best solution for this patient. This atlas allows an enhanced lecture of exams and offer to surgeons a playful map.

For instance, in case of a double kidney, we can offer a reinstatement of a damaged, yet still functioning, moiety or remove it. This is the essential and primary decision that surgeons have to make. For a tumor, we have two different options:

- To remove the tumor and the kidney around, perform a partial nephrectomy, leave a sufficient blood supply for the remaining part of the kidney that is left in place, and reorganize the emptying of this remaining kidney, reconstructing a functional urinary tract. For this option, we need to know much more than the anatomy of the main vessels and we need a precise description of the anatomy of the urinary tract.
- To remove the entire kidney, performing a total nephrectomy.

57.2.2 3D Virtual Model of the Patient

It will help the surgeon to set up a strategy for the procedure and to define the different steps for it and their chronology through the virtual clone of the patient.

It has become possible to very precisely describe each vessel until their final destination. It is then easy to write the storyline for the surgical procedure in a stepwise fashion. The detailed map of the vessels allows to know which one has to be secure and where it has to be done (*a clip applying system: only available on Synapse*™ *from Fuji and Visible patient solution*™).

We take the example of a renal tumor with the aim of performing a partial nephrectomy using Visible Patient™. This surgery has to observe the laws of oncology and leave a part of the normal kidney with a functional urinary tract which can empty the urine.

Consequently, it is necessary to draw a line that will mark out the correct margin on the 3D

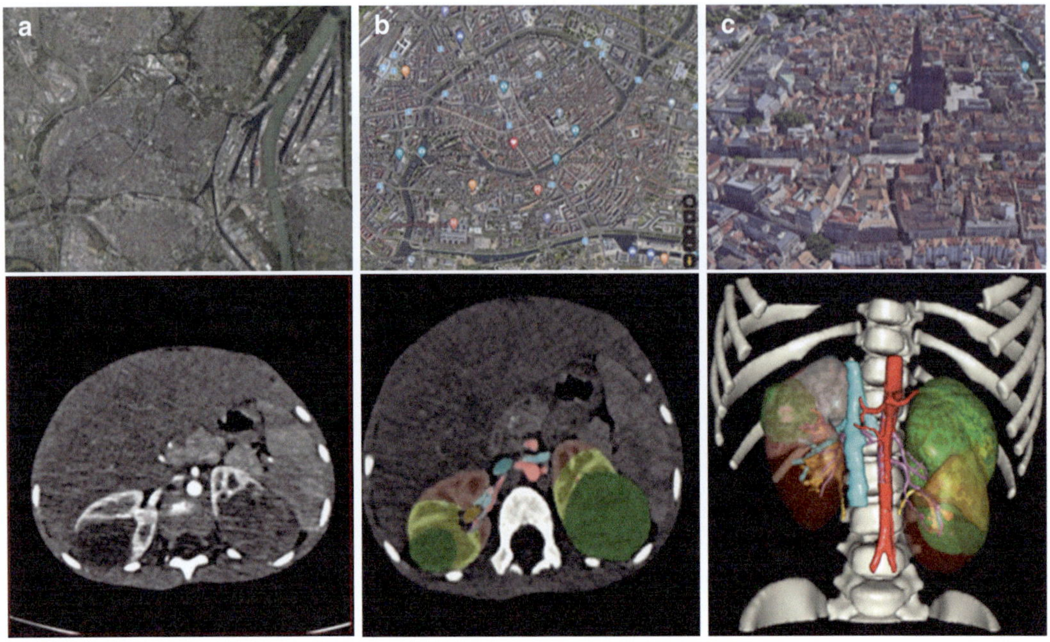

Fig. 57.2 3D reconstruction and mapping. (**a**) Satellite view—original CT scan slice. (**b**) Playful map—anatomical atlas. (**c**) 3D map—3D reconstruction

model in order to ensure a sufficient resection. For this function, the normal kidney is seen in transparency.

Next, we use the clip applying system. When using a virtual clip on an artery of the 3D reconstruction, the corresponding territory will appear in 3D, perfectly defined. The software will immediately provide the volume of the target organ (the kidney), the volume of the simulated remaining part (absolute value and percentage), and the volume of the resected part (absolute value and percentage). Taking into account the margins for a safe resection, one can instantly know if the first simulated ligature of an artery will be sufficient or not. As a result, it is possible to predict the entire procedure in advance and to organize the reconstruction of the urinary tract which can be added to the model.

57.3 Prerequisite

The CT scan or MRI that is needed for a 3D reconstruction has to be of excellent quality, in high resolution, and with different series and notably one during injection of the contrast fluid for an arterial sequence and a second one during the opacification of the veins and a third sequence for the parenchyma.

57.4 Instrumentation

If you use a workstations solution, you need to buy workstation with dedicated software and you need a specific training to learn how to use it (usually 2 days of training). 3D reconstruction is only available on the computer after your own process of organ and pathology delineation.

If you use an online service like Visible Patient Solution, software is free of charge and available on the computer (PC Windows and Mac OS), tablet, and phone (iOS only). The user pays per case, which means a cost per analysis like blood or biological analysis. You only need an Internet connection to send and receive your image from a secured web portal provided by Visible Patient.

57.5 Technique

If you use a workstations solution, a radiologist or the surgeon has to do the delineation himself/herself to obtain the reconstruction. CT scan and MRI images are imported from internal servers. It needs a learning curve to master the software and train the eye. An automatic lung or liver delineation can be expected in 15 min before manual correction. But the process can be much longer if you are looking for more details or if you want nonautomated segmentation, which means other structures. For instance, in pediatric surgery workstation, automation is too much limited to allow efficient 3D modeling of surrounding anatomical or pathological structures (e.g., no automation for pulmonary sequestration, neuroblastoma, diaphragm, etc.). Manual delineation will be then possible but can (and will) take several hours if you need lots of details and vessels. The main benefit of such a long process will be essentially educative, the user having a better understanding of the medical image if he spent this time. But due to the long processing and the lack of automation, such workstation solutions are not frequently used to perform 3D modeling in pediatric procedure.

If you use Visible Patient online service, reconstruction is made by the service after an anonymization and data securing from a web portal stored on a certified medical data protection system. Such security is not always assumed by other online laboratory and will have to be checked before able to guarantee the patient data protection. In the 3D modeling being performed by online laboratories, you only spent time to order, upload the image, and download the result on your PC, Mac, or smartphone. The main benefit is to have access to any organ and pathology 3D modeling without limitation to spend time and to do it yourself. Visible Patient also adds a double check control of the result, the processing being performed by expert radiology technologists specifically educated for image postprocessing analysis. In some other online laboratories, the processing is performed by a computer science engineer.

57.6 Postoperative Period

Discrepancies may occur between the 3D-reconstructed model and the initial analysis of CT scan images. In fact, a simple analysis of the CT scan and the comparison with the patient's anatomy may reveal some differences that could be corrected by 3D reconstruction (e.g., vascular supply or details on the anatomy of the intrarenal urinary tract). These are the advantages of this technique of preoperative 3D modeling. One question may be the following: could it be possible to know how many arteries and veins have to be secured and in which order? What level of precision could be reached for the description prior to each step of the surgical procedure? Were the surgery proceedings consistent with the preoperative workup, using the 3D reconstruction of the patient?

Discrepancies may rarely occur between the 3D reconstructed model and the original patient, and when it arrived it is usually a lack of details. If you use a workstation solution, a manual upgrade of the 3D modeling can be performed by yourself, but if you use an online service, the improvement has to be requested to the online laboratory. The type of feedback is normal and essential in order to improve the results of new technologies.

57.7 Results

Virtual surgical planning with 3D reconstruction provides helpful information which has an impact on the diagnosis and subsequently optimizes the surgical treatment.

Regarding oncological cases, 3D reconstruction provides a high-definition anatomy precisely showing the tumor location, its relationship with adjacent organs, as well as vascularization and urinary tract anatomy. The prognostic interest is twofold, namely, oncological and functional. Indeed, oncological resection margins can be simulated and a precise estimation of the resection volume estimated.

For example, we report the case of a 21-month-old boy with a bilateral Wilms' tumor.

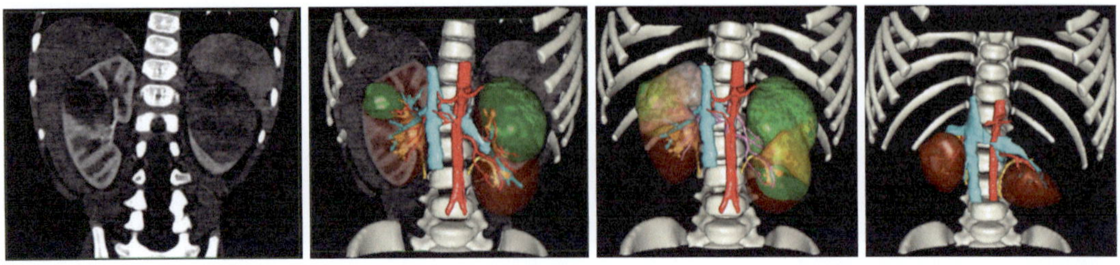

Fig. 57.3 Bilateral Wilms' tumor in a 21-month-old boy

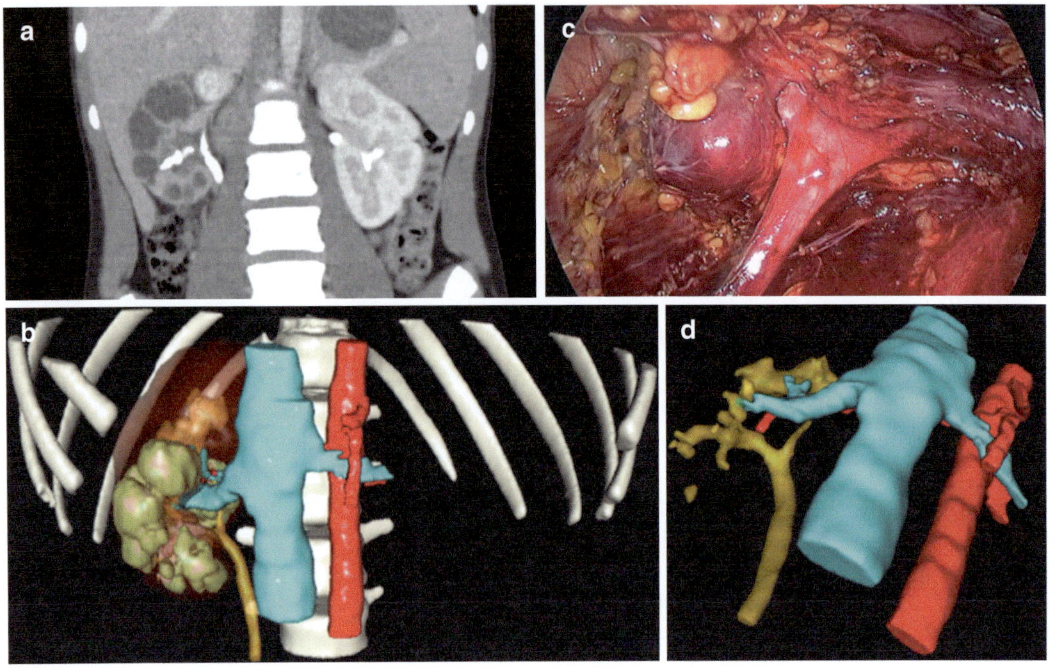

Fig. 57.4 Right pyelic duplication in nonfunctional lower pole kidney. (**a**) CT scan. (**b**) 3D reconstruction view. (**c**) Intraoperative view. (**d**) 3D reconstruction view corresponding to intraoperative view

The vascularization and margin study modeled online by Visible Patient allowed to simulate the resection and to predict the remaining healthy tissue volume in each kidney after resection. As a result, a safe organ-sparing procedure could be performed. Intraoperative observations corresponded to the 3D reconstruction (Fig. 57.3).

In congenital malformation cases, 3D reconstruction provided a better understanding of a complex anatomy.

As an example, we report the case of a 13-year-old girl with chronic and incapacitating right lumbar pain and pyelonephritis. CT scan found a cystic dysplastic middle and inferior pole right kidney with stones. However, due to cystic images, vascularization and urinary tract analysis were challenging. 3D reconstruction performed online by Visible Patient revealed a pelvic duplication obstructed by stones leading to kidney destruction. It was unexplainable with the CT scan alone. We had a precise diagnosis which allowed us to schedule the surgery in a stepwise manner (Fig. 57.4).

Tips and Tricks

- The 3D model has to be used, mobilized, and moved. It is recommended to turn the operative field around as if one were turning the kidney around with a camera, removing and adding different elements, other organs, and other vessels. The first operative step will be the exposure. One has to define how to expose and to detect the difficulties which may be encountered.
- The use of a transparency device is essential to have a good view of the vessels until their final destination and to know the details of the vascular supply for a tumor or a moiety.
- The clip applying system is then tried on vessels which seem to require clipping, coagulation, or ligation. When these maneuvers are experimented, one has to record the procedure step-by-step as if it was a GPS itinerary. A virtual endoscopy of any lumen (e.g., vessels, urinary tract) can be performed to discover any invasive tissue or a thrombus. In case of a tumor, one has to create a virtual dividing line which has to be defined with oncologists along with their corresponding protocols to ensure a perfect resection in terms of oncology.
- Finally, it is possible to simulate port positioning and to add a virtual camera and virtual instruments to the 3D model in order to decide on the perfect placement for each port site.

57.8 Discussion

3D reconstruction allows us to have a personalized approach and plan a stepwise tailored surgery.

In complex Wilms' tumor cases, Schenk et al. demonstrated by using 3D MRI visualization in abdominal tumors that an enhanced anatomy is necessary to prevent injuries to major vessels or to other structures and to decrease the complication rate [1]. The same authors also combined functional information with anatomical data in the treatment of pediatric embryonal abdominal tumors, opening the way to organ-sparing surgery.

Fuchs et al. used 3D reconstruction based on CT scan with a volume rendering software to preoperatively define margins and simulate virtual resection [2].

The main challenge remains the preservation of the remnant kidney vascularization during a partial nephrectomy. In adult patients, in the group without 3D imaging, 80% of patients had global ischemia versus 24% in the 3D imaging group ($p < 0.01$) with comparable tumors (tumor size: 50.9 and 50.8 mm; $p = 0.97$) [3]. Wang et al. demonstrate a significant operative time difference (126.7–36.4 vs. 154.8–34.7, $p = 0.018$) and the occurrence of postoperative urinary leak (0 vs. 4.0% vs. 22.2%, $p = 0.033$) in favor of the virtual surgical planning group in complicated renal tumors [4].

Recently, Raman et al. reported their virtual surgical planning experience in renal tumor on a horseshoe kidney. The preoperative vascularization study revealed the selective clamping sites easily, thereby facilitating the surgery in this unconventional anatomy situation [5].

Some teams have demonstrated the interest of the 3D printing model in urology to plan the surgery, especially in partial nephrectomy cases [6, 7].

Zhang et al. confirmed the process feasibility with CT scan-based images, the influence on the decision-making process during the surgical planning, and the impact on information for patients [8]. The same benefit was observed with MRI-based images [9]. Thanks to 3D printing, a simulation of the intervention can be performed and optimal port placement determined. Souzaki et al. reported three cases of laparoscopic adrenalectomy for neuroblastomas (2 stage IV and 1 stage I) prepared with reconstructions and 3D printing. Two patients had image-defined risk factors (renal vessels). No complications, conversion, or recurrence were reported [10].

Additionally, preoperative simulation is an appealing educational tool. Medical students and residents can have a better understanding of the anatomy and of the disease [11].

Finally, 3D imaging is the first step toward augmented reality surgery. High definition and high precision are required to make a real organ and disease mapping, which imparts the surgeon with an augmented eye.

Recently, Wake et al. reported their experience of a robot-assisted partial nephrectomy and the workflow of the procedure. A kidney model was created using augmented reality and then printed and visualized with specific glasses intraoperatively [12].

Registration type, organ tracking, and tissue deformation issues are ongoing challenges, which need to be solved in order to develop safer and more effective image-guided procedures [13].

Take-Home Messages

- 3D reconstruction allows us to plan a stepwise surgical procedure in order to manage and prevent surgical risks.
- High-quality CT scan or MRI images are required to have a high-definition reconstruction.
- Cases should be discussed with the surgical staff. Discrepancies can occur and have to be reported to the company which provides the 3D reconstruction software.
- 3D reconstruction can be printed in three dimensions for simulation, education, and patient information purposes.

References

1. Schenk JP, Waag K-L, Graf N, Wunsch R, Jourdan C, Behnisch W, et al. [3D-visualization by MRI for surgical planning of Wilms tumors.] ROFO. 2004;176(10):1447–52.
2. Fuchs J, Warmann SW, Szavay P, Kirschner HJ, Schäfer JF, Hennemuth A, et al. Three-dimensional visualization and virtual simulation of resections in pediatric solid tumors. J Pediatr Surg. 2005;40(2):364–70.
3. Porpiglia F, Bertolo R, Checcucci E, Amparore D, Autorino R, Dasgupta P, et al. Development and validation of 3D printed virtual models for robot-assisted radical prostatectomy and partial nephrectomy: urologists' and patients' perception. World J Urol. 2018;36(2):201–7.
4. Wang Z, Qi L, Yuan P, Zu X, Chen W, Cao Z, et al. Application of three-dimensional visualization Technology in Laparoscopic Partial Nephrectomy of renal tumor: a comparative study. J Laparoendosc Adv Surg Tech A. 2017;27(5):516–23.
5. Raman A, Kuusk T, Hyde ER, Berger LU, Bex A, Mumtaz F. Robotic-assisted laparoscopic partial nephrectomy in a horseshoe kidney. A case report and review of the literature. Urology. 2018;114:e3–5.
6. Youssef RF, Spradling K, Yoon R, Dolan B, Chamberlin J, Okhunov Z, et al. Applications of three-dimensional printing technology in urological practice. BJU Int. 2015;116(5):697–702.
7. Colaco M, Igel DA, Atala A. The potential of 3D printing in urological research and patient care. Nat Rev Urol. 2018;15(4):213–21.
8. Zhang Y, Ge H, Li N, Yu C, Guo H, Jin S, et al. Evaluation of three-dimensional printing for laparoscopic partial nephrectomy of renal tumors: a preliminary report. World J Urol. 2016;34(4):533–7.
9. Wake N, Rude T, Kang SK, Stifelman MD, Borin JF, Sodickson DK, et al. 3D printed renal cancer models derived from MRI data: application in pre-surgical planning. Abdom Radiol (NY). 2017;42(5):1501–9.
10. Souzaki R, Kinoshita Y, Ieiri S, Kawakubo N, Obata S, Jimbo T, et al. Preoperative surgical simulation of laparoscopic adrenalectomy for neuroblastoma using a three-dimensional printed model based on preoperative CT images. J Pediatr Surg. 2015;50(12):2112–5.
11. Knoedler M, Feibus AH, Lange A, Maddox MM, Ledet E, Thomas R, et al. Individualized physical 3-dimensional kidney tumor models constructed from 3-dimensional printers result in improved trainee anatomic understanding. Urology. 2015;85(6):1257–61.
12. Wake N, Bjurlin MA, Rostami P, Chandarana H, Huang WC. Three-dimensional printing and augmented reality: enhanced precision for robotic assisted partial nephrectomy. Urology. 2018;116:227–8.
13. Mascagni P, Longo F, Barberio M, Seeliger B, Agnus V, Saccomandi P, et al. New intraoperative imaging technologies: innovating the surgeon's eye toward surgical precision. J Surg Oncol. 2018;118(2):265–82.

Evidence Based Medicine in Minimally Invasive Pediatric Urology

58

S. Garnier, L. Harper, and N. Kalfa

Learning Objectives

- To perform a critical review of the literature with regard to level of evidence for using minimally invasive surgery (MIS) in pediatric urology.
- To present data with significant level of evidence on MIS for nephrectomy, partial nephrectomy, and heminephrectomy.
- To present data with significant level of evidence on MIS for uretero-pelvic junction surgery.
- To present data with significant level of evidence on MIS for uretero-vesical junction surgery, both vesicoureteral reflux and obstructive megaureter.

58.1 Introduction

The use of minimally invasive surgery (MIS), including endoscopic treatment (ET), laparoscopy (LS), and robot-assisted laparoscopic surgery (RALS), has become increasingly common in pediatric urology with the aim to improve recovery and cosmetics, decrease postoperative pain and opioid use, and reduce the risk of postoperative adhesions. However, compared to the adult scientific literature, publications in pediatric urology are still limited, and the level of evidence remains relatively poor as most studies are being retrospective and based on heterogeneous groups of patients.

Evidence-based medicine (EBM) refers to the rational use of scientific data when making decisions about the care of patients. When used appropriately, EBM is a necessary, powerful tool to guide urologists' decision-making for the best care for patients [1].

We performed a critical review of the literature with regard to level of evidence for using MIS in pediatric urology.

58.2 Methods

We first performed a broad PubMed search using the following keywords: "minimally invasive surgery" and pediatric or children or child and urology. Based on these results, we then focused on

S. Garnier · N. Kalfa (✉)
Department of Pediatric Surgery and Urology, Lapeyronie Hospital, CHU, Montpellier, France
e-mail: s-garnier@chu-montpellier.fr; n-kalfa@chu-montpellier.fr

L. Harper
Department of Pediatric Surgery and Urology, Hopital Pellegrin, CHU, Bordeaux, France
e-mail: luke.harper@chu-bordeaux.fr

C. Esposito et al. (eds.), *Minimally Invasive Techniques in Pediatric Urology*,
https://doi.org/10.1007/978-3-030-99280-4_58

five key topics: nephrectomy, heminephrectomy, uretero-pelvic junction (UPJ), vesicoureteral reflux (VUR), and obstructive megaureter. We hence did a PubMed search using the following keywords: "nephrectomy or nephroureterectomy and pediatric or children or child," "heminephroureterectomy or heminephrectomy and pediatric or children or child," "pyeloplasty" or ureteropelvic junction obstruction and surgery and pediatric or children or child," "primary obstructive megaureter" and surgery or "vesico ureteral reflux" and surgery or ureteral reimplantation, and pediatric or children or child. The management of lithiasis was deliberately not included here as another chapter focuses specifically on this topic.

The search was limited to English publications, published in the past 10 years, including human subjects, and we determined a minimum level of evidence (LE) consisting of either cohort studies, case series of more than 30 cases, randomized controlled trials (RCT), meta-analysis, and systematic reviews. Studies including adults (above 18 years of age) or based on less than 30 subjects were excluded. LE was defined according to the Oxford Centre for Evidence-Based Medicine classification (https://www.cebm.net/2009/06/oxford-centre-evidence-based-medicine-levels-evidence-march-2009/). The quality of articles was based on the material and method section, specifically inclusion and exclusion criteria, study type, and patient selection. Absent or insufficient information on these criteria was detrimental to the article's estimated LE.

58.3 Results

A total of 189 studies were identified from the initial search including two systematic reviews [2, 3], one comparative study [4], and one cohort study [5]. Data on laparoscopic single-site surgery (LSS) in pediatric urology came from one systematic review and meta-analysis [6] and two comparative studies [7, 8].

The pediatric nephrectomy (NT)/nephroureterectomy (NUT) search led to 1625 publications of which 14 met all eligibility criteria (Table 58.1). Six papers focused on primary renal neoplasms, seven on nonfunctioning kidneys, and two included both items.

The heminephrectomy (HNT)/heminephroureterectomy (HNUT) for duplex system search led to 1616 publications of which nine were eligible (Table 58.2). Because of a high level of evidence, we included in our analysis the randomized controlled trial by Golebiewski [9] though the sample size was small.

The pyeloplasty (PP)/UPJ search led to 684 publications of which 21 were eligible including 3 RCTs [10–12] (Table 58.3).

The MIS and low ureter surgery search yielded 879 studies of which 18 (Table 58.4), including four RCT [13, 14], were eligible as regards vesicoureteral reflux and five were eligible for primary obstructive megaureter (Table 58.5).

Performing randomized controlled trial for surgical procedures in children remains challenging due to difficulties in ethical approval and limited number of patients, thus good quality observational studies may often be the best evidence we can achieve at the moment.

58.4 Overall Outcomes in Minimally Invasive Pediatric Urology

In a register-based analysis of 70,273 procedures, Tejwani et al. [15] found a lower complication rate for MIS as compared to open surgery (OS). However, as reported by Aksenov et al. [3], complication rates depend on the type of procedure. In this systematic review, NT had a significantly lower rate of complication requiring intervention (1.18%) as compared to PP (3.64%), ureteral reimplantation (UR) (3.65%), or complex reconstruction (11.76%). There was no statistically significant difference in complication rate between PP, partial NT, and UR. Conversion to OS was significantly more frequent for complex reconstructive surgeries (6.62%) than for PP (1%), NT (2.65%), partial NT (3.29%), and UR (1.28%). Partial NT had a significantly higher conversion rate as compared to UR and PP.

Table 58.1 Minimally invasive nephrectomy, summary of characteristics of selected studies

Study (year of issue)	Sample[a]	Study design (LE)	Technique	Indications	Main findings
Fan et al. [6] (2012)	27	SR and meta-analysis 3a-B	TPLS/LSS	NFK and PRN	With level of evidence limitations, LSS offers a safe and efficient alternative to TPLS with less pain, shorter recovery time, and better cosmetic outcome
Malek et al. [23] (2020)	19	SR 3a-B	TPLS/OS	PRT	There is a lack of evidence to support MIS for pediatric renal tumors. Lymph node harvest has been inadequate and there appears to be an increased risk for intraoperative spill
Aminsharifi et al. [19] (2011)	79	Prospective CS 2b-B	TPLS	NFK	TPLS in patients with a history of ipsilateral renal surgery can be done safely
Lee et al. [24] (2011)	303	CS 4-C	RALS/OS	PRT	RALP is a viable option as a nephron-sparing surgical procedure for small renal mass
Kim et al. [16] (2012)	69	CS 4-C	LSS/TPLS/ RALS/OS	NFK	MIS is statistically associated with shorter lengths of hospital stay and decreased postoperative pain medication usage than with OS but with longer surgical time
Mir et al. [72] (2011)	64	CS 4-C	LSS/TPLS	NFK	With appropriate patient selection, almost 50% can be performed using LSS with similar complication rates and outcomes compared to TPLS
Burnand et al. [73] (2018)	54	CS 4-C	TPLS/OS	WT	SIOP criteria indications can be extended for teams experienced after agreement at a multidisciplinary meeting
Romao et al. [20] (2014)	45	CS 4-C	TPLS/OS	PRN	TPLS is an attractive alternative to OS in carefully selected cases. Procedure length and incidence of intraoperative rupture were not increased while postoperative recovery and hospital stay were shorter
Bansal et al. [74] (2014)	32	CS 4-C	LSS/RALS	NFK	LSS has a significantly shorter operative time with comparable postoperative narcotics use as compared to RALS
Duarte et al. [21] (2014)	32	CS 4-C	TPLS/OS	WT	Both techniques showed similar immediate and long-term results
Tam et al. [75] (2013)	30	CS 4-C	RPLS/LSS	NFK	LSS is safe and effective compared to RPLS
Bouty et al. [22] (2020)	50	CSR 4-C	TPLS	WT	Feasible in 20% of WT with oncological outcomes comparable with OS
Harris et al. [76] (2018)	43	CSR 4-C	TPLS	PRN	TPLS approach is likely to be achievable if the volume ratio is at 8.1
Badawy et al. [77] (2011)	35	CSR 4-C	RPLS	NFK	RPLS is safe and feasible

TPLS transperitoneal laparoscopy, *RPLS* retroperitoneal laparoscopy, *OS* open surgery, *LSS* laparoscopic single-site surgery, *RALS* robot-assisted laparoscopic surgery, *CSR* case series report (observational study), *CS* comparative study, *SR* systematic review, *LE* level of evidence, *WT* Wilms' tumor, *NFK* nonfunctioning kidney, *PRN* primary renal neoplasm

[a] Number of patients for clinical trial and number of studies for systematic review

Table 58.2 Minimally invasive heminephrectomy and heminephroureterectomy in duplex system, summary of characteristics of selected studies

Study (year of issue)	Sample	Study design (LE)	Technique	Main findings
Golebiewski et al. [9] (2013)	27	RCT 2b-B	TPLS/OS	MIS should be the preferred option over OS
Escolino et al. [31] (2019)	164	CS 4-C	RPLS Lateral/prone approach	Superiority of one approach over another is not still confirmed
Esposito et al. [29] (2017)	102	CS 4-C	RPLS/TPLS	TPLS is faster, safer, and technically easier to perform compared to RPLS
Neheman et al. [26] (2019)	59	CS 4-C	OS/TPLS/ LSS/RALS	MIS decreases postoperative analgesia and hospital stay in comparison to the OS while demonstrating efficacy and safety
Zhou et al. [7] (2014)	68	CS 4-C	LSS/TPLS	LSS is feasible and safe, although the outcomes were comparable, better subjective cosmetic results LSS
Varda et al. [32] (2018)	43	CS 4-C	RALS/OS	RALS has comparable (if not better) outcomes than OS
Jayram et al. [30] (2011)	142	CSR 4-C	RPLS	Nonfunctioning renal moiety Rate of 5%
Escolino et al. [31] (2015)	52	CSR 4-C	RPLS	RPLS remains a challenging procedure with a long learning curve, performed only in pediatric centers with huge experience in this field
Esposito et al. [27] (2015)	50	CSR 4-C	TPLS	TPLS remains a technically challenging procedure performed only in pediatric centers with high experience MIS

RCT randomized controlled trial

Table 58.3 Minimally invasive pyeloplasty, summary of characteristics of selected studies

Study (year of issue)	Sample	Study design (LE)	Technique	Main findings
Gatti et al. [10] (2017)	98	RCT 1b-A	TPLS/OS	Both are comparable and effective methods, operative time was statistically shorter in the OS, and length of stay is shorter in the TPLS group
Penn et al. [11] (2010)	39	RCT 2b-B	TPLS/OS	TPLS is safe and effective Cost is similar, longer operative times in the laparoscopic group but a shorter overall hospitalization
Badawy et al. [12] (2015)	38	RCT 2b-B	TPLS/RPLS	Both approaches had a high success rate. However, the shorter operative time, shorter length of hospital stay, rapid recovery of intestinal movement, and early resumption of oral feeding are in favor of RPLS
Huang et al. [36] (2015)	15	SR and meta-analysis 3a-B	TPLS/OS	TPLS is associated with shorter length of hospital stay, reduced complications, and equal success rate but prolonged operative time
Chang et al. [41] (2015)	15	SR and meta-analysis 3a-B	RALS/OS	Postoperative success rate was comparable with higher complication rate and costs in the RALS group
Cundy et al. [46] (2014)	12	SR and meta-analysis 3a-B	RALS/TPLS	No significant differences for all primary outcomes Significant differences in favor of RALS for length of hospital stay

Table 58.3 (continued)

Study (year of issue)	Sample	Study design (LE)	Technique	Main findings
Corbett and Mullassery [50] (2015)	15	SR 4-C	Endoscopic treatment	Success rate is lower
Chan et al. [48] (2017)	2219	CS 4-C	RALS/TPLS/OS	Multivariate analysis indicated that surgical approach had minimal effect on the rates of intraoperative and postoperative complications
Piaggio et al. [35] (2017)	30	Prospective CS 2b-B	TPLS/OS	TPLS was a longer procedure than OS. Both procedures had the same efficacy and complication rates, but patients undergoing TPLS needed fewer narcotics for pain control and had a shorter hospitalization
Silay et al. [45] (2016)	575	CS 4-C	TPLS/RALS	Shorter hospitalization time and lower postoperative complication rates with RALS
Polok et al. [38] (2020)	226	CS 4-C	TPLS/OS	Comparable success rates in both groups
Esposito et al. [34] (2019)	67	CS 4-C	RALS/TPLS	Both give excellent results
Neheman et al. [40] (2018)	34	CS 4-C	RALS/TPLS	Results, complication rates, and operative time were comparable while TPLS demonstrated longer hospital stay
Liu et al. [39] (2017)	1750	CSR 4-C	TPLS/RPLS/ LSS/RALS	Four approaches are safe and efficient procedures with equivalent success rates
Kawal et al. [43] (2018)	138	Prospective CSR 4-C	RALS	No significant differences in length of hospital stay and complications or failure rates in infants compared to older children
He et al. [33] (2020)	279	CSR 4-C	TPLS	TPLS has been proven to be safe and effective in children with a low rate of complications. Weight < 10 kg and having intraoperative complications with drainage were risk factors
Minnillo et al. [44] (2011)	155	CSR 4-C	RALS	Long-term surgical success and complication rates were comparable to open surgery
Blanc et al. [37] (2013)	104	CSR 4-C	RPLS	Safe, reliable, and efficient with an excellent outcome in selected children long learning process and remains a challenging task for a teaching center
Chiarenza et al. [49] (2017)	54	CSR 4-C	Vascular hitch	Excellent outcomes in a very selected patient population
Blanc et al. [78] (2019)	50	CSR 4-C	Retroperitoneal-RALPS	Preliminary results suggest that retroperitoneal RALP in children is feasible, safe, and effective
Jacobson et al. [47] (2019)	36	CSR 4-C	Redo RALS	Redo RALS is feasible, efficient, safe, and durable

Table 58.4 Minimally invasive treatment of vesicoureteral reflux, summary of characteristics of selected studies

Study (year of issue)	Sample	Study design (LE)	Technique	Main findings
Nordenström et al. [13] (2017)	77	RCT 1a-B	ET (deflux)	High-grade VUR in infants can be treated with ET and the resolution rate is higher compared with prophylaxis treatment. The complication rate is low and VUR grade 4 and unilateral grade 5 were favorable for resolution and downgrading with ET, whereas, in infants with bilateral grade 5, the results were less encouraging
Garcia-Aparicio et al. [14] (2013)	41	RCT 2b-C	ET (deflux)/ OS	Short- and long-term follow-up shows that multiple endoscopic treatment of VUR grades II, III, and IV with ET is as effective as OS
Deng et al. [59] (2018)	6	SR and meta-analysis 3a-B	RALS/OS	RALS: Longer operation time, fewer days of hospital stay, and postoperative Foley placement but in subgroup analyses, higher rate of short-term postoperative complications No significant differences in success rate, complications, and postoperative analgesia
Harel et al. [58] (2015)	34	Prospective CS 2b-B	RALS/OS	Lower narcotic requirement and lower intensity of postoperative pain for RALS compared to OS
Wang et al. [54] (2016)	76,756	CS 4C	RALS/OS/ LS	Patients who underwent MIS remained more likely to suffer from postoperative urinary complications compared with patients who underwent open OS
Kurtz et al. [62] (2016)	1682	CS 4-C	RALS/OS	Significantly higher rate of complications as well as higher direct costs for RALS
Bustangi et al. [51] (2018)	96	CS 4-C	OS/LS	Both effective in unilateral and bilateral with similar results. LS reduces significantly postoperative pain medication and hospital stay and allows for a faster return to normal activity
Esposito et al. [79] (2019)	151	CS 3b-B	RALS/LS	Short-term bladder dysfunction is a possible complication with no significant difference between both technics Bilaterality, preexisting BBD, and duration of surgery were confirmed on univariate and multivariate analyses as predictors of postoperative bladder dysfunction
Srinivasan et al. [64] (2017)	92	CS 4-C	RALS	Bilateral extravesical ureteral reimplantation is not associated with an increased risk of postoperative morbidity compared with unilateral surgery
Esposito et al. [52] (2016)	90	CS 4-C	OS/LS/ET (no grade 5 and redo)	OS presented significantly more complications and higher morbidity compared to LS and ET Similar success rate with OS and LS
Boysen et al. [57] (2017)	143	Prospective CSR 4-C	RALS	Same radiographic success rate than contemporary series of OS
Boysen et al. [61] (2017)	260	CSR 4-C	RALS	Same low complication rate and almost same radiographic success rate than published series of OS
Soulier et al. [53] (2017)	117	CSR 4-C	LS	The success rate is comparable to OS with the advantages of laparoscopic approach
Grimsby et al. [60] (2015)	61	CSR 4-C	RALS	Lower success rate for RALS More than 10% of patients required at least one reoperation for persistent VUR or a surgical complication = > higher complication rate and lower success rate for RALS compared to the gold standard of OS

Table 58.4 (continued)

Study (year of issue)	Sample	Study design (LE)	Technique	Main findings
Gundeti et al. [80] (2016)	58	CSR 4-C	RALS	There is a need for standardization of technique to facilitate best possible outcomes
Esposito et al. [56] (2018)	55	CSR 4-C	RALS	Safe and effective technique
Herz et al. [63] (2016)	54	CSR 4-C	RALS	Bilateral is associated with higher failure rates, higher complication rates, higher reoperation rates, and more postoperative urinary infections and nonsurgical readmissions compared with unilateral procedure
Akhavan et al. [55] (2014)	50	CSR 4-C	RALS	Effective and safe option

VUR vesicoureteral reflux, *ET* endoscopic treatment

Table 58.5 Minimally invasive treatment of primary obstructive megaureter, summary of characteristics of selected studies

Study (year of issue)	Sample	Study design (LE)	Technique	Main findings
Doudt et al. [65] (2018)	11	SR 3a-B	Endoscopic management	– Modest success rates – Temporizing procedure – Approximately 1/3 of patients require surgical reintervention
Ortiz et al. [66] (2018)	92	CSR 4-C	Endoscopic management	Effective treatment of POM with few complications and good outcomes at long-term follow up. Main complication was secondary VUR that could also be treated endoscopically with a high success rate. => may be considered first-line treatment in POM
Kassite et al. [67] (2018)	42	CSR 4-C	Endoscopic management	Overall success rate of 92%. It avoided reimplantation in 90% of cases
Neheman et al. [69] (2020)	35	CSR 4-C	RALS	Safe and effective (unilateral)
Teklali et al. [68] (2018)	35	CSR 4-C	Endoscopic management	Safe and effective. Proposed as a first-line treatment even under 2 years

POM primary obstructive megaureter

Robotic pediatric urologic procedures are considered technically feasible and safe according to two large sample cohort studies reported by Dangle et al. [5] and Colaco et al. [4] who report similar overall 30- and 90-day complication rates as for LS and OS.

Wider use of LSS in order to confer better esthetic outcome, reduce port-site complications, and postoperative pain [6–8] requires better LE studies to clarify safety and long-term outcomes [2].

58.5 Nephrectomy, Nephroureterectomy, and Partial Nephrectomy

58.5.1 Nonfunctioning Kidney

Recent publications about minimally invasive NT for nonfunctioning kidneys are limited, almost exclusively retrospective, and with very low levels of evidence. MIS for NT or nephroureterectomy in benign diseases is associated with shorter lengths of hospital stay and decreased postoperative pain medication usage when compared to OS [16]. RALS is possible but expensive [17]. The retroperitoneal and transperitoneal approaches can be used equally according to the surgeon's preference and experience as said in the systematic review published in 2009 by Kim et al. [18], as no specific advantage has been proven for either technique. MIS can still be proposed safely in case of prior ipsilateral kidney surgery [19].

58.5.2 Renal Neoplasms

The use of MIS is challenging in renal neoplasm since complete surgical resection without tumor rupture and sufficient lymph node sampling remains the main objective, especially in Wilms' tumors (WT). Many studies showed no difference in tumor ruptures and event-free survival (EFS) despite a lower number of lymph nodes collected. Indeed, Romao et al. [20] showed in a retrospective study comparing OS vs. LS for primary kidney cancer nephrectomy that OS yielded a significantly higher number of lymph nodes, with a median of five lymph nodes (range 2–29) versus two (range 1–14) in MIS. Patients undergoing OS presented larger tumors than their LS counterparts, but operative times were similar. No tumor ruptures occurred with either technique. LS required a shorter use of narcotics and a shorter length of stay. EFS was similar in both groups. Overall recurrences were not more frequent in the LS group though median follow-up was limited (18 months).

Similarly, in the retrospective comparative series of 32 patients with WT by Duarte et al. [21], there were fewer lymph nodes harvested and longer operative times in the LS group but a shorter length of stay. The EFS for both groups were similar, 86.7% (OS) compared to 94.1% (LS) at a median follow-up of 4.29 years. They recommend using MIS only when the tumor's largest dimension is less than 10% of the patient's height. Recently, Bouty et al. [22] retrospectively reported 50 nephrectomies with transperitoneal laparoscopy (TPLS) for WT with no intraoperative rupture and an EFS of 94% at 3 years.

On the other hand, a recent systematic review [23] calls for caution. Based on 19 retrospective studies (two of which are comparative [20, 21]), 104 patients undergoing MIS were compared to 47 patients undergoing OS. The authors show that lymph node harvests have been inadequate in patients undergoing MIS with an increased risk for intraoperative spill/tumor rupture. The overall survival is similar between groups, but follow-up times were inconsistent and patient selection was clearly biased, with only small tumors being selected for MIS.

Nephron-sparing surgery can be proposed for localized small renal masses or bilateral tumors. Lee et al. [24] compare the clinical outcomes between OS and RALS. Intraoperative and postoperative outcomes were comparable between groups. Operative times and kidney ischemia were longer in the RALS group. Positive surgical margins were only reported is the OS group, but this could be due to patient selection bias. Both long-term oncologic outcome and long-term renal function need to be better evaluated.

It should be noted that there are no LE 1 or 2 studies evaluating MIS for pediatric renal tumors. Additionally, subjects were not randomized and the studies do not present standardized outcome data, leading to incomplete data and selective reporting [23]. However, overall, preliminary data suggest that LS for carefully selected patients (small WT with preoperative chemotherapy) is feasible and shows promising results in terms of event-free and overall survival [25].

58.5.3 Heminephrectomy and Heminephroureterectomy for Duplex Systems

Only one study reached a LE 2 thanks to a randomized controlled trial comparing TPLS to OS [9]. TPLS should be the preferred option for HNT/HNUT as it appears to be feasible and safe with lower analgesic requirements and shorter hospital stay in spite of an increased operative time. In this study of 27 patients, no remaining moieties were lost. In a recent comparative study of 59 patients, Neheman et al. [26] confirmed these data.

Regarding the use of robotic surgery, Esposito et al. first reported two case series [27, 28] of 52 LS and 50 RALS and then compared one with the other [29]. He found significantly more complications, reoperation rate, operative time, and hospital stay in the LS group. Furthermore, a negative impact on the remaining moiety resulting in a decreased or nonfunctioning renal moiety occurs in 5% of cases after LS HNT as shown by Jayram et al. [30] (median follow-up of 4.5 years, $n = 142$). Based on 164 patients, Escolino et al. [31] show that there is no superiority of lateral over prone approaches in LS for HNT/HNUT. The prone technique may be faster, and the lateral approach may be more adequate when a longer ureterectomy is required, but the choice of the technique remains dependent on the surgeon's personal preference and experience.

Last, two quite large case series found no differences in surgical outcomes between RALS and OS [32] (except for the hospital stay) and between SSL and TPLS [7].

58.6 Pyeloplasty for Ureteropelvic Junction Obstruction (UPJO)

PP is the topic for which the most data with significant level of evidence is available based on systematic reviews/meta analyses, large cohort, and comparative studies.

58.6.1 Laparoscopic vs. Open Pyeloplasty

Two RCTs compared TPLS and OS PP. One preliminary report from Penn et al. [11] in 2010 and a second one in 2016 from Gatti et al. [10] both reported no difference in success rate, but TPLS was associated with longer operative times and shorter hospitalization. Several descriptive and comparative studies including large samples [33–37] confirmed laparoscopic PP provides comparable success and complications rates than OS with reduced pain and length of stay. In particular, a prospective comparative cohort [35] of 30 patients similar with regard to age found that TPLS, despite being a longer procedure than OS, has the same efficacy and complication rates with fewer narcotics needed. Comparable success rates in both procedures are confirmed in a large retrospective comparative study of 226 patients [38]. EAU/ESPU guidelines are based on these findings but the interest of MIS in very young children remains to be demonstrated and current data is insufficient to defer a cutoff age.

58.6.2 Transperitoneal vs. Retroperitoneal Laparoscopic Pyeloplasty

One randomized controlled trial by Badawy et al. [12] compared trans- vs. retroperitoneal approach for laparoscopic PP in 38 patients. The success rate was comparable, whereas the retroperitoneal laparoscopic (RPLS) approach leads to shorter operative time, earlier oral feeding, and shorter hospital stay. These data are in accordance with the largest case series to date [39] including 451 RPLS, 311 TPLS, 322 LSS, and 805 transumbilical multiport procedures. In this paper, RPLS and TPLS presented comparable complication rates though RPLS was associated with earlier oral feeding and shorter hospital stay. In summary, the choice between RPLS or TPLR remains a matter of surgical preference and personal experience with no definitive EBM evidence for one or another.

58.6.3 Robotic-Assisted Laparoscopy Pyeloplasty

There are no randomized controlled trials or prospective study compared to RALP to open or laparoscopic PP to date. However, several series suggest RALP is effective with reported success rates of 94–100% whether using a transperitoneal or retroperitoneal approach [34, 37, 40–

44]. Hospital stay and duration of stenting were shorter for RALP as compared to LS in a large case series of 575 patients though success and intraoperative complication rates were similar [45]. In a meta-analysis, Cundy et al. [46] found significant advantages for RALP including shortened length of stay, lower analgesia requirement, and lower blood loss though it was associated with a higher cost and longer operative time. The minimum weight for which robotic surgery is possible has been questioned but in a large study of RALP ($n = 138$), Kawal et al. [43] did not find any significant differences in complications or failure rate between infants (median weight 9.9 kg, IQR 8.1, 11.5) and older children. RALP for complex UPJO procedures including anatomic variations (ectopic, malrotated, or horseshoe kidneys), duplex kidney, or recurrent UPJO seems feasible and safe and offers good outcomes [42, 47]. Finally, surgical approach (OS, LS, and RALP PP) may not be the only factor influencing intra- and postoperative complication rates according to a multivariate analysis of 2219 patients from a database of 102 academic institutions. Patient comorbidity may have a greater impact on success rate and length of stay [48].

58.6.4 Other Techniques

The vascular hitch procedure has been proposed as an alternative to dismembered PP in children with an extrinsic compression of the UPJ. Overall results seem favorable as reported in a cohort of 54 selected patients [49]. Comparative studies of vascular hitch vs. other procedures are lacking. The careful selection of patients through intraoperative assessment of anatomical and functional aspects may be a crucial step to confirm the right indication for vascular hitch and maintain a high success rate.

Finally, endourological techniques have been reviewed by Corbett and Mullassery [50] and these cannot be recommended because of a high complication rate (14.8%) and a lower success rate (71%).

58.7 MIS of the Lower Ureter

58.7.1 Vesicoureteral Reflux

The current gold standard surgical option for VUR is open trans-hiatal ureteral reimplantation according to Cohen with a high success rate (95%). MIS such as ET, LS, and RALS reimplantation have been proposed as alternatives.

Endoscopic injection of bulking agents for the treatment of vesicoureteral reflux has become widely used as a therapeutic alternative to ureteral reimplantation. In an RCT comparing Cohen's ureteral reimplantation with ET in children older than 1-year-old, Garcia-Aparicio et al. [14] showed that short- and long-term outcomes were similar for VUR grades II, III, and IV. But the size of the sample was limited and multiple ETs were necessary in 34% of cases. Some authors have even proposed ET in high-grade VUR in infants under 1 year of age. In an RCT, Nordenström et al. [13] showed that infants treated by ET had a higher rate of VUR resolution compared to those with prophylaxis. The complication rate was low and the radioscopic success rate of ET was 100% in unilateral VUR grade 4, 75% in bilateral grade 4, 67% in unilateral grade 5, and 31% in bilateral grade 5. But this study raises questions regarding follow-up which was short and design since it does not compare two operative techniques but rather apply ET to children who may have presented spontaneous regression of VUR.

Ureteral reimplantation using MIS (LS or RALS) has been reported to be safe and feasible but clear EBM is still lacking and data are conflicting. Laparoscopic Lich-Gregoir seems to have a similar success rate to OS in two comparative studies [51, 52] as well as reduced postoperative analgesia, hospital stay, and a faster return to normal activity. These results are in accordance with those from Soulier et al. [53] showing a clinical success rate of 98.3%. However, a large nationwide population-based study of 76,756 patients published by Wang et al. [54] showed that MIS, even if associated with shorter hospital stay, increases the risk of postoperative complications and increases the cost of management of these children.

Similarly, results from RALS are conflicting. Several studies report similar success rates between OS and RALS [52, 55–59] whereas others raise concern about lower success rates and higher complication rates [54, 60–62]. For instance, Grimsby et al. [60] found that more than 10% of patients required at least one reoperation for persistent VUR or complication while Boysen et al. [57], in a prospective observational study, reported a radiographic success rate of 93.8% overall and 94.1% among children with grades III–V VUR. Bilateral MIS reimplantation is also suspected to be a risk factor for complication and postoperative bladder dysfunction. Herz et al. [63] reported an overall surgical success of 84.7% for unilateral reflux, but for bilateral surgery the success rate decreased to 72.2%. On the opposite, Srinivasan et al. [64] found no increased risk in bilateral procedures.

58.7.2 Primary Obstructive Megaureter (POM)

Endoscopic dilation (ED) of POM has been proposed as an alternative treatment to reduce the morbidity associated with OS. However, a systematic review [65] published in 2017 raised concerns about the success rate of ED. Based on previous retrospective studies of limited sample size, the authors showed that the procedure cannot be completed in 10% of cases and that approximately 1/3 of patients require further surgery. On the other hand, a more recent series recommends ED as the first-line treatment for POM. In a cohort of 92 POM, Ortiz et al. [66] found a long-term success rate of 87.3% with a median follow-up of 6 years. Secondary VUR was found in 21.5% and was successfully treated by endoscopic sub-ureteric injection in more than 75% of cases. ED failed in 13% of cases requiring ureteral reimplantation. Failure either occurred early (intraoperative technical problems, double-J stent migration, severe restenosis) or during long-term follow-up (persistent VUR, POM recurrence). Kassite et al. [67] reported a similar overall success rate of 92% in a cohort of 42 POM. In this series, ED avoided reimplantation in 90% of cases but double J stents were associated with significant complications. Based on a series of 35 children, Teklali et al. [68] confirmed this data with results boasting asymptomatic patients and preserved renal function in 91% of cases. Good patient selection (possibility of catheterization of the lower ureter, short stenosis, and good response to the dilation) may help to improve the success rate of ED.

EBM data on RALS for POM is still limited even if this technique was reported more than a decade ago. Only one paper reached our criteria for inclusion [69]. In this study 35 patients with POM underwent dismembered unilateral extravesical cross-trigonal ureteral reimplantation, ten of them with intracorporeal excisional tapering of the obstructed ureter. RALS for POM is thus feasible but either febrile urinary tract infections or grade 3 Clavien complication occurred in more than 10% of patients. Further comparative studies are needed.

58.8 Limits

There are several limits to how we can interpret the existing literature on MIS in pediatric urology. The first has to do with patient age. Though most studies describe their patient population and the age at surgery, the minimum age at which MIS can safely be performed remains to be demonstrated. It is probable that this minimum age, or size, varies according to the type of procedure and technique used. Some authors have, for instance, stated that robotic surgery is feasible above a minimum distance between both anterior superior iliac spines (ASIS) as well as the puboxyphoid distance (PXD) [70]. Recommendations for use of MIS should include this limit.

Several articles have a relatively poor LE even though they are comparative trials or systematic reviews. The main problem with published comparative studies is the absence of clear criteria for choice of technique with a lot of room for selection bias and confounding factors. Many of the systematic reviews published include mainly retrospective case series meaning that though this pool large number of patients they still are equivalent to case series.

Furthermore, MIS is technically demanding, especially in young children. Learning curves show just how difficult these procedures can be, and it is obvious that all surgeons do not possess the same technical skills. A recent paper published in JAMA shows how variation in surgeon's technical skills can explain up to 26% of the variation in postoperative complications. We should always keep this in mind when analyzing published results whether good or bad [71].

Finally, there is an identifiable process to the development of surgical techniques with different questions at different phases of development. These can be summarized by the triad "it can't be done, it can be done, it should be done." Adequate methodology for investigating surgery in all its complex aspects is still lacking. We have yet to find a specific methodology which takes into account the specific nature of surgical development.

58.9 Conclusion

MIS procedures in pediatric urology are feasible in experienced hands with a success rate depending on the type of surgery. However, evidence-based literature reporting MIS in pediatric urology is lacking with few studies showing high level of evidence. Nephrectomy and ureteronephrectomy for benign disease should be performed by TPLS (including SSL) or RPLS rather than OS or RALS. Evidence is lacking to recommend MIS in pediatric kidney cancer even if it seems feasible on carefully selected patients. Heminephrectomy for duplex system may be performed using TPLS or RALS while RPLS shows promising results only in some hands. UPJ may benefit from MIS, especially from RALP that provides similar outcomes, reduced need of analgesia, and shorter hospital stay than OS despite a longer operative time. Transperitoneal or retroperitoneal approach for both laparoscopic and robotic surgery are possible. Last, endoscopic approaches for VUR (subureteric injection) and for POM (endoscopic dilation) are valuable first-line treatments even if their precise indications need to be further clarified. Laparoscopy and robotic-assisted procedures for ureteral reimplantation require larger and comparative studies.

References

1. Routh JC. Evidence-based versus personalized medicine in pediatric urology: the evidence supports evidence-based medicine. J Urol. 2017;197:979–80.
2. Symeonidis EN, Nasioudis D, Economopoulos KP. Laparoendoscopic single-site surgery (LESS) for major urological procedures in the pediatric population: a systematic review. Int J Surg. 2016;29:53–61.
3. Aksenov LI, Granberg CF, Gargollo PC. A systematic review of complications of minimally invasive surgery in the pediatric urological literature. J Urol. 2020;203:1010–6.
4. Colaco M, Hester A, Visser W, Rasper A, Terlecki R. Relative to open surgery, minimally-invasive renal and ureteral pediatric surgery offers no improvement in 30-day complications, yet requires longer operative time: data from the National Surgical Quality Improvement Program Pediatrics. Investig Clin Urol. 2018;59:200.
5. Dangle PP, et al. Ninety-day perioperative complications of pediatric robotic urological surgery: a multi-institutional study. J Pediatr Urol. 2016;12:102.e1–6.
6. Fan X, et al. Laparoendoscopic single-site nephrectomy compared with conventional laparoscopic nephrectomy: a systematic review and meta-analysis of comparative studies. Eur Urol. 2012;62:601–12.
7. Zhou H, et al. Transumbilical single-incision laparoscopic versus conventional laparoscopic upper pole heminephroureterectomy for children with duplex kidney: a retrospective comparative study. Urology. 2014;84:1199–204.
8. Naitoh Y, et al. Laparoendoscopic single-site versus conventional laparoscopic pyeloplasty: a matched pair analysis: laparoendoscopic single-site pyeloplasty. Int J Urol. 2014;21:793–6.
9. Golebiewski A, Losin M, Murawski M, Komasara L, Czauderna P. Laparoscopic versus open upper pole heminephroureterectomy for the treatment of duplex kidneys in children. J Laparoendosc Adv Surg Tech A. 2013;23:942–5.
10. Gatti JM, Amstutz SP, Bowlin PR, Stephany HA, Murphy JP. Laparoscopic vs open pyeloplasty in children: results of a randomized, prospective: controlled trial. J Urol. 2017;197:792–7.

11. Penn HA, et al. Laparoscopic versus open pyeloplasty in children: preliminary report of a prospective randomized trial. J Urol. 2010;184:690–5.
12. Badawy H, Zoaier A, Ghoneim T, Hanno A. Transperitoneal versus retroperitoneal laparoscopic pyeloplasty in children: randomized clinical trial. J Pediatr Urol. 2015;11:122.e1–6.
13. Nordenström J, et al. The Swedish infant high-grade reflux trial: Study presentation and vesicoureteral reflux outcome. J Pediatr Urol. 2017;13(2):130–8.
14. Garcia-Aparicio L, et al. Randomized clinical trial comparing endoscopic treatment with dextranomer hyaluronic acid copolymer and Cohen's ureteral reimplantation for vesicoureteral reflux: long-term results. J Pediatr Urol. 2013;9:483–7.
15. Tejwani R, et al. Open versus minimally invasive surgical approaches in pediatric urology: trends in utilization and complications. J Pediatr Urol. 2017;13:283.e1–9.
16. Kim PH, et al. Early comparison of nephrectomy options in children (open, transperitoneal laparoscopic, laparo-endoscopic single site (LESS), and robotic surgery): early comparison of nephrectomy techniques in children. BJU Int. 2012;109:910–5.
17. Tomaszewski JJ, Casella DP, Turner RM, Casale P, Ost MC. Pediatric laparoscopic and robot-assisted laparoscopic surgery: technical considerations. J Endourol. 2012;26:602–13.
18. Kim C, McKay K, Docimo SG. Laparoscopic nephrectomy in children: systematic review of transperitoneal and retroperitoneal approaches. Urology. 2009;73:280–4.
19. Aminsharifi A, et al. Laparoscopic nephrectomy for nonfunctioning kidneys is feasible after previous ipsilateral renal surgery: a prospective cohort trial. J Urol. 2011;185:930–4.
20. Romao RLP, et al. Comparison between laparoscopic and open radical nephrectomy for the treatment of primary renal tumors in children: single-center experience over a 5-year period. J Pediatr Urol. 2014;10:488–94.
21. Duarte RJ, et al. Wilms tumor: a retrospective study of 32 patients using videolaparoscopic and open approaches. Urology. 2014;84:191–7.
22. Bouty A, et al. Minimally invasive surgery for unilateral Wilms tumors: multicenter retrospective analysis of 50 transperitoneal laparoscopic total nephrectomies. Pediatr Blood Cancer. 2020;67:e28212.
23. Malek MM, et al. Minimally invasive surgery for pediatric renal tumors: a systematic review by the APSA Cancer Committee. J Pediatr Surg. 2020;55(11):2251–9.
24. Lee S, Oh J, Hong SK, Lee SE, Byun S-S. Open versus robot-assisted partial nephrectomy: effect on clinical outcome. J Endourol. 2011;25:1181–5.
25. Warmann SW, et al. Minimally invasive nephrectomy for Wilms tumors in children—data from SIOP 2001. J Pediatr Surg. 2014;49:1544–8.
26. Neheman A, et al. Pediatric partial nephrectomy for upper urinary tract duplication anomalies: a comparison between different surgical approaches and techniques. Urology. 2019;125:196–201.
27. Esposito C, et al. Laparoscopic partial nephrectomy in duplex kidneys in infants and children: results of an European multicentric survey. Surg Endosc. 2015;29:3469–76.
28. Esposito C, et al. Retroperitoneoscopic heminephrectomy in duplex kidney in infants and children: results of a multicentric survey. J Laparoendosc Adv Surg Tech A. 2015;25:864–9.
29. Esposito C, et al. Retroperitoneal and laparoscopic heminephrectomy in duplex kidney in infants and children. Transl Pediatr. 2017;5:245–50.
30. Jayram G, et al. Outcomes and fate of the remnant moiety following laparoscopic heminephrectomy for duplex kidney: a multicenter review. J Pediatr Urol. 2011;7:272–5.
31. Escolino M, et al. Retroperitoneoscopic partial nephrectomy in children: a multicentric international comparative study between lateral versus prone approach. Surg Endosc. 2019;33:832–9.
32. Varda BK, Rajender A, Yu RN, Lee RS. A contemporary single-institution retrospective cohort study comparing perioperative outcomes between robotic and open partial nephrectomy for poorly functioning renal moieties in children with duplex collecting systems. J Pediatr Urol. 2018;14:549.e1–8.
33. He Y, et al. Primary laparoscopic pyeloplasty in children: a single-center experience of 279 patients and analysis of possible factors affecting complications. J Pediatr Urol. 2020;16:331.e1–331.e11.
34. Esposito C, et al. Robot-assisted vs laparoscopic pyeloplasty in children with uretero-pelvic junction obstruction (UPJO): technical considerations and results. J Pediatr Urol. 2019;15:667.e1–8.
35. Piaggio LA, et al. Comparative, prospective, case–control study of open versus laparoscopic pyeloplasty in children with ureteropelvic junction obstruction: long-term results. Front Pediatr. 2017;5:10.
36. Huang Y, Wu Y, Shan W, Zeng L, Huang L. An updated meta-analysis of laparoscopic versus open pyeloplasty for ureteropelvic junction obstruction in children. Int J Clin Exp Med. 2015;8:4922–31.
37. Blanc T, et al. Retroperitoneal laparoscopic pyeloplasty in children: long-term outcome and critical analysis of 10-year experience in a teaching center. Eur Urol. 2013;63:565–72.
38. Polok M, et al. Laparoscopic versus open pyeloplasty in children: experience of 226 cases at one centre. Arch Med Sci. 2020;16:858–62.
39. Liu D, et al. Comparison of laparoscopic approaches for dismembered pyeloplasty in children with ureteropelvic junction obstruction: critical analysis of 11-year experiences in a single surgeon. Urology. 2017;101:50–5.
40. Neheman A, Kord E, Zisman A, Darawsha AE, Noh PH. Comparison of robotic pyeloplasty and standard laparoscopic pyeloplasty in infants: a bi-institutional study. J Laparoendosc Adv Surg Tech A. 2018;28:467–70.

41. Chang S-J, Hsu C-K, Hsieh C-H, Yang SS-D. Comparing the efficacy and safety between robotic-assisted versus open pyeloplasty in children: a systemic review and meta-analysis. World J Urol. 2015;33:1855–65.
42. Esposito C, et al. Robot-assisted laparoscopic pyeloplasty (RALP) in children with complex pelvi-ureteric junction obstruction (PUJO): results of a multicenter European report. World J Urol. 2020; https://doi.org/10.1007/s00345-020-03331-8.
43. Kawal T, et al. Pediatric robotic-assisted laparoscopic pyeloplasty: does age matter? J Pediatr Urol. 2018;14:540.e1–6.
44. Minnillo BJ, et al. Long-term experience and outcomes of robotic assisted laparoscopic Pyeloplasty in children and young adults. J Urol. 2011;185:1455–60.
45. Silay MS, et al. Global minimally invasive pyeloplasty study in children: results from the Pediatric Urology Expert Group of the European Association of Urology Young Academic Urologists working party. J Pediatr Urol. 2016;12:229.e1–7.
46. Cundy TP, et al. Meta-analysis of robot-assisted vs conventional laparoscopic and open pyeloplasty in children: robot-assisted vs laparoscopic and open pyeloplasty in children. BJU Int. 2014;114:582–94.
47. Jacobson DL, et al. Robot-assisted laparoscopic reoperative repair for failed Pyeloplasty in children: an updated series. J Urol. 2019;201:1005–11.
48. Chan YY, Durbin-Johnson B, Sturm RM, Kurzrock EA. Outcomes after pediatric open, laparoscopic, and robotic pyeloplasty at academic institutions. J Pediatr Urol. 2017;13:49.e1–6.
49. Chiarenza SF, et al. Minimally invasive treatment of pediatric extrinsic Ureteropelvic junction obstruction by crossing polar vessels: is vascular hitching a definitive solution? Report of a Multicenter Survey. J Laparoendosc Adv Surg Tech A. 2017;27:965–71.
50. Corbett HJ, Mullassery D. Outcomes of endopyelotomy for pelviureteric junction obstruction in the paediatric population: a systematic review. J Pediatr Urol. 2015;11:328–36.
51. Bustangi N, et al. Extravesical ureteral Reimplantation following lich-Gregoir technique for the correction of Vesico-ureteral reflux retrospective comparative study open vs. laparoscopy. Front Pediatr. 2018;6:388.
52. Esposito C, et al. Surgical management of pediatric vesicoureteral reflux: a comparative study between endoscopic, laparoscopic, and open surgery. J Laparoendosc Adv Surg Tech A. 2016;26:574–80.
53. Soulier V, et al. Laparoscopic vesico-ureteral reimplantation with Lich–Gregoir approach in children: medium term results of 159 renal units in 117 children. World J Urol. 2017;35:1791–8.
54. Wang H-HS, et al. Open versus minimally invasive ureteroneocystostomy: a population-level analysis. J Pediatr Urol. 2016;12:232.e1–6.
55. Akhavan A, Avery D, Lendvay TS. Robot-assisted extravesical ureteral reimplantation: outcomes and conclusions from 78 ureters. J Pediatr Urol. 2014;10:864–8.
56. Esposito C, et al. Robot-assisted extravesical ureteral reimplantation (revur) for unilateral vesico-ureteral reflux in children: results of a multicentric international survey. World J Urol. 2018;36:481–8.
57. Boysen WR, et al. Prospective multicenter study on robot-assisted laparoscopic extravesical ureteral reimplantation (RALUR-EV): outcomes and complications. J Pediatr Urol. 2018;14:262.e1–6.
58. Harel M, et al. Objective pain assessment after ureteral reimplantation: comparison of open versus robotic approach. J Pediatr Urol. 2015;11:82.e1–8.
59. Deng T, et al. Robot-assisted laparoscopic versus open ureteral reimplantation for pediatric vesicoureteral reflux: a systematic review and meta-analysis. World J Urol. 2018;36:819–28.
60. Grimsby GM, et al. Multi-institutional review of outcomes of robot-assisted laparoscopic extravesical ureteral reimplantation. J Urol. 2015;193:1791–5.
61. Boysen WR, et al. Multi-institutional review of outcomes and complications of robot-assisted laparoscopic extravesical ureteral reimplantation for treatment of primary vesicoureteral reflux in children. J Urol. 2017;197:1555–61.
62. Kurtz MP, et al. Robotic versus open pediatric ureteral reimplantation: costs and complications from a nationwide sample. J Pediatr Urol. 2016;12:408.e1–6.
63. Herz D, Fuchs M, Todd A, McLeod D, Smith J. Robot-assisted laparoscopic extravesical ureteral reimplant: a critical look at surgical outcomes. J Pediatr Urol. 2016;12:402.e1–9.
64. Srinivasan AK, Maass D, Shrivastava D, Long CJ, Shukla AR. Is robot-assisted laparoscopic bilateral extravesical ureteral reimplantation associated with greater morbidity than unilateral surgery? A comparative analysis. J Pediatr Urol. 2017;13:494.e1–7.
65. Doudt AD, Pusateri CR, Christman MS. Endoscopic management of primary obstructive megaureter: a systematic review. J Endourol. 2018;32:482–7.
66. Ortiz R, Parente A, Perez-Egido L, Burgos L, Angulo JM. Long-term outcomes in primary obstructive megaureter treated by endoscopic balloon dilation. Experience after 100 cases. Front Pediatr. 2018;6:275.
67. Kassite I, et al. High pressure balloon dilatation of primary obstructive megaureter in children: a multicenter study. Front Pediatr. 2018;6:329.
68. Teklali Y, et al. Endoscopic management of primary obstructive megaureter in pediatrics. J Pediatr Urol. 2018;14:382–7.
69. Neheman A, et al. A novel surgical technique for obstructed megaureter: robot-assisted laparoscopic dismembered extravesical cross-trigonal ureteral reimplantation—short-term assessment. J Endourol. 2020;34:249–54.

70. Finkelstein JB, et al. How to decide which infant can have robotic surgery? Just do the math. J Pediatr Urol. 2015;11:170.e1–4.
71. Stulberg JJ, et al. Association between surgeon technical skills and patient outcomes. JAMA Surg. 2020; https://doi.org/10.1001/jamasurg.2020.3007.
72. Mir SA, et al. Minimally invasive nephrectomy: the influence of laparoendoscopic single-site surgery on patient selection, outcomes, and morbidity. Urology. 2011;77:631–4.
73. Burnand K, et al. Laparoscopic nephrectomy for Wilms' tumor: can we expand on the current SIOP criteria? J Pediatr Urol. 2018;14:253.e1–8.
74. Bansal D, et al. Comparison of pediatric robotic-assisted laparoscopic nephroureterectomy and laparoendoscopic single-site nephroureterectomy. Urology. 2014;83:438–42.
75. Tam YH, et al. Laparoendoscopic single-site nephrectomy and heminephroureterectomy in children using standard laparoscopic setup versus conventional laparoscopy. Urology. 2013;82:430–6.
76. Harris AC, et al. Feasibility of laparoscopic tumour nephrectomy in children. J Pediatr Surg. 2018;53:302–5.
77. Badawy H, Assem A, Saad A, Hanno A, Elsalmy S. Retroperitonoscopic nephrectomy and nephroureterectomy in children and adolescents: analysis of a single-center experience. J Endourol. 2011;25:809–13.
78. Blanc T, et al. Retroperitoneal approach for ureteropelvic junction obstruction: encouraging preliminary results with robot-assisted laparoscopic repair. Front Pediatr. 2019;7:209.
79. Esposito C, et al. Postoperative bladder dysfunction and outcomes after minimally invasive extravesical ureteric reimplantation in children using a laparoscopic and a robot-assisted approach: results of a multicentre international survey: outcome of ureteral reimplantation using mis. BJU Int. 2019;124:820–7.
80. Gundeti MS, Boysen WR, Shah A. Robot-assisted laparoscopic extravesical ureteral reimplantation: technique modifications contribute to optimized outcomes. Eur Urol. 2016;70:818–23.

MIX
Papier aus verantwortungsvollen Quellen
Paper from responsible sources
FSC® C105338

If you have any concerns about our products,
you can contact us on
ProductSafety@springernature.com

In case Publisher is established outside the EU,
the EU authorized representative is:
Springer Nature Customer Service Center GmbH
Europaplatz 3, 69115 Heidelberg, Germany

Printed by Libri Plureos GmbH
in Hamburg, Germany